T0344423

Gastrointestinal Diseases and Their Associated Infections

Gastrointestinal Diseases and Their Associated Infections

GUY D. ESLICK, DrPH, PhD, FACE, FFPH
Professor of Cancer Epidemiology and Medical Statistics
Discipline of Surgery
The University of Sydney
Co-Director, The Whiteley-Martin Research Centre
Director of Research
Nepean Blue Mountains Local Health District (NBMLHD)
Sydney, NSW, Australia

ELSEVIER

GASTROINTESTINAL DISEASES AND THEIR ASSOCIATED
INFECTIONS   ISBN: 978-0-323-54843-4
Copyright © 2019 Elsevier, Inc. All rights reserved.

No part of this publication may be reproduced or transmitted in any form or by any means, electronic or mechanical, including photocopying, recording, or any information storage and retrieval system, without permission in writing from the publisher. Details on how to seek permission, further information about the Publisher's permissions policies and our arrangements with organizations such as the Copyright Clearance Center and the Copyright Licensing Agency, can be found at our website: www.elsevier.com/permissions.

This book and the individual contributions contained in it are protected under copyright by the Publisher (other than as may be noted herein).

Notices

Practitioners and researchers must always rely on their own experience and knowledge in evaluating and using any information, methods, compounds or experiments described herein. Because of rapid advances in the medical sciences, in particular, independent verification of diagnoses and drug dosages should be made. To the fullest extent of the law, no responsibility is assumed by Elsevier, authors, editors or contributors for any injury and/or damage to persons or property as a matter of products liability, negligence or otherwise, or from any use or operation of any methods, products, instructions, or ideas contained in the material herein.

Publisher: Patrick Manley
Acquisition Editor: Kerry Holland
Editorial Project Manager: Jennifer Horigan
Production Project Manager: Sreejith Viswanathan
Cover Designer: Alan Studhome

3251 Riverport Lane
St. Louis, Missouri 63043

Working together
to grow libraries in
developing countries

www.elsevier.com • www.bookaid.org

I would like to dedicate this work to my family: Enid, Marielle, Guillaume, and Éloïse. I would be nowhere without you all by my side, you give reason and meaning to all that I do in this world.

List of Contributors

Susan Adams, MBBS (Hons), FRACS (Paed)
Department of Paediatric Surgery
Sydney Children's Hospital
Sydney, NSW, Australia

Esther Babady, PhD, D (ABMM)
Associate Attending
Laboratory Medicine
Memorial Sloan Kettering Cancer Center
New York, NY, United States

Director of Clinical Operations
Clinical Microbiology Service
Memorial Sloan Kettering Cancer Center
New York, NY, United States

Thomas Borody, MD, PhD, DSc, FRACP, FACP, FACG, AGAF
Professor
Centre for Digestive Diseases
Five Dock, NSW, Australia

Fei Chen, MBBS
St George and Sutherland Clinical School
University of New South Wales
Sydney, NSW, Australia

Jonathan Cher, BMed MD
Department of Paediatric Surgery
Sydney Children's Hospital
Sydney, NSW, Australia

Michael R. Cox, FRACS, MS, MBBS
Professor of Surgery
Department of Surgery
Nepean Hospital
The University of Sydney
Penrith, NSW, Australia

Fatima El-Assaad, PhD (Medicine), BMedSci (HONSI)
Doctor
Microbiome Research Centre
St George and Sutherland Clinical School
St George Hospital
UNSW Sydney
Kogarah, NSW, Australia

Emad M. El-Omar, BSc (Hons), MB ChB, MD (Hons), FRCP (Edin), FRSE, FRACP
Professor of Medicine
St George and Sutherland Clinical School
University of New South Wales
Sydney, NSW, Australia

Director of the Microbiome Research Centre
St George Hospital
Sydney, NSW, Australia

Guy D. Eslick, DrPH, PhD, FACE, FFPH
Professor of Cancer Epidemiology and
Medical Statistics
Discipline of Surgery
The University of Sydney
Co-Director, The Whiteley-Martin Research Centre
Director of Research
Nepean Blue Mountains Local Health District (NBMLHD)
Sydney, NSW, Australia

John Frean, MB BCh, MMed (Path Microbiol), FFSci RCPA, FFTM RCPS (Glasgow), FACTM, MSc (Med Parasitol)
Associate Professor
Centre for Emerging Zoonotic and Parasitic Diseases
National Institute for Communicable Diseases and
University of the Witwatersrand
Johannesburg, South Africa

Carl Freyer, MBBS
St George and Sutherland Clinical School
University of New South Wales
Sydney, NSW, Australia

Andrew Gia, BSc (Advanced) (Honours)
Microbiome Research Centre (MRC)
St George and Sutherland Clinical School
Faculty of Medicine
UNSW Sydney
Kogarah, NSW, Australia

Lan Gong, BSc (Hons), PhD
Doctor
St George and Sutherland Clinical School
University of New South Wales
Kogarah, NSW, Australia

Peter H. Green, MB, BS, MD, FRACP, FACG
Professor
Medicine
Columbia University
New York, NY, United States

Madhusudan Grover, MD
Assistant Professor of Medicine and Physiology
Gastroenterology and Hepatology
Mayo Clinic
Rochester, MN, United States

Sakteesh V. Gurunathan, MD
Doctor
Mount Sinai Health System
Gastroenterology/Genetics & Genomic Sciences
New York, NY, United States

Gerald Holtmann, MD, PhD, MBA, FRACP, FRCP
Professor
Gastroenterology & Hepatology
Princess Alexandra Hospital
Brisbane, QLD, Australia

Mojgan Hosseini, MD
Assistant Professor of Pathology
Department of Pathology
University of California
San Diego, CA, United States

University of California, San Diego
Department of Pathology
San Diego, CA, United States

Karen Helena Keddy, MBBCh, DTM&HBSc (Med), MMed, FCPath (SA), PhD
Doctor
Faculty of Health Sciences
University of the Witwatersrand
Johannesburg, South Africa

Suneeta Krishnareddy, MD
Celiac Disease Center at Columbia
Columbia University Medical Center
New York, NY, United States

Laura W. Lamps, MD
Godfrey Dorr Stobbe Professor of Gastrointestinal Pathology, Gastrointestinal and Hepatobiliary Pathology
Director, Gastrointestinal Pathology
Chief Patient Safety Officer
Anatomic Pathology
Department of Pathology
University of Michigan
Ann Arbor, MI, United States

Janet Mans, PhD, MSc, BSc (Hons), BSc
Senior Lecturer
Department of Medical Virology
University of Pretoria
Pretoria, South Africa

Peter Mead, MD
Infectious Disease Service
Department of Medicine
Memorial Sloan Kettering Cancer Center
New York, NY, United States

Dominique S. Michaud, ScD
Professor
Public Health & Community Medicine
Tufts University Medical School
Boston, MA, United States

Verena Moos, PhD
Doctor
Infectious Diseases
Charité-University Medicine Berlin
Berlin, Germany

Sandrama Nadan, PhD, MSc, BSc (Hons), BSc
Scientist
Centre for Enteric Diseases
National Institute for Communicable Diseases
Sandringham, South Africa

Department of Medical Virology
University of Pretoria
Pretoria, South Africa

Maryam Nesvaderani, MBBS, BSc (Hons)
Doctor
Department of Surgery
Sydney Medical School Nepean
Sydney, NSW, Australia

Yael Nobel, MD
Celiac Disease Center at Columbia
Columbia University Medical Center
New York, NY, United States

Nicola Anne Page, PhD, MPH, MSc (Med), BSc (Agric) (Hons), BSc (Agric)
Senior Scientist
Center for Enteric Diseases
National Institute for Communicable Diseases
Johannesburg, South Africa

Extraordinary Professor
Department of Medical Virology
University of Pretoria
Pretoria, South Africa

Min Young Park, MD, BMusStudies
Doctor
Research Fellow
The Whiteley-Martin Research Centre
The University of Sydney
Sydney, NSW, Australia

Ross Penninkilampi, BMed
The Whiteley-Martin Research Centre
Discipline of Surgery
The University of Sydney
Nepean Hospital
Penrith, NSW, Australia

Ayesha Shah, MBBS, FRACP
Doctor
Department of Gastroenterology & Hepatology
Translational Research Institute
Princess Alexandra Hospital
Brisbane, QLD, Australia

Prapti Shrestha, BMedSc (Hons)
Translational Gastroenterology Laboratory
Western Sydney University
Campbelltown, NSW, Australia

Arunjot Singh, MD, MPH
Assistant Professor of Clinical Pediatrics
Gastroenterology, Hepatology, and Nutrition
Children's Hospital of Philadelphia
Philadelphia, PA, United States

Anthony M. Smith, PhD
Doctor
Faculty of Health Sciences
University of the Witwatersrand
Johannesburg, South Africa

Camille Wu, MBBS, FRACS
Doctor
Department of Paediatric Surgery
Sydney Children's Hospital
Sydney, NSW, Australia

Howard Chi Ho Yim, BSc (Hons), PhD
Doctor
Postdoctoral Fellow
St. George & Sutherland Clinical School
University of New South Wales
Sydney, NSW, Australia

Amany Zekry, MBBS, FRACP, PhD
Associate Professor of Medicine
St George and Sutherland Clinical School
University of New South Wales
Head of Gastroenterology and Hepatology
St George Hospital
Sydney, NSW, Australia

Preface

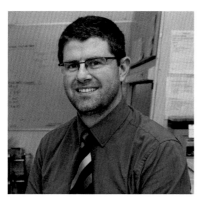

Infections of the gastrointestinal (GI) tract are generally common. Some infections have a long history while others are relatively new on the scene. The importance of understanding these organisms is critical to our overall health. Understanding the "bugs" in our GI tract and their role not only in local infections but ever increasingly on the role that our "gut microbiota" plays in diseases and pathology of other extra GI organ systems appears to be the way of the future. This is very exciting indeed, but we currently only have a rudimentary understanding of the relationship between the multitude of various organisms lining our GI tract and how these organisms may induce, mediate, or halt diseases outside the GI tract. I trust that this volume will provide useful information to the clinician, researcher, and those interested in GI infections. I would sincerely like to thank my esteemed colleagues for taking the time to write chapters in their areas of expertise. This is really just the beginning of what I know will be one of the most exciting fields of medicine over the next few decades. Many thanks to Kerry Holland and Jennifer Horigan from Elsevier for their assistance and support in putting this important volume of work together and publishing it; I hope there will be many updated future editions to come highlighting this exciting field of the gut microbiome.

Guy D. Eslick, DrPH, PhD, FACE, FFPH
Professor of Cancer Epidemiology and Medical Statistics
Discipline of Surgery
The University of Sydney
Co-Director, The Whiteley-Martin Research Centre
Director of Research
Nepean Blue Mountains Local Health District
(NBMLHD)
Sydney, NSW, Australia

Contents

CHAPTER 1

The Esophageal Microbiome: Esophageal Reflux Disease, Barrett's Esophagus, and Esophageal Cancer

PRAPTI SHRESTHA, BMEDSC(HONS) • ROSS PENNINKILAMPI, BMED • GUY D. ESLICK, DRPH, PHD, FACE, FFPH

INFECTIONS OF THE ESOPHAGUS

Infective Esophagitis

The normal flora of the healthy esophagus typically contains species of *Streptococcus, Neisseria, Veillonella, Fusobacterium, Bacteroides, Lactobacillus, Staphylococcus, Prevotella*, Enterobacteriaceae, and yeasts.[1] Infectious esophagitis is rare in those who are not immunocompromised, although some cases of infection with herpes simplex and *Candida albicans* occur on occasion. In the immunosuppressed, often for organ transplantation, chronic inflammatory diseases, or chemotherapy, as well as sufferers of acquired immune deficiency syndrome (AIDS), infective esophagitis becomes more common.[2] It may be caused by cytomegalovirus, herpesvirus, *Candida* species, and others. The typical symptoms of infectious esophagitis are odynophagia, dysphagia, and bleeding. Choice of treatment depends on the particular pathogen implicated.

Chagas Disease or American Trypanosomiasis

Chagas disease, also known as American trypanosomiasis, is a zoonotic disease caused by the protozoan *Trypanosoma cruzi*. Other species of this genus, namely *T. brucei gambiense* and *T. brucei rhodesiense* are responsible for African trypanosomiasis, also known as sleeping sickness. Only Chagas disease exhibits clear esophageal involvement, and hence the discussion here is limited to this disease.

T. cruzi is only found in the Americas, and is harbored by mammals and infected triatomines. Triatomines are a subfamily of Reduviidae insects that are more commonly known as kissing bugs, assassin bugs, or vampire bugs. These insects are the vectors for Chagas disease, able to transfer the protozoans from wild or domestic mammal carriers to humans. Overall, there are more than 150 identified species of insect vectors for Chagas disease, and the parasites have been found to infect over 100 species of mammals.[3] It is estimated that there are eight million individuals with chronic Chagas disease,[4] and that it accounts for approximately 14,000 deaths per year. In Latin America, it represents a significant parasitic cause of morbidity and mortality, and significant efforts have been made to improve control of its spread. Even in nonendemic countries, such as Spain, Canada, the United States, and Australia,[5] Chagas disease has become increasingly visible, especially as it is transmissible vertically, and through both blood and organ transplantation[6] (Fig. 1.1).

Chagas disease acutely presents as a mild febrile illness which usually resolves spontaneously; however, most infected patients will experience an asymptomatic, chronic, subpatent parasitemia, in what is known as the indeterminate phase. Of these cases, a fraction of up to half of patients may experience serious cardiac or gastrointestinal symptoms associated with significant morbidity or mortality.[7] The gastrointestinal complications of chronic Chagas disease may include dilatation of the esophagus (megaesophagus) or colon (megacolon), with the former being responsible for symptoms of dysphagia, odynophagia, and regurgitation. Severe esophageal dysfunction can have grave consequences, particularly by causing aspiration that may lead to aspiration pneumonitis. Hence the symptoms of megaesophagus in chronic Chagas disease may lead to chronic aspiration, weight loss, malnutrition, cachexia, and potentially death (Fig. 1.2).

Two drugs are available for Chagas disease: nifurtimox and benznidazole. However, these drugs have limited efficacy, especially once the clinical course has progressed through to the indeterminate or chronic symptomatic phases. More research from randomized, controlled trials is required to identify more efficacious treatments, and to investigate the usefulness of treatments at each stage of the disease.

Gastrointestinal Diseases and Their Associated Infections. https://doi.org/10.1016/B978-0-323-54843-4.00001-5
Copyright © 2019 Elsevier Inc. All rights reserved.

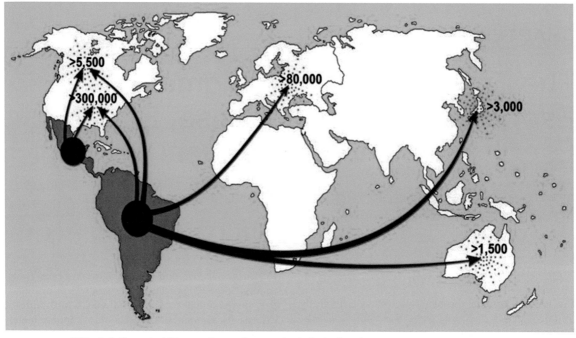

FIG. 1.1 Spread of Chagas disease from endemic Latin America to regions around the world.

Trypanosomiasis, American (Chagas disease)

(Trypanosoma cruzi)

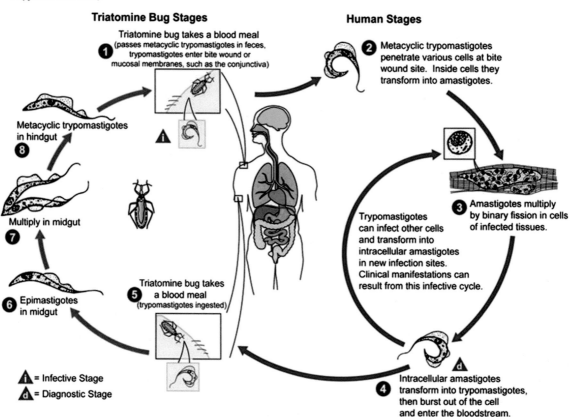

FIG. 1.2 The life cycle for Chagas disease.

GASTROESOPHAGEAL REFLUX DISEASE

Introduction

Gastroesophageal reflux disease (GERD) is defined as a disorder involving the effortless transit of acidic gastric contents into the esophagus or mouth.[8] It is the clinical condition associated with the pathological condition of reflux esophagitis. Although highly prevalent and often associated with significant discomfort, GERD rarely causes serious or fatal sequelae. It hence represents a significant burden in terms of morbidity rather than mortality.[8]

The disorder occurs when lower esophageal sphincter tone, which is responsible for preventing reflux of gastric contents into the esophagus, is compromised. The stratified squamous epithelium of the esophagus is designed to prevent damage during the passing of a bolus, not to resist corrosive acid reflux. Although the esophageal glands secrete mucin and bicarbonate and hence provide some protection, this is insufficient to prevent irritation in cases of recurrent reflux. GERD therefore occurs when two conditions are fulfilled: (1) a transient or prolonged failure of maintenance of appropriate lower esophageal sphincter tone; and, (2) gastric contents are sufficiently acidic such that, when refluxed, will irritate the esophageal mucosa.

Clinical Characteristics

Clinically, GERD typically presents with dysphagia, heartburn, and acid regurgitation. Heartburn typically occurs after meals, and may radiate from the retrosternal region to the neck or back. This pattern is occasionally confused with that of cardiac origin, and hence GERD is an important differential diagnosis when considering chest pain of unknown etiology.[9] Acid regurgitation occurs when the reflux of acidic gastric contents is perceived to reach the pharynx or mouth, and can be quite a troubling symptom. GERD is known to be associated with particular foods: specifically, chocolate, coffee, spicy foods, citrus fruits or other citrus products, and alcohol.[8–10] In typical GERD, sufferers are symptomatic at least twice a week on separate days. It is most common in those over the age of 40, and tobacco use, pregnancy, and obesity represent important risk factors. Other, less common, symptoms include odynophagia, hiccups, nausea, vomiting, and burping.

Importantly, the degree of histological damage is more closely correlated with duration of disease, rather than the severity of the symptomatology. Thus, prolonged GERD, complications such as erosive esophagitis, hematemesis, esophageal strictures, and Barrett's esophagus may arise. However, this condition can often be adequately managed in an outpatient setting and hence such sequelae are uncommon in modern advanced medical systems.

Epidemiology

A recent systematic review article found that the worldwide pooled prevalence of GERD symptoms was approximately 13%, but that this was highly variable dependent on geographical region. The data were consistent with findings from an Australian study reporting a prevalence rate of 12% among a random sample of 1000 individuals from the community.[11] GERD was especially prevalent in India, Pakistan, some Southeast European countries, as well as the United Kingdom and Iceland[8] (Fig. 1.3).

Important risk factors for GERD, with comparisons to those for Barrett's esophagus and esophageal adenocarcinoma, are summarized in Table 1.1. The evidence for these risk factors is adapted from recent meta-analyses for each condition.[12,13] Note that for many of the following reported risk factors, heterogeneity upon statistical meta-analysis was substantial ($I^2 > 75.00$), indicating that there was considerable variation between individual studies.

Moreover, genetic factors have been implicated in GERD symptoms.[14] A twin study in 1057 twin pairs conducted in Minnesota found that the proband concordance in monozygotic twins for GERD was 20.4, with an estimate of genetic variance in GERD given as 13%.[12] Adjusting for anxiety and depression nullified the genetic effect on GERD to statistical nonsignificance. Hence, genetic factors likely play a minor role in GERD, with environmental risk factors being of greater importance.

Helicobacter pylori

Helicobacter pylori (*H. pylori*) is a Gram-negative spiral bacterium previously classified as *Campylobacter pylori*.[15] At least 40% of the world's population, using conservative estimates, have prevalent *H. pylori* infection, which normally occurs in childhood and is carried throughout life. The prevalence of *H. pylori* infection is particularly high in developing countries. In most cases, it is associated with an asymptomatic chronic gastritis, but was famously shown by Warren and Marshall in 1982 to be responsible for the development of peptic ulcers, and its eradication could be effective in allowing such ulcers to heal without relapse.[15,16] It is now known that approximately 70%–80% of gastric ulcers, and an even larger proportion of duodenal ulcers, are the result of *H. pylori* infection.[17] *H. pylori* infection may be diagnosed by urea breath testing, fecal antigen testing, histological examination of biopsy specimens, or by culture in the laboratory.

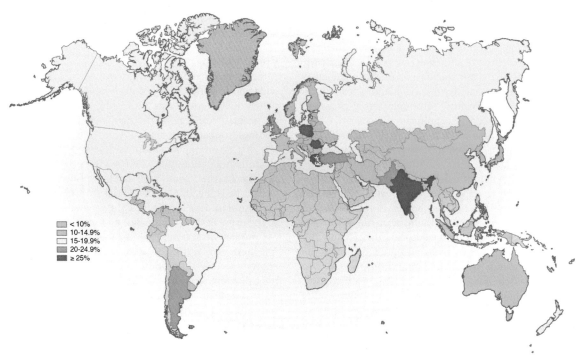

FIG. 1.3 Geographical distribution of gastroesophageal reflux disease. (With permission Rubenstein JH. Risk factors for Barrett's esophagus. Curr Opin Gastroenterol 2014;30(4):408–414.)

TABLE 1.1
Risk Factors Associated With GERD, Barrett's Esophagus, and Esophageal Cancer

Risk Factor	GERD	Barrett's Esophagus	Esophageal Adenocarcinoma
Advancing age	Yes	Yes	
Gender	Yes (Female)	Yes (Male)	Yes (Male)
Smoking	Yes	Yes	Yes
Alcohol use	No	No[11]	
NSAID and/or aspirin use	Yes		
Obesity	Yes	Yes	Yes
Low income	Yes		
Low education	Yes		
Hiatal hernia		Yes	Yes

Epidemiological Associations Between *H. pylori* and GERD

Despite its association with a number of gastrointestinal diseases, *H. pylori* infection has not been implicated as a causative agent for GERD. *H. pylori* colonizes human gastric epithelium, not the stratified squamous epithelium of the esophagus. However, epidemiological studies have shown a curious association: there is a negative correlation between *H. pylori* prevalence and that of GERD. This is most prominent for cytotoxin-associated gene product (CagA) positive strains of *H. pylori*. A systematic review and meta-analysis reported that there was a 22%–53% reduction in GERD prevalence in patients infected with *H. pylori*.[18] The reliability of their results were somewhat questionable, considering the substantial heterogeneity present in the meta-analysis, indicating that the differences in reported effect sizes between studies is highly unlikely to be purely due to chance. They performed a subgroup analysis and found geographical differences in the association between *H. pylori* infection and GERD, which explained some of the observed heterogeneity.

Potential Mechanisms

The mechanism by which *H. pylori* is associated with GERD is yet to be fully elucidated. As previously established, the pathogenesis of GERD involves the reflux of gastric acid into the lower esophagus. The effect of *H. pylori* infection on gastric acid secretion is dependent on the pattern of infection. *H. pylori* infection in the corpus of the stomach can cause atrophic gastritis, which involves depletion of gastric glands. The associated gastric acid hyposecretion may hence have a protective effect against GERD. By contrast, antrum-predominant GERD may be associated with increased gastric acid hypersecretion. In this case, stimulation of production of interleukin-8 (IL-8) and interleukin-1β (IL-1β), which subsequently stimulate the production of gastrin.[19] Gastrin in turn induces further gastric acid secretion by parietal cells. However, increased acid secretion is unlikely to be causative for reflux if the lower esophageal sphincter is functionally intact.

Eradication of *H. pylori*

Generally, eradication of *H. pylori* has been recommended in infected patients to reduce chronic gastric inflammation, and to promote the prevention, remission, or healing of peptic ulcers. The typical treatment strategy involves combination therapy of a proton pump inhibitor (PPI) and two antibiotics such as clarithromycin or metronidazole and amoxicillin. However, some studies have suggested that eradication of *H. pylori* in GERD patients may be counterproductive and increase the severity or risk of disease.

If corpus-predominant *H. pylori* infection protects against GERD via a method involving gastric acid hyposecretion, then it would follow that eradication of *H. pylori* with its subsequent restoration of gastric acid production may cause the emergence of GERD. There is some limited evidence to support this hypothesis. A meta-analysis reported that eradication of *H. pylori* was associated with an increased risk of developing GERD after pooling evidence from 12 randomized controlled trials (pooled risk ratio (RR) = 1.99, 95% CI 1.23–3.22).[20] In a subgroup analysis, this association held true only in Asian studies (pooled RR = 4.53, 95% CI 1.66–12.36); in Western studies, there was a no association between toward a risk of GERD posteradication (pooled RR = 1.22, 95% CI 0.91–1.63). This may be due to the relatively higher prevalence of corpus-predominant *H. pylori* infection in Asian populations compared to Western populations, hence, supporting the acid hyposecretion hypothesis.

As of 2017, the most recent guidelines from the Maastricht V/Florence Consensus Report are that "eradication of *H. pylori* in populations of infected patients, on average, neither causes nor exacerbates [GERD]", and that "the presence of GERD should not dissuade practitioners from *H. pylori* eradication treatment where indicated".[21] Hence, the current paradigm is to proceed with eradication treatment for *H. pylori* in patients with GERD.

Treatment With Proton-Pump Inhibitors in *H. pylori* Infected Patients

A common treatment for GERD is the prescription of proton-pump inhibitors. These drugs inhibit the H^+-K^+-ATPase enzyme, which is involved in the final step of acid secretion. Examples of these drugs include omeprazole, esomeprazole, lansoprazole, pantoprazole, and rabeprazole. In long-term treatment, there is a tendency for *H. pylori* to assume the corpus-predominant pattern that is associated with potentially damaging atrophic gastritis. Hence, current guidelines recommend eradication of *H. pylori* in cases where long-term proton-pump inhibitor use is required.[21]

BARRETT'S ESOPHAGUS

Introduction

Barrett's esophagus is a potential complication of chronic gastroesophageal reflux disease in which there is metaplastic change of the esophageal stratified squamous mucosa. Metaplasia is the process by which one differentiated cell type is replaced by another; in this case, the esophageal mucosa is replaced by the typical columnar epithelium of the intestinal mucosa. This is apparent morphologically in the distal esophagus as alternating "tongues" of deep red metaplastic intestinal mucosa and normal pale lower esophageal mucosa, extending away from the gastroesophageal junction. These morphological changes can be visualized endoscopically, which along with biopsy can identify dysplastic changes histologically. Generally, upon endoscopy the defining characteristic is that the squamocolumnar junction, that is the junction between the esophageal and typical gastric epithelia, lies proximal to the cardioesophageal junction[22,23] (Fig. 1.4).

Barrett's esophagus is most concerning because it is a premalignant condition, conferring increased risk of the development of esophageal adenocarcinoma. The majority of cases of esophageal adenocarcinoma are preceded by Barrett's esophagus; however, it is to be noted that most cases of Barrett's esophagus do not progress to cancer. An important study by Hameeteman and colleagues in 1989 followed 50 patients with Barrett's esophagus over a mean follow-up time of 5.4 years.[24] Six patients had low- or high-grade dysplasia at study entry, and this increased to 13 by the final

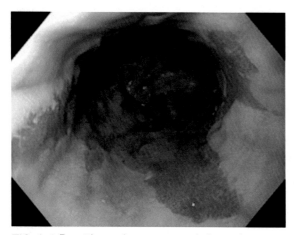

FIG. 1.4 Barrett's esophagus as seen during endoscopy. (With permission Whiteman DC, Appleyard M, Bahin FF, et al. Australian clinical practice guidelines for the diagnosis and management of Barrett's esophagus and early esophageal adenocarcinoma. J Gastroenterol Hepatol 2015;30:804–820.)

follow-up. Furthermore, 5 of the 50 patients developed esophageal adenocarcinoma by the final follow-up. The authors reported that the observed incidence rate in the study of one case in every 52 person-years was more than 125 times the background incidence rate for the general Dutch population at that time. In Barrett's esophagus patients, estimates for the risk of the development of adenocarcinoma of the distal esophagus have ranged from 0.2% to 2.0%.[25,26] As such, individuals with Barrett's esophagus present as an extremely important population for the prevention of esophageal cancer.

Subtypes of Barrett's Esophagus

Barrett's esophagus can be categorized as either long segment or short segment. In short-segment Barrett's esophagus, the distance to which the squamocolumnar junction extends beyond the cardioesophageal junction is <3 cm, while in long-segment Barrett's esophagus it extends to ≥3 cm. Short-segment Barrett's esophagus is more common, and less likely to be associated with severe symptomatology than long-segment Barrett's esophagus. Furthermore, it has been shown that esophageal neoplasia is more prevalent in cases of short-segment Barrett's esophagus than in the long-segment variety. One study found that long-segment Barrett's esophagus was associated with a more than doubling of risk of neoplasia when compared to the short-segment group (OR = 2.55, 95% CI 1.73–3.76).[22]

Clinical Features

Barrett's esophagus develops in stepwise progression from chronic GERD; it has no specific clinical symptoms or signs that allow it to be distinguished from GERD.[23]

Epidemiology

In the United States, the prevalence of Barrett's esophagus has been estimated at 5.6%.[27] Individuals with GERD symptoms who go on to have an endoscopy are found to have Barrett's esophagus in 10%–15% of cases.[22] However, it is also known that of people who develop esophageal cancer, up to 40% of these people did not have any prior reflux symptoms. Therefore, asymptomatic individuals may still develop Barrett's esophagus and progress through to esophageal cancer. One study in male veterans aged over 50 who were undergoing sigmoidoscopy for colorectal cancer screen, who did not have GERD symptoms more than once monthly, found that approximately a quarter of them had detectable Barrett's esophagus.[28] In a Swedish study, a random sample of the adult population (*n* = 3000) in two municipalities were surveyed, and it was found that 1.6% of those which were randomly selected to undergo endoscopy (*n* = 1000) had detectable Barrett's esophagus.[29] As such, the prevalence of Barrett's esophagus even in an asymptomatic population presents a great concern.[23] Risk stratification of an asymptomatic population may facilitate expeditious and effective preventive strategies, but is not currently possible. However, there has been in recent years a growth in the knowledge of the genetic contributors to risk of Barrett's esophagus, with a meta-analysis of genome-wide association studies of Barrett's esophagus and esophageal cancer finding eight new risk loci for the diseases, as well as two loci that increased risk of esophageal cancer independently of Barrett's esophagus.[30]

Helicobacter pylori and Barrett's Esophagus
Evidence for an epidemiological association

In a similar regard to GERD, and perhaps unsurprisingly given the sequential etiologies of these two conditions, *H. pylori* infection has been associated with a reduction in risk of Barrett's esophagus, particularly for the CagA + strains.[27] A meta-analysis of the association between *H. pylori* infection and Barrett's esophagus found an inverse relationship, when those with Barrett's esophagus were compared to healthy controls.[25] That is, those with Barrett's esophagus were less likely to have *H. pylori* than healthy controls, which is suggestive of a protective effect. Interestingly, when comparing individuals who had Barrett's esophagus to controls who were healthy blood donors who had not undergone endoscopic examination, rather than just endoscopically normal, healthy, controls, the risk reduction was no longer observed. The authors of the paper argue that not performing an endoscopic examination of the controls may allow undiagnosed cases of Barrett's esophagus into the control group, potentially confounding the comparison. It is also possible that blood donors have different seropositivity rates for *H. pylori* compared to the rest of the population, which has been supported by a Swedish study.[31] Unfortunately, methodological weaknesses in included studies and heterogeneity within the meta-analysis precludes the drawing of reliable conclusions regarding the association between *H. pylori* infection and risk of Barrett's esophagus. A more recent meta-analysis found that of 49 studies judged eligible for inclusion, only four were sufficiently devoid of selection and other biases to be deemed trustworthy. Quantitative synthesis of only these four included studies showed that *H. pylori* was associated with a reduced prevalence of Barrett's esophagus (pooled RR = 0.49, 95% CI 0.35–0.60).[32] As it stands, the evidential basis for the association is weak, and is insufficient to determine causation.

Potential mechanism

The proposed pathway by which *H. pylori* may reduce the risk of Barrett's esophagus is shared with GERD; atrophy of the corpus of the stomach may cause a depletion of parietal glands, reducing acid secretion. This reduces the degree of acid reflux into the distal esophagus, which may then protect against the erosive esophagitis that instigates the metaplastic change in Barrett's esophagus.[23]

ESOPHAGEAL CANCER

Introduction

Esophageal cancer is one of the deadliest cancers worldwide. It originates as malignant neoplasm within the inner epithelium lining of the esophagus but can rapidly metastasize beyond the mucosa, submucosa, and the muscular tissue into nearby lymph nodes and can also infiltrate other internal organs (trachea, larynx, thyroid glands, lungs, and aorta) that surround the esophagus.[33] Due to the asymptomatic nature of this cancer, diagnosis often remains late until the advanced stage when the tumor has reached superficial or formed secondary malignancies.[34] The 5-year relative survival rate for esophageal cancer ranges from 15% to 25%,[35] compared to 90% for breast cancer[36] and 60% for

bowel cancer on average.[37] Incidences of esophageal cancer is increasing in most of the developing countries,[38–40] as well as in most Western countries[39] with common associated risk factors being tobacco, alcohol,[41–46] low in fruits and vegetables consumption,[47–51] and gastroesophageal reflux disorder (GERD).[39,52,53] Due to its rapid increase in incidence globally,[35] aggressive nature and low survival rate,[54] it is the eighth most common cancer worldwide and ranked as the sixth highest in cancer-related mortality,[55] despite it being a relatively uncommon cancer.

Esophageal Cancer Subtypes and Risk Factors

More than 90% of esophageal cancers are differentiated into two histopathological subtypes, squamous cell carcinoma and esophageal adenocarcinoma, while other types also exist, for instance, melanomas, leiomyosarcomas, carcinoids, and lymphomas.[56] The first subtype originates from the stratified squamous epithelial cells in the mucosa of the esophagus. These malignancies form throughout the mid to distal segments of the esophagus. The consumption of tobacco and alcohol are major risk factors for esophageal squamous-cell carcinoma.[35,39,47,55] These associated risks appear to be linked with the ingestion of carcinogenic substances found in alcohol (aldehyde metabolite), tobacco (nitrosamines),[57] and processed foods.[58] Moreover, patients with achalasia are also at higher risk of developing this cancer, due to chronicity of ingested food retention causing esophagitis and possible noxious compounds.[59] In addition, genetic susceptibility factors in an autosomal dominant condition called Tylosis have been associated with the development of this cancer.[55]

The second subtype, esophageal adenocarcinoma, originates from the mucus-secreting columnar glandular cells in the submucosa of the esophagus. Normally, the esophageal lining is made up of squamous epithelial cells. Due to chronic (weekly or daily) acid exposure in GERD, the squamous cells transform into glandular cells, which in turn raise the risk of developing neoplasm and ultimately adenocarcinoma (by fivefold or sevenfold, respectively).[60] As a result of this, 75% of esophageal adenocarcinoma is found in the distal esophagus of patients diagnosed with Barrett's esophagus.[61] Other risk factors, such as obesity,[62] smoking, and unhealthy diet, appear to exacerbate the acid exposure.[63] In addition, in a genome-wide association study, influence of numerous germline genetic variants has been found to contribute in the risk of Barrett's esophagus and adenocarcinoma.[64]

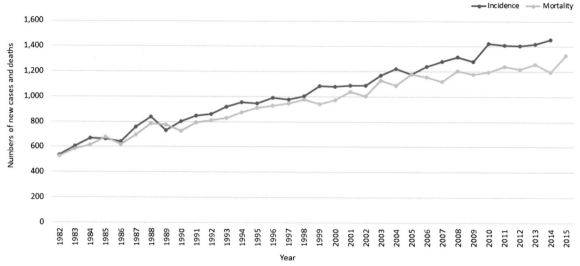

FIG. 1.5 Summary of incidence and mortality trend by year of diagnosis in Australia. The number of new cases and deaths had steady rise from 537 to 1457 and from 527 to 1329, respectively, within 1982–2014. (*Australian Institute of Health and Welfare AIHW 2017. Australian Cancer Incidence and Mortality ACIM books*).[47]

The general consensus of GERD and its sequelae leading to adenocarcinoma exists via intermediate stages including reflux-induced esophagitis, nondysplastic Barrett's esophagus, and low to high grade dysplasia of the esophagus.[65,66] Barrett's esophagus, an acquired condition that transforms esophageal squamous epithelium into intestinal metaplasia or specialized columnar epithelium, is a benign and an asymptomatic condition that is labeled as the "only precursor lesion" and a "strong risk factor" that develops into esophageal adenocarcinoma.[67–71] Despite this link, currently there are no effective strategies for stratifying patients with Barrett's esophagus into risk groups for developing adenocarcinoma.

Epidemiology

The trends of esophageal cancer fluctuate between counties depending upon morphology and anatomical site of the tumor.[39,72] There has been a steady increase in the incidence of esophageal cancer in Australia since 1982, closely followed by the rate of mortality (Fig. 1.5).[73] Nevertheless, over the last decade the new esophageal cancer rates in the Unites States has been declining on average by 1.4% each year, correspondingly a decline in death rates on average by 0.9% per year between the year 2005 and 2014.[74]

Historically, there are higher incidences of squamous cell carcinoma than incidences of adenocarcinoma. Although this remains true in Asia, East Africa, and Middle Eastern countries,[75–77] the predominance of squamous cell carcinoma has been outweighed by adenocarcinoma in the last 4 decades.[77,78] Furthermore, in recent correlation analyses study, countries that are more socioeconomically developed had higher adenocarcinoma to squamous cell carcinoma ratio.[79]

A higher burden of squamous cell carcinoma occurs in the "Asian Esophageal Cancer Belt", which covers Northern Iran, east to China, and north to Russia with more than 100 cases of this cancer occurring per 1000,000 person/year.[39,79] Although cigarette smoking and alcohol consumption both have synergic effect on causing squamous cell carcinoma, risk increases by threefold to sevenfold in smokers than nonsmokers; similarly, chance of cancer is raised by 260%, and 550% who drink 1.5–6 units of alcohol/day and 6+ units of alcohol/day, respectively, as compared to nondrinkers.[80,81] In contrast, a linear decrease in age-standardized incidence has been recorded over the years (1984–2008) and the primary reason for this decrease is believed to be decline in smoking habits.[82]

In Australia and the United States, the incidence of esophageal adenocarcinoma has continued to increase annually over the past 4 decades. However, in a recent cohort study the rate of increase has eventually slowed or plateaued from 8.2% to 1.3% in subsequent years after 1996 ($P = .03$).[83] Additionally, from an age-period-cohort models, age-period and age-cohort effect has shown to be responsible for the trending increase in

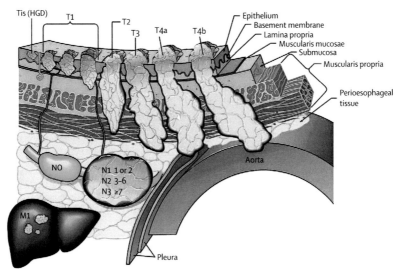

FIG. 1.6 Esophageal Carcinoma according to TNM (tumor, node, metastasis) staging system. Classification of T4 lesions has notable updates as resectable (T4a) or unresectable (T4b), and N status stratified as number of nodes involved. Tis = intraepithelial neoplasia, HGD = high-grade dysplasia.[3]

esophageal adenocarcinoma.[82] Risk factors such as, gastro-esophageal reflux disease, cigarette smoking, and obesity are linked with this cancer, however the specific factor contributing toward the disease is undefined. Evidence of stopping cigarette smoking seemed to have slightly improved in incidence.[84] However, more interventions to these risk factors could further improve the risk to adenocarcinoma.

From a latest genetic-based study, the association of a specific (rs2320615) single nucleotide polymorphisms in the nuclear assembly factor 1 (*NAF1*) gene has demonstrated to reduce the risk of esophageal cancer.[85] The overall impact of genetic variants that has been linked with adenocarcinoma is low. Advance studies to inspect the correlation between the molecular aspects of adenocarcinoma and its risk factors are needed. Although the prognosis for this terminal cancer has marginally improved, screening and surveillance for high-risk patients remain deprived.[86]

Treatment and Survival

According to the 2002 American Joint Committee on Cancer, esophageal cancer is classified based on the tumor-node-metastasis (TNM) classification system (Fig. 1.6). Diagnosis is reliant on imaging modalities such as endoscopic ultrasound, computed tomography, and positron emission tomography scans, while stage-specific treatment relies on multimodality therapies such as surgery, radiotherapy, and chemotherapy are utilized.[87] Most importantly, radiofrequency ablation

has been recommended as an appropriate treatment option as opposed to continuing endoscopic surveillance for a diagnosed low-grade dysplasia.[23,88]

Besides the current TNM staging system, length of the tumor has been considered as an essential prognostic factor in esophageal cancer associated with long-term survival. A retrospective has revealed, on one hand with tumor length of ≤3 cm the patient's survival rate for 1-, 3-, and 5-year was 68%, 51%, and 51%, on the other with tumor length of ≥3 cm the survival rate for similar years was 54%, 29%, and 11%.[89] Additionally, tumor location, histological type, and tumor grade had significant influence in variable survival rates.

Analysis from the Surveillance, Epidemiology, and End results (SEER) database between 1973 and 2007 showed a poor long-term (a decade) survival of only 14% after the diagnosis of esophageal cancer.[90] Nevertheless, in more recent SEER database analyzed study (2016), there was significant improvement in 5-years survival rate (9%–22%, $P < .001$) mainly due to more effective early detection of the disease and application of treatment modalities.[91] Although, the 5-year survival rate for esophageal cancer is poor, trends have improved over the past decade with long-term survival being highly possible in earlier advanced stage.[91,92] Biomarkers, such as HER2 expression, have been shown to have no impact of survival for patients with esophageal adenocarcinoma[93] and a decreased survival rate in squamous cell carcinoma patients.[94]

TABLE 1.2
Alteration of Esophageal Microbiome Between Normal and Diseased Conditions

Studies	Patient Cohorts	Microbial Identification Method	Findings
Macfarlane et al. (2007)[84]	7 controls 7 Barrett's esophagus	16s ribosomal RNA gene sequencing	High levels of *Campylobacter* species in Barrett's esophagus species.
Yang et al. (2009)[83]	12 controls 12 esophagitis 10 Barrett's esophagus	16s ribosomal RNA gene sequencing	Esophageal microbiome classified into Type I (*Streptococcus* species) and Type II (Gram negative/microaerophilic) microbiome.
Liu et al. (2013)[87]	6 controls 6 esophagitis 6 Barrett's esophagus	16s ribosomal DNA gene sequencing	Diverse bacterial communities associated with esophageal diseases.
Blackett et al. (2013)[88]	39 controls 37 GORD 45 Barrett's esophagus 30 Adenocarcinoma	Culture analysis followed by real-time PCR assays	Shift in esophageal biofilm with disease progression. Increased number of *Campylobacter concisus* colonized in GORD and Barrett's esophagus.

MICROBIOME IN THE ESOPHAGEAL HEALTH AND DISEASE

The microbiome population within the human esophagus is relatively simple compared to the rest of the gastrointestinal tract. The transient nature of most content in the esophagus means that the microbiome is not significantly affected by external sources. The first attempt to study the microflora of the healthy esophagus was made two decades ago. *Streptococcus viridans* was the predominant species identified from aspirate saline solution collected from the esophagus and oropharynx.[95] Following the revolutionary development of 16S ribosomal RNA gene sequencing technology in the 1980s, investigations into the human microbiome have grown exponentially. This technology was used to provide a more in-depth analysis of esophageal biopsies collected from four healthy individuals. Six different phyla, *Firmicutes*, *Bacteroides*, *Actinobacteria*, *Proteobacteria*, *Fusobacteria*, and *TM7*, were found in all individuals with higher prevalence of *Streptococcus* (39%), *Prevotella* (17%), and *Veilonella* (14%) species.[96]

Microbial Dysbiosis in Esophageal Diseases

The commensal microbes found in the esophagus have metabolic and immune-regulating roles in maintaining health. Conversely, imbalance in the existing microbial community or dysbiosis has been found to contribute toward etiology of various gastric cancers including esophageal cancer.[97] The association between changes in esophageal microbiome and other esophageal diseases, esophagitis and Barrett's esophagus, was investigated by comparing biopsies and aspirate samples with the control groups (Table 1.2).

The esophageal microbiome was categorized into two types: type I microbiome from genus *Streptococcus* (gram positive) associated with healthy controls whereas type II microbiome had inclusion of gram-negative anaerobes/microaerophiles that were linked with esophagitis and Barrett's esophagus (Table 1.2).[98] It was proposed that these nitrate-reducing anaerobes, only found in type II category, produced nitrite as their metabolic by-product. Nitrite reacts readily with amines, amides, and amino acids to form N-nitroso, a carcinogenic compound that may aggravate the existing diseases to progress toward forming adenocarcinoma.[99–101]

Mechanism of Pathogenesis Induced by Immune Response

A balanced immune system plays a critical role in sustaining the symbiotic relationship between the esophageal mucosa and its commensal microbes.[102,103] An imbalance in this delicate networking leads to inflammatory (innate immunity) and pathogenic infectious (adaptive immunity) responses. Our current understanding of esophageal cancer pathogenesis involves erosive damage of the mucosal lining due to acid reflux followed by chronic inflammation.

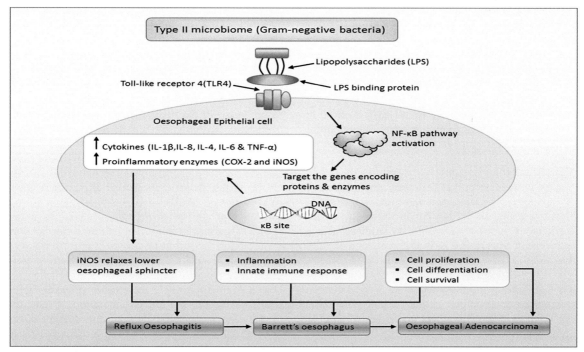

FIG. 1.7 Putative mechanism of activation of NF-κB pathway by Type II microbiome in esophageal epithelial cell.[104]

Essentially, various hypotheses have been proposed to gain further understanding of the disease processes. The major microbial component of Gram-negative (Type II) microbiota, lipopolysaccharide (LPS), activates the proinflammatory cytokines via the stimulation of Toll-like receptor 4 (TLR4) and nuclear factor kappa B cells (NF-κB) pathway (Fig. 1.7).[105,106] A gradual increase in the activation of NF-κB pathway has been reported throughout the spectrum of reflux-disorders: reflux esophagitis, Barrett's esophagus, and adenocarcinoma.[104,107–109] Most proteins associated with the innate immune response—interleukin-1 beta (IL-1β), interleukin-6, interleukin-8, and tumor necrosis factor-alpha (TNF-α)[104,109,110]—are also up-regulated during disease progression. Although the expression of Toll-like receptors 1–5, 7, and 9 in esophageal epithelial cells is more varied between test groups, their role in activation of NF-κB pathway in reflux-related diseases remains undefined.[111,112]

Furthermore, during the activation pathway, the genes that encode proinflammatory enzymes, such as Cyclooxygenase 2 (COX-2) and inducible nitric oxide synthase (iNOS), are up-regulated. An increased expression of COX-2 and iNOS has been reported in the epithelial cells of Barrett's metaplasia and across the progression from low to high-grade dysplasia and adenocarcinoma.[113–116] Similarly, both iNOS and COX-2 have shown to have an elevated expression in inflammatory bowel diseases, for instance in ulcerative colitis[117] and Crohn's disease.[118–120] It has also been hypothesized that the Type II microbiome could promote in gastric reflux, as LPS involves in relaxation of the lower esophageal sphincter through iNOS pathway.[121]

In terms of esophageal cell carcinoma, a molecular pathogenesis finding involving the cell–cell junction adhesion protein called p120-catenin (p120ctn, delta1, or Ctnnd 1) has been discovered. Normally, p120-catenin forms a specific junctional complex with other classical cadherins (Types I and II) at the epithelial cell membrane to create a normal homeostatic cell adhesion.[122] In esophageal cancer, a statistically significant amount of p120-catenin was lost or mislocalized.[123]

Helicobacter pylori and Esophageal Cancer

The role played by gastric microflora, *Helicobacter pylori* (*H. pylori*), in reflux-disorders is controversial. Although *H. pylori* colonization is a known risk factor for gastric cancer development,[124] case–control studies have indicated the bacterium is inversely linked with risk of gastro-esophageal diseases.[125–128] Although the mechanism of protection by the bacterium is yet to be elucidated, the reduced acid secretion during *H. pylori* infected atrophic gastritis may contribute to the inverse relation.[129,130] The eradication of *H. pylori* in clinical intervention trials inferred increasing incidence of reflux esophagitis in patients with existing hiatus hernia and corpus gastritis.[131] On the contrary, another published intervention study found that eradication therapy did not develop any de novo inflammation of the esophagus nor made the existing reflux disease worse.[132]

Eitzen and colleagues aimed to determine the role of *H. pylori* in the development of esophageal squamous cell carcinoma based on a systematic review and quantitative meta-analysis.[133] They conducted a comprehensive literature search and identified 17 studies that met the inclusion criteria. The 17 studies consisted of 2226 cases and 6711 of which 1346 cases and 3364 controls were *H. pylori* positive. Overall, there was no statistically significant protective effect of *H. pylori* infection on esophageal squamous cell carcinoma (OR = 0.82; 95% CI: 0.63–1.06). There was no evidence of publication bias ($P = .53$), but there was significant heterogeneity ($I^2 = 74\%$). Those with *H. pylori* cagA positive strains were associated with an increased risk of developing esophageal squamous cell carcinoma (OR = 1.39; 95% CI: 1.14–1.71). There was no heterogeneity among these studies ($I^2 = 0\%$). This finding was further enforced by the strong relationship demonstrated in developing countries (OR = 1.70; 95% CI: 1.25–2.32). This meta-analysis showed a relationship between *H. pylori* cagA positivity and esophageal squamous cell carcinoma, which has not previously been identified.[133]

Other Associated Microorganisms with Cancer

Recently, a prospective study disclosed an association between specific oral microbiota and esophageal cancers. Assessment of samples from prediagnostic mouthwash of two cohorts (adenocarcinoma and squamous cell carcinoma) using 16S rRNA sequencing found that the periodontal pathogens, *Tannerella forsythia* and *Porphyromonas gingivalis*, demonstrated an increasing trend of adenocarcinoma and squamous cell carcinoma, respectively. In addition, the normal flora of the oral cavity, *Neisseria* and *Streptococcus pneumonia*, was related to the decreased risk of esophageal adenocarcinoma.[134]

CONCLUSION

Over the last 50 years, there has been an increased incidence of esophageal cancer in many countries,

it has ultimately plateaued in some countries. However, the mortality and survival rate still remain poor possibly due to its strong association with long-standing risk factors (smoking, drinking, obesity, and GERD). However, the application of routine endoscopic surveillance strategy and multimodality therapies has resulted in a slight improvement in prognosis of the disease. Although attempts have been made to find potential biomarkers to predict the progression sequence of the disease, none could be recommended for diagnostic purpose (for dysplasia) except for p53 immunohistochemistry. Discovery of antibodies for more verified biomarkers needs to be found.

Alteration of microbiome in the distal esophagus has shown to activate an important hallmark of inflammatory response contributing toward a relation between inflammation and adenocarcinoma formation. Nevertheless, a paradoxical uncertainty exists whether the change in microbiome is due to acid reflux (being the primary factor) or the altered microbiome (being the primary factor) that has induced abnormality of the lower esophageal sphincter to cause reflux-associated diseases, accelerated by LPS–TLR–NFκB pathway. Finally, a future multiomics longitudinal study with further characterization of the esophageal microbiome and their relation to underlying epithelial barrier may provide insights into disease progression, earlier diagnosis, risk stratification, and potential treatments.

REFERENCES

1. Eslick G. Infectious causes of esophageal cancer. *Infect Dis Clin*. 2010;24:845–852.
2. Walsh TJ, Belitsos NJ, Hamilton SR. Bacterial esophagitis in immunocompromised patients. *Arch Intern Med*. 1986;146(7):1345–1348.
3. Coura JR, Viñas PA. Chagas disease: a new worldwide challenge. *Nature*. 2010;465:S6.
4. Rassi A, Rassi A, Marin-Neto JA. Chagas disease. *Lancet*. 2010;375(9723):1388–1402.
5. Gascon J, Bern C, Pinazo M-J. Chagas disease in Spain, the United States and other non-endemic countries. *Acta Trop*. 2010;115(1):22–27.
6. Prata A. Clinical and epidemiological aspects of Chagas disease. *Lancet Infect Dis*. 2001;1(2):92–100.
7. Coura JR, Borges-Pereira J. Chagas disease: 100 years after its discovery. A systemic review. *Acta Trop*. 2010;115(1):5–13.
8. Richter JE, Rubenstein JH. Presentation and epidemiology of gastresophageal reflux disease. *Gastroenterology*. 2018;154:267–276.
9. Eslick GD, Fass R. Noncardiac chest pain: evaluation and treatment. *Gastroenterol Clin N Am*. 2003;32:531–552.

10. Rubenstein JH. Risk factors for Barrett's esophagus. *Curr Opin Gastroenterol.* 2014;30(4):408–414.

11. Eslick GD, Talley NJ. Gastresophageal reflux disease (GERD): risk factors, and impact on quality of life-a population-based study. *J Clin Gastroenterol.* 2009;43:111–117.

12. Eusebi LH, Ratnakumaran R, Yuan Y, Solaymani-Dodaran M, Bazzoli F, Ford AC. Global prevalence of, and risk factors for, gastro-esophageal reflux symptoms: a meta-analysis. *Gut.* 2018;67:430–440.

13. Thrift AP, Cook MB, Vaughan TL, et al. Alcohol and risk of Barrett's esophagus: a pooled analysis from the international BEACON consortium. *Am J Gastroenterol.* 2014;109(10):1586–1594.

14. Lembo A, Zaman M, Jones M, Talley NJ. Influence of genetics on irritable bowel syndrome, gastro-esophageal reflux and dyspepsia: a twin study. *Aliment Pharmacol Ther.* 2007;25(11):1343–1350.

15. Marshall B, Warren JR. Unidentified curved bacilli in the stomach of patients with gastritis and peptic ulceration. *Lancet.* 1984;323(8390):1311–1315.

16. Marshall B, Warren JR, Blincow E, et al. Prospective double-blind trial of duodenal ulcer relapse after eradication of *Campylobacter pylori*. *Lancet*. 1988;332(8626):1437–1442.

17. Kuipers EJ, Thijs JC, Festen HP. The prevalence of *Helicobacter pylori* in peptic ulcer disease. *Aliment Pharmacol Ther.* 1995;9(suppl 2):59–69.

18. Raghunath A, Hungin A, Wooff D, Childs S. Prevalence of *Helicobacter pylori* in patients with gastro-esophageal reflux disease: systematic review. *BMJ.* 2003;326:737.

19. Ramis IB, Vianna JS, Gonçalves CV, von Groll A, Dellagostin OA, da Silva PEA. Polymorphisms of the IL-6, IL-8 and IL-10 genes and the risk of gastric pathology in patients infected with *Helicobacter pylori*. *J Microbiol Immunol Infect.* 2017;50:153–159.

20. Xie T, Cui X, Zheng H, Chen D, He L, Jiang B. Meta-analysis: eradication of *Helicobacter pylori* infection is associated with the development of endoscopic gastresophageal reflux disease. *Eur J Gastroenterol Hepatol.* 2013;25(10):1195–1205.

21. Malfertheiner P, Megraud F, O'Morain CA, et al. Management of *Helicobacter pylori* infection—the Maastricht V/florence consensus Report. *Gut.* 2017;66(1):6–30.

22. Chang J, Fasanella K, Chennat J, Davison J, McGrath K. Prevalence of esophageal neoplasia in short-segment versus long-segment Barrett's esophagus. *Esophagus.* 2016;13(2):151–155.

23. Whiteman DC1, Appleyard M, Bahin FF, et al. Australian clinical practice guidelines for the diagnosis and management of Barrett's esophagus and early esophageal adenocarcinoma. *J Gastroenterol Hepatol.* 2015;30:804–820.

24. Hameeteman W, Tytgat GNJ, Houthoff HJ, van den Tweel JG. Barrett's esophagus; development of dysplasia and adenocarcinoma. *Gastroenterology.* 1989;96(5):1249–1256.

25. Wang C, Yuan Y, Hunt RH. *Helicobacter pylori* infection and Barrett's esophagus: a systematic review and meta-analysis. *Am J Gastroenterol.* 2009;104(2):492–500; quiz 491, 501.

26. Cameron AJ, Ott BJ, Payne WS. The incidence of adenocarcinoma in columnar-lined (Barrett's) esophagus. *N Engl J Med.* 1985;313(14):857–859.

27. Hayeck T, Kong C, Spechler S, Gazelle G, Hur C. The prevalence of Barrett's esophagus in the US: estimates from a simulation model confirmed by SEER data. *Dis Esophagus.* 2010;23:451–457.

28. Gerson LB, Shetler K, Triadafilopoulos G. Prevalence of Barrett's esophagus in asymptomatic individuals. *Gastroenterology.* 2002;123(2):461–467.

29. Ronkainen J, Aro P, Storskrubb T, et al. Prevalence of Barrett's esophagus in the general population: an endoscopic study. *Gastroenterology.* 2005;129(6):1825–1831.

30. Gharahkhani P, Fitzgerald RC, Vaughan TL, et al. Genome-wide association studies in esophageal adenocarcinoma and Barrett's esophagus: a large-scale meta-analysis. *Lancet Oncol.* 2016;17(10):1363–1373.

31. Sorberg M, Nyren O, Granstrom M. Unexpected decrease with age of *Helicobacter pylori* seroprevalence among Swedish blood donors. *J Clin Microbiol.* 2003;41(9):4038–4042.

32. Fischbach LA, Nordenstedt H, Kramer JR, et al. The association between Barrett's esophagus and *Helicobacter pylori* infection: a meta-analysis. *Helicobacter.* 2012;17(3):163–175.

33. Postlethwait RW. Carcinoma of the thoracic esophagus. *Surg Clin.* 1983;63:933–940.

34. Pennathur A, et al. Esophagectomy for T1 esophageal cancer: outcomes in 100 patients and implications for endoscopic therapy. *Ann Thorac Surg.* 2009;87:1048–1054; discussion 1054-5.

35. Pennathur A, Gibson MK, Jobe BA, Luketich JD. Esophageal carcinoma. *Lancet.* 2013;381:400–412.

36. Howlader N, Noone AM, Krapcho M, et al., eds. *SEER Cancer Statistics Review, 1975–2014.* Bethesda, MD: National Cancer Institute; 2017. Available at: https://seer.cancer.gov/csr/1975_2014/.

37. National Cancer Institute. *SEER 18 2007-2013. SEER Cancer Statistics Review;* 2018. Available at: https://seer.cancer.gov/statfacts/html/colorect.html.

38. Pakzad R, et al. The incidence and mortality of esophageal cancer and their relationship to development in Asia. *Ann Transl Med.* 2016;4:29.

39. Eslick GD. Epidemiology of esophageal cancer. *Gastroenterol Clin N Am.* 2009;38:17–25.

40. Ferlay J, Soerjomataram I, Ervik M, et al. *GLOBOCAN 2012 v1.0, Cancer Incidence and Mortality Worldwide: IARC CancerBase No. 11.* Lyon, France: International Agency for Research on Cancer; 2013. Available at: http://globocan.iarc.fr.

41. Lepage CO, Drouillard A, Jouve JL, Faivre J. Epidemiology and risk factors for esophageal adenocarcinoma. *Dig Liver Dis.* 2013;45:625–629.

42. Castellsagué X, et al. Independent and joint effects of tobacco smoking and alcohol drinking on the risk of esophageal cancer in men and women. *Int J Cancer*. 1999;82:657–664.

43. Gao YT, et al. Risk factors for esophageal cancer in Shanghai, China. I. Role of cigarette smoking and alcohol drinking. *Int J Cancer*. 1994;58:192–196.

44. Zambon P, et al. Smoking, type of alcoholic beverage and squamous-cell esophageal cancer in northern Italy. *Int J Cancer*. 2000;86:144–149.

45. Lee C-H, et al. Independent and combined effects of alcohol intake, tobacco smoking and betel quid chewing on the risk of esophageal cancer in Taiwan. *Int J Cancer*. 2005;113:475–482.

46. Hashibe M, et al. Esophageal cancer in central and eastern Europe: tobacco and alcohol. *Int J Cancer*. 2007;120: 1518–1522.

47. Watanabe M. Risk factors and molecular mechanisms of esophageal cancer: differences between the histologic subtype. *J Cancer Metastasis Treat*. 2015;0(0).

48. Vial M, Grande L, Pera M. Epidemiology of adenocarcinoma of the esophagus, gastric cardia, and upper gastric third. *Recent Results Canc Res*. 2010;182:1–17.

49. Brown LM, et al. Dietary factors and the risk of squamous cell esophageal cancer among black and white men in the United States. *Cancer Causes Control*. 1998;9:467–474.

50. Launoy G, et al. Diet and squamous-cell cancer of the esophagus: a French multicentre case-control study. *Int J Cancer*. 1998;76:7–12.

51. De Stefani E, et al. Vegetables, fruits, related dietary antioxidants, and risk of squamous cell carcinoma of the esophagus: a case-control study in Uruguay. *Nutr Cancer*. 2000;38:23–29.

52. Correction: esophageal adenocarcinoma incidence: are we reaching the peak? *Cancer Epidemiol Biomark Prev*. 2010;19:2416.

53. Ferlay J, et al. Cancer incidence and mortality worldwide: sources, methods and major patterns in GLOBOCAN 2012. *Int J Cancer*. 2015;136:E359–E386.

54. Mao W-M, Zheng W-H, Ling Z-Q. Epidemiologic risk factors for esophageal cancer development. *Asian Pac J Cancer Prev*. 2011;12:2461–2466.

55. Arnal MJD, Arenas ÁF, Arbeloa ÁL. Esophageal cancer: risk factors, screening and endoscopic treatment in Western and Eastern countries. *World J Gastroenterol*. 2015;21:7933–7943.

56. Jain S, Dhingra S. Pathology of esophageal cancer and Barrrett's esophagus. *Ann Cardiothorac Surg*. 2017;6:99–109.

57. Lee C-H, et al. Carcinogenetic impact of alcohol intake on squamous cell carcinoma risk of the esophagus in relation to tobacco smoking. *Eur J Cancer*. 2007;43:1188–1199.

58. Song Q, et al. Processed food consumption and risk of esophageal squamous cell carcinoma: a case-control study in a high risk area. *Cancer Sci*. 2012;103:2007–2011.

59. Brücher BLDM, Stein HJ, Bartels H, Feussner H, Siewert JR. Achalasia and esophageal cancer: incidence, prevalence, and prognosis. *World J Surg*. 2001;25:745–749.

60. Rubenstein JH, Taylor JB. Meta-analysis: the association of esophageal adenocarcinoma with symptoms of gastro-esophageal reflux. *Aliment Pharmacol Ther*. 2010;32:1222–1227.

61. Singhi AD, et al. Undifferentiated carcinoma of the esophagus: a clinicopathological study of 16 cases. *Hum Pathol*. 2015;46:366–375.

62. Long E, Beales ILP. The role of obesity in esophageal cancer development. *Therap Adv Gastroenterol*. 2014;7: 247–268.

63. Kubo A, Corley DA, Jensen CD, Kaur R. Dietary factors and the risks of esophageal adenocarcinoma and Barrett's esophagus. *Nutr Res Rev*. 2010;23:230–246.

64. Ek WE, et al. Germline genetic contributions to risk for esophageal adenocarcinoma, barrett's esophagus, and gastresophageal reflux. *J Natl Cancer Inst*. 2013;105:1711–1718.

65. Zhang HY, Spechler SJ, Souza RF. Esophageal adenocarcinoma arising in Barrett esophagus. *Cancer Lett*. 2009;275:170–177.

66. Souza RF. From reflux esophagitis to esophageal adenocarcinoma. *Dig Dis*. 2016;34:483–490.

67. Umar SB, Fleischer DE. Esophageal cancer: epidemiology, pathogenesis and prevention. *Nat Clin Pract Gastroenterol Hepatol*. 2008;5:517–526.

68. Ingelfinger JR, Rustgi AK, El-Serag HB. Esophageal carcinoma. *N Engl J Med*. 2014;371:2499–2509.

69. Rubenstein JH, Shaheen NJ. Epidemiology, diagnosis, and management of esophageal adenocarcinoma. *Gastroenterology*. 2015;149:302–317. e1.

70. Whiteman DC, Kendall BJ. Barrett's esophagus: epidemiology, diagnosis and clinical management. *Med J Aust*. 2016. https://doi.org/10.5694/mja16.00796.

71. Reid BJ, Li X, Galipeau PC, Vaughan TL. Barrett's esophagus and esophageal adenocarcinoma: time for a new synthesis. *Nat Rev Cancer*. 2010;10:87–101.

72. Otterstatter MC, et al. Esophageal cancer in Canada: trends according to morphology and anatomical location. *Can J Gastroenterol*. 2012;26:723–727.

73. Australian Institute of Health and Wellfare (AIHW). *Australian Cancer Incidence and Mortality (ACIM) Books: Esophageal Cancer*; 2016.

74. National Cancer Institute. *Cancer Stat Facts: Esophageal Cancer. Surveillance, Epidemiology, End Results Program*; 2018. Available at: https://seer.cancer.gov/statfacts/html/esoph.html.

75. Gholipour M, et al. Esophageal cancer in Golestan Province, Iran: a review of genetic susceptibility and environmental risk factors. *Middle East J Dig Dis*. 2016;8:249–266.

76. Liang H, Fan J-H, Qiao Y-L. Epidemiology, etiology, and prevention of esophageal squamous cell carcinoma in China. *Cancer Biol Med*. 2017;14:33–41.

77. Abnet CC, Arnold M, Wei W-Q. Epidemiology of esophageal squamous cell carcinoma. *Gastroenterology.* 2018;154:360–373.

78. Blot WJ, McLaughlin JK. The changing epidemiology of esophageal cancer. *Semin Oncol.* 1999;26:2–8.

79. Wong MCS, et al. Global incidence and mortality of esophageal cancer and their correlation with socioeconomic indicators temporal patterns and trends in 41 countries. *Sci Rep.* 2018;8:4522.

80. Islami F, et al. Alcohol drinking and esophageal squamous cell carcinoma with focus on light-drinkers and never-smokers: a systematic review and meta-analysis. *Int J Cancer.* 2011;129:2473–2484.

81. Bagnardi V, et al. Light alcohol drinking and cancer: a meta-analysis. *Ann Oncol.* 2013;24:301–308.

82. Thrift AP, Whiteman DC. The incidence of esophageal adenocarcinoma continues to rise: analysis of period and birth cohort effects on recent trends. *Ann Oncol.* 2012;23:3155–3162.

83. Pohl H, Welch HG. The role of overdiagnosis and reclassification in the marked increase of esophageal adenocarcinoma incidence. *J Natl Cancer Inst.* 2005;97:142–146.

84. Wang Q-L, Xie S-H, Li W-T, Lagergren J. Smoking cessation and risk of esophageal cancer by histological type: systematic review and meta-analysis. *J Natl Cancer Inst.* 2017:109.

85. Yue C, et al. Association between genetic variants and esophageal cancer risk. *Oncotarget.* 2017;8:47167–47174.

86. Coleman HG, Xie S-H, Lagergren J. The epidemiology of esophageal adenocarcinoma. *Gastroenterology.* 2018;154:390–405.

87. Napier KJ, Scheerer M, Misra S. Esophageal cancer: a Review of epidemiology, pathogenesis, staging workup and treatment modalities. *World J Gastrointest Oncol.* 2014;6:112–120.

88. Phoa KN, et al. Radiofrequency ablation vs endoscopic surveillance for patients with Barrett esophagus and low-grade dysplasia. *J Am Med Assoc.* 2014;311:1209.

89. Zeybek A, et al. Significance of tumor length as prognostic factor for esophageal cancer. *Int Surg.* 2013;98:234–240.

90. Polednak AP. Trends in survival for both histologic types of esophageal cancer in U.S. Surveillance, Epidemiology and End Results areas. *Int J Cancer.* 2003;105:98–100.

91. Njei B, Mccarty TR, Birk JW. Trends in esophageal cancer survival in United States adults from 1973 to 2009: a SEER database analysis. *J Gastroenterol Hepatol.* 2016;31:1141–1146.

92. Rustgi AK, El-Serag HB. Esophageal carcinoma. *N Engl J Med.* 2014;371:2499–2509.

93. Nagaraja V, Shaw N, Morey AL, Cox MR, Eslick GD. HER2 expression in oesophageal carcinoma and Barrett's oesophagus associated adenocarcinoma: an Australian study. *Eur J Surg Oncol.* 2016;42:140–148.

94. Dreilich M, et al. HER-2 overexpression (3+) in patients with squamous cell esophageal carcinoma correlates with poorer survival. *Dis Esophagus.* 2006;19:224–231.

95. Gagliardi D, Makihara S, Corsi PR, et al. Microbial flora of the normal esophagus. *Dis Esophagus.* 1998.

96. Pei Z, et al. Bacterial biota in the human distal esophagus. *Proc Natl Acad Sci USA.* 2004;101:4250–4255.

97. Sheflin AM, Whitney AK, Weir TL. Cancer-promoting effects of microbial dysbiosis. *Curr Oncol Rep.* 2014;16:406.

98. Yang L, et al. Inflammation and intestinal metaplasia of the distal esophagus are associated with alterations in the microbiome. *Gastroenterology.* 2009;137:588–597.

99. Macfarlane S, Furrie E, Macfarlane GT, Dillon JF. Microbial colonization of the upper gastrointestinal tract in patients with Barrett's esophagus. *Clin Infect Dis.* 2007;45:29–38.

100. Suzuki H, Iijima K, Scobie G, Fyfe V, McColl KEL. Nitrate and nitrosative chemistry within Barrett's esophagus during acid reflux. *Gut.* 2005;54:1527–1535.

101. Mirvish SS. Role of N-nitroso compounds (NOC) and N-nitrosation in etiology of gastric, esophageal, nasopharyngeal and bladder cancer and contribution to known exposures to NOC. *Cancer Lett.* 1995;93:17–48.

102. Liu N, et al. Characterization of bacterial biota in the distal esophagus of Japanese patients with reflux esophagitis and Barrett's esophagus. *BMC Infect Dis.* 2013;13:130.

103. Blackett KL, et al. Esophageal bacterial biofilm changes in gastro-esophageal reflux disease, Barrett's and esophageal carcinoma: association or causality? *Aliment Pharmacol Ther.* 2013;37:1084–1092.

104. Konturek PC, et al. Activation of NFκB represents the central event in the neoplastic progression associated with Barrett's esophagus: a possible link to the inflammation and overexpression of COX-2, PPARγ and growth factors. *Dig Dis Sci.* 2004;49:1075–1083.

105. Hu J, Jacinto R, McCall C, Li L. Regulation of IL-1 receptor-associated kinases by lipopolysaccharide. *J Immunol.* 2002;168:3910–3914.

106. Pikarsky E, et al. NF-κB functions as a tumour promoter in inflammation-associated cancer. *Nature.* 2004;431:461–466.

107. Lee JS, et al. Involvement of oxidative stress in experimentally induced reflux esophagitis and Barrett's esophagus: clue for the chemoprevention of esophageal carcinoma by antioxidants. *Mutat Res.* 2001;480–481, 189–200.

108. Colleypriest BJ, Ward SG, Tosh D. How does inflammation cause Barrett's metaplasia? *Curr Opin Pharmacol.* 2009;9:721–726.

109. O'Riordan JM, et al. Proinflammatory cytokine and nuclear factor kappa-B expression along the inflammation-metaplasia-dysplasia-adenocarcinoma sequence in the esophagus. *Am J Gastroenterol.* 2005;100:1257–1264.

110. Abdel-Latif MMM, Kelleher D, Reynolds JV. Potential role of NF-κB in esophageal adenocarcinoma: as an emerging molecular target. *J Surg Res.* 2009;153:172–180.

111. Lim DM, Narasimhan S, Michaylira CZ, Wang ML. TLR3-mediated NF-kappa B signaling in human esophageal epithelial cells. *Am J Physiol Liver Physiol.* 2009;297:G1172–G1180.

112. Sheyhidin I, et al. Overexpression of TLR3, TLR4, TLR7 and TLR9 in esophageal squamous cell carcinoma. *World J Gastroenterol.* 2011;17:3745–3751.

113. Wilson KT, Fu S, Ramanujam KS, Meltzer SJ. Increased expression of inducible nitric oxide synthase and cyclooxygenase-2 in Barrett's esophagus and associated adenocarcinomas. *Cancer Res.* 1998;58:2929–2934.

114. Shirvani VN, Ouatu-Lascar R, Kaur BS, Omary MB, Triadafilopoulos G. Cyclooxygenase 2 expression in Barrett's esophagus and adenocarcinoma: ex vivo induction by bile salts and acid exposure. *Gastroenterology.* 2000;118:487–496.

115. Morris CD, Armstrong GR, Bigley G, Green H, Attwood SE. Cyclooxygenase-2 expression in the Barrett's metaplasia-dysplasia- adenocarcinoma sequence. *Am J Gastroenterol.* 2001;96:990–996.

116. Buskens CJ, et al. Prognostic significance of elevated cyclooxygenase 2 expression in patients with adenocarcinoma of the esophagus. *Gastroenterology.* 2002;122:1800–1807.

117. Verma R, Ahuja V, Paul J. Frequency of single nucleotide polymorphisms in NOD1 gene of ulcerative colitis patients: a case-control study in the Indian population. *BMC Med Genet.* 2009;10:82.

118. Hugot JP, et al. Association of NOD2 leucine-rich repeat variants with susceptibility to Crohn's disease. *Nature.* 2001;411:599–603.

119. Ogura Y, et al. A frameshift mutation in NOD2 associated with susceptibility to Crohn's disease. *Nature.* 2001;411:603–606.

120. Strober W, Murray PJ, Kitani A, Watanabe T. Signalling pathways and molecular interactions of NOD1 and NOD2. *Nat Rev Immunol.* 2006;6:9–20.

121. Fan YP, Chakder S, Gao F, Rattan S. Inducible and neuronal nitric oxide synthase involvement in lipopolysaccharide-induced sphincteric dysfunction. *Am J Physiol Gastrointest Liver Physiol.* 2001;280:G32–G42.

122. Davis MA, Ireton RC, Reynolds AB. A core function for p120-catenin in cadherin turnover. *J Cell Biol.* 2003;163:525–534.

123. Stairs DB, et al. Deletion of p120-catenin results in a tumor microenvironment with inflammation and cancer that establishes it as a tumor suppressor gene. *Cancer Cell.* 2011;19:470–483.

124. Eslick GD, Lim LL-Y, Byles JE, Xia HH-X, Talley NJ. Association of *Helicobacter pylori* infection with gastric carcinoma: a meta-analysis. *Am J Gastroenterol.* 1999;94:2373–2379.

125. Loffeld RJ, et al. Colonization with cagA-positive *Helicobacter pylori* strains inversely associated with reflux esophagitis and Barrett's esophagus. *Digestion.* 2000;62:95–99.

126. Rokkas T, Pistiolas D, Sechopoulos P, Robotis I, Margantinis G. Relationship between *Helicobacter pylori* infection and esophageal neoplasia: a meta-analysis. *Clin Gastroenterol Hepatol.* 2007;5.

127. Islami F, Kamangar F. *Helicobacter pylori* and esophageal cancer risk: a meta-analysis. *Cancer Prev Res.* 2008;1:329–338.

128. Gall A, et al. Bacterial composition of the human upper gastrointestinal tract microbiome is dynamic and associated with genomic instability in a Barrett's esophagus cohort. *PLoS One.* 2015;10.

129. Koike T, et al. The prevalence of *Helicobacter pylori* infection and the status of gastric acid secretion in patients with gastresophageal junction adenocarcinoma in Japan. *Inflammopharmacology.* 2007;15:61–64.

130. Sýkora J, et al. Gastric emptying of solids in children with H. pylori-positive and H. pylori-negative non-ulcer dyspepsia. *J Pediatr Gastroenterol Nutr.* 2004;39:246–252.

131. Hamada H, et al. High incidence of reflux oesophagitis after eradication therapy for *Helicobacter pylori*: impacts of hiatal hernia and corpus gastritis. *Aliment Pharmacol Ther.* 2000;14:729–735.

132. Kandulski A, Malfertheiner P. *Helicobacter pylori* and gastresophageal reflux disease. *Curr Opin Gastroenterol.* 2014;30:402–407.

133. Eitzen K, Eslick GD, Cox MR. *Helicobacter pylori* cagA positivity – an important determinant for esophageal squamous cell carcinoma risk: a systematic review and meta-analysis. *J Gastroenterol Hepatol.* 2011;26(suppl 4):81–82.

134. Peters BA, et al. Oral microbiome composition reflects prospective risk for esophageal cancers. *Cancer Res.* 2017;77:6777–6787.

CHAPTER 2

Helicobacter pylori, Peptic Ulcer Disease and Gastric Cancer

FATIMA EL-ASSAAD, PHD (MEDICINE), BMEDSCI (HONSI) •
LAN GONG, BSC (HONS), PHD • ANDREW GIA, BSC (ADVANCED) (HONOURS) •
HOWARD CHI HO YIM, BSC (HONS), PHD • EMAD M. EL-OMAR, BSC (HONS),
MB CHB, MD (HONS), FRCP (EDIN), FRSE, FRACP

INTRODUCTION

Helicobacter pylori Infection

Helicobacter pylori (*H. pylori*) is a highly prevalent gram-negative bacterium that remains a major cause of morbidity and mortality worldwide.[1] *H. pylori* colonizes more than half of the world population, and persistence of this infection remains the strongest risk factor for gastric cancer and peptic ulcer disease (PUD).[1] The incidence of *H. pylori* infection is closely related to exposure to contaminated food or water, use of antibiotics, poor sanitation, and living conditions and thus, varies dramatically across the globe.[2] China, sub-Saharan Africa, South America, and parts of Europe such as Poland and Portugal have the highest incidence,[3] and prevalence is lowest in Europe,[4] the United States, Australia,[5] and Saudi Arabia.[6]

H. pylori originated in Africa, and several strains of *H. pylori* have coevolved with human populations since the beginning of modern time (100 kyr).[7] Previously classed as *Campylobacter pyloridis*, *H. pylori* is a spiral rod-shaped, multiple-flagellate, microaerophilic, fastidious *Proteobacterium* and can be cultured *in vitro* on different solid media containing blood at pH 6–7. Under conditions of stress, particularly through oxygen deprivation,[8] exposure to antibiotics[9] and attachment to gastric epithelium,[10] these spiral rod-shaped *H. pylori* can transform into two types of coccoid cells, viable nonculturable and a degenerate form, to survive in less favorable environments.[11,12]

H. pylori colonizes the mucosal lining of the stomach with patchy distribution predominately in the antrum and less frequently in the fundus. It is able to persistently colonize the stringent gastric microenvironment withstanding the high concentrations of gastric acid and digestive enzymes and low partial oxygen pressure. *H. pylori* penetrates, infiltrates, and proliferates within the gastric mucosa causing chronic tissue damage and impaired acid secretion. This infection persists for life if not effectively treated.

H. pylori almost exclusively infects humans, predominantly male adults and children and induces a wide spectrum of clinical manifestations.[13,14] Acute symptoms of *H. pylori* infection are variable and can include nausea, vomiting, halitosis, dyspepsia, loss of appetite, weight loss, and generalized malaise that subside within 2 weeks.[15] Chronic infection can also lead to the development of primary gastric mucosa associated lymphoid tissue (MALT) lymphoma, dyspepsia, atrophic gastritis, iron deficiency anemia, and idiopathic thrombocytopenia purpura. Interestingly, *H. pylori* infection confers protection against several extragastric immune and inflammatory conditions including gastroesophageal reflux disease (GERD), oesophagitis, asthma and allergy, esophageal adenocarcinoma, coeliac disease, systemic lupus erythematosus, rheumatoid arthritis, multiple sclerosis, and inflammatory bowel disease.[16]

There are three broad presentations of *H. pylori* infection. The first is a benign gastritis where the majority of infected individuals remain asymptomatic. The second is two serious mutually exclusive gastrointestinal (GI) diseases: PUD (10%–15%) and gastric cancer (1%–3%), and the third is non-GI diseases, which have been reviewed previously. Both PUD and gastric cancer are characterized by high gastrin secretion. However, there are marked contrasting differences in acid secretion. Acid secretion in patients with PUD increases but, production decreases in patients with gastric cancer. Individuals that develop PUD are protected from developing gastric cancer. Adult patients infected with *H. pylori* have low gastric microbiota diversity and a dominant abundance of the *Helicobacter* genus. In contrast, children harbor a more diverse gastric microbiota dominated by an abundance of non-*Helicobacter Proteobacteria*.

Gastrointestinal Diseases and Their Associated Infections. https://doi.org/10.1016/B978-0-323-54843-4.00002-7
Copyright © 2019 Elsevier Inc. All rights reserved.

H. pylori transmission involves multiple or single strains of *H. pylori* infecting a single host via as person to person, food and/or water borne, and iatrogenically. To reach the gastric mucosa, it is considered that *H. pylori* is ingested via oro-oral or feco-oral routes and is transmitted via intimate contact and within families (person to person).[17] Environmental reservoirs of *H. pylori* via food and water contamination are possible but isolation of viable bacteria from these sources is rare.[18]

Diagnosis and management of *H. pylori* infection is tailored to the individual patient and aims to relieve symptoms, eradicate the infection, and heal the ulcers.[19] The gold-standard for diagnosis can be made via endoscopy with biopsy as this offers high specificity for *H. pylori* infection. Other tests such as Urease Breath Test (UBT), Fecal Antigen Test (FAT), Serological Test and HpSA, Rapid urease test (RUT), histology, culture, and PCR are also used in diagnosis.[20] The histopathological hallmarks of *H. pylori* infection include markers of active inflammation and most notably neutrophil infiltration in adults and lymphocytes and plasma cell infiltration in children.

H. pylori infection is treated using a combination of acid-suppressing treatment and antibiotics, usually triple therapy using proton-pump inhibitor (PPI), amoxicillin, and clarithromycin. Eradication of *H. pylori* infection heals gastritis and can reduce the risk of developing gastric cancer and peptic ulcer disease. The standard triple therapy was considered the gold standard for treating *H. pylori* infection until the first report of antibiotic resistance in 1990, particularly in patients with treatment failure,[21] as well as, poor patient compliance and reported adverse effects.[22,23] Over-use of clarithromycin has led to resistance against *H. pylori* in Asia–Pacific. Consequently, in 2017, the World Health Organization (WHO) listed clarithromycin resistant-*H. pylori* as a priority pathogen for the development and discovery of new antibiotics. In regions of high clarithromycin resistance, quadruple therapy, a regimen including PPI, bismuth subsalicylate, metronidazole, and tetracycline is used as an alternative treatment.[19]

Pathophysiology of *H. pylori*

In 1983, seminal work by two Australian researchers, Barry Marshall and Robin Warren, uncovered the causative role of *H. pylori* in gastritis and peptic ulcer disease. Until this breakthrough discovery, it was an entrenched belief among the medical fraternity that bacteria could not colonize the stomach and that excessive stomach acid secretion, stress, smoking, alcohol, spicy diet, and susceptible genes caused peptic ulcers. Marshall ingested a culture from a patient with gastritis

and subsequently fulfilled Koch's postulates to demonstrate the causal relationship between *H. pylori* and gastritis.[24] This finding was awarded the Nobel Prize in Physiology and Medicine in 2005 and paved the way for extensive research into the specific virulence factors that enable *H. pylori* to establish persistent colonization of a challenging niche, the stomach.

It remains of immense interest why only 10%–15% of *H. pylori*-infected individuals develop disease. The pathogenesis of *H. pylori* infection is mediated by a complex intricate interplay between bacterial virulence factors, host susceptibility and immune response, and environment exposure.[25] A number of *in vitro*, *in vivo* and new generation *ex vivo* experimental models of *H. pylori*-induced gastric pathology have shed light on disease development.[26] Endoscopic access for gastric tissue sampling and interdisciplinary collaboration among basic scientists, gastroenterologists, pathologists, and microbiologists has also accelerated our understanding of the pathophysiology of *H. pylori*.

Gastric resistance and colonization

Following entry into the stomach, successful colonization by *H. pylori* requires sophisticated means of gastric resistance.[27] The microenvironment of the stomach is acidic (pH 1–2), and survival of *H. pylori* is dependent on its ability to escape the bactericidal acidic milieu of the gastric lumen. At the beginning of infection, *H. pylori* neutralizes its local microenvironment by producing potent intracellular urease, an essential factor in gastric resistance. The production of urease enables hydrolysis of gastric urea to generate ammonia and carbon dioxide buffering the local pH, and consequently, neutralizing the pH around the bacterium. To increase urease production, *H. pylori* can recruit host immune cells to the site to produce urease. Urease and urease-derived ammonia support the survival of *H. pylori* in macrophages.[28]

Attachment, motility, penetration, and chemotaxis

The subsequent presence of ammonia decreases mucous viscosity, thus slowing down the mucous flow rate. This enables *H. pylori* adhesions to attach to the surface gastric epithelial mucosal lining via interactions to host cell receptors, avoid dislodgement by peristalsis and gastric emptying and subsequently, propel deeply into the mucosa and reach deeper nutrient rich layers of the stomach.

The helix morphology and polar motility of *H. pylori* via flagella and flagellin provides a mechanical advantage for deeper penetration via screw-like movements into the host epithelium and successful persistent gastric colonization.[29] Sensing and responding to pH is essential for *H. pylori* survival.[30,31] *H. pylori* actively swims away from acidic stomach lumen and localizes close to the alkaline epithelial surface. *H. pylori* is driven toward the gastric epithelium via chemo-attraction to various metabolites such as amino acids glutamine, histidine, lysine, and alanine as well as mucin, urea, sodium bicarbonate, and sodium chloride. This strategy facilitates the growth and multiplication of the bacteria within the mucosa.

H. pylori has over 30 genes dedicated to the expression of adhesins and can express several on their outer membrane.[31] Some of the well-studied *H. pylori*-adhesins include lipopolysaccharide (LPS), blood-antigen binding protein A (BabA), sialic acid-binding adhesion (SabA), neutrophil-activating protein (NAP), heat shock protein 60 (Hsp60), adherence associated proteins (AlpA and AlpB), *H. pylori* outer membrane protein (HopZ), and lacdiNAc-binding adhesion (LabA), none of which are essential for *H. pylori* attachment.[31] During gastritis, gastric mucin and epithelial receptors such as sialoglycoconjugates, sulfated glycoconjugates, sulfatides, and various sialylated and nonsialylated glycolipids are upregulated. The intimate interactions between *H. pylori*, mucin, and epithelial receptors induce inflammation, promote invasion and replication of *H. pylori* and ultimately disease progression.[16,25,31,32]

Gastric inflammation and tissue damage

H. pylori elicits a vigorous host immune response and failure by the host to eradicate it leads to mucosal damage and subsequent pathology. The long-term persistence of *H. pylori* in the host is dependent on modulation and evasion of the innate and adaptive immune system.[16,33]

Host innate immune response

Following penetration into the gastric epithelium, *H. pylori* needs to evade killing by phagocytes to cause chronic gastritis. The innate immune response provides the first line of defense against any pathogen. Gastric epithelial cells express pattern recognition receptors (PRRs) such as toll-like receptors (TLRs), nucleotide-binding oligomerization domain (NOD)-like receptors (NLRs), retinoic acid-inducible gene-I (RIG-I)-like receptors (RLRs), and C-type lectin receptors (CLRs) that recognize *H. pylori* pathogen-associated molecular patterns (PAMPs). Interaction between *H. pylori* PAMPs and TLRs induces cell signaling cascades and the subsequent inflammatory onslaught via the release of proinflammatory cytokines, chemokines, and recruitment of phagocytes to the gastric mucosa.

Several TLRs including TLR2, 4, 5, and 9 have been shown to detect *H. pylori*-ligands flagellin, LPS, Hsp60, NAP, nucleic acids, peptidyl prolyl cis-, trans-isomerase HP0175.[34] The flagellar protein flagellin can evade recognition by TLR,[35] and *H. pylori*-LPS can be modified to resist antimicrobial calprotectin and the TLR4-mediated inflammatory response.[36,37] Polymorphisms in TLR genes can affect the magnitude of response to *H. pylori* infection and encourage the development of malignancy.[38]

Cytotoxin-associated gene A (CagA) toxin

H. pylori secretes toxins and proteins directly into cells to affect host cellular pathways and consequently, damage tissue. Oncoprotein cytotoxin-associated gene A (CagA) is an *H. pylori* virulence factor encoded by *Cag*-pathogenicity Island (*cag*PAI), found on the most virulent strains of *H. pylori*.[39–41] It is one of the most well-characterized pathogenicity factors of *H. pylori*, and its presence is associated with severe clinical presentation. Not all *H. pylori* isolates from Western countries carry CagA (*CagA*-negative) but all *H. pylori* isolates from East-Asian countries do (*CagA*-positive). Low amounts of CagA are translocated to host gastric epithelial cells via bacterial type IV secretion system (T4SS) and are phosphorylated by cellular oncogenes at the Glu-Pro-IIe-Tyr-Ala (EPIYA) motifs.[31,42–44] Cag-A manipulates intracellular signaling to disrupt normal epithelial differentiation and promote the development of gastric cancer. In addition, *H. pylori* can induce mitochondrial cell death in macrophages, protect itself from nitric oxide (NO) by producing peroxiredoxin, and inhibit killing by neutrophils and monocytes by activating CagA.

Vacuolating cytotoxin A (VacA)

Vacuolating cytotoxin A (VacA) encoded by the *vacA* gene is a pore forming toxin that causes vacuolization of cells by binding to target cells and inserting into endosomes.[45,46] It is found in all strains and can induce cell apoptosis, inhibit T and B cell activation,[47] and invade chloride channels and target mitochondria.[48] The most virulent strain is *H. pylori*. Type I: cagA+ vacA+.

Host adaptive immune response

The adaptive immune response is recruited later in the *H. pylori* infection and is highly specific and targeted. *H. pylori* modulates T cell responses by inducing proinflammatory Th17 and Th1 and antiinflammatory regulatory T cells (Tregs). Both Th1 and Th17 cells promote inflammation by secreting cytokines, chemokines, and triggering the expression of antimicrobial peptides and reactive oxygen species.[16] However, *H. pylori* can evade T cell immunity by inducing a Treg response to persist within the host. It is able to influence dendritic cell Th17/Treg differentiation toward a Treg skewed response independent of *H. pylori* VacA or CagA.[49]

Several other bacterial virulence factors contribute to colonization, persistence, and pathogenesis of *H. pylori* infection. *H. pylori* sheds outer membrane vesicles that package *H. pylori* virulence factors such as cagA to enable survival and persistence of infection.[50] In addition, secreted virulence factors include serine protease HtrA, duodenal ulcer promoting gene A (DupA),[51] induced-by-contact-with epithelium gene (IceA1),[52] outer membrane protein (oipA),[53] and noncoding RNA for example short RNA, miRNA, and piRNA as previously reviewed.[54]

GASTRIC CANCER AND *H. PYLORI* INFECTION

Gastric cancer is a global health issue, being the fifth most common malignancy and the third leading cause of cancer death worldwide.[55] Lifestyle factors such as iron deficiency, a high salt diet, or smoking have been implicated as risk factors for gastric cancer development.[56,57] However, it is *H. pylori* infection that is considered to be the greatest risk factor for noncardia gastric cancer.[58] More specifically, it is the *H. pylori*-induced corpus-dominant gastritis phenotype that disposes to noncardia gastric cancer. This phenotype is characterized by chronic inflammation, gastric atrophy, and hypo- or achlorhydria.[31]

Epidemiology

H. pylori is implicated as the most important risk factor in both intestinal and diffuse histological types of gastric adenocarcinoma.[59] In a prospective, epidemiological study of 1228 gastric cancer cases from 12 studies found *H. pylori* infection was associated with a twofold increase in noncardia gastric cancer risk.[60] This risk is amplified by 1.64-fold with CagA-positive *H. pylori* infection.[61] Incidence rates of gastric cancer vary remarkably geographically, with the Southeast Asian population representing over half of the total gastric cancer cases.[62] In this population, the high rates of gastric cancer are associated with high *H. pylori* seroprevalence.[63] However, India and Thai populations have low gastric cancer incidence despite high rates of *H. pylori* carriage.[63] Together with the fact that remarkably, only 1%–3% of *H. pylori* seropositive individuals progress to gastric cancer,[64] this suggests that bacterial presence alone is insufficient for carcinogenesis. Rather, the clinical outcome of *H. pylori* infection is dictated by a complex interplay between host and pathogen genetics, and environmental factors.

From Infection to Cancer

The oncogenic potential of *H. pylori* infection is primarily attributed to the action of the CagA oncoprotein. In a transgenic mouse model, it was demonstrated that the systemic and stomach-localized expression of CagA led to carcinoma development.[65] In comparison to its Western counterpart, the CagA isoform expressed by East Asian *H. pylori* strains has been shown to have a greater oncogenic potential[66] and has been clinically associated with severe gastric mucosal atrophy and gastritis.[67] These isoforms differ structurally, with the Western CagA carrying EPIYA-A, EPIYA-B and usually repeated EPIYA-C segments while the East Asian CagA possess EPIYA-A, EPIYA-B, and EPIYA-D segments.[62] Mechanistically, the oncogenicity of CagA is derived from its ability to interact and disturb multiple host signaling pathways once delivered into host cells.[62] In conjunction with other pathogenicity factors, *H. pylori* is able to alter host processes to induce chronic inflammation and oncogenic signaling pathways as well as suppress tumor suppressor genes. This includes disruption of tight cell–cell junctions and cell polarity via CagA-mediated dissociation of E-cadherin/β-catenin complexes,[68] the suppression of the c-Met/phosphatidylinositol (PI)3 kinase/Akt antitumor signaling pathway[69] and the downregulation of relevant genes via promoter hypermethylation.[70] Overall, this results in cellular proliferation, the breakdown and disorganization of the gastric epithelium, and reprogramming of cellular expression that together favors the formation of precancerous lesions, gastritis, and ultimately gastric cancer.

Inflammation

Chronic inflammation is a potent driver of carcinogenesis.[71] It is well documented that *H. pylori* infection can result in prolonged and potentially severe gastric inflammation. Initiation of host inflammation is dependent on the recognition of microbial patterns, such as LPS and peptidoglycan by host innate immune receptors including Toll-like receptors (TLRs), NOD1 and NOD2.[72] Engagement of these receptors leads to the activation of the transcription factors NF-κB and AP-1, which then translocate to nucleus.[73] This process has been shown to be type 4 secretion system (T4SS)-dependent.[73] Once in the nucleus, NF-κB and AP-1 induce the expression of target genes. The consequences of which include increased proinflammatory cytokine and chemokine secretion, mutagenic reactive oxygen species (ROS) accumulation as well as mitogenic and antiapoptotic activity.[74] Ultimately, a persistent *H. pylori*-induced inflammatory environment results in severe mucosal damage that can progress to gastritis, gastric atrophy, and carcinogenesis.[75]

Host Genetics and Inflammation

Host genetics is a key predisposing factor to *H. pylori*-associated gastric cancer. Single nucleotide polymorphisms (SNPs) and variable number tandem repeats (VNTRs) in genes involved in innate pathogen recognition and inflammation are able to attenuate or accentuate host responses to infection. Thus, host genotype is a crucial factor in determining gastric cancer risk and patient clinical outcome.[76] Considerable research focus has been placed on the polymorphisms that accentuate inflammation and atrophic gastritis to be used as susceptibility biomarkers for *H. pylori*-associated carcinogenesis.[31,77]

Interleukin-1 beta

Interleukin-1 beta (IL-1β) is a crucial candidate due to its dual role as both a proinflammatory signaling molecule and an inhibitor of gastric acid secretion.[78] IL-1β, its corresponding receptor antagonist Interleukin Receptor Antagonist-1 (IL-1RA), and Interleukin 1 alpha (IL-1α) are encoded by the genes *IL-1B*, *IL-1RN*, and *IL-1A* respectively, as constituents of the Interleukin 1 (IL-1) gene cluster.[79] Multiple functionally relevant polymorphisms that affect IL-1β and IL-1RA secretion have been identified within this gene cluster.[76] In a landmark study, El-Omar et al. associated the genotypes *IL1B-31*C*, *IL1β-511*T*, and *IL1RN*2/*2* with a twofold to threefold increased risk of *H. pylori*-induced hyperchlorydia and noncardia gastric cancer in a Caucasian population.[80] This result has been corroborated by other human studies that confirm a significant, positive association between gastric cancer risk and IL-1 variants, particularly in Caucasian populations.[81–84]

The importance of IL-1β was further demonstrated in animal studies. Stomach-specific overexpression of IL-1β in a transgenic mouse model led to stomach carcinogenesis.[85] This model closely resembled the development of human cancer, with a step-wise progression from spontaneous inflammation to metaplasia and carcinoma in a process that was accelerated by *Helicobacter felis* infection. *H. pylori*-induced tumorigenesis is at least in part, IL-1β-dependent. In an IL-1β-null mouse model, inflammation in response to *H. pylori* infection was heavily attenuated,[86] suggesting that carcinogenesis is, at least in part, IL-1β dependent. Reduced tumor load in the IL-1β-null mice compared to wild-type mice was a result of a lack of NF-κβ activation.

However, it is important to note that there is a marked interethnic and geographical discordance between IL-1 allele status and clinical outcome. Some studies, particularly those focused on Asian populations, found either no or the inverse relationship between IL-1 genetic markers and gastric cancer risk. For instance, in Japanese and Algerian patient cohorts, there was no association between the *IL1β-511*T* allele and gastric cancer,[87,88] while other Asian population cohort studies associated the *IL1B-31*C* and *IL1β-511*T* polymorphisms with a reduced gastric cancer risk.[89] Although it is possible that such variation arises due to inherent differences in study design and statistical power, these trends were observed even when weaker studies were excluded.[89] Undoubtedly, IL-1β is still considered an essential cytokine in *H. pylori*-associated gastric carcinogenesis as concluded by multiple meta-analyses.[79,89,90] The variability in the reports, however, highlights the importance of considering potential confounders such as ethnicity, geography, and disease subtypes as well as *H. pylori* infection status when searching for genetic susceptibility markers.[78]

Other cytokines

Numerous other cytokine gene polymorphisms have been reported to increase *H. pylori*-associated gastric cancer risk. SNPs in the genes encoding IL-2,[91] IL-10, and TNF[82] have been significantly associated with increased risk of gastric cancer. For instance, in two independent studies of a Korean and Indian cohort, carriage of the *IL8-251 A/A* SNPs was linked to an increased risk of gastric cancer development in comparison to healthy controls.[92,93] Due to its proinflammatory and acid suppressive properties, TNF polymorphisms are particularly potent modulators of gastric cancer risk.[76]

Similarly, IL-2 polymorphisms *–330 GG* and *+114 TT* in Caucasians[91] and *IL10-592* in a South Korean[94] population also conferred an increased risk of gastric cancer development. However, this contrasts with other studies, including a large meta-analysis, that were unable to observe any significant association between IL-6, IL-8, and IL-10 polymorphisms with *H. pylori*-associated gastric cancer risk.[89,95] With a multitude of studies that are heterogenous in their approach, it still remains inconclusive if IL-2, IL-6, IL-8, and IL-10 gene polymorphisms confer an increased risk of gastric cancer in *H. pylori*-positive patients.

Innate immune recognition receptors

The recognition of pathogen-associated molecular patterns (PAMPs) by host pattern recognition receptors (PRRs) is essential for the initiation of the innate immune response. It is thus plausible that polymorphisms in the genes encoding these receptors also influence the magnitude of inflammatory responses against *H. pylori* and influence the development of gastric carcinogenesis. Toll-like receptor 4 (TLR4) is one such cell-surface receptor involved in the recognition of *H. pylori* infection. TLR4 engagement with microbial PAMPs activates signal transduction via Myeloid differentiation primary response 88 (MyD88), Toll/IL-1, and TNF Receptor Associated Factor 6 (TRAF6). This ultimately leads to the promotion of proinflammatory gene expression via the transcription factor NF-κB.[96] Functional polymorphism *TLR4+ 896A > G* is associated with the increased risk of severe chronic inflammation.[96] In a Caucasian cohort, it was found that carriers of this polymorphism had an increased risk of gastric atrophy hypochlorhydria in the presence of *H. pylori*. As these are key precancerous hallmarks, it is thus feasible that the TLR4 variant is relevant to the development of gastric carcinogenesis.

NOD-like receptors (NLRs) are also key receptors involved in the detection and response against microbial pathogens. NLRs are intracellular receptors capable of binding a variety of PAMPs including flagellin and LPS. Nucleotide-binding oligomerization domain-containing protein (NOD)-1 and NOD2 are well characterized members of the NLR family. These receptors activate kinase receptor interacting protein 2 (RIP2), which in turn activates mitogenic and inflammatory signaling via the ERK and NF-κβ, respectively.[97] Associations between NOD1 and NOD2 genetic variants have been observed in numerous studies. In a Chinese population-based study, the *NOD2 rs718226* polymorphism was associated with an increased risk of dysplasia or gastric cancer in the presence of *H. pylori*, while the *NOD2 rs2111235 C* and *rs7205423 G* alleles were associated with decreased risk.[98] In relation to NOD1, *NOD1 rs7789045 TT* and *NOD1 rs2907749 G* were associated with increased and decreased risk of gastric cancer, respectively.[99] The biological consequences of these SNPs have yet to be conclusively elucidated. However, it has been suggested that an overall reduction in the NOD1/2-mediated innate immune response results in *H. pylori* persistence, which then triggers chronic inflammation via other signaling pathways. There is also a proposed role of the inflammasome and autophagy, which both require NLR receptors, in propagating inflammation and bestowing a susceptibility to gastric cancer.[97]

Prevention and Management

As *H. pylori* is evidently the greatest risk factor for non-cardia gastric cancer, there has been an increasing interest to eradicate the pathogen as a means to prevent gastric cancer. The Japanese national health insurance scheme approved *H. pylori* eradication treatment for patients with chronic gastritis.[100] The most common treatment used is a PPI-based triple therapy consisting of a PPI in conjunction with amoxicillin and clarithromycin.[100] This in conjunction with routine gastric cancer screening to detect early, precancerous lesions[101] has been instrumental in curbing the high rates of gastric cancer incidence and deaths in Japan. With 1.5 million prescriptions written annually since the treatment's approval in 2013, gastric cancer death rates have decreased significantly from 2013 to 2016.[100] Similar successes have been reported in a Western population, with the risk of noncardia adenocarcinoma sharply decreasing from 5 years post eradication treatment.[102]

Assessing the effectiveness and the magnitude of benefit for such an approach has been the cause of much debate. When evaluating the effectiveness, it is important to consider confounders such as the geographical and ethnic variability in baseline gastric cancer risk. Whether *H. pylori* eradication is still effective once atrophic gastritis or intestinal metaplasia has already developed is also an important consideration.[103] There is conflicting evidence from randomized controlled trials (RCT) in this regard. One RCT suggested that there is a point of no return, whereby eradication was only protective of gastric cancer in individuals without atrophic gastritis[104] while others demonstrated that eliminating *H. pylori* in subjects with atrophic gastric or early gastric cancer was able to reduce recurrent cancer incidence.[105,106] A systematic review and meta-analyses of 24 studies carried out by Lee et al.[103] resolved this dissonance. After adjusting for baseline gastric cancer incidence individuals who underwent *H. pylori* eradication had a lower gastric cancer incidence than those who did not. This benefit was enhanced in those with higher baseline incidence. Furthermore, eradication was also beneficial for high-risk individuals, with a reduced gastric cancer risk in those with atrophic gastritis and intestinal metaplasia. Therefore, *H. pylori* eradication treatment provides benefit across all baseline gastric cancer risks in both asymptomatic and high-risk individuals. Although, other factors such as long-term PPI use can increase the risk of gastric cancer in patients who have received eradication therapy.[107]

PEPTIC ULCER DISEASE AND *H. PYLORI* INFECTION

PUD is a break in the mucosal lining of upper gastrointestinal (GI) tract, which is usually larger than 5 mm in diameter with depth to the submucosa.[108] The diagnosis is typically based on the presenting symptoms including chronic, upper abdominal pain related to eating a meal (dyspepsia), with confirmation by either barium swallow or endoscopy that may show an ulcer in the stomach (gastric ulcer), proximal duodenum (duodenal ulcer), or the lower esophagus (esophageal ulcer). PUD is present in around 4% of the population worldwide. It results from an imbalance of factors that promote mucosal damage, including gastric acid, pepsin, *H. pylori* infection, nonsteroidal antiinflammatory drug (NSAID) use, and the host mechanisms involved in gastroduodenal defense, including prostaglandins, mucus, bicarbonate, and mucosal blood flow.[108]

H. pylori infection is the leading cause of PUD, although NSAID-related ulcers are also common in *H. pylori*-infected patients.[109] For decades, a decline in PUD incidence has been observed in developing countries. This has been linked to a decrease in the prevalence of *H. pylori* infection,[110] as well as the prolific use of antisecretory agents such as PPI.[111] This decline is largely limited to uncomplicated PUD, while rates of complicated PUD characterized by bleeding ulcers and perforation remain unchanged.[112]

H. pylori eradication is an effective treatment for PUD and reducing rates of relapse, but dyspeptic symptoms may persist in up to 30% of patients.[111,113] *H. pylori*-infected patients have a 3%–25% risk of developing PUD over their lifetime. The benefit of antibiotics treatment normally lasts for at least 6 years during which most patients no longer need antisecretory medication.[114] The interaction between *H. pylori* infection and the usage of NSAID or aspirin in PUD patients remains unclear with several studies giving conflicting results.[115] Current guidelines recommend a *"H. pylori* test and treat strategy" for naïve NSAID users to prevent PUD occurrence.[113]

H. pylori infection may have different effects on the production of hydrochloric acid in gastric secretions: acute infection causes hypochlorhydria (increased secretion) while chronic infection leads to either hypo- or hyperchlorhydria (reduced secretion) depending on the anatomic site of infection.[116] Hypochlorhydria in acute infection facilitates *H. pylori* survival in the stomach. Chronically infected patients can present with pangastritis with hyperchlorhydria, gastric atrophy, metaplasia, dysplasia, and carcinoma. Ten percent of patients manifest an antral predominant gastritis with hypochlorhydria due to a decrease in somatostatin and increase in gastrin secretion, leading to a potential development of PUD.[116]

There is a small percentage of PUD characterized as idiopathic PUD (IPUD) with *H. pylori* negative NSAID negative ulcers localized predominantly in the antrum.[117] IPUD usually has severe clinical outcomes including delayed ulcer healing, higher rates of re-bleeding after initial healing, more refractory to treatment, and higher mortality than that of *H. pylori*-related

PUD, which may be associated with the lack of *H. pylori* infection in these patients.[118]

Pathophysiology of *H. pylori*-mediated PUD

H. pylori usually colonizes gastric or duodenal mucosa and induces vigorous immune responses, leading to development of various GI diseases such as gastritis, PUD and gastric cancer.[3] The prevalence of PUD varies with geographical location and ethnicity due to differences in host genetic diversity, the phylogeographic origin of *H. pylori*, infection rates and environmental exposures. Interestingly, although it is an important cause, *H. pylori* infection is not one of the main contributors to the recurrence of PUD. Patients that are older, male, or those with chronic kidney disease are more at risk of suffering recurrent PUD.[119] Reinfection with *H. pylori* following successful eradication treatment is also associated with an increased risk of PUD recurrence.[120]

The exact mechanism behind *H. pylori*-mediated PUD development is yet to be fully understood. However, *H. pylori*-induced chronic inflammation of the gastric mucosa may play a role in the severe damage of the stomach epithelium and the subsequent manifestation of PUD.[121] As discussed earlier, the development of GI diseases including PUD and gastric carcinoma is linked to a few *H. pylori* virulence factors including cytotoxin VacA, secreted antigen CagA and its export apparatus bacterial type IV secretion system (T4SS).[43] The *H. pylori*-mediated immune response includes an increased level of CD3+CD4+ T cells in the gastric lamina propria (LP), which may play an important role in the pathogenesis of persistent infection.[122] *H. pylori* also manipulates T cell function by eliciting Foxp3+ regulatory T cells (Tregs) that are negatively associated with PUD.[123] Tregs are positively associated with *H. pylori* virulence factors VacA and outer inflammatory protein A (OipA) of *H. pylori* as well as histological grade but negatively associated with PUD.[124] These findings suggest that *H. pylori* specific Tregs contribute to the persistence of *H. pylori* colonization in gastric mucosa via suppressing the immune response and then lead to PUD development.

INTERACTIONS BETWEEN *H. PYLORI* AND THE MICROBIOME

More than 100 trillion symbiotic microorganisms live on and within humans and play a pivotal role in health and disease.[125] The highest density of microbes colonizes the GI tract and collectively forms the gut microbiota. Several factors such as diet, environment, and lifestyle can profoundly change the composition of the microbiome. This imbalance of microbial composition, known as dysbiosis, has been implicated in several infectious diseases, liver diseases, GI diseases, metabolic diseases, respiratory diseases, autoimmune diseases, coronary heart disease, and neurological disorders.[126] The interaction between gut microbiome and GI diseases is discussed in detail in Chapter 21 of this book.

The composition of the gut microbiome is influenced by acid suppression, gastric inflammation, and *H. pylori* infection.[127,128] The predominant gastric bacteria belong to the phyla of *Firmicutes, Actinobacteria, Bacteroidetes, Proteobacteria* (which include *H. pylori*), and the genus of *Streptococcus, Lactobacillus,* and *Propionibacterium*.[128] Higher levels of *Streptococci* are found in the gut microbiome of PUD patients.[129] *H. pylori*-infected PUD patients have higher levels of *Porphyromonas gingivalis, Prevotella intermedia,* and *Fusobacterium nucleatum,* and decreased levels of *Aggregatibacter actinomycetemcomitans*,[130] suggesting that *H. pylori* infection may aggravate the progress of chronic periodontitis. A recent study demonstrated alterations in the gastric microbiome in patients with various stages of gastric cancer following *H. pylori* eradication.[131] This suggests that *H. pylori* colonization in these patients induces dysbiosis and a reduction in microbial diversity, which can be restored by antimicrobial therapy.

Some non-*H. pylori* bacteria in GI may play a role in the transformation of gastric epithelial cells, leading to PUD and gastric carcinoma.[132] It was demonstrated that the lack of commensal bacteria in *H. pylori*-infected hypergastrinemic Insulin-Gastrin (INS-GAS) mice led to mild gastric pathology including reduced gastritis and delayed intraepithelial neoplasia.[133] Furthermore, the accelerated phenotype in the *H. pylori*-infected INS-GAS mouse model of gastric cancer is linked to a shifted gastric microbial profile with an increased level of *Firmicutes* and a decreased level of *Bacteroidetes*.[133] Colonization of germ-free INS-GAS mice with a restricted commensal microbiota (altered Schaedler's flora) prior to challenge with *H. pylori* causes severe gastric pathology including gastric corpus inflammation, neoplastic lesion formation, epithelial hyperplasia, and dysplasia.[134]

In mouse models, it has been demonstrated that non-gastric gut microbes can also affect *H. pylori*-mediated gastric carcinogenesis. For example, precolonization with different enterohepatic *Helicobacter* species (non-*H. pylori*) in *H. pylori*-infected mice had mixed consequences on proinflammatory *H. pylori*-induced gastric pathology.[135,136] *H. hepaticus* was shown to promote gastric inflammation while *H. bilis* and *H. muridarum*

attenuated it. These results demonstrate that the GI microbiota is capable of interacting with *H. pylori* and can influence the clinical outcome of *H. pylori*-associated disorders.

The efficiency of *H. pylori* eradication therapy using antibiotics is mediated by the effects of anti-*H. pylori* antibiotics on non-*H. pylori* microbes in the GI tract.[137] In addition, *H. pylori* infection suppresses acid secretion in the stomach, which can allow the survival of ingested microorganisms, facilitating their transition through the stomach and their colonization of the distal intestine and colon. Treatment with antisecretory agents like PPI could also result in microbial overgrowth in the stomach. The resulting gut dysbiosis may have further impacts on GI health and disease.[116]

CONCLUSION

H. pylori establishes persistent infection with extremely high prevalence rates globally. Although the majority of infected individuals remain asymptomatic, *H. pylori* is able to lead to severe GI diseases. The bacterium is the strongest causative factor for two distinct, mutually exclusive conditions, PUD and gastric cancer. PUD is characterized by antral predominant gastritis and hyperchlorhydria, while gastric cancer is characterized by corpus-predominant gastritis and hypo- or achlorhydria. Although different, both conditions are a result of *H. pylori*-mediated changes in host acid secretion and inflammatory pathways in conjunction with other predisposing factors such as NSAID use, host genetics, and diet modulating the risk of developing either clinical outcome. *H. pylori* in the context of PUD and gastric cancer is an interesting case whereby a complex interplay between virulence factors, host genetics, microbial ecology, and environmental factors can dictate whether infection can result in one of three vastly different clinical outcomes.

REFERENCES

1. Mitchell H, Katelaris P. Epidemiology, clinical impacts and current clinical management of *Helicobacter pylori* infection. *Med J Aust*. 2016;204(10):376–380.
2. Eusebi LH, Zagari RM, Bazzoli F. Epidemiology of *Helicobacter pylori* infection. *Helicobacter*. 2014;19(suppl 1):1–5.
3. O'Connor A, O'Morain CA, Ford AC. Population screening and treatment of *Helicobacter pylori* infection. *Nat Rev Gastroenterol Hepatol*. 2017;14(4):230–240.
4. Roberts SE, Morrison-Rees S, Samuel DG, Thorne K, Akbari A, Williams JG. Review article: the prevalence of *Helicobacter pylori* and the incidence of gastric cancer across Europe. *Aliment Pharmacol Ther*. 2016;43(3):334–345.

5. Pandeya N, Whiteman DC. Prevalence and determinants of *Helicobacter pylori* sero-positivity in the Australian adult community. *J Gastroenterol Hepatol.* 2011;26(8):1283–1289.

6. Hanafi MI, Mohamed AM. *Helicobacter pylori* infection: seroprevalence and predictors among healthy individuals in Al Madinah, Saudi Arabia. *J Egypt Publ Health Assoc.* 2013;88(1):40–45.

7. Moodley Y, Linz B, Bond RP, et al. Age of the association between *Helicobacter pylori* and man. *PLoS Pathogens.* 2012;8(5):e1002693.

8. Eaton KA, Catrenich CE, Makin KM, Krakowka S. Virulence of coccoid and bacillary forms of *Helicobacter pylori* in gnotobiotic piglets. *J Infect Dis.* 1995;171(2):459–462.

9. Berry V, Jennings K, Woodnutt G. Bactericidal and morphological effects of amoxicillin on *Helicobacter pylori*. *Antimicrob Agents Chemother.* 1995;39(8):1859–1861.

10. Segal ED, Falkow S, Tompkins LS. *Helicobacter pylori* attachment to gastric cells induces cytoskeletal rearrangements and tyrosine phosphorylation of host cell proteins. *Proc Natl Acad Sci USA.* 1996;93(3):1259–1264.

11. Azevedo NF, Almeida C, Cerqueira L, Dias S, Keevil CW, Vieira MJ. Coccoid form of *Helicobacter pylori* as a morphological manifestation of cell adaptation to the environment. *Appl Environ Microbiol.* 2007;73(10):3423–3427.

12. Saito N, Konishi K, Sato F, et al. Plural transformation-processes from spiral to coccoid *Helicobacter pylori* and its viability. *J Infect.* 2003;46(1):49–55.

13. Ibrahim A, Morais S, Ferro A, Lunet N, Peleteiro B. Sex-differences in the prevalence of *Helicobacter pylori* infection in pediatric and adult populations: systematic review and meta-analysis of 244 studies. *Dig Liver Dis.* 2017;49(7):742–749.

14. Burucoa C, Axon A. Epidemiology of *Helicobacter pylori* infection. *Helicobacter.* 2017;22(suppl 1).

15. White JR, Winter JA, Robinson K. Differential inflammatory response to *Helicobacter pylori* infection: etiology and clinical outcomes. *J Inflamm Res.* 2015;8:137–147.

16. Robinson K. *Helicobacter pylori*-mediated protection against extra-gastric immune and inflammatory disorders: the evidence and controversies. *Diseases.* 2015;3(2):34–55.

17. Didelot X, Nell S, Yang I, Woltemate S, van der Merwe S, Suerbaum S. Genomic evolution and transmission of *Helicobacter pylori* in two South African families. *Proc Natl Acad Sci USA.* 2013;110(34):13880–13885.

18. Zamani M, Vahedi A, Maghdouri Z, Shokri-Shirvani J. Role of food in environmental transmission of *Helicobacter pylori*. *Caspian J Intern Med.* 2017;8(3):146–152.

19. Malfertheiner P, Megraud F, O'Morain CA, et al. Management of *Helicobacter pylori* infection–the Maastricht IV/florence consensus report. *Gut.* 2012;61(5):646–664.

20. Kalali B, Formichella L, Gerhard M. Diagnosis of *Helicobacter pylori*: changes towards the future. *Diseases.* 2015;3(3):122–135.

21. Weil J, Bell GD, Powell K, et al. *Helicobacter pylori* and metronidazole resistance. *Lancet (London, England).* 1990;336(8728):1445.

22. Graham DY, Lew GM, Malaty HM, et al. Factors influencing the eradication of *Helicobacter pylori* with triple therapy. *Gastroenterology.* 1992;102(2):493–496.

23. Kuo YT, Liou JM, El-Omar EM, et al. Primary antibiotic resistance in *Helicobacter pylori* in the Asia-Pacific region: a systematic review and meta-analysis. *Lancet Gastroenterol Hepatol.* 2017;2(10):707–715.

24. Marshall BJ. The pathogenesis of non-ulcer dyspepsia. *Med J Aust.* 1985;143(7):319.

25. Kao CY, Sheu BS, Wu JJ. *Helicobacter pylori* infection: an overview of bacterial virulence factors and pathogenesis. *Biomed J.* 2016;39(1):14–23.

26. Burkitt MD, Duckworth CA, Williams JM, Pritchard DM. *Helicobacter pylori*-induced gastric pathology: insights from in vivo and ex vivo models. *Dis Models Mech.* 2017;10(2):89–104.

27. Miller EF, Maier RJ. Ammonium metabolism enzymes aid *Helicobacter pylori* acid resistance. *J Bacteriol.* 2014;196(17):3074–3081.

28. Schwartz JT, Allen LA. Role of urease in megasome formation and *Helicobacter pylori* survival in macrophages. *J Leukoc Biol.* 2006;79(6):1214–1225.

29. Gu H. Role of flagella in the pathogenesis of *Helicobacter pylori*. *Curr Microbiol.* 2017;74(7):863–869.

30. Schreiber S, Konradt M, Groll C, et al. The spatial orientation of *Helicobacter pylori* in the gastric mucus. *Proc Natl Acad Sci USA.* 2004;101(14):5024–5029.

31. Amieva MR, El-Omar EM. Host-bacterial interactions in *Helicobacter pylori* infection. *Gastroenterology.* 2008;134(1):306–323.

32. Dunne C, Dolan B, Clyne M. Factors that mediate colonization of the human stomach by *Helicobacter pylori*. *World J Gastroenterol.* 2014;20(19):5610–5624.

33. Gobert AP, Wilson KT. Human and *Helicobacter pylori* interactions determine the outcome of gastric diseases. *Curr Top Microbiol Immunol.* 2017;400:27–52.

34. Smith SM. Role of Toll-like receptors in *Helicobacter pylori* infection and immunity. *World J Gastrointestinal Pathophysiol.* 2014;5(3):133–146.

35. Gewirtz AT, Yu Y, Krishna US, Israel DA, Lyons SL, Peek Jr RM. *Helicobacter pylori* flagellin evades toll-like receptor 5-mediated innate immunity. *J Infect Dis.* 2004;189(10):1914–1920.

36. Pachathundikandi SK, Lind J, Tegtmeyer N, El-Omar EM, Backert S. Interplay of the gastric pathogen *Helicobacter pylori* with toll-like receptors. *BioMed Research International.* 2015;2015:192420.

37. Gaddy JA, Radin JN, Cullen TW, et al. *Helicobacter pylori* resists the antimicrobial activity of calprotectin via lipid a modification and associated biofilm formation. *mBio.* 2015;6(6):e01349–e01315.

38. El-Omar EM, Ng MT, Hold GL. Polymorphisms in Toll-like receptor genes and risk of cancer. *Oncogene.* 2008;27(2):244–252.

39. Censini S, Lange C, Xiang Z, et al. cag, a pathogenicity island of *Helicobacter pylori*, encodes type I-specific and disease-associated virulence factors. *Proc Natl Acad Sci USA*. 1996;93(25):14648–14653.

40. Tummuru MK, Cover TL, Blaser MJ. Cloning and expression of a high-molecular-mass major antigen of *Helicobacter pylori*: evidence of linkage to cytotoxin production. *Infect Immun*. 1993;61(5):1799–1809.

41. Covacci A, Censini S, Bugnoli M, et al. Molecular characterization of the 128-kDa immunodominant antigen of *Helicobacter pylori* associated with cytotoxicity and duodenal ulcer. *Proc Natl Acad Sci USA*. 1993;90(12):5791–5795.

42. Tegtmeyer N, Wessler S, Necchi V, et al. *Helicobacter pylori* employs a unique basolateral type IV secretion mechanism for CagA delivery. *Cell Host Microbe*. 2017;22(4):552–560.e555.

43. Amieva M, Peek Jr RM. Pathobiology of *Helicobacter pylori*-induced gastric cancer. *Gastroenterology*. 2016;150(1):64–78.

44. Jimenez-Soto LF, Haas R. The CagA toxin of *Helicobacter pylori*: abundant production but relatively low amount translocated. *Sci Rep*. 2016;6:23227.

45. Leunk RD, Johnson PT, David BC, Kraft WG, Morgan DR. Cytotoxic activity in broth-culture filtrates of *Campylobacter pylori*. *J Med Microbiol*. 1988;26(2):93–99.

46. Cover TL, Blaser MJ. Purification and characterization of the vacuolating toxin from *Helicobacter pylori*. *J Biol Chem*. 1992;267(15):10570–10575.

47. Torres VJ, VanCompernolle SE, Sundrud MS, Unutmaz D, Cover TL. *Helicobacter pylori* vacuolating cytotoxin inhibits activation-induced proliferation of human T and B lymphocyte subsets. *J Immunol*. 2007;179(8):5433–5440.

48. Palframan SL, Kwok T, Gabriel K. Vacuolating cytotoxin A (VacA), a key toxin for *Helicobacter pylori* pathogenesis. *Front Cell Infect Microbiol*. 2012;2:92.

49. Kao JY, Zhang M, Miller MJ, et al. *Helicobacter pylori* immune escape is mediated by dendritic cell-induced Treg skewing and Th17 suppression in mice. *Gastroenterology*. 2010;138(3):1046–1054.

50. Parker H, Keenan JI. Composition and function of *Helicobacter pylori* outer membrane vesicles. *Microb Infect*. 2012;14(1):9–16.

51. Lu H, Hsu PI, Graham DY, Yamaoka Y. Duodenal ulcer promoting gene of *Helicobacter pylori*. *Gastroenterology*. 2005;128(4):833–848.

52. Peek Jr RM, Thompson SA, Donahue JP, et al. Adherence to gastric epithelial cells induces expression of a *Helicobacter pylori* gene, iceA, that is associated with clinical outcome. *Proc Assoc Am Phys*. 1998;110(6):531–544.

53. Yamaoka Y, Kwon DH, Graham DY. A M(r) 34,000 proinflammatory outer membrane protein (oipA) of *Helicobacter pylori*. *Proc Natl Acad Sci USA*. 2000;97(13):7533–7538.

54. Backert S, Neddermann M, Maubach G, Naumann M. Pathogenesis of *Helicobacter pylori* infection. *Helicobacter*. 2016;21(suppl 1):19–25.

55. Ferlay J, Soerjomataram I, Dikshit R, et al. Cancer incidence and mortality worldwide: sources, methods and major patterns in GLOBOCAN 2012. *Int J Cancer*. 2015;136(5):E359–E386.

56. Hartgrink HH, Jansen EPM, van Grieken NCT, van de Velde CJH. Gastric cancer. *Lancet*. 2009;374(9688):477–490.

57. Megraud F, Bessede E, Varon C. *Helicobacter pylori* infection and gastric carcinoma. *Clin Microbiol Infect*. 2015;21(11):984–990.

58. Hunt RH, Camilleri M, Crowe SE, et al. The stomach in health and disease. *Gut*. 2015;64(10):1650–1668.

59. Correa P, Piazuelo MB. *Helicobacter pylori* infection and gastric adenocarcinoma. *US Gastroenterol Hepatol Rev*. 2011;7(1):59–64.

60. Group HaCC. Gastric cancer and *Helicobacter pylori*: a combined analysis of 12 case control studies nested within prospective cohorts. *Gut*. 2001;49(3):347–353.

61. Huang JQ, Zheng GF, Sumanac K, Irvine EJ, Hunt RH. Meta-analysis of the relationship between cagA seropositivity and gastric cancer. *Gastroenterology*. 2003;125(6):1636–1644.

62. Hatakeyama M. *Helicobacter pylori* CagA and gastric cancer: a paradigm for hit-and-run carcinogenesis. *Cell Host Microbe*. 2014;15(3):306–316.

63. Fock KM, Ang TL. Epidemiology of *Helicobacter pylori* infection and gastric cancer in Asia. *J Gastroenterol Hepatol*. 2010;25(3):479–486.

64. Uemura N, Okamoto S, Yamamoto S, et al. *Helicobacter pylori* infection and the development of gastric cancer. *N Engl J Med*. 2001;345(11):784–789.

65. Ohnishi N, Yuasa H, Tanaka S, et al. Transgenic expression of *Helicobacter pylori* CagA induces gastrointestinal and hematopoietic neoplasms in mouse. *Proc Natl Acad Sci USA*. 2008;105(3):1003.

66. Miura M, Ohnishi N, Tanaka S, Yanagiya K, Hatakeyama M. Differential oncogenic potential of geographically distinct *Helicobacter pylori* CagA isoforms in mice. *Int J Cancer*. 2009;125(11):2497–2504.

67. Azuma T, Ohtani M, Yamazaki Y, Higashi H, Hatakeyama M. Meta-analysis of the relationship between CagA seropositivity and gastric cancer. *Gastroenterology*. 2004;126(7):1926–1927; author reply 1927-1928.

68. Zhang XY, Zhang PY, Aboul-Soud MA. From inflammation to gastric cancer: role of *Helicobacter pylori*. *Oncol Lett*. 2017;13(2):543–548.

69. Suzuki M, Mimuro H, Kiga K, et al. *Helicobacter pylori* CagA phosphorylation-independent function in epithelial proliferation and inflammation. *Cell Host Microbe*. 2009;5(1):23–34.

70. Servetas SL, Bridge DR, Merrell DS. Molecular mechanisms of gastric cancer initiation and progression by *Helicobacter pylori*. *Curr Opin Infect Dis*. 2016;29(3):304–310.

71. Hanahan D, Weinberg RA. Hallmarks of cancer: the next generation. *Cell*. 2011;144(5):646–674.

72. Backert S, Naumann M. What a disorder: proinflammatory signaling pathways induced by *Helicobacter pylori*. *Trends Microbiol*. 2010;18(11):479–486.

73. Naumann M, Sokolova O, Tegtmeyer N, Backert S. *Helicobacter pylori*: a paradigm pathogen for subverting host cell signal transmission. *Trends Microbiol*. 2017;25(4):316–328.

74. Baltimore D. NF-κB is 25. *Nat Immunol*. 2011;12:683.

75. Rossi AFT, Cadamuro ACT, Biselli-Périco JM, et al. Interaction between inflammatory mediators and miR-NAs in *Helicobacter pylori* infection. *Cell Microbiol*. 2016;18(10):1444–1458.

76. Wroblewski LE, Peek RM, Wilson KT. *Helicobacter pylori* and gastric cancer: factors that modulate disease risk. *Clin Microbiol Rev*. 2010;23(4):713–739.

77. Lochhead P, El-Omar EM. Gastric cancer. *Br Med Bull*. 2008;85(1):87–100.

78. McLean MH, El-Omar EM. Genetics of gastric cancer. *Nat Rev Gastroenterol Hepatol*. 2014;11(11):664–674.

79. Xue H, Lin B, Ni P, Xu H, Huang G. Interleukin-1B and interleukin-1 RN polymorphisms and gastric carcinoma risk: a meta-analysis. *J Gastroenterol Hepatol*. 2010;25(10):1604–1617.

80. El-Omar EM, Carrington M, Chow WH, et al. Interleukin-1 polymorphisms associated with increased risk of gastric cancer. *Nature*. 2000;404(6776):398–402.

81. Raza Y, Khan A, Khan AI, et al. Combination of interleukin 1 polymorphism and *Helicobacter pylori* infection: an increased risk of gastric cancer in pakistani population. *Pathol Oncol Res*. 2017;23(4):873–880.

82. El-Omar EM, Rabkin CS, Gammon MD, et al. Increased risk of noncardia gastric cancer associated with proinflammatory cytokine gene polymorphisms. *Gastroenterology*. 2003;124(5):1193–1201.

83. Machado JC, Pharoah P, Sousa S, et al. Interleukin 1B and interleukin 1RN polymorphisms are associated with increased risk of gastric carcinoma. *Gastroenterology*. 2001;121(4):823–829.

84. Li C, Xia HHX, Xie W, et al. Association between interleukin-1 gene polymorphisms and *Helicobacter pylori* infection in gastric carcinogenesis in a Chinese population. *J Gastroenterol Hepatol*. 2007;22(2):234–239.

85. Tu S, Bhagat G, Cui G, et al. Overexpression of interleukin-1beta induces gastric inflammation and cancer and mobilizes myeloid-derived suppressor cells in mice. *Cancer Cell*. 2008;14(5):408–419.

86. Shigematsu Y, Niwa T, Rehnberg E, et al. Interleukin-1beta induced by *Helicobacter pylori* infection enhances mouse gastric carcinogenesis. *Cancer Lett*. 2013;340(1):141–147.

87. Kato S, Onda M, Yamada S, Matsuda N, Tokunaga A, Matsukura N. Association of the interleukin-1 beta genetic polymorphism and gastric cancer risk in Japanese. *J Gastroenterol*. 2001;36(10):696–699.

88. Drici Ael M, Moulessehoul S, Tifrit A, et al. Effect of IL-1beta and IL-1RN polymorphisms in carcinogenesis of the gastric mucosa in patients infected with *Helicobacter pylori* in Algeria. *Libyan J Med*. 2016;11:31576.

89. Persson C, Canedo P, Machado JC, El-Omar EM, Forman D. Polymorphisms in inflammatory response genes and their association with gastric cancer: a HuGE systematic review and meta-analyses. *Am J Epidemiol*. 2011;173(3):259–270.

90. Ying HY, Yu BW, Yang Z, et al. Interleukin-1B 31 C>T polymorphism combined with *Helicobacter pylori*-modified gastric cancer susceptibility: evidence from 37 studies. *J Cell Mol Med*. 2016;20(3):526–536.

91. Melchiades JL, Zabaglia LM, Sallas ML, et al. Polymorphisms and haplotypes of the interleukin 2 gene are associated with an increased risk of gastric cancer. The possible involvement of *Helicobacter pylori*. *Cytokine*. 2017;96:203–207.

92. Kang JM, Kim N, Lee DH, et al. The effects of genetic polymorphisms of IL-6, IL-8, and IL-10 on *Helicobacter pylori*-induced gastroduodenal diseases in Korea. *J Clin Gastroenterol*. 2009;43(5):420–428.

93. Kumar S, Kumari N, Mittal RD, Mohindra S, Ghoshal UC. Association between pro-(IL-8) and anti-inflammatory (IL-10) cytokine variants and their serum levels and *H. pylori*-related gastric carcinogenesis in northern India. *Meta Gene*. 2015;6:9–16.

94. Kim J, Cho YA, Choi IJ, et al. Effects of interleukin-10 polymorphisms, *Helicobacter pylori* infection, and smoking on the risk of noncardia gastric cancer. *PLoS One*. 2012;7(1):e29643.

95. Ramis IB, Vianna JS, Goncalves CV, von Groll A, Dellagostin OA, da Silva PEA. Polymorphisms of the IL-6, IL-8 and IL-10 genes and the risk of gastric pathology in patients infected with *Helicobacter pylori*. *J Microbiol Immunol Infect*. 2017;50(2):153–159.

96. Hold GL, Rabkin CS, Chow WH, et al. A functional polymorphism of toll-like receptor 4 gene increases risk of gastric carcinoma and its precursors. *Gastroenterology*. 2007;132(3):905–912.

97. Mommersteeg MC, Yu J, Peppelenbosch MP, Fuhler GM. Genetic host factors in *Helicobacter pylori*-induced carcinogenesis: emerging new paradigms. *Biochim Biophys Acta Rev Canc*. 2018;1869(1):42–52.

98. Li Z-X, Wang Y-M, Tang F-B, et al. NOD1 and NOD2 genetic variants in association with risk of gastric cancer and its precursors in a Chinese population. *PLoS One*. 2015;10(5):e0124949.

99. Wang P, Zhang L, Jiang JM, et al. Association of NOD1 and NOD2 genes polymorphisms with *Helicobacter pylori* related gastric cancer in a Chinese population. *World J Gastroenterol*. 2012;18(17):2112–2120.

100. Tsuda M, Asaka M, Kato M, et al. Effect on *Helicobacter pylori* eradication therapy against gastric cancer in Japan. *Helicobacter*. 2017;22(5).

101. Lin JT. Screening of gastric cancer: who, when, and how. *Clin Gastroenterol Hepatol*. 2014;12(1):135–138.

102. Doorakkers E, Lagergren J, Engstrand L, Brusselaers N. *Helicobacter pylori* eradication treatment and the risk of gastric adenocarcinoma in a Western population. *Gut*. Published Online First: 30 January 2018. doi: 10.1136/gutjnl-2017-315363.

103. Lee YC, Chiang TH, Chou CK, et al. Association between *Helicobacter pylori* eradication and gastric cancer incidence: a systematic review and meta-analysis. *Gastroenterology*. 2016;150(5):1113.

104. Ford AC, Forman D, Hunt RH, Yuan Y, Moayyedi P. *Helicobacter pylori* eradication therapy to prevent gastric cancer in healthy asymptomatic infected individuals: systematic review and meta-analysis of randomised controlled trials. *Br Med J*. 2014;348.

105. Li WQ, Ma JL, Zhang L, et al. Effects of *Helicobacter pylori* treatment on gastric cancer incidence and mortality in subgroups. *J Natl Cancer Inst*. 2014;106(7).

106. Fukase K, Kato M, Kikuchi S, et al. Effect of eradication of *Helicobacter pylori* on incidence of metachronous gastric carcinoma after endoscopic resection of early gastric cancer: an open-label, randomised controlled trial. *Lancet*. 2008;372(9636):392–397.

107. Cheung KS, Chan EW, Wong AYS, Chen L, Wong ICK, Leung WK. Long-term proton pump inhibitors and risk of gastric cancer development after treatment for *Helicobacter pylori*: a population-based study. *Gut*. 2018;67(1):28.

108. Malfertheiner P, Chan FK, McColl KE. Peptic ulcer disease. *Lancet (London, England)*. 2009;374(9699):1449–1461.

109. Tabiri S, Akanbong P, Abubakari BB. Assessment of the environmental risk factors for a gastric ulcer in northern Ghana. *Pan Afr Med J*. 2016;25:160.

110. Zhang H, Xue Y, Zhou LY, Liu X, Suo BJ. [The changes of main upper gastrointestinal diseases and *Helicobacter pylori* infection status in the past thirty five years]. *Zhonghua nei ke za zhi*. 2016;55(6):440–444.

111. McJunkin B, Sissoko M, Levien J, Upchurch J, Ahmed A. Dramatic decline in prevalence of *Helicobacter pylori* and peptic ulcer disease in an endoscopy-referral population. *Am J Med*. 2011;124(3):260–264.

112. Lanas A, Garcia-Rodriguez LA, Polo-Tomas M, et al. The changing face of hospitalisation due to gastrointestinal bleeding and perforation. *Aliment Pharmacol Ther*. 2011;33(5):585–591.

113. Malfertheiner P, Megraud F, O'Morain CA, et al. Management of *Helicobacter pylori* infection-the Maastricht V/florence consensus report. *Gut*. 2017;66(1):6–30.

114. Sung JJ, Kuipers EJ, El-Serag HB. Systematic review: the global incidence and prevalence of peptic ulcer disease. *Aliment Pharmacol Ther*. 2009;29(9):938–946.

115. Huang JQ, Sridhar S, Hunt RH. Role of *Helicobacter pylori* infection and non-steroidal anti-inflammatory drugs in peptic-ulcer disease: a meta-analysis. *Lancet (London, England)*. 2002;359(9300):14–22.

116. Smolka AJ, Schubert ML. *Helicobacter pylori*-induced changes in gastric acid secretion and upper gastrointestinal disease. *Curr Top Microbiol Immunol*. 2017;400:227–252.

117. Iijima K, Kanno T, Abe Y, et al. Preferential location of idiopathic peptic ulcers. *Scand J Gastroenterol*. 2016;51(7):782–787.

118. Kanno T, Iijima K, Abe Y, et al. *Helicobacter pylori*-negative and non-steroidal anti-inflammatory drugs-negative idiopathic peptic ulcers show refractoriness and high recurrence incidence: multicenter follow-up study of peptic ulcers in Japan. *Dig Endosc*. 2016;28(5):556–563.

119. Seo JH, Hong SJ, Kim JH, et al. Long-term recurrence rates of peptic ulcers without *Helicobacter pylori*. *Gut Liver*. 2016;10(5):719–725.

120. Zhou LY, Song ZQ, Xue Y, Li X, Li YQ, Qian JM. Recurrence of *Helicobacter pylori* infection and the affecting factors: a follow-up study. *J Digest Dis*. 2017;18(1):47–55.

121. Rhee KH, Park JS, Cho MJ. *Helicobacter pylori*: bacterial strategy for incipient stage and persistent colonization in human gastric niches. *Yonsei Med J*. 2014;55(6):1453–1466.

122. Eaton KA, Mefford M, Thevenot T. The role of T cell subsets and cytokines in the pathogenesis of *Helicobacter pylori* gastritis in mice. *J Immunol*. 2001;166(12):7456–7461.

123. Cheng HH, Tseng GY, Yang HB, Wang HJ, Lin HJ, Wang WC. Increased numbers of Foxp3-positive regulatory T cells in gastritis, peptic ulcer and gastric adenocarcinoma. *World J Gastroenterol*. 2012;18(1):34–43.

124. Bagheri N, Shirzad H, Elahi S, et al. Downregulated regulatory T cell function is associated with increased peptic ulcer in *Helicobacter pylori*-infection. *Microb Pathog*. 2017;110:165–175.

125. Young VB. The role of the microbiome in human health and disease: an introduction for clinicians. *Br Med J*. 2017;356:j831.

126. Lynch SV, Pedersen O. The human intestinal microbiome in health and disease. *N Engl J Med*. 2016;375(24):2369–2379.

127. Wroblewski LE, Peek Jr RM. *Helicobacter pylori*, cancer, and the gastric microbiota. *Adv Exp Med Biol*. 2016;908:393–408.

128. Ianiro G, Molina-Infante J, Gasbarrini A. Gastric microbiota. *Helicobacter*. 2015;20(suppl 1):68–71.

129. Khosravi Y, Dieye Y, Poh BH, et al. Culturable bacterial microbiota of the stomach of *Helicobacter pylori* positive and negative gastric disease patients. *Sci World J*. 2014;2014:610421.

130. Hu Z, Zhang Y, Li Z, et al. Effect of *Helicobacter pylori* infection on chronic periodontitis by the change of microecology and inflammation. *Oncotarget*. 2016;7(41):66700–66712.

131. Li TH, Qin Y, Sham PC, Lau KS, Chu KM, Leung WK. Alterations in gastric microbiota after *H. pylori* eradication and in different histological stages of gastric carcinogenesis. *Sci Rep*. 2017;7:44935.

132. Abreu MT, Peek Jr RM. Gastrointestinal malignancy and the microbiome. *Gastroenterology*. 2014;146(6):1534–1546.e1533.

133. Lofgren JL, Whary MT, Ge Z, et al. Lack of commensal flora in *Helicobacter pylori*-infected INS-GAS mice reduces gastritis and delays intraepithelial neoplasia. *Gastroenterology*. 2011;140(1):210–220.

134. Lertpiriyapong K, Whary MT, Muthupalani S, et al. Gastric colonisation with a restricted commensal microbiota replicates the promotion of neoplastic lesions by diverse intestinal microbiota in the *Helicobacter pylori* INS-GAS mouse model of gastric carcinogenesis. *Gut.* 2014;63(1):54–63.

135. Lemke LB, Ge Z, Whary MT, et al. Concurrent Helicobacter bilis infection in C57BL/6 mice attenuates proinflammatory *H. pylori*-induced gastric pathology. *Infect Immun.* 2009;77(5):2147–2158.

136. Ge Z, Feng Y, Muthupalani S, et al. Coinfection with Enterohepatic Helicobacter species can ameliorate or promote *Helicobacter pylori*-induced gastric pathology in C57BL/6 mice. *Infect Immun.* 2011;79(10):3861–3871.

137. Ma JL, Zhang L, Brown LM, et al. Fifteen-year effects of *Helicobacter pylori*, garlic, and vitamin treatments on gastric cancer incidence and mortality. *J Natl Cancer Inst.* 2012;104(6):488–492.

CHAPTER 3

The Role of Infections and the Microbiome in Gallbladder Diseases

GUY D. ESLICK, DRPH, PHD, FACE, FFPH • MICHAEL R. COX, FRACS, MS, MBBS

BENIGN DISEASE

Acute Calculous Cholecystitis

Gallstones are the most common cause of acute cholecystitis, and a large proportion of patients (~90%) are asymptomatic having gallstone disease for many years even decades before surgical treatment.[1] Indeed up to 80% of people with gallstones never become symptomatic and require gallbladder surgery. Problems can arise when a gallstone becomes impacted in the neck of the gallbladder or the cystic duct causing obstruction, which subsequently results in acute inflammation. This inflammation is due in part to bile stasis that leads to the release of inflammatory enzymes such as phospholipase A, which transforms lecithin to lysolecithin leading to inflammation. The resulting damage to the gallbladder mucosa from distention escalates into the release of additional inflammatory molecules such as prostaglandins, causing ischemia leading to a cycle of ever increasing inflammation. This is where infection can play a role in not only increasing inflammation but also in the later stages necrosis and gallbladder perforation.

Previous studies have identified the types of organisms associated with acute calculous cholecystitis as *Escherichia coli* (41%), enterococci (23%), *Salmonella typhi* (2%–5%), and *Pseudomonas* (1%).[2,3] It has previously been hypothesized that bacteria may augment the development of cholesterol gallstones.[4] These bacteria make work in a symbiotic relationship with the bile to produce gallstones but have no direct effect on the gallbladder itself unless an inflammatory cascade is initiated within the gallbladder. There can be additional complications associated with some bacterial infections where the organisms produce gas (e.g., *Clostridium, E. coli*) that can enter the wall of the gallbladder (i.e., emphysematous cholecystitis) (Fig. 3.1).

Some studies suggest the routine use of antibiotics for patients with acute cholecystitis until their gallbladder is removed or until the resolution of the cholecystitis. However, the evidence for the use of antibiotics for uncomplicated acute cholecystitis is conflicting.[5-9] Moreover, antibiotics are indicated for gallbladder gangrene/necrosis, rupture, or emphysematous cholecystitis, as well as for at-risk individuals (e.g., frail, diabetic, immunocompromised patients) with uncomplicated acute cholecystitis.[7] It is also important to ensure that the antibiotics selected for treatment achieve adequate concentrations in bile.

In 2003 the Infectious Diseases Society of America (IDSA) produced the guidelines for antibiotic use among patients with acute cholecystitis.[7]

For patients with community-acquired acute cholecystitis of mild-to-moderate severity: cefazolin, cefuroxime, or ceftriaxone.

For patients with community-acquired acute cholecystitis of severe physiologic disturbance, advanced age, or immunocompromised state: imipenem-cilastatin,

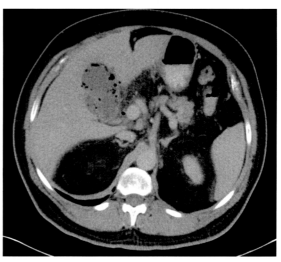

FIG. 3.1 A CT scan showing emphysematous cholecystitis.

Gastrointestinal Diseases and Their Associated Infections. https://doi.org/10.1016/B978-0-323-54843-4.00003-9
Copyright © 2019 Elsevier Inc. All rights reserved.

TABLE 3.1
The Different Antibiotic Options Recommended Depending on the Grade of Acute Cholecystitis

Grade 1	Grade 2	Grade 3
Ampicillin/sulbactam	Piperacillin/tazobactam	Piperacillin/tazobactam
Piperacillin/tazobactam	Ceftriaxone, cefotaxime, cefepime, cefozopran, or ceftazidime ± metronidazole	Cefepime, ceftazidime, or cefozopran ± metronidazole
Cefazolin, cefotiam, cefuroxime, ceftriaxone, or cefotaxime ± metronidazole	Cefoperazone/sulbactam	Imipenem/cilastatin, meropenem, doripenem, ertapenem
Ceftazidime	Ertapenem	Aztreonam ± metronidazole
Cefozopran	Levofloxacin	
Cefmetazole	Ciprofloxacin	
Cefoxitin	Pazufloxacin/metronidazole	
Flomoxef	Moxifloxacin	
Cefoperazone/sulbactam		
Ertapenem		
Levofloxacin		
Ciprofloxacin		
Pazufloxacin ± metronidazole		
Moxifloxacin		

meropenem, doripenem, piperacillin-tazobactam, ciprofloxacin plus metronidazole, levofloxacin plus metronidazole, or cefepime plus metronidazole.

For patients with healthcare-associated biliary infection of any severity: imipenem-cilastatin, meropenem, doripenem, piperacillin-tazobactam, ciprofloxacin plus metronidazole, levofloxacin plus metronidazole, or cefepime plus metronidazole, with vancomycin added to each regimen.

The Tokyo Guidelines for antimicrobial therapy for acute cholangitis and cholecystitis were published.[10,11] These guidelines recommended different possible antibiotics for patients with different grades of acute cholecystitis (Table 3.1).

The flowcharts for each grade of acute cholecystitis show the potential paths for patients depending on their clinical presentation (Figs. 3.2–3.4).

Cholecystectomy on the index admission should be the preferred approach for all patients presenting with acute cholecystectomy. Best practice evidence has shown that early cholecystectomy is safe with less complications, less days in hospital, and a low conversion rate compared with delayed cholecystectomy.[12,13]

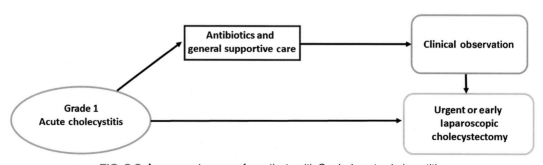

FIG. 3.2 Assessment process for patients with Grade 1 acute cholecystitis.

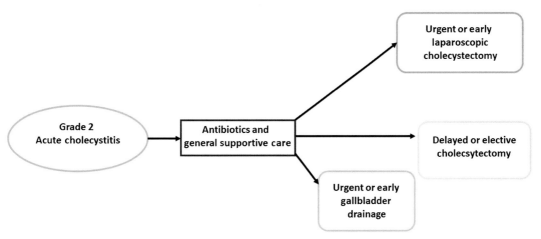

FIG. 3.3 Assessment process for patients with Grade 2 acute cholecystitis.

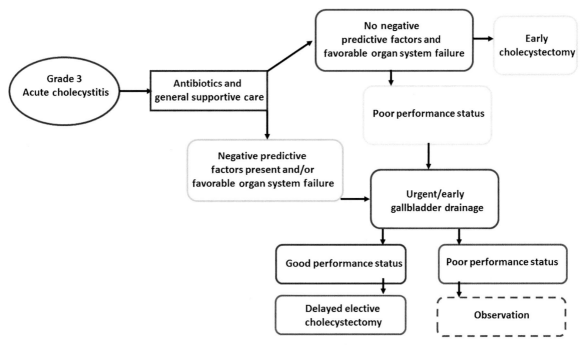

FIG. 3.4 Assessment process for patients with Grade 3 acute cholecystitis.

Acute Acalculous Cholecystitis

A minority of patients (5%–10%) present with acute acalculous cholecystitis (cholecystitis with no gallstones). These patients are usually hospitalized and critically ill, although acute acalculous cholecystitis may also occur among individuals at risk in an outpatient setting. It predominantly affects males aged 50 years, those in the postoperative period after major surgery, burn patients with sepsis, and patients with diabetes mellitus, vasculitis (including polyarteritis nodosa), multisystem organ failure, and prolonged use of parenteral nutrition.[14] It should also be noted that those

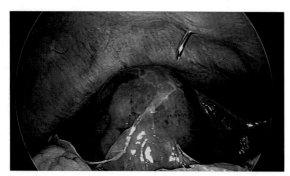

FIG. 3.5 A gangrenous gallbladder at cholecystectomy.

with acute acalculous cholecystitis are at a substantially increased risk of developing gangrenous cholecystitis (Fig. 3.5). A retrospective review of 27 cases of acalculous cholecystitis reported high rates of gangrenous cholecystitis (63%), gallbladder perforation (15%), and mortality (41%).[15]

The pathophysiology of this condition is mainly due to bile stasis and/or gallbladder ischemia. Bile stasis may be the result of a major illness, medications, total parental nutrition, and surgery, and this is turn leads to the production of inflammatory enzymes (e.g., phospholipase) that injure the gallbladder mucosa and produce fluids, resulting in distension and a cycle of inflammatory responses.[16]

A major complication associated with acute acalculous cholecystitis is secondary bacterial infection. As with acute calculous cholecystitis, antibiotics should be initiated early and treatment should follow the IDSA or Tokyo guidelines.[7,10,11] The types of organisms associated with acute acalculous cholecystitis are shown in Table 3.2. These may include viruses (e.g., cytomegalovirus), with viral infections acquired by immunocompromised patients, or parasites, such as those causing helminthic infection (e.g., ascariasis), which is a major cause of biliary disease in developing countries such as Asia, southern Africa, and Latin America (Fig. 3.6). Moreover, infections with *Clonorchis sinensis* may lead to cholecystitis,[17] inducing eosinophilic cholecystitis. A meta-analysis reported that infections with liver fluke were strongly associated with cholangitis, cholecystitis, cholelithiasis, hepatocellular carcinoma, and cholangiocarcinoma.[18]

Acute Cholangitis

Acute cholangitis is an inflammation of the bile duct that is clinically associated with fever, jaundice, and

TABLE 3.2
Types of Infections Associated With Acute Acalculous Cholecystitis
BACTERIAL
• Typhoid[34,35]
• *Salmonella paratyphi* B[36]
• *Salmonella* virchow[37]
• *Campylobacter*[38]
• *Streptococcus agalactiae*[39]
• Tuberculosis[40]
• Leptospirosis[41]
• *Eikenella corrodens*[42]
• Q fever[43,44]
• *Lactococcus garvieae*[45]
• *Lactobacillus plantarum*[46]
VIRAL
• Human immunodeficiency virus[47,48]
• Epstein-Barr virus[49–51]
• Hepatitis A[52–54]
• Hepatitis C[55]
• Dengue virus[56–58]
• Mumps[59]
• Hantavirus[60]
• Cytomegalovirus[61]
• Crimean-Congo fever[62]
PARASITIC
• Malaria[63,64]
• Scrub typhus[65]
• Tapeworm[66]
FUNGI
• Candida infection[67]

From Su'a B, Hill AG, Poole GH. Acute acalculous cholecystitis. In: Cox MR, Eslick GD, Padbury R, eds. *The Management of Gallstone Disease. A Practical and Evidence-based Approach.* Springer International Publishing; 2018, with permission.

abdominal pain and is due to bacterial infection of the biliary tract. It is more likely to occur if the bile duct is already partially or completely obstructed by gallstones, a benign stricture, or a malignant stricture. The risk of infection is higher when there has been a

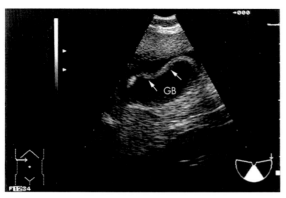

FIG. 3.6 Sagittal ultrasound image of the gall bladder shows a ribbon-like (worm), non-shadowing echogenic region (arrows) within the gallbladder (GB).

previous intervention on the common bile duct that causes contamination of the bile. There are three types of cholangitis: (1) primary sclerosing,[19] (2) secondary (acute),[20] and IgG4-associated cholangitis.[21]

There are some defensive mechanisms to prevent cholangitis. First, the bile salts have bacteriostatic activity and the biliary epithelium secretes IgA and mucus, which prevent organisms from adhering to the mucosa. Moreover, Kupffer cells on the biliary epithelium and the small space between the cholangiocytes stop translocation of bacteria from the hepatobiliary system into the portal venous system. In addition, normal bile flow removes bacteria into the duodenum.

When biliary obstruction occurs leading to bile stasis and increases the intraductal pressure, the pressure (i.e., choledochal pressure) is a very important factor in the pathogenesis of acute cholangitis. If the pressure increases substantially then cholangiovenous and cholangiolymphatic reflux can occur, which can lead to bacteremia and endotoxemia. This leads to an increase in the levels of inflammatory mediators (i.e., tumor necrosis factor [TNF], soluble TNF receptors, and interleukin [IL]-1, IL-6, and IL-10).

The pathogenic organisms that occur in acute cholangitis are similar to those isolated in both acute calculous cholecystitis and acute acalculous cholecystitis. They consist of predominantly *E. coli* (25%–50%), *Klebsiella* species (15%–20%), *Enterococcus* species (10%–20%), and *Enterobacter* species (5%–10%).[22] In addition, anaerobic organisms such as *Bacteroides fragilis* and *Clostridium perfringens* are also associated with acute cholangitis.[23] As mentioned previously, parasites

are also linked to blockage of the biliary tract and these can induce acute cholangitis; pathogens responsible include the liver flukes *C. sinensis*, *Opisthorchis viverrini* and *Opisthorchis felineus*, and *Ascaris lumbricoides*.[24] Management of infections should be as per the IDSA or the Tokyo guidelines.[7,10,11]

MALIGNANT DISEASES

Gallbladder Cancer

There are several organisms associated with the development of gallbladder cancer. The organisms with the strongest evidence supporting a relationship between chronic infection and the subsequent development of gallbladder cancer are *S. typhi* and *Salmonella paratyphi*.[25] A meta-analysis of 17 studies assessing chronic *S. typhi* carrier state with gallbladder cancer found a substantially increased risk (odds ratio [OR], 4.28; 95% confidence interval [CI], 1.84–9.96) (Fig. 3.7). The majority of studies were from India and China (Asia), which had an increased risk compared with non-Asian countries (OR, 4.13; 95% CI, 2.87–5.94). This evidence highlights chronic *S. typhi* carrier state as an important risk factor for the development of gallbladder cancer.

In addition, the potential role of various *Helicobacter* species in the development of gallbladder cancer has been emerging.[26] These predominantly include *Helicobacter bilis* and *Helicobacter pylori*, which have been isolated from human bile samples of more than 75% of patients with gallbladder cancer and more than 50% of patients with chronic cholecystitis.[27–30] These early studies produced very large relative risks (RRs) ranging from RR: 2.6 (95% CI, 0.6–4.6) to RR: 9.9 (95% CI, 1.4–70.5). There is an urgent need for additional research into the role of helicobacter infection in the development of gallbladder cancer, as this is a preventable disease.

Currently, there is no evidence supporting the potential role of any viruses or fungi, including yeasts, in the development of gallbladder cancer. However, a case of concomitant infection with *A. lumbricoides* and gallbladder carcinoma highlighted the potential of chronic infections that may lead to cancer development.[31] This case involved a 73-year-old female who presented to hospital with right-sided upper abdominal pain, nausea, and vomiting. She had slightly elevated liver function test results, with a normal bilirubin level. A computed tomography examination of her abdomen revealed a dilated gallbladder with a mass (Fig. 3.8). At cholecystectomy

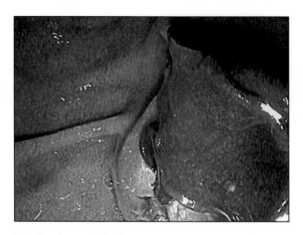

Study name	Statistics for each study				Odds ratio and 95% confidence interval
	Odds ratio	Lower limit	Upper limit	P value	
Nath et al.1997	4.80	0.23	98.93	0.31	
Sharma et al.	0.86	0.41	1.80	0.69	
Shukla et al.	7.19	2.21	23.43	0.00	
Csendes et al.	6.03	0.31	115.37	0.23	
Hazrah et al.	1.02	0.05	22.32	0.99	
Dutta et al.	14.00	1.96	100.09	0.01	
Nath et al. 2008	4.42	0.61	32.14	0.14	
Welton et al.	6.55	3.07	14.00	0.00	
Tewari et al.	2.52	1.11	5.75	0.03	
Strom et al.	12.70	0.27	598.00	0.20	
Roa et al.	2.11	0.11	40.24	0.62	
Pandey et al.	1.30	0.86	1.97	0.21	
Safaeian et al.	11.90	4.55	31.10	0.00	
Yagyu et al.	2.10	0.50	8.76	0.31	
Singh et al.	4.90	0.90	26.74	0.07	
Caygill et al.	167.00	71.69	389.00	0.00	
Serra et al.	0.50	0.20	1.22	0.13	
	4.28	1.84	9.96	0.00	

0.01   0.1   1   10   100

FIG. 3.7 A Forest plot showing the studies linking *Salmonella typhi* infection with gallbladder cancer development.

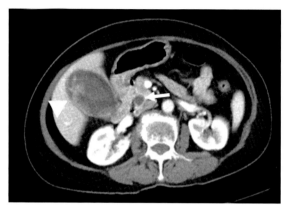

FIG. 3.8 Axial computed tomography (CT) showing dilated heterogeneous gallbladder (arrowhead) with distended common bile duct (arrow).

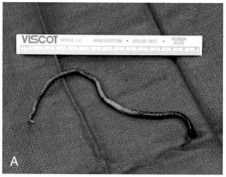

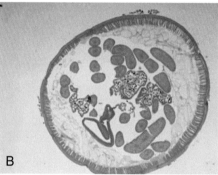

FIG. 3.9 Ex vivo image of Ascaris lumbricoides (A) and cross-sectional image after hematoxylin and eosin (H&E) staining (B).

the common bile duct was found to be obstructed by a worm (Fig. 3.9). The patient's pathology returned as T1bN0 gallbladder carcinoma with negative margins. The common bile duct intraluminal mass was a female A. lumbricoides.

The Gallbladder Microbiome

This is a new field of research in terms of classifying and identifying organisms from the gallbladder.[32] There have been studies that have isolated organisms from the gallbladder itself and from bile contained within the gallbladder; however, isolating these organisms does not confer any pathogenic potential or provide any link with the development of any gallbladder pathology. The gallbladder may contain commensal or nonpathogenic organisms.

In a metagenomics study of 15 Chinese patients with gallstone disease, whole-metagenome shotgun (WMS) sequencing and 16S ribosomal RNA (rRNA) sequencing of bile samples were performed.[32] Organisms were clustered into oral or intestinal, oral and intestinal, or other groups. The analysis revealed that organisms were more likely to come from the oral or respiratory tracts and that many bacteria were patient specific. A total of 13 novel biliary bacteria were identified using WMS sequencing (Fig. 3.10). The study showed the extreme complexity associated with the microecology of the biliary tract.

Another metagenomic study from South America aimed to determine the microorganisms in the gallbladder bile of patients with gallbladder cancer ($n = 7$) and cholelithiasis ($n = 30$).[33] Genomic DNA was extracted from bile and the V3–V4 region of 16S rRNA was amplified. The sequencing results were compared with the 16S database, and the bacteria were identified by homology searches and phylogenetic analysis. Interestingly, no S. typhi and Helicobacter sp. were identified from any of the bile samples. The main organisms identified in the gallbladder cancer bile samples were Fusobacterium nucleatum, E. coli, and Enterobacter sp., whereas those identified in the cholecystitis bile samples were E. coli, Salmonella sp., and Enterococcus gallinarum. Obviously, the role of these organisms in causing any gallbladder disease needs further research.

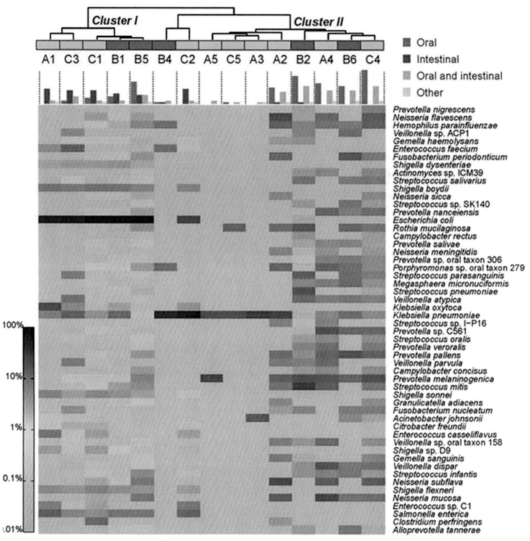

FIG. 3.10 Distributions of WMS sequencing reads and microbial communities within bile samples. Hierarchical clustering of samples based on microbial community, distribution of bacterial origin and heatmap of species abundances. Individuals are denoted by coloured blocks. Bacterial origins were classified as oral (referring to the oral cavity/respiratory tract), intestinal, both oral and intestinal, and other (environmental or unknown). For bacteria with ≥ 0.1% abundance in at least three individuals, the distribution of their origin in each individual is reflected by the histogram above the heatmap. The heatmap colour scale quantifies the log10 relative abundance of species, from grey (none or low abundance) to dark red (high abundance).

CONCLUSION

The gallbladder is a fascinating organ and there is an unbelievable amount of knowledge yet to be gained regarding the role of infections and the microbiome. There is need for greater understanding of the organisms associated with gallbladder disease as well as how other gut organisms may be linked or play roles in gallbladder disease. The developing technology will only take us so far in terms of identifying these organisms, making advances into the causal pathway (e.g., Koch postulates, Bradford Hill criteria) are at an entirely different level of understanding and complexity, which may take many decades before solutions are identified. Continued research is the key for finding the answers to these problems; let us hope that governments and funding organizations are prepared to pave the way to find solutions.

REFERENCES

1. Cox MR, Eslick GD, Padbury R. *The Management of Gallstone Disease. A Practical and Evidence-based Approach.* Springer International Publishing; 2018.
2. Csendes A, Burdiles P, Maluenda F, et al. Simultaneous bacteriologic assessment of bile from gallbladder and common bile duct in control subjects and patients with gallstones and common duct stones. *Arch Surg.* 1996;131:389–394.
3. Eslami G, Nowruzi J, Fllah F, et al. Detection of bacteria responsible for gallbladder inflammation and gallstones. *Iran J Clin Infect Dis.* 2007;2:139–141.
4. Vitetta L, Best SP, Sali A. Single and multiple cholesterol gallstones and the influence of bacteria. *Med Hypotheses.* 2000;55:502–506.
5. Fuks D, Cossé C, Régimbeau JM. Antibiotic therapy in acute calculous cholecystitis. *J Vis Surg.* 2013;150:3.
6. Strasberg SM. Clinical practice. Acute calculous cholecystitis. *N Engl J Med.* 2008;358:2804.
7. Solomkin JS, Mazuski JE, Bradley JS, et al. Diagnosis and management of complicated intra-abdominal infection in adults and children: guidelines by the Surgical Infection Society and the Infectious Diseases Society of America. *Clin Infect Dis.* 2010;50:133.
8. Kanafani ZA, Khalifé N, Kanj SS, et al. Antibiotic use in acute cholecystitis: practice patterns in the absence of evidence-based guidelines. *J Infect.* 2005;51:128.
9. Mazeh H, Mizrahi I, Dior U, et al. Role of antibiotic therapy in mild acute calculus cholecystitis: a prospective randomized controlled trial. *World J Surg.* 2012;36:1750.
10. Gomi H, et al. Tokyo Guidelines: antimicrobial therapy for acute cholangitis and cholecystitis. *J Hepatobiliary Pancreat Sci.* 2018;25:3–16.
11. Okamoto K, et al. Tokyo Guidelines 2018: flowchart for the management of acute cholecystitis. *J Hepatobiliary Pancreat Sci.* 2018;25:55–72.
12. Cao AM, Eslick GD, Cox MR. Early cholecystectomy is superior to delayed cholecystectomy for acute cholecystitis: a meta-analysis. *J Gastrointest Surg.* 2015;19:848–857.
13. Cao AM, Eslick GD, Nagaraja V, Ma D, Cox MR. Early laparoscopic cholecystectomy is superior to delayed acute cholecystitis: a meta-analysis of case-control studies. *Surg Endosc.* March 2016;30(3):1172–1182.
14. Gu MG, Kim TN, Song J, Nam YJ, Lee JY, Park JS. Risk factors and therapeutic outcomes of acute acalculous cholecystitis. *Digestion.* 2014;90:75–80.
15. Kalliafas S, Ziegler DW, Flancbaum L, et al. Acute acalculous cholecystitis: incidence, risk factors, diagnosis, and outcome. *Am Surg.* 1998;64:471–475.
16. Orlando III R, Gleason E, Drezner AD. Acute acalculous cholecystitis in the critically ill patient. *Am J Surg.* 1983;145(4):472–476.
17. Ishikawa T, Meier-Stephenson V, Heitman SJ. Biliary obstruction caused by the liver fluke, *Fasciola hepatica. Can Med Assoc J.* 2016;188:524–526.
18. Xia J, Jiang S-C, Peng H-J. Association between liver fluke infection and hepatobiliary pathological changes: a systematic review and meta-analysis. *PLoS One.* 2015;10:e0132673.
19. Dyson JK, Beuers U, Jones EJ, Lohse AW, Hudson M. Primary sclerosing cholangitis. *Lancet.* 2018;391:2547–2559.
20. Ahmed M. Acute cholangitis – an update. *World J Gastrointest Pathophysiol.* 2018;9:1–7.
21. Hubers LM, Maillette de Buy Wenniger LJ, Doorenspleet ME, et al. IgG4-associated cholangitis: a comprehensive review. *Clin Rev Allergy Immunol.* 2015;48:198–206.
22. van den Hazel SJ, Speelman P, Tytgat GN, Dankert J, van Leeuwen DJ. Role of antibiotics in the treatment and prevention of acute and recurrent cholangitis. *Clin Infect Dis.* 1994;19:279–286.
23. Jain MK, Jain R. Acute bacterial cholangitis. *Curr Treat Options Gastroenterol.* 2006;9:113–121.
24. Kinney TP. Management of ascending cholangitis. *Gastrointest Endosc Clin N Am.* 2007;17:289–306.
25. Nagaraja V, Eslick GD. Systematic review with meta-analysis: the relationship between *Salmonella typhi* Carrier status and gallbladder cancer. *Aliment Pharmacol Ther.* 2014;39:745–750.
26. de Martel C, Plummer M, Parsonnet J, van Doorn L-J, Franceschi S. Helicobacter species in cancers of the gallbladder and extrahepatic biliary tract. *Br J Cancer.* 2009;100:194–199.
27. Cen L, Pan J, Zhou B, et al. Helicobacter Pylori infection of the gallbladder and the risk of chronic cholecystitis and cholelithiasis: a systematic review and meta-analysis. *Helicobacter.* 2018. https://doi.org/10.1111/hel.12457.
28. Matsukura N, Yokomuro S, Yamada S, et al. Association between *Helicobacter bilis* in bile and biliary tract malignancies: *H. bilis* in bile from Japanese and Thai patients with benign and malignant diseases in the biliary tract. *Jpn J Canc Res.* 2002;93:842–847.
29. Bulajic M, Maisonneuve P, Schneider-Brachert W, et al. *Helicobacter pylori* and the risk of benign and malignant biliary tract disease. *Cancer.* 2002;95:1946–1953.
30. Murata H, Tsuji S, Tsujii M, et al. *Helicobacter bilis* infection in biliary tract cancer. *Aliment Pharmacol Ther.* 2004;20(suppl 1):90–94.
31. Lyons R, Schneider J. Gallbladder carcinoma in association with *Ascaris lumbricoides* infection. *Surg Infect Case Rep.* 2017;2(1):52–54.
32. Shen H, Ye F, Xie L, et al. Metagenomic sequencing of bile from gallstone patients to identify different microbial community patterns and novel biliary bacteria. *Sci Rep.* 2015;5:17450. https://doi.org/10.1038/srep17450.

33. Tsuchiya Y, Loza E, Villa-Gomez G, et al. Metagenomics of microbial communities in gallbladder bile from patients with gallbladder cancer or cholelithiasis. *Asian Pac J Cancer Prev.* 2018;19:961–967.

34. Abdur-Rahman OL, Adeniran OJ, Nasir AA. Outcome of acalculous cholecystitis from typhoid in Nigerian children. *J Natl Med Assoc.* 2009;101(7):717–719.

35. Axelrod D, Karakas SP. Acalculous cholecystitis and abscess as a manifestation of typhoid fever. *Pediatr Radiol.* 2007;37(2):237.

36. Benjelloun el B, et al. A case report of acute acalculous cholecystitis due to *Salmonella paratyphi* B complicated by biliary peritonitis. *Pan Afr Med J.* 2013;16:127.

37. Commons R, Dimitriou J, Campbell I. Acalculous cholecystitis caused by Salmonella virchow. *ANZ J Surg.* 2008;78(6):514.

38. Udayakumar D, Sanaullah M. Campylobacter cholecystitis. *Int J Med Sci.* 2009;6(6):374–375.

39. Brewer L, et al. Streptococcus agalactiae endocarditis presenting as acalculous cholecystitis in a previously well woman. *BMJ Case Rep.* 2013. https://doi.org/10.1136/bcr-2012-008278.

40. Chen PL, et al. Respiratory failure and acalculous cholecystitis in a patient with AIDS and disseminated tuberculosis: masking effect of fluoroquinolone monotherapy and immune restoration syndrome. *Int J Infect Dis.* 2009;13(4):e165–e168.

41. Chong VH, Goh SK. Leptospirosis presenting as acute acalculous cholecystitis and pancreatitis. *Ann Acad Med Singapore.* 2007;36(3):215–216.

42. Dezsi CA, et al. Empyema thoracis, hemorrhagic pericarditis and acalculous cholecystitis caused by *Eikenella corrodens* sepsis. *Orv Hetil.* 2013;154(47):1873–1876.

43. Ergas D, Abdul-Hai A, Sthoeger ZM. Acalculous cholecystitis: an unusual presentation of acute Q fever masquerading as infectious endocarditis. *Am J Med Sci.* 2008;336(4):356–357.

44. Figtree M, et al. Q fever cholecystitis in an unvaccinated butcher diagnosed by gallbladder polymerase chain reaction. *Vector Borne Zoonotic Dis.* 2010;10(4):421–423.

45. Kim JH, et al. First report of human acute acalculous cholecystitis caused by the fish pathogen *Lactococcus garvieae*. *J Clin Microbiol.* 2013;51(2):712–714.

46. Tena D, et al. Acute acalculous cholecystitis complicated with peritonitis caused by *Lactobacillus plantarum*. *Diagn Microbiol Infect Dis.* 2013;76(4):510–512.

47. Agholi M, et al. First detection of acalculous cholecystitis associated with Sarcocystis infection in a patient with AIDS. *Acta Parasitol.* 2014;59(2):310–315.

48. Alave J, et al. Acalculous cholecystitis caused by *Histoplasma capsulatum* in a severely immunosuppressed HIV-infected patient. *J Infect Dev Ctries.* 2011;5(3):235–238.

49. Arya SO, et al. Epstein Barr virus-associated acute acalculous cholecystitis: a rare occurrence but favourable outcome. *Clin Pediatr.* 2010;49(8):799–804.

50. Attilakos A, et al. Acute acalculous cholecystitis in children with Epstein-Barr virus infection: a role for Gilbert's syndrome? *Int J Infect Dis.* 2009;13(4):e161–e164.

51. Chalupa P, Kaspar M, Holub M. Acute acalculous cholecystitis with pericholecystitis in a patient with Epstein-Barr virus infectious mononucleosis. *Med Sci Mon Int Med J Exp Clin Res.* 2009;15(2):CS30-3.

52. Basar O, et al. An unusual cause of acalculous cholecystitis during pregnancy: hepatitis A virus. *Dig Dis Sci.* 2005;50(8):1532.

53. Bouyahia O, et al. Hepatitis A: a rare cause of acalculous cholecystitis in children. *Med Maladies Infect.* 2008;38(1):34–35.

54. Fuoti M, et al. Acute acalculous cholecystitis as a complication of hepatitis A: report of 2 pediatric cases. *Pediatr Med e Chir.* 2008;30(2):102–105.

55. Tresallet C, et al. Hepatitis C virus infection revealed by an acute acalculous cholecystitis. *J Radiol.* 2010;91(7–8):813–815.

56. Berrington WR, Hitti J, Casper C. A case report of dengue virus infection and acalculous cholecystitis in a pregnant returning traveler. *Trav Med Infect Dis.* 2007;5(4):251–253.

57. Bhatty S, et al. Acute acalculous cholecystitis in dengue fever. *J Pakistan Med Assoc.* 2009;59(8):519–521.

58. Goh BK, Tan SG. Case of dengue virus infection presenting with acute acalculous cholecystitis. *J Gastroenterol Hepatol.* 2006;21(5):923–924.

59. Brent AJ, et al. Acute cholecystitis complicating mumps. *Clin Infect Dis.* 2006;42(2):302–303.

60. Frohlich R, Rommele U. Acalculous cholecystitis in hantavirus infections. *Dtsch Med Wochenschr.* 2013;138(23):1255–1258.

61. Gora-Gebka M, et al. Acute acalculous cholecystitis of viral etiology—a rare condition in children? *J Pediatr Surg.* 2008;43(1):e25–e27.

62. Guner R, et al. A case of Crimean Congo hemorrhagic fever complicated with acalculous cholecystitis and intraabdominal abscess. *J Clin Virol.* 2011;50(2):162–163.

63. Abreu C, et al. Acute acalculous cholecystitis in malaria: a review of seven cases from an adult cohort. *Infection.* 2013;41(4):821–826.

64. Carvalho D, et al. Acute acalculous cholecystitis in a patient with severe malaria. *Acta Med Port.* 2011;24(suppl 3):631–634.

65. Hayakawa K, et al. A case of scrub typhus with acalculous cholecystitis, aseptic meningitis and mononeuritis multiplex. *J Med Microbiol.* 2012;61(Pt 2):291–294.

66. Malik AA, Wani RA, Bari S. Acute acalculous cholecystitis due to *Taenia saginata*. *Ann Saudi Med.* 2008;28(5):388–389.

67. Grosser J, Solomon H, Sotelo-Avila C. Acalculous candidal cholecystitis after pediatric renal transplant. *Pediatr Transplant.* 2011;15(4):E71–E75.

CHAPTER 4

Hepatitis B Virus, Hepatitis C Virus, the Microbiome, and Hepatocellular Carcinoma

FEI CHEN, MBBS • CARL FREYER, MBBS • LAN GONG, BSC (HONS), PHD • AMANY ZEKRY, MBBS, FRACP, PHD

HEPATITIS B INFECTION AND THE ROLE IN HEPATOCELLULAR CARCINOMA

Discovery

The hepatitis B virus (HBV) was discovered more than 50 years ago; however, descriptions of "endemic hepatitis" by Hippocrates, likely attributable to viral hepatitis, date back to the 5th century BC. The term hepatitis B was first introduced in 1947 by MaCallum after observing that "infectious hepatitis" (hepatitis A) and "serum hepatitis" (hepatitis B) resulted from different routes of transmission, namely, fecal-oral and parenteral, respectively.[1] Blumberg and Alter[2] serendipitously discovered the hepatitis B surface antigen (HBsAg) in 1963 while analyzing blood samples collected from various global indigenous populations in work unrelated to hepatitis . The antigen was initially named the "Australia antigen" after its identification in the serum of Australian Aborigines and it was subsequently shown to be a specific marker of "serum hepatitis."[3–5] Studies in the 1970s determined the structure of the hepatitis B virion, with identification of the Australia antigen as a component of the outer HBsAg along with the discovery of the core antigen.[6] The molecular composition of HBV and its genome have since been determined and effective vaccination is now available. The discovery of the Australia antigen was a watershed moment in the history of viral hepatitis and opened the door for modern research into this field.

Epidemiology

HBV is estimated to affect 3.5% of the total global population, i.e., 257 million people.[7] The prevalence of HBV varies widely by geographic region. Areas with low prevalence (<2%) include Western Europe, United States, Canada, and Australia. Intermediate-prevalence areas (2%–7%) include the Middle East, Mediterranean, and Russia, and high-prevalence areas (>8%)

include parts of Africa and the Western Pacific. South Sudan has the highest estimated prevalence in the world (22.8%).[7,8] Indigenous populations in many nations have higher prevalence rates, including Australian Aboriginal and Torres Strait Islanders, New Zealand Maori, and Native North Americans. The majority of the global disease burden arises from Africa and the Western Pacific regions.[7]

The risk of developing chronic HBV infection following acute infection decreases with increasing age and plateaus in early adulthood.[9] Perinatal infection will result in chronic infection in 90% of cases, whereas infection in immune-competent adults will only progress to chronic infection in up to 5% of cases.[10,11] In highly endemic regions, vertical transmission and horizontal spread among children are the main routes of infection. Horizontal transmission beyond childhood is thought to be a major contributor of incident cases of HBV in intermediate-prevalence cases; however, vertical transmission still plays a significant role. In low-prevalence countries, vertical transmission is rare and the majority of new infections are due to horizontal transmission in adolescence and adulthood.[12] A significant proportion of patients with chronic HBV infection will develop hepatic cirrhosis and hepatocellular carcinoma (HCC), with an estimated 15%–25% dying of these complications.[8] In 2013, there were an estimated 686,000 deaths globally directly attributable to HBV infection.[13]

Transmission

Hepatitis B is highly infectious and transmission occurs via exposure to infected body fluids. The main routes of transmission are perinatal (vertical) and horizontal.

Perinatal transmission accounts for the majority of transmission worldwide, particularly in highly endemic countries. Perinatal transmission can occur before,

Gastrointestinal Diseases and Their Associated Infections. https://doi.org/10.1016/B978-0-323-54843-4.00004-0
Copyright © 2019 Elsevier Inc. All rights reserved.

during, or after birth. Transmission risk from mother to child is related to maternal hepatitis e antigen (HBeAg) status and HBV viral load.

Horizontal transmission is common in countries with intermediate–low prevalence, with common routes of exposure being injecting drug, sexual contact, and healthcare exposure.[14]

Virology

HBV is a hepadnavirus containing a circular partially double-stranded DNA genome. There are 10 known genotypes (named A-J) that differ based on divergence in their complete genotype by at least 8% and more than 4% at the level of the S gene (see later discussion).[15] HBV genotypes exhibit geographic variation.[16] Genotype A is prevalent in North America, Western Europe, and Africa; genotypes B and C are prevalent in Asia; genotype D is prevalent in India, the Mediterranean, and the Middle East; genotype E is found in sub-Saharan Africa; genotype F in Central America; genotype G in France, Germany, and the United States; genotype H is found in Central and South America; and genotype I in Vietnam. Genotype J is the most recently discovered genotype and has been found in the Ryukyu Islands of Japan.[16,17] Some clinically significant associations have been observed between genotypes. Response to interferon (IFN) therapy appears to be superior in genotypes A and B, compared with C and D[18]; disease activity and progression of liver disease is greater in genotype C than in B[19]; and HBeAg seroconversion occurs earlier in genotype B than in C.[20]

The HBV virion is 40–42 nm in diameter with an outer envelope made up of surface antigen lipoproteins and an inner core nucleocapsid containing the viral genome.[6,21] The genome contains four open reading frames encoding four viral genes: the pre-S-S (presurface/surface), pre-C-C (precore/core), X, and polymerase genes. The surface gene encodes the pre-S1, pre-S2, and S proteins (small [S], middle [M], and large [L] proteins). The "S protein" is the most abundant of these and is known as the HBsAg. The core gene produces the nucleocapsid, as well as the e antigen, which is not involved in replication. The X gene encodes the X protein, the function of which is not completely clear. However, the X protein has been implicated in hepatic carcinogenesis. The polymerase gene encodes a large protein involved in DNA replication and packaging.[22]

Multiple mutant forms of the HBV exist, with the most common occurring in the precore or basal core regions. A single nucleotide change at position 1896 in the precore region results in a stop codon, eliminating production of HBeAg. A double nucleotide change in the basal core region at positions 1762 and 1764 results in decreased HBeAg production.[23,24] These mutations do not diminish the replicative ability of HBV.

Mutations in the HBsAg can occur from mutations in the surface gene or the overlapping polymerase gene. Alterations in amino acids from positions 124–127 may result in an altered "a" epitope, which is the binding site for the neutralizing hepatitis B surface antibody (HBsAb). These mutants may result in a patients testing negative for HBsAg but having detectable viral DNA in the serum. Furthermore, hepatitis B core antibody (HBcAb) should be positive. These mutations may lead to failure of vaccination and immune escape.[25]

Natural History
Acute hepatitis B

Age of acquisition influences the clinical presentation of acute HBV infection. Neonates and young children are usually asymptomatic, whereas one-third of adults develop clinically apparent hepatitis. Up to 1% of acute infections will result in acute liver failure.[26] Serum HBsAg will appear between 2 and 10 weeks after infection, and with clearance, it will disappear with the emergence of anti-HBs. Persistence of HBsAg beyond the 6 months indicates chronic infection.

Chronic hepatitis B

Chronic hepatitis B is often asymptomatic, unless decompensated cirrhosis or extrahepatic manifestations are present. The chronic disease course of HBV infection can be described in various phases that reflect the interaction between viral replication and the host immune response. The latest nomenclature divides infection into five phases, based on the patients HBV DNA levels, alanine aminotransferase (ALT) levels, and serologic status. The phases described do not necessarily occur chronologically and patients may not fit into a specific phase at a given time. This highlights the need for serial monitoring and individualizing decision making with regard to treatment.[27]

Phase 1 is characterized by HBeAg positivity, markedly elevated HBV DNA levels, and normal range of ALT levels. Liver histologic finding is notable for the absence of fibrosis or significant necroinflammation. This phase was previously termed "immune tolerant" and is more common in patients infected perinatally or in early childhood.

Phase 2 is characterized by HBeAg positivity, high HBV DNA levels, and an elevated ALT level. Liver histologic examination reveals marked necroinflammation. This phase may be reached rapidly in patients infected in adulthood, or after year to decades if infected in early life. A majority of patients will achieve HBeAg seroconversion and adequate viral suppression.

Phase 3 is characterized by HBeAg negativity, hepatitis B e antibody (HBeAb) positivity, low or undetectable HBV DNA levels, and normal range of ALT levels. This phase was previously termed the "inactive carrier" phase. Liver histologic examination shows low necroinflammatory activity and minimal fibrosis. Progression to cirrhosis and HCC is low if patients remain in this phase. Spontaneous loss of HBsAg occurs at a rate of 1%–3% per year.

Phase 4 is characterized by HBeAg negativity, HBeAb positivity, fluctuating or persistently elevated moderate to high HBV DNA levels, and fluctuating or persistently elevated ALT levels. Liver histologic examination is notable for active necroinflammation and the presence of fibrosis. Spontaneous disease remission is rare in this phase and the presence of precore and/or basal core mutations (see Virology section) is common.

Phase 5 is characterized by negative HBsAg and HBsAb, positive HBcAb, and normal range of ALT levels in the serum. Serum HBV DNA level is usually very low (<2000 IU/mL) or undetectable; however, the HBV DNA level is detectable in the liver. If this stage is reached prior to the development of advanced fibrosis/cirrhosis, the prognosis is excellent. If advanced fibrosis/cirrhosis is already established, patients will require monitoring accordingly[27] (see Treatment section).

Extrahepatic manifestations

Extrahepatic manifestations of HBV infection occur in 10%–20% of patients and are likely due to circulating immune complexes that subsequently activate complement pathways. These include arthritis-dermatitis, glomerulonephritis (both membranous and membranoproliferative), cryoglobulinemia, and polyarteritis nodosa.[28,29]

Diagnosis

The presence of HBsAg in the serum is the hallmark of HBV infection. Serologic markers for HBV infection include HBsAg, anti-HBs, anti-HBc, HBeAg, and anti-HBe. Serum HBsAg appears 2–10 weeks after initial exposure, followed 1–2 weeks later by IgM anti-HBc. Persistent infection will result in production of IgG anti-HBc. Suppression of HBV can be detected by disappearance of HBsAg and the appearance of anti-HBs. Anti-HBc will persist in whom the infection has cleared, whereas a patient who is immune due to vaccination will only have positive anti-HBs. HBeAg and anti-HBe are useful to determine the phase of infection that a patient is in (see earlier discussion). HBV DNA level is a direct measure of viral load, and its quantification can be used to determine the need for and response to antiviral treatment.[26] Interpretation of serologic markers can be seen in Table 4.1.

Management of Hepatitis B
Indications for therapy

The decision to commence treatment for hepatitis B is based on three parameters: serum HBV DNA levels, serum ALT levels, and severity of liver disease (presence or absence of fibrosis/cirrhosis). This applies to both e antigen–negative and e antigen–positive patients.[27,30]

TABLE 4.1 Interpretation of Hepatitis B Serology				
	HBsAg	**Anti-HBs**	**Anti-HBc IgG**	**Anti-HBc IgM**
Acute hepatitis B	Positive	Negative	Negative	Positive
Resolved infection[a]	Negative	Positive	Positive	Negative
Vaccinated	Negative	Positive	Negative	Negative
Chronic hepatitis B	Positive	Negative	Positive	Negative
Not infected	Negative	Negative	Negative	Negative

[a]Requires hepatitis B virus DNA testing to exclude occult infection.
Anti-HBc, hepatitis B surface antibody; *anti-HBs*, hepatitis B surface antibody; *HBsAg*, hepatitis B surface antigen.

In patients in whom the serum HBV DNA level is >20,000 IU/mL, treatment should be initiated if their serum ALT level exceeds two times the upper limit of normal, regardless of their degree of fibrosis. Treatment should be considered for patients whose serum HBV DNA level is >2000 IU/mL, whose serum ALT level exceeds the upper limit of normal (usually around 40 IU/mL), and who have at least moderate fibrosis or necroinflammation assessed traditionally by liver biopsy. Treatment may also be initiated in patients with serum HBV DNA levels exceeding 2000 IU/mL with at least moderate fibrosis, regardless of their serum ALT levels. In patients reluctant to undergo liver biopsy, noninvasive markers of fibrosis, such as transient elastography, may be utilized to determine the degree of fibrosis. It is recommended that treatment for hepatitis B be commenced in certain patients regardless of their serum ALT levels. This includes patients with compensated or decompensated cirrhosis with detectable HBV DNA levels, e antigen–negative and e antigen–positive patients with a family history of HCC or cirrhosis, as well as in patients with extrahepatic manifestations of hepatitis B.

Monitoring of patients on and off treatment
In patients who do not meet the criteria for treatment with antiviral therapy, serum ALT and HBV DNA levels, as well as assessment of liver fibrosis severity, should be performed periodically. Ideally, e antigen–positive patients who do not meet the treatment criteria should be followed up every 3–6 months, and every 6–12 months for e antigen–negative patients whose HBV DNA level is less than 2000 IU/mL and who do not meet the treatment criteria.[27]

Treatment strategies
The current available options for hepatitis B treatment include treatment with nucleos(t)ide analogue (NA) and pegylated interferon α (PegIFN-α).[27,30] The NAs that have been approved for use in Australia include lamivudine and adefovir dipivoxil, which have low barrier against HBV resistance, and NAs with high barrier to HBV resistance include entecavir (ETV), tenofovir disoproxil fumarate (TDF), and tenofovir alafenamide (TAF). The main advantages of treatment with NAs include the following:
- Predictable high long-term antiviral resistance.
- Higher tolerability, with minimal side effects.
- Minimal contraindications, including use in several patient subgroups such as those with decompensated liver disease, those with acute hepatitis B, liver transplant recipients, or those with extrahepatic manifestations.

However, treatment with NAs are usually long term (even lifelong in some cases). As such, treatment with PegIFN-α may be considered in selected cases to induce long-term immune control within a finite duration (48 weeks). The main drawbacks to treatment with PegIFN-α are its high variability of response and its unfavorable safety profile, making a large proportion of patients ineligible or unwilling to undertake this treatment.

Goals of therapy
The main goal of hepatitis B treatment is to prevent disease progression and HCC development, thus improving survival and quality of life for patients. Other goals of hepatitis B treatment depend on the clinical setting and can include prevention of mother-to-child transmission during pregnancy, prevention of hepatitis B reactivation in patients receiving immunosuppressive therapy or chemotherapy, prevention of acute or subacute liver failure in patients with acute hepatitis B, and treatment of extrahepatic manifestations of hepatitis B. In patients with hepatitis B–related HCC, treatment goals include virus suppression to stabilize HBV-induced liver disease and hence prevent disease progression, as well as to prevent HCC recurrence after potentially curative HCC treatment.[27,30]

The main endpoint in all treatment strategies is to achieve long-term suppression of HBV replication and in turn reducing necroinflammatory activity and fibrotic liver processes, leading to reduced risk for HCC development. Suppression of HBV DNA to undetectable levels is usually associated with normalization of ALT levels, unless there is a secondary cause to this, which is most commonly alcoholic or nonalcoholic liver disease. This persistence of ALT elevation is associated with lower chance of fibrosis regression. HBeAg loss is not a reliable endpoint, given that HBeAg seroreversion or development of HBeAg-negative chronic hepatitis B may occur when treatments are stopped after HBeAg loss. Loss of HBsAg is regarded as the optimal treatment endpoint, or "functional cure." Unfortunately, with the currently available treatment options, this is very rarely achieved. In the rare event that HBsAg occurs, treatment in these patients can safely be discontinued.[27] However, it is unclear if loss of HBsAg will prevent long-term complications associated with HBV, such as HCC development, given that chronic HBV infection cannot be completely eradicated because of the covalently closed circular DNA (cccDNA) of HBV and the integrated HBV DNA.

Special Population

Patients with acute hepatitis B

Most patients with acute hepatitis B recover spontaneously without any specific treatment. Only patients with severe acute hepatitis B, characterized by prolonged course (more than 4 weeks), coagulopathy (international normalized ratio > 1.5), and signs of acute liver failure, require antiviral treatment. Studies have supported the early use of highly potent NAs, including TDF and ETV, to prevent progression to acute liver failure and subsequent liver transplantation and mortality.[27] The use of glucocorticoids in acute hepatitis B has only been studied in older studies, which did not include the use of current antiviral drugs.

Management of hepatitis B in pregnancy

HBeAg-positive mothers transmit the virus to their infants in up to 85%–90% of cases.[31,32] Prophylactic vaccination fails in a significant proportion of women with high viral loads (>200,000 IU/mL).[33,34] Further reduction of transmission can be achieved with antiviral therapy in the third trimester,[35] and antiviral therapy should be offered to women with high viral loads.[30] All pregnant women should therefore be screened for HBsAg in the first trimester of pregnancy. Treatment of hepatitis B in pregnancy with TDF is only recommended in patients with advanced fibrosis or cirrhosis, and patients with high HBV load, starting at week 24–28 of gestation until up to 12 weeks after delivery.[35,36] In patients already on NA therapy, only TDF is recommended, given its extensive safety data in pregnant women with HBV infection. PegIFN-α is contraindicated during pregnancy. Antiviral commencement should be delayed in women of childbearing age without advanced fibrosis who plans to fall pregnant soon until the child is born.[27] Children born from mothers with e antigen–positive chronic hepatitis B with high HBV load (>200,000 IU) should receive a combination of hepatitis B immunoglobulin and vaccination within 12 h of birth to reduce the risk of perinatal transmission.[37] Breastfeeding is not contraindicated in women treated with TDF.[38,39]

Management of hepatitis B in patients undergoing immunosuppressive therapy or chemotherapy

Hepatitis B reactivation in the setting of immunosuppressive therapy or chemotherapy carries a morbidity and mortality risk. The risk of hepatitis B reactivation varies depending on the virologic profile, the underlying disease, and the type and duration of immunosuppression, and it is highest in patients treated with

rituximab, either alone or in combination with steroids. Therefore all patients who are candidates for chemotherapy, immunosuppressive therapy, and biologic immunomodulator therapy should be screened for HBV markers including HBsAg, HBcAb, and HBV DNA. Prophylaxis treatment with ETV, TDF, or TAF is recommended in all patients with positive HBsAg during therapy and should continue for at least 12 months (or 18 months in the setting of rituximab) after therapy completion.[40] Treatment may be continued for a longer period if the underlying disease has not achieved remission. Liver function and HBV DNA levels should be monitored every 3–6 months until at least 12 months after NA therapy withdrawal, as large proportions of hepatitis B reactivation occurs following NA therapy discontinuation.[27]

In patients with negative HBsAg but positive HBcAb, prophylaxis with ETV, TDF, or TAF is recommended only in the high-risk group, including those treated with rituximab or those undergoing stem cell transplantation. Otherwise, preemptive therapy, not prophylaxis, is recommended in patients with low to moderate risk with negative HBsAg but positive HBcAb. This involves monitoring of HBsAg and/or HBV DNA levels every 1–3 months during and after therapy, and commencing NA therapy with ETV, TDF, or TAF in the case of detectable HBV DNA levels or HBsAg seroreversion, regardless of the ALT levels. However, in the setting of unknown risk for new biologicals, long duration of immunosuppression, or limited compliance to monitoring, universal prophylaxis is recommended.[27]

Hepatocellular Carcinoma Risk in Patients With Chronic Hepatitis B

Chronic hepatitis B is now recognized as one of the most important cause for the development of HCC, accounting for over 50% of the HCC cases worldwide. However, it was not until the mid-1970s that scientists recognized the causative role of chronic hepatitis B in HCC development. This was following the discovery of the hepatitis-associated antigen, now known as the HBsAg, which has been reported to persist in patients with chronic hepatitis B with or without cirrhosis, leading to HCC development in a significant proportion of patients.[41] Various mechanisms have been proposed in the pathogenesis of HCC in patients with chronic HBV infection. Integration of the HBV DNA into the hepatocyte genome and the epigenetic regulation of the minichromosome cccDNA result in chromosomal instability and activation of cancer-related genes along with inactivation of cancer-suppressive genes through interference with various cellular transcription and signal transduction processes.[42] In addition, chronic hepatitis B results in release of cytokines and growth factors as part of the adaptive immune response, leading to hepatocyte necrosis and fibroblast proliferation, resulting in liver fibrosis/cirrhosis.[43]

There are many risk factors associated with the increased risk of HCC development in patients with chronic hepatitis B. These include patients from certain areas of the world such as Asia and Africa, male gender, older age (more than 40 years old), presence of cirrhosis, positive family history of HCC, high HBV load count (with the HBV load following a linear pattern to the risk of HCC development), having genotype C HBV infection, presence of precore mutation, heavy alcohol consumption, coinfection with other viruses such as hepatitis C virus (HCV) or hepatitis D virus and human immunodeficiency virus (HIV), and exposure to aflatoxin (Table 4.2).[44–47] A study in Taiwan investigated the role of metabolic risk factors and smoking in the development of HCC in male patients with chronic hepatitis B. The study demonstrated a significantly higher risk of HCC in patients with high burden of metabolic risk factors (having three or more metabolic risk factors) than those with a low metabolic risk profile or none. Smoking was also demonstrated to have a significant effect on this association.[48]

Although high HBV load is associated with increased risk of HCC development, data regarding the effect of viral suppression using antivirals on the risk of HCC development has not been very impressive. Patients who achieve loss of HBsAg with antiviral treatments may benefit from some reduction, but there is no elimination of the risk of HCC development. The risk of HCC development in patients with undetected HBV load remains considerably high, especially in males of older age and patients with cirrhosis. This may be explained with the prolonged survival and extended exposure of patients to HBsAg with antiviral treatments.[41] A retrospective study from Taiwan observed the association between low-level viremia (HBV DNA level < 2000 IU/mL) while on ETV and the risk of HCC development. This study demonstrated that low-level viremia is not harmless and still has a significant risk of HCC development, albeit lower than those who did not achieve virologic response on ETV. This risk is more evident in patients with cirrhosis.[49]

As such, patients with chronic hepatitis B, especially those at high risk, should be continuously screened for HCC, regardless of the virologic remission (Table 4.3).[27]

TABLE 4.2
Factors Associated With Increased Risk of HCC Development in Patients With Chronic Hepatitis B

Viral Factors	Patient Factors
Genotype C hepatitis B	Male
High viral load	Age >40 years
Coinfection with other viruses	Asian or African origin
Precore mutation	Presence of cirrhosis
	Family history of HCC
	Heavy alcohol consumption
	High metabolic risk factor profile
	Smoking

HCC, hepatocellular carcinoma.

TABLE 4.3
Patients With Chronic Hepatitis B Recommended for HCC Surveillance[30]

All patients with cirrhosis
All patients with a history of HCC
Patients with chronic hepatitis B (positive HBsAg)
Family history of HCC
Asian men >40 years old, Asian women >50 years old
African/North American black >20 years old

HBsAg, hepatitis B surface antigen; HCC, hepatocellular carcinoma.

HEPATITIS C AND ITS ROLE IN HEPATOCELLULAR CARCINOMA
Discovery

In 1989 the HCV was identified by molecular cloning and confirmed to be the cause of the vast majority of non-A and non-B hepatitis associated with posttransfusion and injecting drug use.[50,51]

HCV is a blood-borne virus transmitted primarily through contact with contaminated blood and blood-derived fluids. Blood transfusion was the main route of infection for posttransfusion hepatitis before HCV identification.[51] Historically, prevalence was increasing in every region until routine blood screening started in the early to mid-1990s, significantly reducing the risk of HCV transmission through blood transfusion.[52]

Currently in the majority of developed countries, people who inject drugs and men who have sex with men represent most of the new cases of HCV. In contrast, blood transfusion and unsafe medical practices are still a major route of HCV transmission in developing countries.[53]

Virology

HCV is a single-stranded RNA virus that belongs to the family Flaviviridae. It encodes a protein chain of 3010 amino acids and contains structural and nonstructural proteins. HCV consist of a 9.6-kb single-stranded positive-sense RNA genome with a 5′ untranslated region that functions as an internal ribosome entry site, a single long open reading frame encoding a polyprotein of approximately 3000 amino acids, and a 3′ untranslated region. Using the host's ribosome, HCV creates a single polyprotein, which is then cleaved by host cell peptidases (proteases) to yield three structural proteins named E1, E2, core, and p7 and by viral proteases, which generate the six nonstructural proteins named as NS2, NS3, NS4a, NS4b, N4a, and NS5B.[54]

HCV is a very heterogeneous virus with at least seven well-characterized genotypes defined as genotypes 1–7 based on phylogenetic and sequence analyses of whole viral genomes. Within these genotypes, there may be further division into subtypes, which is best demonstrated in HCV genotype 1a and genotype 1b.[54] The geographic distribution of genotypes varies by region. Overall, genotype 1 and genotype 3 are the most observed genotypes globally, accounting for 46% and 30% of cases, respectively. Genotype 2 and genotype 6 are most commonly found in East Asia, whereas genotype 4 and genotype 6 are in North Africa and the Middle East and genotype 5 is mostly in South Africa. It is estimated that genotypes 2, 4, and 6 together account for nearly one-quarter of all HCV cases globally.[55,56]

Epidemiology

Based on anti-HCV antibody data, it is estimated that the global prevalence of HCV is at 1.6% (range, 1.3%–2.1%), which corresponds to 115 million individuals infected with HCV. However, in 2015, a lower global prevalence of 1·0% was estimated, based on HCV viremia (HCV RNA positive), thus corresponding to 71.1 million (62·5–79·4) viremic infections.[57]

There is significant variation in the prevalence of HCV infection globally between countries, ranging from 0.3% in Europe to 8.5% in Egypt. The largest viremic populations were in Egypt, with 6,358,000 cases in 2008. Furthermore, the highest prevalence (accounting for 80% of the infected population globally) was reported in China, Pakistan, India, Egypt, and Russia.

In most countries, males had a higher rate of infections, likely due to higher rates of injection drug use.[58]

Natural History of Hepatitis C Virus

Acute infection after exposure to a risk factor is clinically mild and typically infrequently diagnosed, particularly in those who progress to chronic hepatitis. After 6 months of persistence of HCV RNA within the blood the infection is defined as being chronic. The transition from acute to chronic hepatitis C is usually subclinical. However, a small proportion of infected individuals may become symptomatic and exhibit clinical and biochemical evidence of acute hepatitis.[58]

Spontaneous resolution of chronic hepatitis C is relatively rare but can occur. Based on retrospective studies of posttransfusion hepatitis, in 15%–40% of people acute HCV infection clears spontaneously. In one international prospective study including 632 participants with acute HCV, in 25% of infected individuals the HCV infection cleared after an acute infection. Among those with clearance, the median time to clearance was around 12–16 weeks. Female sex, favorable IL28B genotype, and HCV genotype 1 were independent predictors of spontaneous clearance.[59]

Chronic HCV infection is the most common outcome after acute infection. The natural history of the disease remains incompletely defined, and our knowledge and understanding of this infection is likely to change with the current availability of effective curative therapy for chronic HCV infection.

In general, however, chronic HCV infection has been recognized as the leading cause of end-stage liver disease, HCC, and liver-related death. In most cases, chronic hepatitis follows an indolent asymptomatic course and individuals come to recognize their infection and liver disease status mostly through incidental testing. The progression of the disease is generally slow, with persistent hepatic inflammation resulting in cirrhosis occurring in around 10%–20% of infected individuals after 20–30 years.[58] However, the progression rate of chronic HCV infection to cirrhosis is highly variable among individuals, varying from 2% to 51% after 22 years of infection.[59] At an individual level, the rate of progression of liver disease from fibrosis to cirrhosis is increased by other coexistent variables such as age at infection, male gender, genetics, alcohol intake, and metabolic factors including obesity, insulin resistance, and type II diabetes mellitus. In addition, coinfection with other viruses, such as HBV or HIV, has been shown to accelerate the course of disease progression. Even after viral eradication with treatment, these coexistent factors can still contribute to the progression of liver disease.

With the establishment of liver cirrhosis, the annual risk of developing hepatic decompensation and HCC has been estimated to be 3%–6% and 1%–5%, respectively.

In the current era where effective curative therapy for HCV infection is available, it is likely that these treatment regimens will favorably alter the natural history of chronic HCV infection.

Hepatitis C Virus and Hepatocellular Carcinoma

The incidence of HCV-related HCC varies with both geographic location and ethnicity. HCV is the leading cause of HCC in the United States, Europe, Australia, Japan, and South America, whereas HBV is the major cause of HCC in the majority of Asia and Africa.[60]

Chronic infection with HCV is associated with an increased risk of HCC (Table 4.4). In a large, population-based study of 12,008 Taiwanese men who were followed up for 9.2 years, individuals who were seropositive for anti-HCV antibodies had a 20-fold increased risk of HCC compared with seronegative individuals.[61] Age and the hepatic fibrosis stage are key time-dependent risks for the development of HCC with chronic HCV infection. In particular, cirrhosis is associated with an annual incidence of 1%–7% per year.[62]

Various host genetic polymorphisms associated with the immune system and metabolic functions have also been identified to be associated with HCV-induced HCC.[63] The results however remain inconsistent across the studied cohorts in this area of research. In this regard, a large genomic study from Japan identified several single nucleotide polymorphism (SNP) in major histocompatibility complex (MHC) class I polyptide-related sequence A (MICA, rs2596542), which is involved in the response of dendritic cells to type I IFN in chronic hepatitis C. Another SNP in the MICA promoter (rs2596538) was associated with increased levels of serum soluble MICA protein. A subsequent study in Caucasian patients with hepatitis C in Switzerland did not replicate the association with HCC for this locus, but for a nearby locus in human leukocyte antigen complex P5 (HCP5) (rs2244546), suggesting that the MICA/HCP5 region contains a potential susceptibility locus. An IL28B variant (rs12979860), initially identified as an IFN response predictor, may be associated with the increased risk of HCV-related HCC.[64,65]

SNPs in genes associated with metabolic functions have also been weakly associated with HCV-induced HCC. For instance, an SNP in the patatin-like phospholipase domain-containing protein 3 (PNPLA3) gene

TABLE 4.4
Factors Associated With Increased Risk of Hepatocellular Carcinoma With Chronic Hepatitis C
Age
Male gender
Fibrosis stage
Immune and metabolic host genetic polymorphisms
Metabolic risk factors such as type II diabetes mellitus and obesity
Genotype 3

(rs738409) associated with alcoholic and nonalcoholic steatohepatitis (NASH) may have a weak association with HCV-related HCC.[66,67]

Men are at increased risk for HCC partly because they have a greater incidence of viral hepatitis. A cross-sectional study reported total serum testosterone levels to be associated with an increased risk of both advanced hepatic fibrosis and advanced hepatic inflammatory activity in HCV-infected men; however, the association with HCC was not examined.[68]

Metabolic risk factors such as type II diabetes mellitus and obesity in individuals with HCV contribute to an increased risk of HCC. HCV infection has high comorbidity with diabetes mellitus, which confers a two-- to threefold increase in HCC risk.[69]

As for viral factors, clinical studies have associated HCV genotype 3 with increased steatosis, increased fibrosis progression rate and hence risk of HCC development.[70] Further, a study from Taiwan reported a correlation between level of HCV RNA and the risk of HCC,[64] but this was not replicated in other studies from the United States and Europe.

Treatment of Chronic Hepatitis C Virus

Although HCV causes persistent hepatitis, the RNA viral genome does not integrate into the host genome and a virologic cure is achievable by treatment. Accepted cure is defined as undetectable HCV RNA in serum at 12–24 weeks following completion of treatment (sustained virologic response [SVR]).

Over the past two decades the development of infectious HCV cell culture models has increased our understanding of the HCV lifecycle and has led to dramatic improvements in the treatment of HCV infection. Unlike HBV and HIV, the goal of HCV treatment is viral clearance or "cure," due to the absence of a latent host reservoir (Wang et al., 2016a). Virus clearance with treatment is identified by an SVR, defined as the absence of detectable levels of virus in the blood 12 weeks after the end of therapy (SVR12).

Treatment of chronic HCV infection started in 1991 with subcutaneous IFN-α, resulting in low SVR rates of less than 16%. Addition of ribavirin to the regimen increased the SVR rate to 28% in genotype 1 patients and up to 66% in other genotypes.[39,71] PegIFN was subsequently developed, which had a longer half-life, allowing weekly dosing instead of every 1–2 days, which, in combination with ribavirin, increased the SVR rate to approximately 44% for genotype 1 patients and 70%–80% for genotype 3.[39,71] However, treatment with these regimens had multiple intolerable adverse side effects, which made it difficult to cure chronic HCV infection in many cases.

A major breakthrough in HCV research and hence treatment came with the discovery of the first HCV strain capable of producing infectious viral particles in vitro. Wakita and colleagues[72] isolated a genotype 2a replicon (JFH1) from a Japanese patient with fulminant hepatitis C. The complete JFH1 genome was cloned into a DNA plasmid, allowing transcription of HCV RNA in vitro. When HuH7 cells were transfected with this RNA, viral replication was established and infectious viral particles were produced, which could infect naive HuH7 cells in vitro, as well as infect chimpanzees.[73] For the first time, this allowed researchers to study the entire HCV lifecycle in vitro. Subsequently, direct-acting antiviral agents (DAAs) targeting different steps of HCV replications were developed.

Direct-Acting Antiviral Agents in the Treatment of Chronic Hepatitis C Virus Infection

Agents that target the nonstructural 3/4A (NS3/4A) serine protease, the NS5B RNA-dependent RNA polymerase, and the NS5A protein have been developed and approved for clinical use.[74] Although initial approvals of DAAs involved regimens administered in combination with PegIFN, approvals since 2016 in Australia have been exclusively for IFN-free treatment regimens. Given the markedly improved efficacy, tolerability, and safety of regimens that combine various DAAs compared with regimens containing IFN, all patients would benefit from IFN-free therapy. Therefore IFN-free regimens are recommended as first-line therapy for all indications.[75]

Current DAAs for chronic HCV infection are effective and safe treatment, achieving SVR rates of more than 90% across genotypes, is possible in patients with liver cirrhosis. By achieving an SVR, DAAs are generally predicted to be associated with a reduction in the incidence of HCC. Furthermore, the ability to treat patients

with cirrhosis has meant that those most at risk of developing HCC can benefit from achieving a cure. A full review of the Australian recommendations for the current treatment of chronic HCV infection is available online.[75]

Effect of a Sustained Virologic Response on Risk of Hepatocellular Carcinoma

In many studies, achieving an SVR has been shown to reduce all-cause mortality and liver-related mortality.[76–78] Long-term follow-up studies after IFN-based therapies reported that achieving an SVR was associated with reduced risk of HCC. Compared with non-SVR, patients who achieved an SVR demonstrated HCC incidence rates of 1.1/1000 person-years, whereas an incidence of 7.2/1000 person-years was noted in the non-SVR group.[73,78,79]

Evidence however continues to emphasize that the risk of HCC is not entirely eliminated by achieving an SVR. Age, presence of type II diabetes mellitus, alcohol intake, and low platelet count at the time of treatment appear to be associated with increased risk of HCC development. In this setting, among patients with cirrhosis over the age of 60 years, the 8-year risk of HCC was 12.2%.[80,81]

Risk of Hepatocellular Carcinoma After Direct-Acting Antiviral Agent Treatment

There is ongoing controversy in the literature regarding the risk of HCC with, and after, DAA. Some groups reported an unexpected increase in the incidence of HCC, and more aggressive faster progression of HCC in patients with liver cirrhosis receiving DAAs.[82,83]

However, not all reports have managed to clearly separate incident HCC versus de novo HCC. In studies focusing on de novo HCC occurrence, incidence rates of 7.6%–9% within 6 months of treatment was reported. Child-Pugh class B, more severe hepatic fibrosis, low platelet count, and previous HCC were significantly associated with HCC development. Another large study from Egypt, where a large number of patients have been treated with DAAs, reported an incidence ratio of 3.83% after a median follow-up period of 23 months.[84]

Further to these findings, another analysis from Japan of over 1000 treated patients treated for HCV infection has reported the incidence of HCC after SVR in the DAA group to be more than twofold higher than in the IFN-based therapy group.[85]

In contrast to these data, findings from other studies and large database analysis have dismissed the notion of increased risk of HCC with DAAs; rather, they demonstrated a reduction in HCC risk. In a large analysis by Innes et al.,[86] it was concluded that the higher risk of HCC development with DAAs is related to baseline risk factors and patient selection, rather than the use of DAAs per se . Similarly, analysis of a large Veterans Affairs national healthcare system cohort including 63,354 patients who started antiviral therapy between January 1999 and December 2015 reported a significant decline in HCC risk with SVR, irrespective of whether the antiviral therapy was DAA or IFN based. In fact, in this analysis, the DAA-induced SVR was associated with a 71% reduction in HCC risk compared with treatment with IFN-based therapy. Similar findings were reported by other authors.[87]

In support, a French study combined data from three prospective multicenter studies including more than 6000 patients treated with DAA. In this study the investigators focused on patients with HCC who underwent curative procedures before DAA treatment. They reported the rates of HCC recurrence to be similar in treated and untreated patients, which was around 2.2%.[88]

This subject remains debatable in the literature; however, it has not negated the practice of treating advanced liver disease with HCC, but emphasized the importance of ongoing surveillance for HCC among cirrhotic patients, even after achieving an SVR.

CONCLUSIONS

Significant advances have been made in the treatment of HCV infection, with a global aim to eliminate the virus with the new therapeutic regimens. In patients with liver cirrhosis, achieving an SVR with treatment has been shown to reduce all-cause mortality and liver-related complications including HCC. There is however a persistent risk of HCC achieving an SVR, and hence, ongoing surveillance is recommended.

There has been controversy in the literature with respect to the increased risk of de novo HCC with DAAs. The evidence however is not firm and no conclusive recommendations have been made based on the current literature. This issue remains unresolved; however, it has not precluded treating patients with cirrhosis, but has emphasized the need for ongoing surveillance and for close monitoring of HCC after successful treatment outcomes.

ROLE OF GUT MICROBIOTA IN HEPATOCELLULAR CARCINOMA

HCC is usually the result of chronic liver diseases (CLDs) such as nonalcoholic fatty liver disease (NAFLD), NASH, liver fibrosis, and liver cirrhosis,[89] as more than 80% of HCC develops in the microenvironment of liver injury, inflammation, fibrosis, or cirrhosis.[90] As discussed earlier, chronic hepatitis B and C also represent a high risk factor for HCC development compared with autoimmune hepatitis and alcoholic liver disease with a relatively low HCC risk.[91] In addition to hepatitis viruses (HBV and HCV), many other microorganisms in gut microbiota play important roles in disease progression of HCC and CLDs at various stages.[89] The interaction between gut microbiome and gastrointestinal health is discussed in detail in Chapter 21. Significant changes in the gut microbiota composition have been observed in patients with different CLDs such as NAFLD, NASH, and liver cirrhosis,[92-94] and this gut dysbiosis contributes to CLD progression and even promotes HCC by contributing to hepatic inflammation through a failing gut barrier with increased intestinal permeability and the activation of pattern-recognition receptors such as toll-like receptor (TLR) 4 via microbe-associated molecular patterns (MAMPs) such as endotoxin lipopolysaccharide (LPS).[48] The multilayer intestinal barrier is usually well maintained and protects liver with minimum exposure to gut-derived factors including bacteria, metabolites, and proinflammatory MAMPs via the gut–liver axis.[95] The failure of intestinal barrier resulting in a leaky gut has been reported in patients with CLDs due to multiple factors including decreased bile acid secretion, enteric dysbiosis, intestinal inflammation, and increased permeability of gut–vascular barrier,[96] which then leads to increased blood LPS levels, endotoxemia, bacterial overgrowth, and translocation. Furthermore, this increased exposure of the chronically injured liver to the TLR4 ligand LPS and bacterial metabolites contributes to hepatic inflammation and hepatocarcinogenesis in animal models and patients.[97-99] Indeed, high levels of blood LPS detected in HCC mouse model[97] promote HCC induced by diethylnitrosamine (DEN) and carbon tetrachloride (CCl4), which can be attenuated in germ-free, antibiotic-treated, or TLR4-deficient mice.[98] Interestingly, treatment of dextran sulfate sodium is able to increase LPS levels via damaging intestinal barrier and then promotes HCC in mice.[100] The LPS–TLR4 axis promotes DEN-induced HCC via nuclear factor κB–mediated upregulation of the hepatomitogen epiregulin,[98] as well as tumor necrosis factor α–dependent and interleukin 6–dependent compensatory hepatocyte proliferation with reduced oxidative stress and apoptosis.[97] Moreover, LPS induces epithelial–mesenchymal transition, tumor cell invasion, and metastasis in HCC model by activating TLR4/JNK/MAPK signaling pathway.[101,102]

Alterations of gut microbiota have been observed in many kinds of liver diseases,[103] in which certain patterns are detected, such as increased levels of Enterobacteriaceae and decreased levels of Lachnospiraceae and *Bifidobacterium* species. Gut dysbiosis can lead to endotoxemia via endotoxins and bacterial metabolites through bacterial translocation, which then induce immune dysfunction, leading to further hepatocyte necrosis and liver failure in patients with advanced CLDs[104] and even HCC.[48] Indeed, disruption of intestinal homeostasis and gut eubiosis by antibiotics, such as penicillin, promotes protumorigenic inflammation and DEN-induced HCC in rats, which could be suppressed by probiotics such as *Lactobacillus, Bifidobacterium,* and *Enterococcus* species.[105] It was reported that the obesity-induced gut microbial metabolite deoxycholic acid (DCA) promotes HCC through senescence secretome in a mouse model of NASH-induced HCC with exposure to the chemical carcinogen 7,12-dimethylbenz[*a*] anthracene (DMBA) followed by high-fat diet (HFD).[99] In this study, following DMBA-HFD treatment, obesity-induced alterations of the gut microbiota, including a strong increase in gram-positive bacterial strains, in particular *Clostridium* clusters; increased serum levels of DCA, a gut bacterial metabolite known to cause DNA damage; and increased levels of a secondary bile acid whose production depends on 7α-dehydroxylation of primary bile acids by the microbiota especially *Clostridium* clusters were observed. These provoke senescence-associated secretory phenotype (SASP), which in turn secretes various inflammatory and tumor-promoting factors in the liver, thus facilitating HCC development.[99] Signs of SASP were also observed in the area of HCC arising in patients with NASH, indicating that a similar pathway may contribute to at least certain aspects of obesity-associated HCC development in humans.[106] It was reported that the hepatic translocation of obesity-induced lipoteichoic acid, a gram-positive bacterial component, promotes HCC by enhancing SASP collaboratively with DCA to upregulate the expression of SASP factors and cyclooxygenase-2 (COX2) through TLR2, which in turn suppresses the antitumor immunity via a prostaglandin E_2 (PGE_2)-dependent pathway.[107] Moreover, COX2 overexpression and excess PGE_2 production were detected in human HCC with noncirrhotic NASH, indicating that a similar mechanism could also function in humans.[107] Furthermore, many new therapeutic strategies have been developed and tested in animal models or clinical studies for the prevention and treatment of HCC and CLDs by interrupting the gut microbiota-LPS-TLR4-liver axis, including antibiotics, probiotics, prebiotics, fecal microbiota transplantation, and TLR antagonists.[89] Besides, accumulating evidence that the gut microbiome influences efficiency of cancer therapy,[108] especially programed cell death protein 1–dependent immunotherapy,[109] suggests a potential role of gut microbiota in HCC treatment because the B7-H1/PD-1 axis also contributes to immune suppression in human HCC.[110]

REFERENCES

1. MacCallum FO. Homologous serum hepatitis. *Proc Roy Soc Med.* 1946;39:655–657.
2. Blumberg BS, Alter HJ, Visnich S. A "New" antigen in leukemia sera. *J Am Med Assoc.* 1965;191:541–546.
3. Blumberg BS, Sutnick AI, London WT. Australia antigen and hepatitis. *J Am Med Assoc.* 1969;207(10): 1895–1896.
4. Prince AM. An antigen detected in the blood during the incubation period of serum hepatitis. *Proc Natl Acad Sci U S A.* 1968;60(3):814–821.
5. Okochi K, Murakami S. Observations on Australia antigen in Japanese. *Vox Sang.* 1968;15(5):374–385.
6. Dane DS, Cameron CH, Briggs M. Virus-like particles in serum of patients with Australia-antigen-associated hepatitis. *Lancet.* 1970;1(7649):695–698.
7. World Health Organization. *Global Hepatitis Report, 2017.* 2017: France.
8. Gupta N, Goyal M, Wu CH, Wu GY. The Molecular and Structural Basis of HBV-resistance to Nucleos(t)ide Analogs. *J Clin Transl Hepatol.* 2014;2(3):202–211.
9. Edmunds WJ, et al. The influence of age on the development of the hepatitis B Carrier state. *Proc Biol Sci.* 1993;253(1337):197–201.
10. McMahon BJ, et al. Acute hepatitis B virus infection: relation of age to the clinical expression of disease and subsequent development of the carrier state. *J Infect Dis.* 1985;151(4):599–603.
11. Hyams KC. Risks of chronicity following acute hepatitis B virus infection: a review. *Clin Infect Dis.* 1995;20(4): 992–1000.
12. MacLachlan JH, Cowie BC. Hepatitis B virus epidemiology. *Cold Spring Harb Perspect Med.* 2015;5(5): a021410.
13. Collaborators GMaCoD. Global, regional, and national age-sex specific all-cause and cause-specific mortality for 240 causes of death, 1990-2013: a systematic analysis for the Global Burden of Disease Study 2013. *Lancet.* 2015;385(9963):117–171.
14. Iqbal K, et al. Epidemiology of acute hepatitis B in the United States from population-based surveillance, 2006–2011. *Clin Infect Dis.* 2015;61(4):584–592.
15. Kramvis A, Kew M, François G. Hepatitis B virus genotypes. *Vaccine.* 2005;23(19):2409–2423.
16. Lin CL, Kao JH. The clinical implications of hepatitis B virus genotype: recent advances. *J Gastroenterol Hepatol.* 2011;26(suppl 1):123–130.

17. Sunbul M. Hepatitis B virus genotypes: global distribution and clinical importance. *World J Gastroenterol.* 2014;20(18):5427–5434.

18. Janssen HL, et al. Pegylated interferon alfa-2b alone or in combination with lamivudine for HBeAg-positive chronic hepatitis B: a randomised trial. *Lancet.* 2005;365(9454):123–129.

19. Kao JH, et al. Hepatitis B genotypes correlate with clinical outcomes in patients with chronic hepatitis B. *Gastroenterology.* 2000;118(3):554–559.

20. Chu CJ, Hussain M, Lok AS. Hepatitis B virus genotype B is associated with earlier HBeAg seroconversion compared with hepatitis B virus genotype C. *Gastroenterology.* 2002;122(7):1756–1762.

21. Robinson WS, Lutwick LI. The virus of hepatitis, type B (first of two parts). *N Engl J Med.* 1976;295(21):1168–1175.

22. Ganem D, Prince AM. Hepatitis B virus infection—natural history and clinical consequences. *N Engl J Med.* 2004;350(11):1118–1129.

23. Okamoto H, et al. Hepatitis B virus with mutations in the core promoter for an e antigen-negative phenotype in carriers with antibody to e antigen. *J Virol.* 1994;68(12):8102–8110.

24. Li J, et al. Mechanism of suppression of hepatitis B virus precore RNA transcription by a frequent double mutation. *J Virol.* 1999;73(2):1239–1244.

25. Coppola N, et al. Clinical significance of hepatitis B surface antigen mutants. *World J Hepatol.* 2015;7(27):2729–2739.

26. Trépo C, Chan HL, Lok A. Hepatitis B virus infection. *Lancet.* 2014;384(9959):2053–2063.

27. European Association for the Study of the Liver. European association for the study of the, EASL 2017 clinical practice guidelines on the management of hepatitis B virus infection. *J Hepatol.* 2017;67(2):370–398.

28. Johnson RJ, Couser WG. Hepatitis B infection and renal disease: clinical, immunopathogenetic and therapeutic considerations. *Kidney Int.* 1990;37(2):663–676.

29. Cacoub P, Terrier B. Hepatitis B-related autoimmune manifestations. *Rheum Dis Clin N Am.* 2009;35(1):125–137.

30. Terrault NA, et al. AASLD guidelines for treatment of chronic hepatitis B. *Hepatology.* 2016;63(1):261–283.

31. Beasley RP, et al. The e antigen and vertical transmission of hepatitis B surface antigen. *Am J Epidemiol.* 1977;105(2):94–98.

32. Stevens CE, et al. Vertical transmission of hepatitis B antigen in Taiwan. *N Engl J Med.* 1975;292(15):771–774.

33. Wiseman E, et al. Perinatal transmission of hepatitis B virus: an Australian experience. *Med J Aust.* 2009;190(9):489–492.

34. Pan CQ, et al. An algorithm for risk assessment and intervention of mother to child transmission of hepatitis B virus. *Clin Gastroenterol Hepatol.* 2012;10(5):452–459.

35. Brown RS, et al. Antiviral therapy in chronic hepatitis B viral infection during pregnancy: a systematic review and meta-analysis. *Hepatology.* 2016;63(1):319–333.

36. Lin YJ, et al. Chronic hepatitis C virus infection and the risk for diabetes: a community-based prospective study. *Liver Int.* 2017;37(2):179–186.

37. World Health Organization. *Global Hepatitis Programme, Guidelines for the Prevention, Care, and Treatment of Persons with Chronic Hepatitis B Infection.* Geneva, Switzerland: World Health Organization; 2015:1. Online resource (1 PDF file (xxx, 134 pages)).

38. Beasley RP, et al. Evidence against breast-feeding as a mechanism for vertical transmission of hepatitis B. *Lancet.* 1975;2(7938):740–741.

39. Fried MW, et al. Peginterferon alfa-2a plus ribavirin for chronic hepatitis C virus infection. *N Engl J Med.* 2002;347(13):975–982.

40. Pattullo V. Prevention of hepatitis B reactivation in the setting of immunosuppression. *Clin Mol Hepatol.* 2016;22(2):219–237.

41. Rapti I, Hadziyannis S. Risk for hepatocellular carcinoma in the course of chronic hepatitis B virus infection and the protective effect of therapy with nucleos(t)ide analogues. *World J Hepatol.* 2015;7(8):1064–1073.

42. Neuveut C, Wei Y, Buendia MA. Mechanisms of HBV-related hepatocarcinogenesis. *J Hepatol.* 2010;52(4):594–604.

43. Guerrieri F, et al. Molecular mechanisms of HBV-associated hepatocarcinogenesis. *Semin Liver Dis.* 2013;33(2):147–156.

44. Fattovich G, Bortolotti F, Donato F. Natural history of chronic hepatitis B: special emphasis on disease progression and prognostic factors. *J Hepatol.* 2008;48(2):335–352.

45. Chen G, et al. Past HBV viral load as predictor of mortality and morbidity from HCC and chronic liver disease in a prospective study. *Am J Gastroenterol.* 2006;101(8):1797–1803.

46. Chan HL, et al. Genotype C hepatitis B virus infection is associated with an increased risk of hepatocellular carcinoma. *Gut.* 2004;53(10):1494–1498.

47. Kao JH, et al. Basal core promoter mutations of hepatitis B virus increase the risk of hepatocellular carcinoma in hepatitis B carriers. *Gastroenterology.* 2003;124(2):327–334.

48. Yu MW, et al. Influence of metabolic risk factors on risk of hepatocellular carcinoma and liver-related death in men with chronic hepatitis B: a large cohort study. *Gastroenterology.* 2017.

49. Kim JH, et al. Low-level viremia and the increased risk of hepatocellular carcinoma in patients receiving entecavir treatment. *Hepatology.* 2017;66(2):335–343.

50. Choo QL, et al. Identification of the major, parenteral non-A, non-B hepatitis agent (hepatitis C virus) using a recombinant cDNA approach. *Semin Liver Dis.* 1992;12(3):279–288.

51. Prati D. Transmission of hepatitis C virus by blood transfusions and other medical procedures: a global review. *J Hepatol.* 2006;45(4):607–616.

52. Coste J, et al. Implementation of donor screening for infectious agents transmitted by blood by nucleic acid technology: update to 2003. *Vox Sang.* 2005;88(4):289–303.

53. Simonsen L, et al. Unsafe injections in the developing world and transmission of bloodborne pathogens: a review. *Bull World Health Organ.* 1999;77(10):789–800.

54. Kim CW, Chang KM. Hepatitis C virus: virology and life cycle. *Clin Mol Hepatol.* 2013;19(1):17–25.

55. Sievert W, et al. A systematic review of hepatitis C virus epidemiology in Asia, Australia and Egypt. *Liver Int.* 2011;31(suppl 2):61–80.

56. Messina JP, et al. Global distribution and prevalence of hepatitis C virus genotypes. *Hepatology.* 2015;61(1):77–87.

57. Shepard CW, Finelli L, Alter MJ. Global epidemiology of hepatitis C virus infection. *Lancet Infect Dis.* 2005;5(9):558–567.

58. Westbrook RH, Dusheiko G. Natural history of hepatitis C. *J Hepatol.* 2014;61(suppl 1):S58–S68.

59. Aisyah DN, et al. Assessing hepatitis C spontaneous clearance and understanding associated factors-A systematic review and meta-analysis. *J Viral Hepat.* 2018;25(6):680–698.

60. Yang JD, Roberts LR. Hepatocellular carcinoma: a global view. *Nat Rev Gastroenterol Hepatol.* 2010;7(8):448–458.

61. Lee MH, et al. Hepatitis C virus seromarkers and subsequent risk of hepatocellular carcinoma: long-term predictors from a community-based cohort study. *J Clin Oncol.* 2010;28(30):4587–4593.

62. Freeman AJ, et al. Estimating progression to cirrhosis in chronic hepatitis C virus infection. *Hepatology.* 2001;34(4 Pt 1):809–816.

63. Walker AJ, et al. Host genetic factors associated with hepatocellular carcinoma in patients with hepatitis C virus infection: a systematic review. *J Viral Hepat.* 2018;25(5):442–456.

64. Lange CM, et al. Comparative genetic analyses point to HCP5 as susceptibility locus for HCV-associated hepatocellular carcinoma. *J Hepatol.* 2013;59(3):504–509.

65. Kumar V, et al. Genome-wide association study identifies a susceptibility locus for HCV-induced hepatocellular carcinoma. *Nat Genet.* 2011;43(5):455–458.

66. Takeuchi Y, et al. The impact of patatin-like phospholipase domain-containing protein 3 polymorphism on hepatocellular carcinoma prognosis. *J Gastroenterol.* 2013;48(3):405–412.

67. Corradini SG, et al. Patatin-like phospholipase domain containing 3 sequence variant and hepatocellular carcinoma. *Hepatology.* 2011;53(5):1776; author reply 1777.

68. White DL, et al. Higher serum testosterone is associated with increased risk of advanced hepatitis C-related liver disease in males. *Hepatology.* 2012;55(3):759–768.

69. Huang TS, et al. Diabetes, hepatocellular carcinoma, and mortality in hepatitis C-infected patients: a population-based cohort study. *J Gastroenterol Hepatol.* 2017;32(7):1355–1362.

70. Kanwal F, et al. HCV genotype 3 is associated with an increased risk of cirrhosis and hepatocellular cancer in a national sample of U.S. Veterans with HCV. *Hepatology.* 2014;60(1):98–105.

71. Manns MP, et al. Peginterferon alfa-2b plus ribavirin compared with interferon alfa-2b plus ribavirin for initial treatment of chronic hepatitis C: a randomised trial. *Lancet.* 2001;358(9286):958–965.

72. Wakita T, et al. Production of infectious hepatitis C virus in tissue culture from a cloned viral genome. *Nat Med.* 2005;11(7):791–796.

73. van der Meer AJ, Berenguer M. Reversion of disease manifestations after HCV eradication. *J Hepatol.* 2016;65(suppl 1):S95–S108.

74. Suwanthawornkul T, et al. Efficacy of second generation direct-acting antiviral agents for treatment naive hepatitis C genotype 1: a systematic review and network meta-analysis. *PLoS One.* 2015;10(12):e0145953.

75. Thompson AJ. Australian recommendations for the management of hepatitis C virus infection: a consensus statement. *Med J Aust.* 2016;204(7):268–272.

76. Tada T, et al. Viral eradication reduces all-cause mortality, including non-liver-related disease, in patients with progressive hepatitis C virus-related fibrosis. *J Gastroenterol Hepatol.* 2017;32(3):687–694.

77. van der Meer AJ, et al. Risk of cirrhosis-related complications in patients with advanced fibrosis following hepatitis C virus eradication. *J Hepatol.* 2017;66(3):485–493.

78. Nahon P, et al. Eradication of hepatitis C virus infection in patients with cirrhosis reduces risk of liver and non-liver complications. *Gastroenterology.* 2017;152(1):142–156.e2.

79. Bruno S, et al. Improved survival of patients with hepatocellular carcinoma and compensated hepatitis C virus-related cirrhosis who attained sustained virological response. *Liver Int.* 2017;37(10):1526–1534.

80. Cardoso H, et al. High incidence of hepatocellular carcinoma following successful interferon-free antiviral therapy for hepatitis C associated cirrhosis. *J Hepatol.* 2016;65(5):1070–1071.

81. Lee MH, et al. Clinical efficacy and post-treatment seromarkers associated with the risk of hepatocellular carcinoma among chronic hepatitis C patients. *Sci Rep.* 2017;7(1):3718.

82. Reig M, Boix L, Bruix J. The impact of direct antiviral agents on the development and recurrence of hepatocellular carcinoma. *Liver Int.* 2017;37(suppl 1):136–139.

83. Ravi S, et al. Unusually high rates of hepatocellular carcinoma after treatment with direct-acting antiviral therapy for hepatitis C related cirrhosis. *Gastroenterology.* 2017;152(4):911–912.

84. El Kassas M, et al. Increased recurrence rates of hepatocellular carcinoma after DAA therapy in a hepatitis C-infected Egyptian cohort: a comparative analysis. *J Viral Hepat.* 2018;25(6):623–630.

85. Toyoda H, et al. Differences in background characteristics of patients with chronic hepatitis C who achieved sustained virologic response with interferon-free versus interferon-based therapy and the risk of developing hepatocellular carcinoma after eradication of hepatitis C virus in Japan. *J Viral Hepat.* 2017;24(6):472–476.

86. Innes H, et al. The risk of hepatocellular carcinoma in cirrhotic patients with hepatitis C and sustained viral response: role of the treatment regimen. *J Hepatol.* 2017.

87. El-Serag HB, et al. Risk of hepatocellular carcinoma after sustained virological response in Veterans with hepatitis C virus infection. *Hepatology.* 2016;64(1):130–137.

88. ANRS collaborative study group on hepatocellular carcinoma. Lack of evidence of an effect of direct-acting antivirals on the recurrence of hepatocellular carcinoma: data from three ANRS cohorts. *J Hepatol.* 2016;65(4):734–740.

89. Yu LX, Schwabe RF. The gut microbiome and liver cancer: mechanisms and clinical translation. *Nat Rev Gastroenterol Hepatol.* 2017.

90. El-Serag HB. Hepatocellular carcinoma. *N Engl J Med.* 2011;365(12):1118–1127.

91. Singal AG, El-Serag HB. Hepatocellular carcinoma from epidemiology to prevention: translating knowledge into practice. *Clin Gastroenterol Hepatol.* 2015;13(12):2140–2151.

92. Leung C, et al. The role of the gut microbiota in NAFLD. *Nat Rev Gastroenterol Hepatol.* 2016;13(7):412–425.

93. Boursier J, et al. The severity of nonalcoholic fatty liver disease is associated with gut dysbiosis and shift in the metabolic function of the gut microbiota. *Hepatology.* 2016;63(3):764–775.

94. Qin N, et al. Alterations of the human gut microbiome in liver cirrhosis. *Nature.* 2014;513(7516):59–64.

95. Giannelli V, et al. Microbiota and the gut-liver axis: bacterial translocation, inflammation and infection in cirrhosis. *World J Gastroenterol.* 2014;20(45):16795–16810.

96. Spadoni I, et al. A gut-vascular barrier controls the systemic dissemination of bacteria. *Science.* 2015;350(6262):830–834.

97. Yu LX, et al. Endotoxin accumulation prevents carcinogen-induced apoptosis and promotes liver tumorigenesis in rodents. *Hepatology.* 2010;52(4):1322–1333.

98. Dapito DH, et al. Promotion of hepatocellular carcinoma by the intestinal microbiota and TLR4. *Cancer Cell.* 2012;21(4):504–516.

99. Yoshimoto S, et al. Obesity-induced gut microbial metabolite promotes liver cancer through senescence secretome. *Nature.* 2013;499(7456):97–101.

100. Achiwa K, et al. DSS colitis promotes tumorigenesis and fibrogenesis in a choline-deficient high-fat diet-induced NASH mouse model. *Biochem Biophys Res Commun.* 2016;470(1):15–21.

101. Li H, et al. LPS promotes epithelial-mesenchymal transition and activation of TLR4/JNK signaling. *Tumour Biol.* 2014;35(10):10429–10435.

102. Jing YY, et al. Toll-like receptor 4 signaling promotes epithelial-mesenchymal transition in human hepatocellular carcinoma induced by lipopolysaccharide. *BMC Med.* 2012;10:98.

103. Schnabl B, Brenner DA. Interactions between the intestinal microbiome and liver diseases. *Gastroenterology.* 2014;146(6):1513–1524.

104. Henao-Mejia J, et al. Inflammasome-mediated dysbiosis regulates progression of NAFLD and obesity. *Nature.* 2012;482(7384):179–185.

105. Zhang HL, et al. Profound impact of gut homeostasis on chemically-induced pro-tumorigenic inflammation and hepatocarcinogenesis in rats. *J Hepatol.* 2012;57(4):803–812.

106. Sun B, Karin M. Obesity, inflammation, and liver cancer. *J Hepatol.* 2012;56(3):704–713.

107. Loo TM, et al. Gut microbiota promotes obesity-associated liver cancer through PGE2-mediated suppression of antitumor immunity. *Cancer Discov.* 2017.

108. Roy S, Trinchieri G. Microbiota: a key orchestrator of cancer therapy. *Nat Rev Cancer.* 2017;17(5):271–285.

109. Routy B, et al. Gut microbiome influences efficacy of PD-1-based immunotherapy against epithelial tumors. *Science.* 2017.

110. Wu K, et al. Kupffer cell suppression of CD8+ T cells in human hepatocellular carcinoma is mediated by B7-H1/programmed death-1 interactions. *Cancer Res.* 2009;69(20):8067–8075.

UNCITED REFERENCE

1. Seeger C, Ganem D, Varmus HE. Biochemical and genetic evidence for the hepatitis B virus replication strategy. *Science.* 1986;232(4749):477–484.

CHAPTER 5

Infectious Causes of Acute Pancreatitis

MARYAM NESVADERANI, MBBS, BSC (HONS) • GUY D. ESLICK, DRPH, PHD, FACE, FFPH • MICHAEL R. COX, FRACS, MS, MBBS

INTRODUCTION

Epidemiology

Infection is an uncommon cause of pancreatitis. Gallstones and alcohol are the two most common causes worldwide, responsible for 60%–80% of all cases.[1,2] In 10% of patients, pancreatitis is due to miscellaneous causes including toxins, drugs, malignancy, metabolic abnormalities, trauma, ischemia, autoimmune disease, and infection.[3,4] Idiopathic pancreatitis makes up 15%–25% of cases, and there is evidence that idiopathic pancreatitis may also include pancreatitis of viral cause.[5] The incidence of infectious pancreatitis is unclear for a number of reasons. A criterion for determining whether a particular microorganism causes pancreatitis was suggested by Parenti et al. in 1996, and the determination requires histologic evidence of pancreatitis from autopsy or surgery and/or radiographic evidence of pancreatitis combined with identification of the offending organism in pancreatic tissue by stain or culture.[6] This leads to difficulty in identifying infectious pancreatitis, as the majority of cases of pancreatitis are mild and pancreatic tissue would not be available for analysis.[6] Advancements in molecular methods of microbiology identification, such as polymerase chain reaction (PCR), have made diagnosis of microbial infection easier; however, there are a few studies that have examined the incidence of infection in this way. Infection was found to responsible for 0.09%–2% of cases of acute pancreatitis in a few cohort studies.[7–10] However, only one of these studies adequately described how infection was diagnosed in cases of acute pancreatitis.

Infectious Agents

The most common group of infections associated with pancreatitis are caused by viruses, including mumps virus, coxsackievirus type B (CVB), hepatitis viruses, cytomegalovirus (CMV), varicella-zoster virus (VZV), herpes simplex virus (HSV), and human immunodeficiency virus (HIV). Other microbial agents that have been definitively proven to cause pancreatitis include bacteria such as *Mycoplasma*, *Salmonella*, *Leptospira*, *Legionella*, and *Mycobacterium*. Fungi and parasites, including *Aspergillus*, *Ascaris*, *Clonorchis*, *Echinococcus*, *Toxoplasma*, and *Cryptosporidium*, have also been shown to cause pancreatitis (Table 5.1).[6]

Viruses

Viruses implicated in pancreatitis are thought to cause disease via direct cytopathic effects from infection of pancreatic cells or secondary to edema of the pancreatic duct due to infection of adjacent structures, such as the liver or biliary tree.

Mumps

Mumps virus was the first infectious agent found to cause pancreatitis, based on the studies performed in 1817.[6] Mumps virus is a single-stranded DNA paramyxovirus that causes parotitis, which can be complicated by orchitis, meningoencephalitis, arthritis, and pancreatitis.[3,6] It most commonly occurs among young children and adolescents and typically begins with fever, myalgia, and headache followed by parotitis. The clinical picture in pancreatitis is abdominal pain and diarrhea occurring 4–8 days after onset of mumps illness.[6] Most cases are self-limiting and resolve without complications.[6] Treatment of mumps is supportive, and there is no specific antiviral therapy available.

The diagnosis of mumps pancreatitis relies on laboratory confirmation with antiviral antibodies, reverse transcription polymerase chain reaction (RT-PCR), or oral/buccal culture together with a diagnosis of pancreatitis and exclusion of other causes.[11]

The incidence of pancreatitis secondary to mumps is difficult to determine, as few studies have examined this and the incidence of mumps has sharply fallen after the introduction of the measles, mumps, and rubella (MMR) vaccine. In a series of 1068 adult patients with pancreatitis, one case was caused by mumps virus (0.09%).[7]

Gastrointestinal Diseases and Their Associated Infections. https://doi.org/10.1016/B978-0-323-54843-4.00005-2
Copyright © 2019 Elsevier Inc. All rights reserved.

TABLE 5.1
Infectious Causes of Acute Pancreatitis

	Pathogen	Evidence for Causation[a]	Mechanism of Causation	Diagnosis	Treatment
Viruses	Mumps	1	Direct infection	Serologic testing, RT-PCR, oral/buccal culture	Supportive
	Coxsackievirus type B	1	Direct infection	Serologic testing	Supportive
	Hepatitis B	1	Direct infection, obstruction of pancreatic duct due to edema at ampulla of Vater	Serologic testing	Supportive, lamivudine may improve outcomes[b]
	Hepatitis C, A, and E	2	Direct infection, obstruction of pancreatic duct due to edema at ampulla of Vater	Serologic testing	Supportive
	Cytomegalovirus	1	Direct infection	PCR, cell culture, immunohistochemistry	Supportive, antiviral medication may improve outcomes[b]
	Varicella-zoster virus	1	Direct infection	Clinical	Supportive, antiviral medication may improve outcomes[b]
	Herpes simplex virus	2	Direct infection	Tissue culture, PCR, immunofluorescence staining, serologic testing	Supportive
Bacteria	*Mycoplasma pneumoniae*	2	Systemic immune response/distant cytokines	Cold hemagglutinin test, PCR	Limited evidence
	Salmonella typhimurium	1	Direct infection	Cell culture	IV antibiotics
	Leptospira	2	Local immune response resulting in small vessel vasculitis and ishcemia	Microscopic agglutination test	IV antibiotics
	Legionella pneumophila	2	Direct infection, effects of *Legionella* toxin, local and systemic immune response	Cell culture, urine antigen testing, serologic testing	IV antibiotics
	Mycobacterium tuberculosis	1	Direct infection	Acid-fast bacilli stain from pancreatic tissue, PCR pancreatic tissue	Antituberculosis therapy
	Mycobacterium avium	1	Direct infection	Acid-fast bacilli stain from pancreatic tissue, PCR pancreatic tissue	Antituberculosis therapy

		[a]	Direct infection	Histologic testing or cell culture from pancreatic tissue	
Fungi	*Aspergillus*	1			Antifungal therapy may improve outcomes[b]
Parasites	*Ascaris lumbricoides*	1	Mass effect causing pancreatic duct obstruction, ascending infection	Ultrasonography, duodenoscopy, MRCP, ERCP	Antihelminthic medications +/− ERCP and sphincterotomy
	Clonorchis	1	Mass effect causing pancreatic duct obstruction, ascending infection	Ultrasonography, duodenoscopy, MRCP, ERCP	Antihelminthic medications +/− ERCP and sphincterotomy
	Echinococcus	1	Mass effect causing pancreatic duct obstruction, rupture of cyst into biliary tree, ascending infection	Ultrasonography, MRCP, ERCP	Antihelminthic medications +/− ERCP +/− open surgical treatment
	Toxoplasma gondii	1	Direct infection	Cell culture, serologic testing	Limited evidence
	Cryptosporidium parvum	1	Direct infection, mass effect causing pancreatic duct obstruction	Serologic testing, stool antigen testing	Supportive management

ERCP, endoscopic retrograde cholangiopancreatography; *MRCP*, magnetic resonance cholangiopancreatography; *PCR*, polymerase chain reaction; *RT-PCR*, reverse transcription polymerase chain reaction.

[a]1 = Histologic evidence of pathogen in pancreatic tissue or pathogen has been cultured from pancreatic tissue in patient with confirmed acute pancreatitis, 2 = serologic diagnosis or culture from nonpancreatic tissue in patient with acute pancreatitis.

[b]Limited evidence.

A 1977 study found 3 patients in a series of 116 (3%) patients had rising antibody titers to mumps, consistent with acute infection.[12] A different study found mumps to be a significant cause of pancreatitis in children, responsible for 18/49 cases (37%), but this was not replicated in a different study that only found 1/211 (0.5%) cases of childhood pancreatitis due to mumps.[13,14] Historical studies have shown that 0.3%–5.1% of patients with mumps go on to develop pancreatitis.[6] Most of these studies did not describe how mumps was diagnosed, and the diagnostic criteria for pancreatitis have also changed since the historical studies were performed, making interpretation of this data difficult. Interestingly, there have been six case reports of pancreatitis associated with administration of the MMR vaccine.[15]

Coxsackievirus type B

CVB is an RNA enterovirus with six serotypes.[6] It was first identified in 1958 as a cause for pancreatitis.[16] CVB most commonly manifests as fever or mild upper respiratory tract or gastrointestinal symptoms; however, in rare cases, it can be complicated by aseptic meningitis, pericarditis, and pancreatitis.[5] The majority of cases are self-limited; however, in neonates, there is increased risk of disseminated illness that is severe and often fatal.[6] Diagnosis of CVB requires clinical feature of disease together with positive serologic test results.[17] The treatment of CVB is largely supportive, as in most cases, CVB is self-limited. In cases of pericarditis and meningitis, antiviral medications play a limited role.

Evidence for the role of CVB in pancreatitis mostly comes from case reports and serologic studies, with CVB4 and CVB3 serotypes most commonly implicated.[5,6] Two cases of pancreatitis secondary to CVB have been documented in neonates, where CVB was isolated in pancreatic tissue.[6] A case report described an adult with acute pancreatitis where CVB was isolated in a skin biopsy, and the patient had an elevated antibody titer against CVB.[18] Another case report has documented a case of a patient with pericarditis, hepatitis, and pancreatitis, with antibody titers suggestive of CVB.[17] The majority of studies rely on serologic evidence, and a variety of such studies have shown that the incidence of CVB-associated pancreatitis is 0%–11%.[6] A study of 40 patients with alcoholic pancreatitis used RT-PCR to investigate the presence of enteroviruses; however, no enterovirus RNA was found to indicate acute viremia in this sample of patients.[19] Interestingly, serologic studies have also shown an association between CVB and type 1 diabetes, suggesting CVB affects both the exocrine and endocrine pancreas.[5] Animal models also support the role of CVB in pancreatitis, as mouse models of CVB-induced pancreatitis share many pathologic features with human disease.[5] Different serotypes of CVB have been shown to result in different forms of pancreatitis in animal models; CVB4-P infection in mice was found to cause a transient, acute pancreatitis, whereas CVB4-V induces a severe pancreatitis that progresses to chronic pancreatitis.[5]

Hepatitis viruses

The literature indicates a strong association between hepatitis and pancreatitis. Acute pancreatitis has been most strongly associated with fulminant hepatitis, with a frequency of up to 30% in three different studies.[20] The occurrence of acute pancreatitis in nonfulminant hepatitis is much less common.

There is evidence that acute pancreatitis may be caused by viral hepatitis. There are five hepatitis viruses: A, B, C, D, and E. The best evidence exists for an association between hepatitis B and pancreatitis, and weaker evidence exists for an association among hepatitis A, C, and E viruses. The diagnosis of hepatitis-related pancreatitis is made using serologic tests specific to the different hepatitis antigens and antibodies, together with radiologic and/or biochemical evidence for pancreatitis. There are two main proposed mechanisms for pancreatitis-associated hepatitis; edema at the ampulla of Vater may cause obstruction of pancreatic fluid outflow, resulting in pancreatitis, or there may be a direct cytopathic effect on pancreatic cells by the virus.[21]

Hepatitis B is a single-stranded DNA virus.[6] Early evidence for the role of hepatitis B in pancreatitis came from studies in liver transplant patients; in a series of 27 chronic hepatitis B carriers who underwent liver transplant, 6 developed acute hepatitis and among them 4 developed acute pancreatitis.[6] Hepatitis B antigens have also been found in pancreatic acinar cells and pancreatic juice, demonstrating the ability of hepatitis B virus to infect the pancreas directly.[6] It is difficult to determine the incidence of hepatitis B–related pancreatitis, but most studies find that it is a rare event. A prospective study following 54 patients with acute hepatitis B found that 1 patient developed acute pancreatitis within 4 weeks.[20] Interestingly, one study suggests that lamivudine may play a role in treating hepatitis-related pancreatitis; a patient with chronic hepatitis B had repeated episodes of pancreatitis and it was found that these episodes could be controlled with lamivudine therapy.[22]

There is limited evidence for the role of other hepatitis viruses in causing pancreatitis. A systemic review found an association between hepatitis A and acute pancreatitis in an Asian population, with an estimated frequency of 0%–0.1%.[23] Another systematic review has found 55 cases of acute pancreatitis associated with hepatitis E reported in the literature.[24] There are only two case reports of patients who have been diagnosed with concurrent acute hepatitis C and acute pancreatitis, making it a rare cause.[20]

Cytomegalovirus

CMV is a ubiquitous double-stranded DNA virus in the Herpesviridae family, with a seroprevalence of 60%–100% worldwide.[6,25] In immunocompetent hosts, infection is asymptomatic or results in a self-limiting mononucleosis syndrome.[6] However, in immunocompromised hosts, it can cause hepatitis, meningitis, encephalitis, myelitis, colitis retinitis, and pneumonitis.[6] Reliable methods of diagnosing CMV infection include PCR, cell culture, and immunohistochemistry.[26] The role of serologic assays is limited, as studies have shown poor correlation of results obtained from different kits and IgM can persist for months after a primary infection has resolved.[26]

Definitive evidence of CMV causing pancreatitis comes from studies that have shown intracytoplasmic or intranuclear inclusions of CMV in pancreatic tissue, together with a diagnosis of pancreatitis. There are 10 case reports that have demonstrated this, and the majority of patients had necrotizing pancreatitis.[6,27–29] Seven of these patients were immunocompromised, and two had HIV/AIDS infection. Owing to the ubiquitous nature of CMV infection, CMV inclusions have also been found in the pancreatic tissue of individuals at autopsy who did not have pancreatitis. CMV was noted in 4 of 4000 autopsied acinar pancreatic cells.[6] However, the data suggests that CMV does play a role in the development of pancreatitis, particularly in immunocompromised hosts. There are a few case reports of patients with hyperimmunoglobulin E syndrome,[30] systemic lupus erythematosus, and AIDS with CMV pancreatitis.[28,29]

There are a few case reports of CMV causing pancreatitis in immunocompetent hosts. One study, using DNA PCR to diagnose acute CMV, found a case of hepatitis and pancreatitis due to CMV in an immunocompetent 29-year-old male.[25] Interestingly, this patient was treated with ganciclovir that resulted in clinical improvement, suggesting a role for antiviral drugs in CMV pancreatitis. There are two other case reports of CMV pancreatitis in immunocompetent hosts.[27,31] The majority of studies however implicate a role for CMV in patients with immunocompromised states.

Varicella-zoster virus

VZV is a DNA virus and member of the Herpesviridae family. It causes two different forms of disease: varicella (chicken pox) and herpes zoster (shingles). Chicken pox in children is usually benign and self-limiting, starting with a prodromal phase of fever, malaise, or pharyngitis followed by the appearance of characteristic skin lesions.[32] Varicella infection can cause severe disease in adults or immunocompromised individuals, resulting in disseminated infection and encephalitis, pneumonia, or rarely pancreatitis.[32] Diagnosis is usually clinical, based on the presence of characteristic vesicular lesions that are present in a widespread distribution in chicken pox or in a dermatomal distribution in shingles. The mechanism of VZV pancreatitis is thought to be direct injury to pancreatic acinar cells as a result of viral inclusions in cells.[33]

Evidence for VZV causing pancreatitis comes from three case reports of VZV in children, who had an acute varicella infection and pancreatitis. Histopathologic examination demonstrated viral inclusions in the pancreas.[6] VZV associated with pancreatitis occurs most commonly in children and immunocompromised individuals. There have been case reports of VZV pancreatitis in patients admitted to intensive care unit (ICU), with AIDS, receiving long-term immunosuppression, and who underwent organ transplant.[34] A case has been described of a 50-year-old male who underwent renal transplant 3 years ago. He was diagnosed with pancreatitis, hepatitis, and disseminated VZV infection concurrently. This patient was treated with acyclovir, which led to resolution of his condition.[35] VZV is less likely to cause pancreatitis in immunocompetent hosts, yet several cases have been described in the literature. There have been four case reports of VZV pancreatitis in immunocompetent children.[33] One child died of respiratory failure,[36] two recovered after receiving supportive treatment, and one recovered after receiving a course of acyclovir.[33,37,38] There are fewer case reports of VZV pancreatitis in immunocompetent adults.[34]

The treatment of VZV pancreatitis is largely supportive. The use of acyclovir has been shown to improve resolution of symptoms in a few case reports; however, no studies have not yet been performed to evaluate this.[33]

Herpes simplex virus (HSV)

HSV is a double-stranded DNA virus that causes infection of mucosal surfaces and can lead to disseminated infection in immunocompromised states. Both HSV-1 and HSV-2 have been associated with pancreatitis.[6] The evidence for HSV causing pancreatitis is relatively weak compared with other viruses. The strongest evidence for this association comes from a case report of disseminated HSV-2 infection resulting in an HIV-infected patient; this patient had HSV DNA in the pancreas

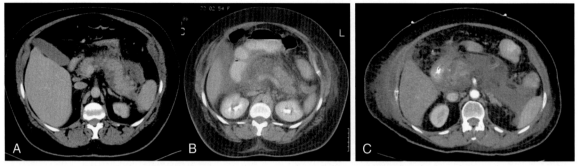

FIG. 5.1 The progression of pancreatic necrosis on (**A**) day 7, (**B**) day 8, and (**C**) day 9.

demonstrated by in situ hybridization, but the patient did not have clinical features of pancreatitis.[6] The diagnosis of HSV is largely based on tissue culture, PCR, immunofluorescence staining, or serologic testing. The role of serologic tests is limited, as the presence of IgM antibodies does not correlate well with acute infection. There are five case reports to date in the literature; however, only two of these use reliable methods to diagnose acute HSV infection. Two of these reports are from immunocompromised patients with allergic granulomatous angiitis and invasive pulmonary aspergillosis with disseminated HSV-1; in both cases the pancreas showed inclusions of virus.[39] In the other three reports, one is from a child with pancreatitis who tested positive for anti-HSV IgM,[40] another describes an immunocompetent 22-year-old man with pancreatitis and IgM-positive serologic test result, and the final report found HSV-1 isolated from gastric contents of a man with idiopathic pancreatitis. [41,42]

HIV
The annual incidence of pancreatitis in the general population is relatively low, at 17–30 cases per 100,000, compared with the incidence of HIV/AIDS.[43] Different studies have estimated the annual incidence of AIDS/HIV to be 6–140 per 1000 person years.[43] The reasons for an increased incidence of pancreatitis in HIV/AIDS are multifactorial. The most common cause is the use of nucleoside reverse transcriptase inhibitors, as well as some medications used to treat opportunistic infections.[6,43] Other reasons include comorbidities that are more commonly found in patients with HIV/AIDS, such as hyperlipidemia, gallstones, and alcohol use.[6] Lastly, certain opportunistic infections have been directly shown to cause acute pancreatitis, such as CMV, HSV, *Cryptococcus*, and *Mycoplasma* infections.[6] To date, there has been no evidence linking HIV directly to pancreatitis, with no studies demonstrating HIV in the

pancreas by using PCR or in situ hybridization.[3] Interestingly, the risk of pancreatitis is increased in patients with lower CD4 cell counts and higher viral loads.[43] A likely reason for this is that these patients are more prone to opportunistic infections that are associated with pancreatitis and are more likely to use medications such as pentamidine or trimethoprim/sulfamethoxane, which have been shown to result in pancreatitis.[43] CD4 lymphocytes have also been shown to play an important role in preventing acinar cell necrosis, which leads to acute pancreatitis (Fig. 5.1).[43]

Other viruses
There have been fewer case reports of pancreatitis associated with Epstein-Barr, vaccinia, and rubella viruses, and the evidence for these associations are weaker than those for the viruses described earlier.[6]

Bacteria
The mechanism of bacterial infection resulting in pancreatitis is an ascending infection from the small bowel or biliary tree to the pancreatic duct, effects of the immune response to infection at a distant organ, or seeding from hematogenous or lymphatic sources.[6]

Mycoplasma
Mycoplasma pneumoniae is the cause of up to 30% cases of community-acquired pneumonia and can result in extrapulmonary complications in up to 25% of cases.[44,45] The proposed mechanism of extrapulmonary disease, including pancreatitis, is the production of cytokines in distant organs due to bacterial lipoproteins or altered immune modulation due to infection, causing an inflammatory response in distant organs.[44]

 M. pneumoniae was first associated with pancreatitis based on case reports and case series of patients from historical studies performed in the 1970s–1980s, which demonstrated that 32%–33% of patients with pancreatitis had increased antibody titers to *M. pneumoniae*.[6] However, in many cases, these patients did not have respiratory disease and no temporal relationship could be established between the timing of infection with *M. pneumoniae* and pancreatitis. There have been no studies to date to show the evidence of *Mycoplasma* infection within pancreatic specimens; therefore, the evidence for *M. pneumonia* causing pancreatitis is not definitive.[6] A 2017 study reviewed the literature and found 15 cases of patients with serologic evidence of *M. pneumoniae* infection during an admission with acute pancreatitis, but in 3 of the patients, there were no signs of respiratory infection or the diagnostic criteria for pancreatitis were not met.[44] Two of these case reports were in patients with acute necrotizing pancreatitis.[44]

Salmonella

Typhoid fever is an infection primarily caused by *Salmonella typhi* that results in fever, abdominal pain, and constipation. Typhoid fever can result in a severe multisystemic illness and in rare cases can cause pancreatitis.[46] The evidence for the role of *Salmonella* in pancreatitis comes from studies that demonstrate *S. typhi* in pancreatic tissue of patients with concurrent acute pancreatitis and *Salmonella* infection.[6] Salmonellosis has also been shown to cause elevated lipase levels in 16%–23% of patients without evidence of clinical pancreatitis.[47,48] The majority of case reports involving *Salmonella* pancreatitis are mild; however, in cases in which *Salmonella* causes severe pancreatitis or local complications, the microorganism responsible is usually *S. typhi*, rather than *Salmonella enterica*.[48] The mechanism of pancreatitis is direct infection of the pancreas by bacteria travelling from the blood or lymphatic tissue or by an ascending infection from the small bowel.[46] There have been two case reports of *S. typhi* resulting in rhabdomyolysis, renal failure, and pancreatitis.[46,49] *S. typhi* has also been shown to cause acute pancreatitis in children.[50] In one report a 64-year-old woman had necrotizing pancreatitis with pancreatic tissue growing *S. typhi* and was successfully treated with intravenous (IV) ciprofloxacin.[48]

Leptospirosis

Leptospirosis is a zoonotic tropical disease caused by the spirochete bacteria *Leptospira*.[51] It is most commonly found in India, Sri Lanka, Thailand, and Malaysia.[52] In symptomatic infection, patients will develop fever, arthralgia, pharyngitis, cough, and rash, which usually resolves after 3–7 days in 90% of cases.[51] A minority of patients will develop a severe form of infection, also known as Weil disease, which can result in

hepatitis, myocarditis, and rarely pancreatitis.[51] The exact incidence of leptospirosis causing pancreatitis is unknown, but a case series showed that 3 of 88 patients with leptospirosis had concurrent acute pancreatitis.[3] The mechanism for leptospirosis pancreatitis is likely to be small vessel vasculitis and ischemic injury leading to autodigestion of the organ as a result of the immunologic response to infection.[51]

Leptospirosis is diagnosed by microscopic agglutination test (MAT), which is the gold standard, or serologic enzyme-linked immunosorbent assay (ELISA). To diagnose leptospirosis pancreatitis a diagnosis of acute pancreatitis is required together with a positive MAT or ELISA result. To date, leptospires have not been isolated from pancreatic tissue, but in blood, intra-abdominal fluid, and bile on microscopic examination from patients with acute pancreatitis and concurrent leptospirosis.[6,53] There have been numerous case reports and case series describing the cases of leptospirosis pancreatitis. A case series of six patients with severe leptospirosis admitted to an ICU in a Sri Lankan hospital showed that four patients also suffered concurrent pancreatitis, and two further case reports of leptospirosis pancreatitis have been described in this region.[51] There are also several case reports of leptospirosis pancreatitis from other countries.[53–58] *Leptospira* has been associated with necrotizing pancreatitis in a few reports.[6,52,59]

The treatment of leptospirosis pancreatitis includes IV antibiotic therapy, usually with penicillin G or ceftriaxone in severe cases, together with supportive management for pancreatitis.[53]

Legionellosis

Legionella pneumophila is a common cause of community-acquired pneumonia, also known as legionnaires' disease, that is more likely to result in severe pneumonia requiring ICU admission compared with other bacterial pathogens.[60] *L. pneumophila* can also cause extrapulmonary complications such as rhabdomyolysis, acute renal failure, hepatitis, and rarely pancreatitis.[61] Legionnaires' disease is diagnosed by sputum culture, urine antigen testing, or serologic assays.[61] This diagnosis of pancreatitis secondary to legionnaires' disease is usually made when a test for *Legionella* is positive together with a diagnosis of pancreatitis. To date, there have been no reports of *L. pneumophila* being isolated or detected in pancreatic tissue; however, autopsy reports have found the pathogen in the spleen, liver, kidney, myocardium, and bones of patients with legionnaires' disease.[60] It is likely that pancreatitis is caused by hematologic spread to the organ, *Legionella* toxin release affecting the organ, or cell-mediated inflammation as a response to infection.[61,62] To date, there have been 15 case reports of legionella pancreatitis.[6,60-62] The incidence of pancreatitis in legionnaires' disease is unknown, but a small case series found that 3 out of 14 patients hospitalized in ICU for severe legionnaires' disease developed pancreatitis.[61] The treatment for legionella pancreatitis is with IV macrolides, quinolones, or a combination of one of these two antibiotics together with rifampicin, and this has been shown to lead to resolution of the condition in several studies.[60-62]

Mycobacteria

There is evidence that both *Mycobacterium tuberculosis* and *Mycobacterium avium* can cause acute pancreatitis.

M. tuberculosis

The incidence of abdominal tuberculosis is 11%–16% and most commonly involves the ileocecal region.[62] About 29% of these patients will have concurrent active pulmonary disease, however isolated tuberculosis of the pancreas is rare.[63] Tuberculosis of the pancreas can occur in the context of military tuberculosis or as an isolated tubercular abscess of the pancreas.[6] The incidence of pancreatic tuberculosis has been found to be 2.1%–4.7% in autopsies of patients with military tuberculosis and is more common in immunocompromised patients such as those with HIV.[64] It has been shown that pancreatic enzymes confer resistance to invasion by *M. tuberculosis*; therefore, the pancreas is not commonly affected as other intra-abdominal organs.[63] The mechanism of pancreas involvement is thought to be by hematogenous spread, the ingestion of microbes from sputum, or direct spread from adjacent organs.[63]

Tuberculosis of the pancreas is difficult to diagnose and most commonly presents with abdominal pain, weight loss, and/or fever.[65] Patients will usually have a reactive Mantoux test. Computed tomographic (CT) findings will show a mass in the head of the pancreas, and the diagnosis is often confused with pancreatic cancer.[6] Laboratory markers are usually not indicative of pancreatitis and amylase level is frequently normal.[6,65] The diagnosis cannot usually be confirmed without resection or biopsy of the pancreatic lesion for histologic assessment, which should demonstrate granuloma formation and a positive acid-fast bacilli stain.[64] PCR is superior to smear and culture in detecting *M. tuberculosis* and provides faster results.[63] Tuberculosis of the pancreas can result in obstructive jaundice, gastrointestinal bleeding, acute or chronic pancreatitis, portal hypertension, or pancreatobiliary fistula.[63] Treatment is usually 6–9 months of antituberculosis therapy in drug-susceptible cases and 12 months in drug-resistant cases.[64,65] The mortality is 7% in immunocompetent individuals.[64,65] There have been approximately 116 cases of pancreatic tuberculosis identified in the literature from 1966 to 2004.[63] A case report described a man with tuberculosis of the pancreas who developed pancreatitis. He had a history of recurrent pancreatitis and was diagnosed with tuberculosis after a positive Mantoux test. Imaging revealed a mass in the head of the pancreas, and biopsy result was consistent with pancreatic tuberculosis. The pancreatic mass regressed in size after treatment with isoniazid, pyrazinamide, and pyridoxine and the patient recovered from pancreatitis.[65] In another case report, a 28-year-old male presented with abdominal pain, nausea, and vomiting, but amylase and lipase levels were not elevated. CT demonstrated edema of the pancreas, consistent with pancreatitis, and a midabdominal mass composed of lymph nodes. *M. tuberculosis* was grown from an endoscopic ultrasound–fine-needle aspiration sample taken from the intra-abdominal nodes. The patient was treated for tuberculosis and recovered.[66]

M. avium

M. avium is the most common cause of nontuberculous mycobacterial infection.[67] *M. avium* has been isolated in the pancreas in disseminated *M. avium* infection in both nonimmunocompromised and immunocompromised hosts; however, it usually occurs in patients with HIV infection.[6] There are usually no typical signs of acute pancreatitis and on histologic examination, granulomatous inflammation of the pancreas is seen. *M. avium* has been cultured from the pancreatic tissue in affected patients.[6] The likely mechanism of infection is hematogenous spread from disseminated infection.[6] Interestingly, it has been shown that patients can be infected with both *M. tuberculosis* and *M. avium*. A case describes a 40–year-old HIV-infected man presenting with epigastric pain. CT revealed a mass in the pancreatic head, and cultures from the mass grew *M. tuberculosis* and *M. avium*. He was treated with antituberculosis antibiotics and his condition resolved.[67]

Other bacteria

There are case reports of pancreatitis being caused by *Campylobacter jejuni*, *Yersinia enterocolitica*, *Yersinia pseudotuberculosis*, *Brucella*, *Nocardia*, and *Actinomyces*.[3,6]

Fungi

There is limited evidence for fungi causing acute pancreatitis. *Aspergillus* has been shown to cause pancreatitis in one case report, where a 62-year-old man with lymphoma developed pancreatitis, and autopsy findings revealed *Aspergillus* invading the pancreas causing necrosis.[6] *Cryptococcus neoformans, Candida, Coccidiiodes immitis, Paracoccidioides brasiliensis, Histoplasma capsulatum*, and *Pneumocystis carinii* are yeasts that have been noted to cause abscesses in the pancreas but there is no direct evidence that they cause pancreatitis.[6]

Parasites

Ascaris

The parasite that most frequently causes pancreatitis is *Ascaris lumbricoides*, a soil-transmitted intestinal roundworm.[6] It is most commonly found in tropical and subtropical regions and infection is associated with poor sanitary conditions.[68] In India, 70% of children are infected with *A. lumbricoides* and it is the second most common cause of pancreatitis in this region, responsible for 23% of cases.[6,69] Hepatobiliary and pancreatic ascariasis can result in biliary colic or acute cholangitis, which are the most common presentations,[70] but can also cause acute pancreatitis.[69] The mechanism of acute pancreatitis is by obstruction of the common bile duct (CBD) or pancreatic duct, and infection may also cause abscess formation by migration into the distal pancreas.[6] About 90% of patients with pancreatitis caused by ascariasis will have mild disease, and 10% will develop necrotizing pancreatitis.[69]

Patients typically present with abdominal pain, vomiting, and raised levels of pancreatic enzymes.[6] Diagnosis of ascariasis pancreatitis can be made by ultrasonography, duodenoscopy, endoscopic retrograde cholangiopancreatography (ERCP), or magnetic resonance cholangiopancreatography.[69] Ultrasonography is the last invasive diagnostic test but cannot detect small worm loads, whereas ERCP cannot detect worms in the gallbladder.[69] The treatment of choice is antihelminthic medications such as albendazole, mebendazole, pyrantel pamoate, or levamisole.[69,70] ERCP and sphincterotomy should be performed if symptoms do not resolve with medical management.[69]

Clonorchis

Clonorchis sinensis, also known as the Chinese liver fluke, has also been thought to cause pancreatitis by obstructing the CBD or pancreatic duct. It is a less common cause of pancreatitis compared with ascariasis infection.[6] Treatment is also with antihelminthic medications. There is limited evidence for other trematodes causing pancreatitis, namely, *Fasciola hepatica, Opisthorchis* species, and *Dicrocoelium dendriticum*.[6]

Echinococcus

Echinococcosis is an infection caused by the tapeworm *Echinococcus granulosus*, which forms hydatid cysts, most commonly in the liver.[71] It is a rare cause of pancreatitis, with 17 cases described in the literature.[71-82] The hydatid cysts that are formed cause pancreatitis by compression on the biliary tree or pancreatic duct, or cysts may directly rupture into the biliary tree.[6] Intrabiliary rupture of a cyst occurs in 1%–25% of cases of infection and can also result in hydatid abscess or cholangitis.[71]

One case report describes a patient with a hydatid cyst in the liver, which ruptured in the biliary tree causing necrotizing pancreatitis.[71] The patient had open surgery for drainage of cyst and removal of hydatid debris from the CBD, following a failed ERCP.[71] Another case report describes a man with recurrent episodes of acute pancreatitis due to a large hydatid hepatic cyst.[72] The patient was treated with albendazole for 2 weeks prior to open surgery for removal of the cyst.[72] The treatment of choice for cystobiliary communication causing pancreatitis is ERCP, although in most published cases, patients will require open surgical treatment with drainage of cyst and T-tube drainage of the CBD to adequately manage infection.[71,72]

Protozoa

Toxoplasma

Toxoplasma gondii is a protozoan parasite that most commonly causes asymptomatic infection in humans with a life cycle that requires development in cat intestinal epithelia.[6] Humans become infected through contact with cysts shed in cat feces, which may be ingested via contact with contaminated soil, water, or food.[83] Severe toxoplasmosis occurs most commonly in immunocompromised individuals or organ transplant recipients.[83] Toxoplasmosis has been associated with pancreatitis in a few case reports, and this usually occurs in the setting of disseminated infection in patients with HIV infection.[6] There is one case report of toxoplasmosis causing severe necrotizing pancreatitis, where toxoplasmal cysts were found in the pancreas associated with necrosis on autopsy.[84] Pancreas transplant recipients are also at increased risk of toxoplasmosis due to immunosuppressive medications.[83]

Cryptosporidium

Cryptosporidium parvum is a protozoan pathogen that mostly infects the small intestine. In immunocompetent hosts, it causes a self-limited diarrheal illness, whereas in immunocompromised hosts, it can result in severe disseminated infection.[85] *C. parvum* can also infect the biliary tract and this has been well described in patients with HIV infection, resulting in cholecystitis, sclerosing cholangitis, and rarely pancreatitis.[6] *C. parvum* has also been incidentally found in the pancreas on autopsy of HIV-infected patients; however, there is usually minimally inflammatory change of the parenchyma. There have been limited case reports of *C. parvum* causing acute pancreatitis; there are two reports of patients presenting with pancreatitis who were also found to have active *C. parvum* infection based on serologic results and stool antigen testing.[85] These cases resolved with supportive management.[85]

CONCLUSION

Viruses are the most common agent shown to cause pancreatitis; however, numerous bacteria, fungi, and parasites have also been definitely shown to cause this disease. The mechanism of disease varies in each case but usually results from direct infection of the pancreas from hematologic, lymphatic, or direct spread from adjacent organs; an immune-based reaction as a result of the host's response to the initial infection; or the compression or mass effect from infected structures adjacent to the pancreas. The treatment of infectious pancreatitis also varies in each case depending on the pathogen, with antimicrobial, antiviral, or anthelminthic medications shown to improve patient outcomes in case reports. In certain cases, such as infection with parasites, endoscopic or open surgery is indicated to maintain control of the infectious agent.

As idiopathic pancreatitis makes up 15%–25% of all causes, it is highly likely that a portion of idiopathic pancreatitis is actually due to infectious agents. Future directions for research should focus on testing of idiopathic cases with PCR or newer sequencing technology such as RNA/DNA sequencing to identify transcripts from infectious agents. Specific treatments for microbes identified may improve the morbidity and mortality in idiopathic pancreatitis, which some studies find to have higher mortality than with other causes.[1,86]

REFERENCES

1. Nesvaderani M, Eslick GD, Vagg D, Faraj S, Cox MR. Epidemiology, aetiology and outcomes of acute pancreatitis: a retrospective cohort study. *Int J Surg.* 2015;23:68–74.
2. Roberts SE, Morrison-Rees S, John A, Williams JG, Brown TH, Samuel DG. The incidence and aetiology of acute pancreatitis across Europe. *Pancreatology.* 2017;17(2):155–165.
3. Economou M, Zissis M. Infectious cases of acute pancreatitis. *Ann Gastroenterol.* 2000;13(2):98–101.
4. Sakorafas GH, Tsiotou AG. Aetiology and pathogenesis of acute pancreatitis: current concepts. *J Clin Gastroenterol.* 2000;30(4):343–356.
5. Huber S, Ramsingh AI. Coxsackievirus-induced pancreatitis. *Viral Immunol.* 2004;17:358–369.
6. Parenti DM, Steinberg W, Kang P. Infectious causes of acute pancreatitis. *Pancreas.* 1996;13(4):356–371.
7. Gullo M, Migliori M, Olah A, et al. Acute pancreatitis in five European countries: aetiology and mortality. *Pancreas.* 2002;24(3):223–227.
8. Thomson SR, Hendry WS, McFarlane GA, Davidson AI. Epidemiology and outcome of acute pancreatitis. *Br J Surg.* 1987;74(5):398–401.
9. Jarnagin WR. *Blumgart's Surgery of the Liver, Pancreas and Biliary Tract.* 5th ed. Philadelphia, PA: Elsevier Inc.; 2012.
10. Birgisson H, Moller PH, Birgisson S, et al. Acute pancreatitis: a prospective study of its incidence, aetiology, severity and mortality in Iceland. *Eur J Surg.* 2002;168(5):278–282.
11. Centers for Disease Control and Prevention. Mumps: Questions and Answers about Lab Testing. http://www.cdc.gov/mumps/lab/qa-lab-test-infect.html.
12. Imrie CW, Ferguson JC, Sommerville RG. Coxsackie and mumps virus infection in a prospective study of acute pancreatitis. *Gut.* 1977;18(1):53–56.
13. Haddock G, Coupar G, Youngson GG, MacKinlay GA, Raine PA. Acute pancreatitis in children: a 15 year review. *J Pediatr Surg.* 1994;29(6):719–722.
14. Lautz TB, Chin AC, Radhakrishnan J. Acute pancreatitis in children: spectrum of disease and predictors of severity. *J Pediatr Surg.* 2011;46(6):1144–1149.
15. Toovey S, Jamieson A. Pancreatitis complicating adult immunization with a combined mumps measles rubella vaccine. A case report and literature review. *Travel Med Infect Dis.* 2003;1(30):189–192.
16. Kibrick S, Benirschke K. Severe generalized disease occurring in the newborn period and due to infection with Coxsackie virus, group B; evidence of intrauterine infection with this agent. *Pediatrics.* 1958;22(5):857–875.
17. Persichino J, Garrison R, Krishnan R, Sutjita M. Effusive-constrictive pericarditis, hepatitis and pancreatitis in a patient with possible coxsackievirus B infection: a case report. *BMC Infect Dis.* 2016;16:375.
18. Chrysos G, Kokkoris S, Protopsaltis J, Korantzopoulos P, Giannoulis G. Coxsackievirus infection associated with acute pancreatitis. *JOP.* 2004;5(5):384–387.
19. Khan J, Nordback I, Seppanen H, et al. Is alcoholic pancreatitis associated with enteroviral infection? *World J Gastroenterol.* 2013;19(24):3819–3823.
20. Khedmat H, Ghamar-Chehreh ME, Agah S, Aghaei A. Pancreatitis developing in the context of acute hepatitis: a literature review. *JOP.* 2015;16(2):104–109.
21. Mishra A, Saigal S, Gupta R, Sarin SK. Acute pancreatitis associated with viral hepatitis: a report of six cases with review of literature. *Am J Gastroenterol.* 1999;94(8):2292–2295.

22. Chen CH, Changchien CS, Lu SN, Wang JH, Hung CH, Lee CM. Lamivudine treatment for recurrent pancreatitis associated with reactivation of chronic B hepatitis. *Dig Dis Sci*. 2002;47(3):564–567.

23. Haffar S, Bazerbachi F, Prokop L, Watt KD, Murad MH, Chari ST. Frequency and prognosis of acute pancreatitis associated with fulminant or non-fulminant acute hepatitis A: a systematic review. *Pancreatology*. 2017;17(2):166–175.

24. Haffar S, Bazerbachi F, Garg S, Lake JR, Freeman ML. Frequency and prognosis of acute pancreatitis associated with acute hepatitis E: a systematic review. *Pancreatology*. 2015;15(4):321–326.

25. Chan A, Bazerbachi F, Hanson B, Alraies MC, Duran-Nelson A. Cytomegalovirus hepatitis and pancreatitis in the immunocompetent. *Ochsner J*. 2014;14(2):295–299.

26. Ross SA, Novak Z, Pati S, Boppana SB. Diagnosis of cytomegalovirus infections. *Infect Disord - Drug Targets*. 2013;11(5):466–473.

27. Terada T. Cytomegalovirus-associated severe fatal necrotizing pancreatitis in a patient with interstitial pneumonitis treated with steroids. An autopsy case. *JOP*. 2011;12(2):158–161.

28. Ikura Y, Matsuo T, Ogami M, et al. Cytomegalovirus-associated pancreatitis in a patient with systemic lupus erythematosis. *J Rheumatol*. 2000;27(11):2715–2717.

29. Gonzalez-Reimers E, Santolaria-Fernadez F, Gomez-Sirvent JL, Mendez-Medina R, Martinez-Riera A. Cytomegalovirus-associated pancreatitis in acquired immunodeficiency syndrome. *HPB Surg*. 1992;5(3):181–184.

30. Watanabe T, Joko K, Yokota T, et al. Pancreatitis and cholangitis due to cytomegalovirus in a patient with hyperimmunoglobulin E syndrome. *Pancreas*. 2010;39(6):940–942.

31. Oku T, Maeda M, Waga E, et al. Cytomegalovirus cholangitis and pancreatitis in an immunocompetent patient. *J Gastroenterol*. 2005;40(10):987–992.

32. Arvin AM. Varicella-zoster virus. *Clin Microbiol Rev*. 1996;9(3):361–381.

33. Kulasegaran S, Wilson EJ, Vasquez L, Hulme-Moir M. Varicella zoster virus: a rare cause of acute pancreatitis in an immunocompetent child. *BMJ Case Rep*. 2016. https://doi.org/10.1136/bcr-2015-213581. Published online 2016 Jan 13.

34. Wang Z, Ye J, H Y. Acute pancreatitis associated with herpes zoster: case report and literature review. *World J Gastroenterol*. 2014;20(47):18053–18056.

35. Chhabra P. Simultaneous occurrence of varicella zoster virus-induced pancreatitis and hepatitis in a renal transplant recipient: a case report and review of literature. *Perm J*. 2017;21:16–083.

36. Kumar S, Jain AP, Pandit AK. Acute pancreatitis: rare complication of chicken pox in an immunocompetent host. *Saudi J Gastroenterol*. 2007;13(3):138–140.

37. Torre J, Martin JJ, Garcia CB, Polo ER. Varicella infection as a cause of acute pancreatitis in an immunocompetent child. *Pediatr Infect Dis J*. 2000;19(12):1218–1219.

38. Franco J, Fernandes R, Oliveira M, Alves AD, Braga M, Soares I. Acute pancreatitis associated with varicella infection in an immunocompetent child. *J Paediatr Child Health*. 2009;45(9):547–548.

39. Shintaku M, Umehara Y, Iwaisako K, Tahara M, Adachi Y. Herpes simplex pancreatitis. *Arch Pathol Lab Med*. 2003;127(2):231–234.

40. Olivieri C, Nanni L, Taddei A, Manzoni C, Pintus C. Acute pancreatitis associated with herpes simplex virus infection in a child. *Pancreas*. 2012;41(2):330–331.

41. Konstantinou G, Liatsos C, Patelaros E, Karangiannis S, Karnesis L, Mavrogiannis C. Acute pancreatitis associated with herpes simplex virus infection: report of a case and review of the literature. *Eur J Gastroenterol Hepatol*. 2009;21(1):114–116.

42. Rand KH. Isolation of herpes simplex virus type 1 from gastric contents of a patient with acute pancreatitis. *South Med J*. 1981;74(4):489–491.

43. Dragovic G. Acute pancreatitis in HIV/AIDS patients: an issue of concern. *Asian Pac J Trop Biomed*. 2013;3(6):422–425.

44. Valdes Lacasa T, Duarte Borges MA, Garcia Marin A, Gomez Cuervo C. Acute pancreatitis caused by Mycoplasma pneumonia: an unusual etiology. *Clin J Gastroenterol*. 2017;10(3):279–282.

45. Waites KB, Talkington DF. Mycoplasma pneumonia and its role as a human pathogen. *Clin Microbiol Rev*. 2004;17(4):697–728.

46. Khan FY, Al-ani A, Ali HA. Typhoid rhabdomyolysis with acute renal failure and acute pancreatitis: a case report and review of the literature. *Int J Infect Dis*. 2009;13(5):282–285.

47. Dean R, Gill D, Buchan D. Salmonella colitis as an unusual cause of elevated serum lipase. *Am J Emerg Med*. 2017;35(5):800.

48. Blank A, Maybody M, Isom-Batz G, Roslin M, Dillon EH. Necrotizing acute pancreatitis induced by *Salmonella typhimurium*. *Dig Dis Sci*. 2003;48(8):1472–1474.

49. Ali M, Abdalla H. *Salmonella typhi* infection complicated by rhabdomyolysis, pancreatitis and polyneuropathy. *Arab J Nephrol Transplant*. 2011;4(2):91–93.

50. Asano T, Kuwabara K, Takagi A, et al. Acute pancreatitis complicating typhoid fever in a 4-year old girl. *Pediatr Int*. 2007;49(6):1004–1006.

51. Herath NJ, Kamburapola CJ, Agampodi SB. Severe leptospirosis and pancreatitis; A case series from a leptospirosis outbreak in Anuradhapura district, Sri Lanka. *BMC Infect Dis*. 2016;16(1):644.

52. Lim SM, Hoo F, Sulaiman WA, Ramachandran V, Siew-Mooi C. Acute necrotising pancreatitis and acalculous cholecystitis: a rare presentation of leptospirosis. *J Pak Med Assoc*. 2014;64(8):958–959.

53. Kaya E, Dervisoglu A, Eroglu C, Polat C, Sunbul M, Ozkan K. Acute pancreatitis caused by leptospirosis: report of two cases. *World J Gastroenterol*. 2005;11(28):4447–4449.

54. Yew KL, San Go C, Razali F. Pancreatitis and myopericarditis complication in leptospirosis infection. *J Formos Med Assoc*. 2015;114(8):785–786.

55. Panagopoulos P, Terzi I, Karanikas M, Galanpoulos N, Maltezos E. Myocarditis, pancreatitis, polyarthritis, mononeuritis multiplex and vasculitis with symmetrical peripheral gangrene of the lower extremities as a rare presentation of leptospirosis: a case report and review of the literature. *J Med Case Rep*. 2014;8:150.

56. Ranawaka N, Jeevagan V, Karunanavake P, Javasinghe S. Pancreatitis and myocarditis followed by pulmonary haemorrhage, a rare presentation of leptospirosis – a case report and literature survey. *BMC Infect Dis.* 2013;13:38.

57. Silva AP, Burg LB, Locatelli JF, Manes J, Crispim M. Leptospirosis presenting as ascending progressive leg weakness and complicating with acute pancreatitis. *Braz J Infect Dis.* 2011;15(5):493–497.

58. Baburai P, Antony T, Louis F, Harikrishnan BL. Acute abdomen due to acute pancreatitis; a rare presentation of leptospirosis. *J Assoc Phys India.* 2008;56:911–912.

59. Jain AK, Mohan LN. Acute necrotising pancreatitis associated with leptospirosis- a case report. *Indian J Surg.* 2013;75(3):245–246.

60. Franchini S, Marinosci A, Ferrante L, Sabbadini MG, Tresoldi M, Dagna L. Pancreatic involvement in Legionella pneumonia. *Infection.* 2015;43(4):367–370.

61. Mégarbane B1, Montambault S, Chary I, Guibert M, Axler O, Brivet FG. Acute pancreatitis caused by severe *Legionella pneumophila* infection. *Infection.* 2000;28(5):329–331.

62. Hadef H1, Bilbault P, Arzouq H, Berna C, Phelipot JY, Jaeger A. Violent abdominal pain: severe *Legionella pneumophila* lung infection with acute pancreatitis. *Am J Emerg Med.* 2006;24(3):371–372.

63. Salahuddin A, Saif MW. Pancreatic tuberculosis or autoimmune pancreatitis. *Case Rep Med.* 2014. https://doi.org/10.1155/2014/410142. Published online 2014 Apr 15.

64. Chen CH, Yang CC, Yeh YH, Yang JC, Chon DA. Pancreatic tuberculosis with obstructive jaundice- a case report. *Am J Gastroenterol.* 1999;94(9):2534–2536.

65. Redha S, Suresh RL, Subramaniam J, Merican I. Pancreatic tuberculosis presenting with recurrent acute pancreatitis. *Med J Malaysia.* 2001;56(1):95–97.

66. Netherland NA1, Chen VK, Eloubeidi MA. Intra-abdominal tuberculosis presenting with acute pancreatitis: diagnosis by endoscopic ultrasound-guided fine-needle aspiration. *Dig Dis Sci.* 2006;51(2):247–251.

67. Albu E, Yousuf AM, Swaminathan K, Parikh V, Gerst PH. Tuberculous and nontuberculous mycobacterial infection of the pancreas in a patient with AIDS. *Pancreas.* 1996;12(4):412–413.

68. Guzman GE, Teves PM, Monge E. Ascariasis as a cause of recurrent abdominal pain. *Dig Endosc.* 2010;22(2):156–157.

69. Khuroo MS, Rather AA, Khuroo NS, Khuroo MS. Hepatobiliary and pancreatic ascariasis. *World J Gastroenterol.* 2016;22(33):7507–7517.

70. Tortajada-Laureiro L, Olveira-Martín A, Marín-Serrano E, Ruiz-Fernández G, Eun JH, Segura-Cabral JM. Biliary parasite (Ascaris) as a cause of acute pancreatitis. Ultrasound diagnosis. *Rev Esp Enferm Dig.* 2012;104(7):389–390.

71. Sıkar HE, Kaptanoğlu L, Kement M. An unusual appearance of complicated hydatid cyst: necrotizing pancreatitis. *Ulus Travma Acil Cerrahi Derg.* 2017;23(1):81–83.

72. Kitchens WH, Liu C, Ryan ET, Fernandez-del Castillo C. Hepatic hydatid cyst: a rare cause of recurrent pancreatitis. *J Gastrointest Surg.* 2014;18(11):2057–2059.

73. Makni A, Jouini M, Kacem M, Safta ZB. Acute pancreatitis due to pancreatic hydatid cyst: a case report and review of the literature. *World J Emerg Surg.* 2012. https://doi.org/10.1186/1749-7922-7-7. Published online 2012 Mar 24.

74. Mohamed H, Azza S, Chrif A, Karim S, Adnen C. Hydatid cyst of the pancreas revealed by acute pancreatitis: report of a case. *Pan Afr Med J.* 2015. https://doi.org/10.11604/pamj.2015.22.166.6242. Published online 2015 Oct 21.

75. Mahmoudi A, Zouari K. A rare complication of hydatid cyst of the liver: acute pancreatitis. *Pan Afr Med J.* 2015. https://doi.org/10.11604/pamj.2015.21.247.7600. Published online 2015 Aug 6.

76. Mattous M, Belabbes S. Acute pancreatitis revealing a hydatid cyst of the pancreas. *Pan Afr Med J.* 2015. https://doi.org/10.11604/pamj.2015.20.429.6734. Published online 2015 Apr 29.

77. Karaman B, Battal B, Sari S, Verim S. US diagnosis of acute pancreatitis caused by ruptured hydatid disease to the biliary system. *JBR-BTR.* 2014;97(4):269.

78. Belkouch A, Mouhsine A. Hydatid cyst ruptured in the biliary duct: an exceptional cause of acute pancreatitis. *Pan Afr Med J.* 2014. https://doi.org/10.11604/pamj.2014.18.298.5147. Published online 2014 Aug 4.

79. Ozcaglayan O, Halefoglu AM, Ozcaglayan T, Sumbul HA. Ultrasonographic diagnosis of acute pancreatitis caused by ruptured hydatid disease to the biliary system. *JBR-BTR.* 2014;97(1):33–35.

80. Chaudhary A, Upadhyaya AC, Kankanala VV, et al. Intrabiliary rupture of hepatic hydatid cyst with impacted hydatid membranes at ampulla of Vater presenting as acute pancreatitis. *Trop Gastroenterol.* 2013;34(1):251–253.

81. Cakir OO, Ataseven H, Demir A. Hydatid acute pancreatitis. *Turkiye Parazitol Derg.* 2012;36(4):251–253.

82. Rodríguez-Sicilia MJ, González-Artacho C, Cabello-Tapia MJ, de-la-Torre-Rubio P, de-Teresa-Galván J. Recurrent acute pancreatitis as clinical presentation of hydatid disease of the liver. *Rev Esp Enferm Dig.* 2012;104(8):441–442.

83. Oz HS. Toxoplasmosis, pancreatitis, obesity and drug discovery. *Pancreat Disord Ther.* 2014;4(2):138.

84. Ahuja SK1, Ahuja SS, Thelmo W, Seymour A, Phelps KR. Necrotizing pancreatitis and multisystem organ failure associated with toxoplasmosis in a patient with AIDS. *Clin Infect Dis.* 1993;16(3):432–434.

85. Norby SM, Bharucha AE, Larson MV, Temesgen Z. Acute pancreatitis associated with Cryptosporidium parvum enteritis in an immunocompetent man. *Clin Infect Dis.* 1998;27(1):223–224.

86. De Beaux AC, Palmer KR, Carter DC. Factors influencing morbidity and mortality in acute pancreatitis; an analysis of 279 cases. *Gut.* 1995;37:121–126.

CHAPTER 6

Clinical Conditions Associated With Bacterial Overgrowth

AYESHA SHAH, MBBS, FRACP •
GERALD HOLTMANN, MD, PHD, MBA, FRACP, FRCP

INTRODUCTION

The human microbiome is a diverse microbial community composed mainly of bacteria, as well as archaea, viruses, fungi, and protozoa. The microbes colonizing the human digestive tract play an important role in the digestion of food, absorption of micronutrients, production of vitamins,[1] immune hemostasis,[2] and maintaining the gut barrier function.[3] Using culture-independent techniques, we now acknowledge that virtually all segments of the human gastrointestinal (GI) tract are colonized by bacteria,[4] including segments that were traditionally considered "sterile" because of the hostile environment with low pH (stomach) or high concentration of aggressive digestive enzymes and bile acids (duodenum).[5] There is growing evidence that dysbiosis (alteration in the composition, density, and function of the intestinal microbes) of the gut microbiota is associated with the pathogenesis of both intestinal and extraintestinal disorders.[6,7]

The most recognized dysbiosis is small intestinal bacterial overgrowth (SIBO). This is a condition characterized by both increased bacterial density and small intestinal dysbiosis.[8-10] SIBO is frequently associated with GI symptoms such as bloating, distension, flatulence, abdominal discomfort, diarrhea, and weight loss[11] and may even cause structural changes such as atrophy of small intestinal villi[12] with subsequent alterations to the small intestinal absorption. SIBO overlaps with other GI disorders and symptoms, often making it unclear if it is the cause of, consequence of, or an epiphenomenon in relation to the other disorder.[13,14] Antibiotic treatment of SIBO targets the dysbiosis and potentially improves symptoms[15] or other consequences of the altered mucosal or luminal bacterial colonization. Indeed, previous studies[16] have shown a link between meal-related symptoms and the density of the bacterial colonization of the small intestine. This may suggest that normalization of the mucosal bacterial colonization is a potential target for

therapy. To appropriately target therapy, it is important to reliably diagnose SIBO. However, the available noninvasive tests such as breath test lack sensitivity and specificity,[17,18] whereas other tests such as those based on microbial culture of intestinal aspirates[19] are rarely used in the clinical setting. Limited data are available regarding the influence of SIBO on GI functions such as the permeability or the symptom response to a standardized nutrient challenge. While an increased intestinal permeability is believed to play a role in irritable bowel syndrome (IBS), chronic liver disease[20,21] or nonalcoholic fatty liver disease,[22-24] sensory function is critical for functional gastrointestinal disorders (FGIDs) such IBS.[25]

Several studies have now shown a role for dysbiosis of the duodenal microbiota in IBS[26,27] and celiac disease.[28] Similarly, the role of intestinal microbiota in the pathogenesis of irritable bowel disease (IBD) is well recognized. Gut microbiota are now considered an essential factor in driving mucosal inflammation in IBD,[29,30] and gut microbial dysbiosis and decreased diversity of the gut microbial ecosystem are common features in these patients.[31] Hepatobiliary manifestations constitute one of most common extraintestinal manifestations in IBD,[32] with primary sclerosing cholangitis (PSC) being the most common hepatobiliary manifestation.[33] This association is particularly interesting, as 70%–80% of patients with PSC have concomitant IBD,[34] and there is increasing evidence that gut microbial dysbiosis (via the gut–liver cross talk) plays an important role in the pathogenesis and outcome of PSC.[35] The gut is ultimately to be responsible for what happens to the bile ducts. However, studies so far have focused on the stool and colonic mucosa-associated microbiome (MAM). None have focused on characterizing the MAM in the proximal duodenum and the distal ileum, both of which form a very important link in the bidirectional axis between the gut and the liver, the so-called enterohepatic circulation.

Gastrointestinal Diseases and Their Associated Infections. https://doi.org/10.1016/B978-0-323-54843-4.00006-4
Copyright © 2019 Elsevier Inc. All rights reserved.

Noninvasive and simple breath tests based on the measurement of exhaled gases, such as hydrogen and methane, following a glucose or lactulose challenge have been advocated because they are safe and easy to perform.[36,37] Compared with the direct aspiration method, the glucose-hydrogen (H_2) breath test has a sensitivity of 62.5% and a specificity of 81.7%. The lactulose-H_2 breath test has a sensitivity of 52.4% and a specificity of 85.7% when compared with the direct aspiration method.[38] Nevertheless, there is lack of consensus as to the appropriate thresholds to diagnose bacterial overgrowth if breath tests are used. There is agreement neither on the optimal duration of the breath tests nor on the cutoff levels that define a positive result. Moreover, 8%–27% of humans do not have detectable H_2 production from their GI microbiota, instead produce methane (CH_4).[39] Therefore if H_2 is analyzed in isolation, the test result may not be positive even in the presence of high densities of non–H_2-producing bacteria. This clearly limits the practical value in the clinical setting.

Against this background, research regarding the bacterial colonization of the GI tract in health and disease is required to better understand the role of the GI microbiome and dysbiosis in the manifestation of various diseases.

Characterization of the Gut Microbiome

The gut microbiome can be characterized by the composition of the bacteria colonizing the mucosa, the density of bacterial colonization, and the metabolic products produced by the bacteria. It is widely believed that culture methods and the quantification of colony-forming units (CFUs) or the metabolic characterization of metabolic products of cultured bacteria are most appropriate to characterize the microbiome. Thus conventional culture-based methods were used to assess the intestinal microbes. However, culture-based methods have proven to be inadequate in determining the true microbial diversity of the intestinal microbiota because a large fraction of the microbiota remains uncultivated.[40] Human studies utilizing a variety of culture-independent molecular assays demonstrate a hitherto unimagined complexity of the human gut microbiota with hundreds of phylotypes, of which 80% remain uncultured.[41] So far, most studies have focused on the fecal microbiota, partially because fecal samples are relatively easy to obtain; however, fecal material is predominantly composed of those microbes resident in the intestinal lumen, which does not accurately reflect the composition of the MAM.[42–45]

The above-mentioned limitations of culture-based direct tests have triggered the development of indirect tests in the clinical setting to identify patients with altered (increased) bacterial colonization of the intestine. The most widely available indirect tests to diagnose SIBO are breath tests[37] based on the fermentation of carbohydrates by bacteria, to produce acids, water, and gases. The substrate is orally administered and the level of hydrogen (H_2), methane (CH_4), or carbon dioxide (CO_2) is measured in the exhaled breath. Substrates can be glucose lactulose, xylose, or bile acids. Depending on the detection protocol, substrates may also be labeled with radioactive or stable isotopes and the alveolar exhaled breath is measured with appropriate detectors (e.g., solid-state electrochemical detectors [H_2 and CH_4], scintillation devices [^{14}C], or infrared spectroscopy [^{13}C]). Alternatively, metabolic products such as H_2, CH_4, and CO_2 can be measured utilizing gas chromatography or solid-state sensors. The substances used for hydrogen and methane testing include glucose[46,47] or lactulose.[48] These breath tests are now widely used in the clinical setting to diagnose bacterial overgrowth.

DIRECT TESTS: QUALITATIVE CULTURE OF PROXIMAL SMALL BOWEL ASPIRATES

Jejunal fluid aspirate culture is the "gold standard" for studying jejunal microflora and establishing the diagnosis of SIBO.[8] However, there are significant drawbacks with using culture for the diagnosis of SIBO.

METHODOLOGICAL LIMITATIONS OF DIRECT TESTS

Lack of Standardization of Collection Technique

Jejunal fluid can be aspirated by endoscopic suction, by intestinal intubation with a catheter, by a capsule biopsy, or intraoperatively.[49] The appropriate technique of specimen collection for culture has not been defined[8,50,51] and there is no clear consensus on this. Some authors have employed a fluoroscopically positioned tube for specimen collection and others have used a sterile wash catheter passed through the instrument channel of an upper endoscope as means of collecting a specimen free of contamination by saliva and other luminal secretions. Contamination from oral flora or saliva during oral intubation is always a major concern, and it may result in false-positive results and an overestimation of SIBO.[52] Despite the vigorous attempts to minimize cross-contamination during intubation by using oral antiseptics, by simultaneous culture of saliva and aspirate,[52] by using sterile gloves, and by placing a sterile catheter under aseptic conditions in the small intestine, the risks cannot be completely eliminated. Moreover, gram-positive bacterial overgrowth is mainly due to upper respiratory flora and is a frequent finding in the upper part of the small bowel of healthy elderly people[53] and has not been correlated with symptoms of SIBO.[54-57] Aspiration of the jejunal fluid is technically challenging, as it increases endoscopy time and is unsuccessful at times because of the sparseness of the jejunal fluid aspirate.[58]

Lack of Standardization of Culture Methods

Culture techniques on aspirated specimen also vary. The sample can be plated on nonselective media in a fashion analogous to quantitative urine culture. It is important that the specimen be transported promptly to the laboratory for both aerobic and anaerobic cultures. However, small bowel culturing methodology, sample handling, and microbiological techniques were highly variable in the 50 published studies (diagnosing SIBO based on culture) in the systematic review by Khoshini et al. Furthermore, compared with genomic methods, culturing reveals only a fraction (20%) of the microbiota.[40]

Lack of Diagnostic Cutoff Values

Also, the review by Khoshini et al.,[19] has clearly highlighted that the definition of SIBO based on the cutoff level of 10^5 CFU bacteria/mL is more diagnostic of the stagnant loop condition rather than SIBO itself. This stems from their observation that when SIBO was defined by investigators in 1960s and 1970s, it was in the context of abnormal or postsurgical anatomy.[59,60] However, over the years, there is increasing suspicion of bacterial growth–like entity in many other GI and medical conditions. They also concluded that many GI conditions have increased bacterial counts in the small intestine, but less than 10^5 CFU/mL. Hence, we need studies to first define the normal level of bacteria in the small bowel in the healthy controls and then redefine SIBO. There are only studies [50,61,62] on the validation of SIBO as a diagnostic test that tried to validate culture against controls but were conducted in three very diverse groups of population.

Lack of Standardization of Location for Sampling Site in the Small Intestine

Khoshini et al. reported that there was significant heterogeneity in the 50 studies that used culture for SIBO diagnosis, especially in sampling with many studies not mentioning the location of sampling site in the small intestine, with consensus on the location of sampling being beyond the ligament of Treitz.

Although the literature suggests sampling from the proximal jejunum, most physicians who perform luminal aspirations obtain samples from the duodenum using a standard upper endoscope, despite using the same colony count bacteria.[63] A lower cutoff value of $\geq 10^3$ CFU/mL may be more clinically relevant for aspirates obtained from the third and fourth parts of the duodenum, given their proximal location, relative protection from translocation of bacteria from the colon, and frequent exposure to acid from stomach, all of which would decrease the risk of SIBO.[64-66]

False-Negative Culture Results

Cultures may be false negative, particularly in cases of overgrowth by obligate anaerobes.[67] Cultures from several different jejunal sites revealed that the overgrowth may be noncontinuous or patchy in the upper GI tract, leading to false-negative results when only one culture site is assessed.[68] Other concerns that have been addressed include the ability to access only upper small bowel and hence more distal bacterial overgrowth can be overlooked.[8,69,70] However, the clinical implications of distal SIBO remain unclear.

Despite these numerous problems, culturing remains the "gold standard"; however, this makes it very difficult to assess the validity of breath test and other strategies used for the diagnosis of SIBO.

CULTURE OF SPECIMENS OBTAINED BY MUCOSAL BIOPSY VERSUS ASPIRATION

As microorganisms are present in the mucous layer, which overlies the intestinal epithelium, culture of the mucosal biopsy, which is endoscopically more easy, fast, and efficient than aspiration, could be an alternative to study the jejunal microflora.[49] Only two studies have compared the culture of mucosal biopsies and aspiration for the diagnosis of SIBO and found significant correlation between the two methods (Table 6.1).

The first study that compared the culture of unwashed biopsy and luminal fluid found significant correlation in relation to the total bacterial counts and the type of

TABLE 6.1
Comparison of Small Bowel Biopsy and Aspiration for the Diagnosis of SIBO

Bacterial Counts and Organisms Compared Using Culture of Unwashed Small Bowel Biopsy and Aspirate	Year	Sensitivity (%)	Specificity (%)	Positive Predictor Value (%)	Negative Predictor Value (%)
Chandra et al.[71]	2010	83.5	97.3	94.7	91.6
Riordan et al.[58]	1995	90.3	100	100	

organisms recovered. Culture of the biopsy was found to have a very high sensitivity, specificity, and predictive value of 90.3%, 100%, and 100%, respectively.[58]

Similarly a study by Chandra et al.[71] showed culture of unwashed endoscopic jejunal mucosal biopsy yields similar results to fluid with respect to presence of growth, nature of organisms, and presence or absence of SIBO. The sensitivity, specificity, and positive and negative predictor values of culture in diagnosing SIBO were 83.5%, 97.3%, 94.7%, and 91.6%, respectively. However, while these data suggest that mucosal biopsies are not inferior to the current gold standard of aspiration of small intestinal fluid, it is evident that contamination of the working channel of the endoscope ultimately will affect the sensitivity and specificity of biopsy-based tests, unless precautions are taken to avoid cross-contamination.

MOLECULAR TECHNIQUES TO CHARACTERIZE THE SMALL INTESTINE MICROBIOME

To address these methodological constraints, we plan to obtain mucosal biopsies from the GI tract that are not cross-contaminated by oral or luminal content by using a novel aseptic biopsy device (the Brisbane Aseptic Biopsy Device [BABD]). This comprises sterile forceps encased by a sheath with a plug at the tip, allowing targeted aseptic sampling of the mucosa (Fig. 6.1). A pilot study comparing duodenal mucosal biopsies collected in six patients with iron deficiency anemia using BABD and standard forceps confirmed that BABD allowed collection of samples more representative of the MAM by precluding luminal cross-contamination.[72]

INDIRECT TESTS: BREATH TESTS

To overcome the limitations and challenges of direct tests in the diagnosis of SIBO, several indirect tests have

been developed. The most widely available indirect tests to diagnose SIBO are breath tests.[37,46]

They are all based on the same principle. A substrate is orally administered and a metabolic product is measured in the exhaled air. Substrates can be glucose, lactulose, xylose, or bile acids labeled with radioactive or stable isotopes. The radioactive or stable isotopes can be measured with appropriate detectors in the exhaled air (e.g., via scintillation devices or infrared spectroscopy). The measured gases can include labeled carbon dioxide (CO_2), hydrogen (H_2), and methane (CH_4). For hydrogen and methane testing the substances include glucose[46,47] or lactulose (Fig. 6.2).[48]

Many bacteria produce hydrogen or methane. Thus this metabolic product can be used to diagnose an increased bacterial density. Although H_2 production appears more ubiquitous, predominant methane production (CH_4 producers) is seen in 36%–50% of healthy subjects.[73-76] The predominant methanogenic bacteria in humans is *Methanobrevibacter smithii*,[77-79] although certain *Clostridium* and *Bacteroides* species can also produce CH_4.[80] There has been considerable interest in the role of methane as a cause of constipation[81] and this may even predict a differential treatment in IBS with constipation.[82] Methanogenic bacteria comprise a group of colonic anaerobic organisms that rely on the production of methane from H_2 and CO_2 as their sole source of energy.[83] Methane generally has not been found to have a physiologic role in humans[84] and it must be excreted, either as flatus (80%) or in the breath (20%), after its absorption into the circulation through the intestinal mucosa.[83]

HYDROGEN AND METHANE BREATH TEST

Quantification of hydrogen and methane in breath samples remains the most inexpensive, noninvasive, and widely available test for the diagnosis of SIBO.[19]

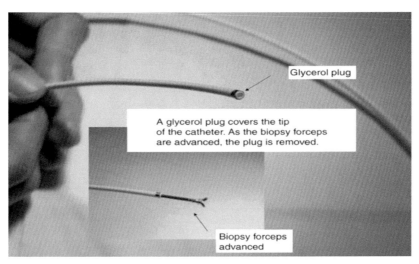

FIG. 6.1 Image of the Brisbane Aseptic Biopsy Device (BABD).

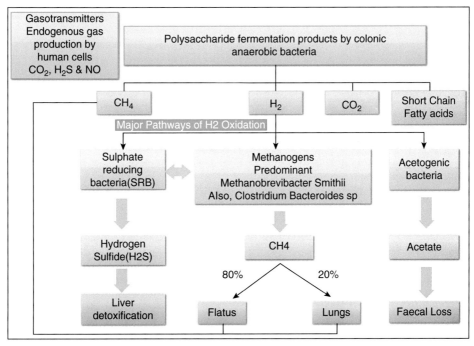

FIG. 6.2 During the fermentation of polysaccharides by anaerobic bacteria in the gastrointestinal tract, methane (CH_4), carbon dioxide (CO_2), and hydrogen (H_2), as well as short-chain fatty acids, are produced. The H_2 is competitively utilized by specialized bacteria (sulfate-reducing, methanogenic, or acetogenic bacteria) to produce hydrogen sulfide (H_2S), methane (CH_4), and acetate, respectively.

Human cells are not capable of producing H_2 or CH_4 gas,[85] so the presence of these gases in the human breath indicates the metabolism of (nondigested) carbohydrates by gut bacteria.[18] After oral ingestion of various substrates, H_2 can be measured in exhaled breath using gas chromatography or other techniques and reported in parts per million (ppm);[86] CH_4 can be measured similarly (Fig. 6.3).

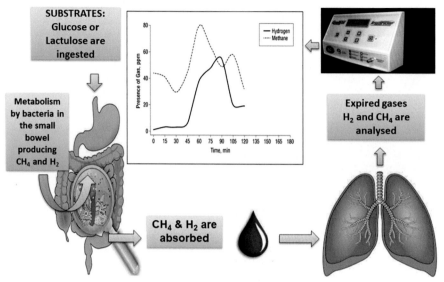

FIG. 6.3 The principles behind breath tests.

BREATH TESTS: SENSITIVITY AND SPECIFICITY

Even in patients with SIBO, gas production is variable and is clearly dependent on the concentration and the type of colonizing bacteria in the small bowel (hydrogen- or methane-predominant overgrowth, as discussed earlier), the absorptive capacity of the small bowel, and the availability of carbohydrate residues.

CAUSES OF FALSE-POSITIVE AND FALSE-NEGATIVE BREATH TEST RESULTS

False-positive results can be seen in subjects with carbohydrate malabsorption (chronic pancreatitis and celiac disease), because of colonic fermentation and gas production.[87–90] Alterations in GI motility can alter intestinal transit and the results of breath test. GI motor disorders, where delayed gastric emptying may cause false-negative test results,[91] and rapid transit through the small bowel will produce false-positive breath test results.[88,92–94] False-positive results may also be due to the oral bacterial flora and if the subject has failed to adhere to a low-fiber diet the day before the test.[90] Smoking raises and exercise lowers hydrogen concentrations and is therefore not allowed during the test.[95] High fasting concentrations (increased basal level of H_2) may be due to SIBO, but this is a

very unspecific finding that may also be due to slow intestinal transit, leaving a residue of poorly absorbable carbohydrates remaining in the colon.[96] Different tests are performed in the fasting state after at least 1 day of a low-fiber diet.

GLUCOSE BREATH TEST

Glucose breath test (GBT) was first introduced in 1976 for the assessment of SIBO.[97] Glucose is readily absorbed in the proximal small bowel, and in the absence of severe transit abnormalities, it rarely reaches the colon,[93,98] making it a suitable substrate to detect at least proximal SIBO. However, a negative GBT cannot exclude an SIBO affecting the distal small bowel. This means that GBT favors specificity over sensitivity.[18,99,100] The glucose hydrogen breath test is considered positive if there is a clearly recognizable single "early" hydrogen peak, exceeding 10–20 ppm.[46,97,101]

LACTULOSE BREATH TEST

The increase in hydrogen level after lactulose ingestion was first described by Bond and Levitt.[98] Lactulose is a nonabsorbable substance that is normally metabolized by gut bacteria in the colon with the production of hydrogen and/or methane. Lactulose passes unabsorbed through the small bowel and into the colon. Therefore, apart from detecting SIBO, it can also be used as a measure of orocecal transit.[102] As ingested lactulose is nonabsorbed, it theoretically should be able to detect bacterial overgrowth anywhere along the length of the small bowel, including ileum.[48] This means that unlike GBT, lactulose breath test (LBT) favors sensitivity over specificity.

LACK OF UNIVERSALLY ACCEPTED CUTOFF VALUES FOR LACTULOSE BREATH TESTS

A variety of end points have been used to define a positive LBT; however, owing to the several reasons discussed in the following, there is no universally recognized and validated standard for a positive study. The original definition of a positive lactulose test (that is, indicating SIBO) is to look for a "double peak effect," an easily detected early hydrogen peak (>20 ppm), due to small intestinal bacteria, occurring at least 15 min before the later prolonged peak, corresponding to the passage of the remaining lactulose into the colon,[48] but this is seldom seen in practice.[103] Moreover, detection of two easily distinguishable hydrogen peaks is not a safe criterion, as it has been shown in transit studies that a bolus can reach the cecum, imitating the first peak followed by the body of lumen contents, producing a second peak, thus yielding false-positive results.[104,105]

Another concern is that the early peak in hydrogen or methane may be a result of rapid transit[105,106] and importantly lactulose itself accelerates small bowel transit.[107] This also highlights that without a clear second peak in the LBT, it is impossible to distinguish SIBO from colonic fermentation.

Some studies have used restrictive definitions, such as a rise in H_2 levels within 90 min.[108–111] This has not been validated and should be compared with the fact that the mean orocecal transit time assessed with LBT in healthy controls is slightly above 90 min, which would give rise to high chances of false-positive results. A solution to this problem would be simultaneous measurement of transit by using an independent test such as scintigraphy.[105,112]

However, the sensitivity and the specificity of breath tests in the diagnosis of SIBO remain unclear because of the heterogeneity of the patient populations examined and methodological issues including use of different substrates and different doses of

TABLE 6.2
Specificity and Sensitivity of Breath Test[19]

Breath Test	Sensitivity (%)	Specificity (%)
Bile acid breath test	33–70	76–100
^{14}C-D-xylose breath test	30–95	40–94
Glucose breath test	62.5	81.8
Lactulose breath test	52.5	85.7

substrates, the length of the test, the sampling intervals, and the definition of a normal and abnormal breath test (Table 6.2).

CHARACTERISTICS OF THE GUT MICROBIOME IN HEALTHY SUBJECTS

In humans the GI tract represents a large microbial ecosystem, housing several trillion microbial cells. Collectively, the number of intestinal microbial cells is 10 times greater than the number of human body cells.[113] The composition and diversity of the intestinal microbiota has a tremendous potential to impact our physiology, both in health and in disease.

The number of bacterial cells present in the mammalian gut shows a continuum that goes from 10^1 to 10^3 bacteria CFU/mL of content in the stomach and duodenum, progressing to 10^4–10^7 bacteria CFU/mL in the jejunum and ileum, and culminating in 10^{11}–10^{12} CFU/mL in the colon.[114] Additionally, the microbial composition varies between these sites. In addition to the longitudinal heterogeneity displayed by the intestinal microbiota, there is also a great deal of latitudinal variation in the microbiota composition. The intestinal epithelium is separated from the lumen by a thick and physiochemically complex mucous layer. The microbiota present in the intestinal lumen differ significantly from the microbiota attached and embedded in this mucous layer as well as the microbiota present in the immediate proximity of the epithelium (Fig. 6.4).[72,115,116]

In comparison to the colon, the upper GI tract harbors only a relatively small number of bacteria. A variety of factors seem to contribute to this, including the composition of chyme with relatively high concentrations of bile and high concentrations of

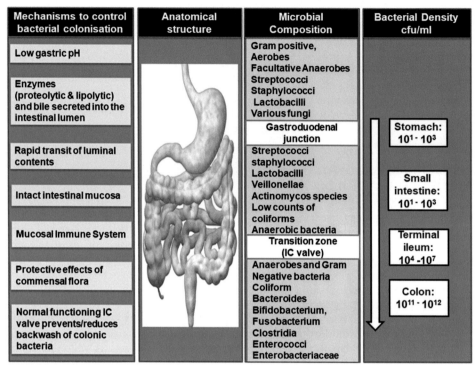

Mechanisms to control bacterial colonisation	Anatomical structure	Microbial Composition	Bacterial Density cfu/ml
Low gastric pH		Gram positive, Aerobes Facultative Anaerobes Streptococci Staphylococci Lactobacilli Various fungi	
Enzymes (proteolytic & lipolytic) and bile secreted into the intestinal lumen		**Gastroduodenal junction**	Stomach: 10^1- 10^3
Rapid transit of luminal contents		Streptococci staphylococci Lactobacilli Veillonellae Actinomycos species Low counts of coliforms Anaerobic bacteria	Small intestine: 10^1- 10^3
Intact intestinal mucosa			
Mucosal Immune System		**Transition zone (IC valve)**	Terminal ileum: 10^4 -10^7
Protective effects of commensal flora		Anaerobes and Gram Negative bacteria Coliform Bacteroides Bifidobacterium, Fusobacterium Clostridia Enterococci Enterobacteriaceae	Colon: 10^{11}- 10^{12}
Normal functioning IC valve prevents/reduces backwash of colonic bacteria			

FIG. 6.4 Composition of the gut microbiota in the different parts of the gastrointestinal tract and the factors that influence the density and composition of bacterial colonization. *IC*, ileocecal.

digestive enzymes that may adversely affect growth of microorganisms. In additions, luminal content is rapidly moved toward the ileum with an intestinal transit time of minutes or rarely more than an hour, whereas the transit time through the colon may take days. All these factors result in relatively low density of bacteria in the small intestine.[5] The upper GI tract thus might be seen as a somehow hostile environment and bacteria must overcome the barriers of mucus and antimicrobial defenses in the stomach and duodenum to colonize these sites.[117] Other protective factors include the integrity of the intestinal mucosa and its protective mucous layer; the enzymatic activities of intestinal, pancreatic, and biliary secretions; the protective effects of some of the commensal flora, such as lactobacilli; the mechanical and physiologic properties of the ileocecal valve[118,119]; and local and systemic immunity.[120]

The microflora of the stomach are gram positive and aerobic, and the most commonly isolated species are various gram-positive aerobes such as streptococci, staphylococci, lactobacilli, and various fungi and facultative anaerobes, reflecting the flora of the oropharynx.[121] The small intestine constitutes a zone of transition between the sparsely populated stomach and the luxuriant bacterial flora of the colon. Under normal conditions the microflora of the proximal small bowel is like that of the stomach. The predominant species include streptococci, staphylococci, and lactobacilli. *Veillonella* and *Actinomyces* sp. are also frequently isolated, whereas coliforms and other anaerobic bacteria are found in lower concentrations.

In the distal ileum, gram-negative bacteria outnumber gram-positive organisms. Coliforms are consistently present, and anaerobic bacteria such as *Bacteroides*, *Bifidobacterium*, *Fusobacterium*, and *Clostridium* are found in substantial concentrations.[121–123] Thus, in the terminal ileum distal to the ileocecal sphincter, bacterial concentrations increase sharply. Within the colon, the bacterial concentration is 10^{11}–10^{12} CFU/mL, and anaerobic bacteria outnumber aerobes by 1000-fold. The predominant isolates are *Bacteroides*, *Bifidobacterium*, and *Eubacterium*.[121,124–127] Anaerobic gram-positive cocci, clostridia, enterococci, and various species of Enterobacteriaceae are also common.

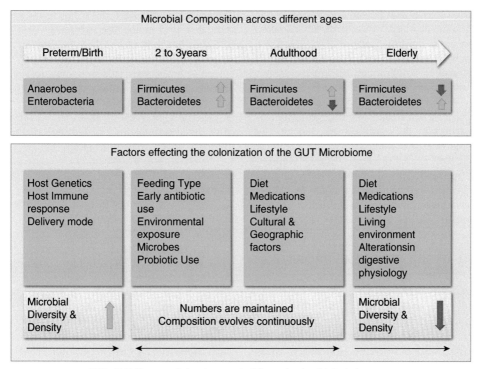

FIG. 6.5 Temporal development of the gut microbiota in humans.

GUT MICROBIOME AND ENVIRONMENTAL FACTORS

There is ample evidence that the composition and density of human GI microbiome respond to a variety of environmental factors.

Immediately after birth, the GI tract is sterile but is rapidly colonized by bacteria acquired from the immediate environment; this starts during the passage through the vaginal birth channel when the newborn is exposed to lactobacilli from the mother's vagina, subsequently the newborn is exposed to and ingests bacteria from parents and siblings.[128] The first 2 years after birth are characterized by a succession of bacteria within the intestine that partly reflects the exposure and partly reflects the changes in the diet of neonates and infants; however, while the relative composition may change, the diversity and the type of bacteria found in the GI tract thereafter more or less remain constant (Fig. 6.5).

It is believed that once the flora is established in the early years, it generally continues to exist unchanged through life,[129] until older age (>65 years), which is characterized by declines in microbiome stability and diversity.[130,131] Endogenous and exogenous factors have varying influence on the gut microbiota (fecal microbiome), including mode of delivery of a neonate,[132] host

genetic features,[133] host immune response,[134] diet[135] (including dietary supplements, breastfeeding, and formula feeding), xenobiotics (including antibiotics) and other drugs,[136,137] infections,[138] diurnal rhythm,[139] and environmental microbial exposures.[6,140] However, their effect on the MAM remains largely unknown.

GUT MICROBIOME IN GASTROINTESTINAL DISEASES

The changes in the gut microbiome have been implicated as relevant for the manifestation or progression of various GI and non-GI diseases.[6] Historically, the stomach was thought to be sterile by the gastric acid, but there was a change in the belief with the discovery of *Helicobacter pylori* by Warren and Marshall in 1982, which has evolved to colonize an acidic stomach and caused chronic active gastritis.[117]

While traditionally gastric *H. pylori* colonization was diagnosed utilizing histologic examination or rapid urease testing, new developments have allowed mapping of normal gastric mucosa using broad-range polymerase chain reaction (PCR) and 16S ribosomal RNA (rRNA) sequence analysis.[4] Similarly, the duodenum and most parts of the small bowel have long been considered sterile, with bacteria only present due to cross-contamination, or overgrowth.[65] Characterization of the small intestine, including the duodenal microbiome, is plagued by the methodology, as the collection is beset by contamination from the mouth oropharynx and the stomach.[141]

Utilizing real-time PCR and 16S rRNA gene sequencing, studies have shown a role for gut microbiota dysbiosis (imbalances in the composition, density, and function of the intestinal microbes) of the duodenal microbiota in IBS[26,27] and in celiac disease.[28] Characterization of the duodenal and intestinal MAM and the associated gut microbiota dysbiosis might be critical for the understanding of the pathophysiologic conditions of various FGIDs and inflammatory GI disorders.

MICROBIAL DYSBIOSIS IN THE PROXIMAL SMALL INTESTINE
Small Intestinal Bacterial Overgrowth as an Example of Small Intestinal Dysbiosis
The role of the GI microbiome in a variety of disorders has become an area of considerable interest. However, even before that, SIBO has been identified as a condition that is defined by excessive and/or abnormal type of bacterial growth in the small bowel.[8–10]

In SIBO the overall density of bacteria (e.g., expressed as number of CFUs per milliliter of an intestinal aspirate) is increased. The contaminating flora seen in SIBO has the features of both oropharyngeal and colonic bacteria, but these occur in SIBO at different levels than those in their original location. The main bacteria recovered were *Streptococcus* (71%), *Escherichia coli* (69%), *Staphylococcus* (25%), *Micrococcus* (22%), *Klebsiella* (20%), and *Proteus* (11%) for microaerophilic bacteria and *Lactobacillus* (75%), *Bacteroides* (29%), *Clostridium* (25%), *Veillonella* (25%), *Fusobacterium* (13%), and *Peptostreptococcus* (13%) for anaerobic bacteria.[10]

While the conceptual framework of SIBO is now widely accepted, there is a gap in relation to the generally accepted definitions of SIBO or the universally established and accepted diagnostic criteria. This stems from the lack of universally accepted and applied gold standard for the diagnosis of SIBO. Indeed, the validity of the traditional "gold standard," jejunal cultures >10^5 CFU/mL with colonic bacteria, has been challenged, largely because this cutoff was established from samples following surgical diversion.[50,142]

Khoshini et al.[19] found a wide spectrum of bacterial counts in various GI conditions compared with healthy controls in the small bowel but below 1×10^5 CFU/mL. They suggested that various cutoff levels proposed in

literature have not been uniformly tested or adequately validated and many are arbitrary. Also, the review showed that studies in which healthy adults without any GI symptoms were used as controls, the counts were 0–10^3 CFU/mL. This systematic review and subsequent studies have questioned the validity of ≥10^5 CFU/mL as the cutoff for SIBO diagnosis.[19,64,66] Currently, a bacterial concentration of ≥10^3 CFU/mL is generally considered significant.[64,143] However, it might be that these thresholds are still too high.

Concept of "Classical SIBO" and "SIBO in FGIDs"
To complicate matters further, Quigley et al.[13,144,145] have proposed the concept of "classical" SIBO and SIBO in "functional" GI complaints and other diseases.

The "classical SIBO" refers to a situation in which clinical features can be pathophysiologically explained by SIBO and subsequent alterations of gut morphology. This may refer to patients with SIBO presenting with maldigestion and/or malabsorption linked to atrophy of intestinal villi caused by SIBO. These patients typically have other structural abnormalities of the GI tract, such as resection of the ileocolonic valve or enteroenteral fistula. In this more restrictive concept of SIBO, jejunal fluid culture remains a valuable benchmark, as abnormal results correlate with clinical and pathologic consequences. In the second concept involving "SIBO in FGIDs," there is no maldigestion and/or malabsorption, and in this group, symptoms are linked to SIBO. It remains to be elucidated if SIBO is a cause, a consequence, or an epiphenomenon in these situations.[144]

Thus there is a paradigm shift in our understanding of the concept of SIBO and its association with other GI disorders and medical conditions.

Prevalence of Small Intestinal Bacterial Overgrowth in Healthy Subjects and Patient Cohorts
Against the background of a lack of universally accepted diagnostic criteria for SIBO, the so-far published data on the prevalence of SIBO in general population are somehow questionable.[146] The lack of a generally accepted and validated diagnostic test has limited the ability to define the prevalence of SIBO in the population.[19] In addition, attempts to link SIBO with specific disorders or symptoms are also hampered by the lack of appropriately defined thresholds or reference ranges for small intestinal bacterial colonization in healthy subjects. It thus has been questioned if SIBO is the cause, consequence, or an epiphenomenon in relation to the other disorders.[13,14]

TABLE 6.3
Prevalence of SIBO in Various Gastrointestinal Disorders

Gastrointestinal Disorders	Prevalence of SIBO (%)	References
Irritable bowel syndrome[a]	9.52–84 11.11–30.77 2.01–21.43	LHBT[106,110,147–150] GHBT[151–155] Culture[143,156–159]
Functional dyspepsia	5.3–56.5	160,161
Ulcerative colitis	6.5–17.8	162–165
Crohn disease	15.38–45.2	162,164,166–170
Celiac disease	9.3–66.66	23,171–173
Gastroparesis	39–60	174,175
Postchole-cystectomy syndrome	46.8	176

[a]Only case control studies reporting the prevalence of SIBO in inflammatory bowel syndrome have been included.
GHBT, glucose hydrogen breath test; LHBT, lactulose hydrogen breath test; SIBO, small intestinal bacterial overgrowth.

Against this background, a systematic review by Grace et al.,[11] revealed a considerable variability of SIBO in the general population, ranging from 0% to 20%. In addition, many studies aimed to define the prevalence of SIBO in a variety of patient cohorts. Also, a variety of cohort studies have assessed the prevalence of SIBO in several GI disorders with various methods (Table 6.3). Overall the data suggest that the prevalence of SIBO is increased in a variety of FGIDs and organic GI disorders.

Symptoms in Patients with Small Intestinal Bacterial Overgrowth

Clinical symptoms in patients with SIBO are variable. A systematic review by Grace et al.[11] reported diarrhea as the predominant symptom in SIBO, followed by abdominal pain and bloating. A wide range of symptoms have been described in SIBO, but most studies have not used validated questionnaire. The more serious manifestations of SIBO include signs of nutrient malabsorption,[177] namely, weight loss, steatorrhea, fat-soluble vitamin deficiencies, and deficiency of B_{12}, folate, and iron and serum bile acids.

A study by Jacobs et al.[64] was unable to identify a single symptom or cluster of symptoms that can clinical recognize patients with either SIBO or small intestinal fungal overgrowth. Thus symptoms were generally poor predictors of bacterial and/or fungal overgrowth, hence testing is essential.

FUTURE RESEARCH

Diagnostic Uncertainty and the Need for More Sensitive and Specific Diagnostic Tests

There is emerging evidence that the bacterial colonization of the GI tract plays a critical role in various GI and non-GI disorders. Interventions targeting the GI microbiome may even provide opportunities to prevent the manifestation or progression of a variety of diseases. The bacterial colonization of the GI mucosa can be characterized by the type of bacteria and/or the density of bacteria. In the routine clinical practice, breath tests are used to diagnose an increase in bacterial density by measuring the production of volatile gases after standardized administration of a substrate (e.g., glucose or lactulose). However, these breath tests have many limitations including poor sensitivity and sensitivity, lack of substrates used, and uncertainty regarding the most appropriate cutoff values.

However, contrasting these opportunities, there is a lack of appropriate, established, and universally accepted diagnostic measures. The obvious gaps relate to diagnostic approaches that allow to precisely quantitate the bacterial density and approaches to characterize the bacteria colonizing the mucosa utilizing molecular techniques. This will enable research that better characterize the link between the GI microbiome and specific disorders.

REFERENCES

1. Resta SC. Effects of probiotics and commensals on intestinal epithelial physiology: implications for nutrient handling. *J Physiol.* 2009;587:4169–4174.
2. Wu HJ, Wu E. The role of gut microbiota in immune homeostasis and autoimmunity. *Gut Microb.* 2012;3:4–14.
3. Camilleri M, Madsen K, Spiller R, Van Meerveld BG, Verne GN. Intestinal barrier function in health and gastrointestinal disease. *Neuro Gastroenterol Motil.* 2012;24:503–512.
4. Bik EM, Eckburg PB, Gill SR, et al. Molecular analysis of the bacterial microbiota in the human stomach. *Proc Natl Acad Sci USA.* 2006;103:732–737.
5. Guarner F, Malagelada JR. Gut flora in health and disease. *Lancet (Lond Engl).* 2003;361:512–519.
6. Lynch SV, Pedersen O. The human intestinal microbiome in health and disease. *N Engl J Med.* 2016;375:2369–2379.

7. Carding S, Verbeke K, Vipond DT, Corfe BM, Owen LJ. Dysbiosis of the gut microbiota in disease. *Microb Ecol Health Dis.* 2015;26.

8. Corazza GR, Menozzi MG, Strocchi A, et al. The diagnosis of small bowel bacterial overgrowth. Reliability of jejunal culture and inadequacy of breath hydrogen testing. *Gastroenterology.* 1990;98:302–309.

9. American Gastroenterological Association medical position statement: guidelines for the evaluation and management of chronic diarrhea. *Gastroenterology.* 1999;116:1461–1463.

10. Bouhnik Y, Alain S, Attar A, et al. Bacterial populations contaminating the upper gut in patients with small intestinal bacterial overgrowth syndrome. *Am J Gastroenterol.* 1999;94:1327–1331.

11. Grace E, Shaw C, Whelan K, Andreyev HJ. Review article: small intestinal bacterial overgrowth–prevalence, clinical features, current and developing diagnostic tests, and treatment. *Aliment Pharmacol Ther.* 2013;38:674–688.

12. Riordan SM, McIver CJ, Wakefield D, Duncombe VM, Thomas MC, Bolin TD. Small intestinal mucosal immunity and morphometry in luminal overgrowth of indigenous gut flora. *Am J Gastroenterol.* 2001;96:494–500.

13. Quigley EM, Abu-Shanab A. Small intestinal bacterial overgrowth. *Infect Dis Clin N Am.* 2010;24:943–959, viii-ix.

14. Ghoshal U, Ghoshal UC, Ranjan P, Naik SR, Ayyagari A. Spectrum and antibiotic sensitivity of bacteria contaminating the upper gut in patients with malabsorption syndrome from the tropics. *BMC Gastroenterol.* 2003;3:9.

15. Shah SC, Day LW, Somsouk M, Sewell JL. Meta-analysis: antibiotic therapy for small intestinal bacterial overgrowth. *Aliment Pharmacol Ther.* 2013;38:925–934.

16. Zhong L, Shanahan ER, Raj A, et al. Dyspepsia and the microbiome: time to focus on the small intestine. *Gut.* 2016;66(6):1168–1169.

17. Sachdev AH, Pimentel M. Gastrointestinal bacterial overgrowth: pathogenesis and clinical significance. *Ther Adv Chronic Dis.* 2013;4:223–231.

18. Simrén M, Stotzer PO. Use and abuse of hydrogen breath tests. *Gut.* 2006;55:297–303.

19. Khoshini R, Dai SC, Lezcano S, Pimentel M. A systematic review of diagnostic tests for small intestinal bacterial overgrowth. *Dig Dis Sci.* 2008;53:1443–1454.

20. Berg RD. Bacterial translocation from the gastrointestinal tract. *J Med.* 1992;23:217–244.

21. Guarner C, Soriano G. Bacterial translocation and its consequences in patients with cirrhosis. *Eur J Gastroenterol Hepatol.* 2005;17:27–31.

22. Duseja A, Chawla YK. Obesity and NAFLD: the role of bacteria and microbiota. *Clin Liver Dis.* 2014;18:59–71.

23. Miele L, Valenza V, La Torre G, et al. Increased intestinal permeability and tight junction alterations in nonalcoholic fatty liver disease. *Hepatology.* 2009;49:1877–1887.

24. Wigg AJ, Roberts-Thomson IC, Dymock RB, McCarthy PJ, Grose RH, Cummins AG. The role of small intestinal bacterial overgrowth, intestinal permeability, endotoxaemia, and tumour necrosis factor alpha in the pathogenesis of non-alcoholic steatohepatitis. *Gut.* 2001;48:206–211.

25. Camilleri M, Gorman H. Intestinal permeability and irritable bowel syndrome. *Neuro Gastroenterol Motil.* 2007;19:545–552.

26. Kerckhoffs AP, Samsom M, van der Rest ME, et al. Lower Bifidobacteria counts in both duodenal mucosa-associated and fecal microbiota in irritable bowel syndrome patients. *World J Gastroenterol.* 2009;15:2887–2892.

27. Kerckhoffs AP, Ben-Amor K, Samsom M, et al. Molecular analysis of faecal and duodenal samples reveals significantly higher prevalence and numbers of *Pseudomonas aeruginosa* in irritable bowel syndrome. *J Med Microbiol.* 2011;60:236–245.

28. Wacklin P, Kaukinen K, Tuovinen E, et al. The duodenal microbiota composition of adult celiac disease patients is associated with the clinical manifestation of the disease. *Inflamm Bowel Dis.* 2013;19:934–941.

29. Sartor RB. Microbial influences in inflammatory bowel diseases. *Gastroenterology.* 2008;134:577–594.

30. Guarner F. What is the role of the enteric commensal flora in IBD? *Inflamm Bowel Dis.* 2008;14(suppl 2):S83–S84.

31. Manichanh C, Borruel N, Casellas F, Guarner F. The gut microbiota in IBD. *Nat Rev Gastroenterol Hepatol.* 2012;9:599–608.

32. Venkatesh PG, Navaneethan U, Shen B. Hepatobiliary disorders and complications of inflammatory bowel disease. *J Dig Dis.* 2011;12:245–256.

33. Bernstein CN, Blanchard JF, Rawsthorne P, Yu N. The prevalence of extraintestinal diseases in inflammatory bowel disease: a population-based study. *Am J Gastroenterol.* 2001;96:1116–1122.

34. Loftus Jr EV, Sandborn WJ, Lindor KD, Larusso NF. Interactions between chronic liver disease and inflammatory bowel disease. *Inflamm Bowel Dis.* 1997;3:288–302.

35. Karlsen TH. Primary sclerosing cholangitis: 50 years of a gut-liver relationship and still no love? *Gut.* 2016;65:1579–1581.

36. Jones HF, Davidson GP, Brooks DA, Butler RN. Is small-bowel bacterial overgrowth an underdiagnosed disorder in children with gastrointestinal symptoms? *J Pediatr Gastroenterol Nutr.* 2011;52:632–634.

37. Romagnuolo J, Schiller D, Bailey RJ. Using breath tests wisely in a gastroenterology practice: an evidence-based review of indications and pitfalls in interpretation. *Am J Gastroenterol.* 2002;97:1113–1126.

38. Gasbarrini A, Corazza GR, Gasbarrini G, et al. Methodology and indications of H2-breath testing in gastrointestinal diseases: the Rome Consensus Conference. *Aliment Pharmacol Ther.* 2009;29(suppl 1):1–49.

39. Bjorneklett A, Jenssen E. Relationships between hydrogen (H2) and methane (CH4) production in man. *Scand J Gastroenterol.* 1982;17:985–992.

40. Eckburg PB, Bik EM, Bernstein CN, et al. Diversity of the human intestinal microbial flora. *Science.* 2005;308:1635–1638.

41. Zoetendal EG, Rajilic-Stojanovic M, de Vos WM. High-throughput diversity and functionality analysis of the gastrointestinal tract microbiota. *Gut.* 2008;57:1605–1615.

42. Gevers D, Kugathasan S, Denson LA, et al. The treatment-naive microbiome in new-onset Crohn's disease. *Cell Host Microbe.* 2014;15:382–392.

43. Gorkiewicz G, Thallinger GG, Trajanoski S, et al. Alterations in the colonic microbiota in response to osmotic diarrhea. *PLoS One.* 2013;8:e55817.

44. Li G, Yang M, Zhou K, et al. Diversity of duodenal and rectal microbiota in biopsy tissues and luminal contents in healthy volunteers. *J Microbiol Biotechnol.* 2015;25:1136–1145.

45. Sundin J, Rangel I, Fuentes S, et al. Altered faecal and mucosal microbial composition in post-infectious irritable bowel syndrome patients correlates with mucosal lymphocyte phenotypes and psychological distress. *Aliment Pharmacol Ther.* 2015;41:342–351.

46. Kerlin P, Wong L. Breath hydrogen testing in bacterial overgrowth of the small intestine. *Gastroenterology.* 1988;95:982–988.

47. Metz G, Gassull MA, Drasar BS, Jenkins DJ, Blendis LM. Breath-hydrogen test for small-intestinal bacterial colonisation. *Lancet (Lond Engl).* 1976;1:668–669.

48. Rhodes JM, Middleton P, Jewell DP. The lactulose hydrogen breath test as a diagnostic test for small-bowel bacterial overgrowth. *Scand J Gastroenterol.* 1979;14:333–336.

49. Plaut AG, Gorbach SL, Nahas L, Weinstein L, Spanknebel G, Levitan R. Studies of intestinal microflora. 3. The microbial flora of human small intestinal mucosa and fluids. *Gastroenterology.* 1967;53:868–873.

50. Bardhan PK, Gyr K, Beglinger C, Vogtlin J, Frey R, Vischer W. Diagnosis of bacterial overgrowth after culturing proximal small-bowel aspirate obtained during routine upper gastrointestinal endoscopy. *Scand J Gastroenterol.* 1992;27:253–256.

51. Leon-Barua R, Gilman RH, Rodriguez C, et al. Comparison of three methods to obtain upper small bowel contents for culture. *Am J Gastroenterol.* 1993;88:925–928.

52. Hamilton I, Worsley BW, Cobden I, Cooke EM, Shoesmith JG, Axon AT. Simultaneous culture of saliva and jejunal aspirate in the investigation of small bowel bacterial overgrowth. *Gut.* 1982;23:847–853.

53. Husebye E, Skar V, Hoverstad T, Melby K. Fasting hypochlorhydria with gram positive gastric flora is highly prevalent in healthy old people. *Gut.* 1992;33:1331–1337.

54. Holt PR, Rosenberg IH, Russell RM. Causes and consequences of hypochlorhydria in the elderly. *Dig Dis Sci.* 1989;34:933–937.

55. Lipski PS, Kelly PJ, James OF. Bacterial contamination of the small bowel in elderly people: is it necessarily pathological? *Age Ageing.* 1992;21:5–12.

56. MacMahon M, Lynch M, Mullins E, et al. Small intestinal bacterial overgrowth–an incidental finding? *J Am Geriatr Soc.* 1994;42:146–149.

57. Saltzman JR, Kowdley KV, Pedrosa MC, et al. Bacterial overgrowth without clinical malabsorption in elderly hypochlorhydric subjects. *Gastroenterology.* 1994;106:615–623.

58. Riordan SM, McIver CJ, Duncombe VM, Bolin TD. Bacteriologic analysis of mucosal biopsy specimens for detecting small-intestinal bacterial overgrowth. *Scand J Gastroenterol.* 1995;30:681–685.

59. King CE, Toskes PP. Small intestine bacterial overgrowth. *Gastroenterology.* 1979;76:1035–1055.

60. Hamilton JD, Dyer NH, Dawson AM, et al. Assessment and significance of bacterial overgrowth in the small bowel. *Q J Med.* 1970;39:265–285.

61. Omoike IU, Abiodun PO. Upper small intestinal microflora in diarrhea and malnutrition in Nigerian children. *J Pediatr Gastroenterol Nutr.* 1989;9:314–321.

62. Bode JC, Bode C, Heidelbach R, Durr HK, Martini GA. Jejunal microflora in patients with chronic alcohol abuse. *Hepato-Gastroenterology.* 1984;31:30–34.

63. Bohm M, Siwiec RM, Wo JM. Diagnosis and management of small intestinal bacterial overgrowth. *Nutr Clin Pract.* 2013;28:289–299.

64. Jacobs C, Coss Adame E, Attaluri A, Valestin J, Rao S. Dysmotility and ppi use are independent risk factors for small intestinal bacterial and/or fungal overgrowth. *Aliment Pharmacol Ther.* 2013;37:1103–1111.

65. Walker MM, Talley NJ. Review article: bacteria and pathogenesis of disease in the upper gastrointestinal tract–beyond the era of *Helicobacter pylori*. *Aliment Pharmacol Ther.* 2014;39:767–779.

66. Erdogan A, Rao SS. Small intestinal fungal overgrowth. *Curr Gastroenterol Rep.* 2015;17:16.

67. Tabaqchali S. The pathophysiological role of small intestinal bacterial flora. *Scand J Gastroenterol Suppl.* 1970;6:139–163.

68. Tillman R, King C, Toskes P. Continued experience with the xylose breath test-evidence that the small bowel culture as the gold standard for bacterial overgrowth may Be Tarnished. In: *Gastroenterology: WB Saunders Co-Elsevier Inc 1600 John F Kennedy Boulevard, Ste 1800, Philadelphia, PA 19103-2899 USA.* 1981:1304.

69. Lin HC. Small intestinal bacterial overgrowth: a framework for understanding irritable bowel syndrome. *J Am Med Assoc.* 2004;292.

70. Fan X, Sellin JH. Review article: small intestinal bacterial overgrowth, bile acid malabsorption and gluten intolerance as possible causes of chronic watery diarrhoea. *Aliment Pharmacol Ther.* 2009;29:1069–1077.

71. Chandra S, Dutta U, Noor MT, et al. Endoscopic jejunal biopsy culture: a simple and effective method to study jejunal microflora Indian. *J Gastroenterol.* 2010;29:226–230.

72. Shanahan ER, Zhong L, Talley NJ, Morrison M, Holtmann G. Characterisation of the gastrointestinal mucosa-associated microbiota: a novel technique to prevent cross-contamination during endoscopic procedures. *Aliment Pharmacol Ther.* 2016;43:1186–1196.

73. Peled Y, Weinberg D, Hallak A, Gilat T. Factors affecting methane production in humans. Gastrointestinal diseases and alterations of colonic flora. *Dig Dis Sci.* 1987;32:267–271.

74. McKay LF, Eastwood MA, Brydon WG. Methane excretion in man–a study of breath, flatus, and Faeces. *Gut.* 1985;26:69–74.

75. Melcher EA, Levitt MD, Slavin JL. Methane production and bowel function parameters in healthy subjects on low- and high-fiber diets. *Nutr Cancer.* 1991;16:85–92.

76. Levitt MD, Furne JK, Kuskowski M, Ruddy J. Stability of human methanogenic flora over 35 years and a review of insights obtained from breath methane measurements. *Clin Gastroenterol Hepatol.* 2006;4:123–129.

77. Miller TL, Wolin MJ. Enumeration of Methanobrevibacter smithii in human feces. *Arch Microbiol.* 1982;131:14–18.

78. Weaver GA, Krause JA, Miller TL, Wolin MJ. Incidence of methanogenic bacteria in a sigmoidoscopy population: an association of methanogenic bacteria and diverticulosis. *Gut.* 1986;27:698–704.

79. Pochart P, Lemann F, Flourie B, Pellier P, Goderel I, Rambaud JC. Pyxigraphic sampling to enumerate methanogens and anaerobes in the right colon of healthy humans. *Gastroenterology.* 1993;105:1281–1285.

80. McKay LF, Holbrook WP, Eastwood MA. Methane and hydrogen production by human intestinal anaerobic bacteria. *Acta Pathol Microbiol Immunol Scand B.* 1982;90:257–260.

81. Attaluri A, Jackson M, Valestin J, Rao SS. Methanogenic flora is associated with altered colonic transit but not stool characteristics in constipation without IBS. *Am J Gastroenterol.* 2010;105:1407–1411.

82. Pimentel M, Chang C, Chua KS, et al. Antibiotic treatment of constipation-predominant irritable bowel syndrome. *Dig Dis Sci.* 2014;59:1278–1285.

83. Sahakian AB, Jee SR, Pimentel M. Methane and the gastrointestinal tract. *Dig Dis Sci.* 2010;55:2135–2143.

84. Bond Jr JH, Engel RR, Levitt MD. Factors influencing pulmonary methane excretion in man. An indirect method of studying the in situ metabolism of the methane-producing colonic bacteria. *J Exp Med.* 1971;133:572–588.

85. Levitt MD. Production and excretion of hydrogen gas in man. *N Engl J Med.* 1969;281:122–127.

86. Christman NT, Hamilton LH. A new chromatographic instrument for measuring trace concentrations of breath-hydrogen. *J Chromatogr.* 1982;229:259–265.

87. Riordan SM, McIver CJ, Duncombe VM, Bolin TD, Thomas MC. Factors influencing the 1-g 14C-D-xylose breath test for bacterial overgrowth. *Am J Gastroenterol.* 1995;90:1455–1460.

88. Corazza GR, Strocchi A, Gasbarrini G. Fasting breath hydrogen in celiac disease. *Gastroenterology.* 1987;93:53–58.

89. Kerlin P, Wong L, Harris B, Capra S. Rice flour, breath hydrogen, and Malabsorption. *Gastroenterology.* 1984;87:578–585.

90. Riordan SM, McIver CJ, Bolin TD, Duncombe VM. Fasting breath hydrogen concentrations in gastric and small-intestinal bacterial overgrowth. *Scand J Gastroenterol.* 1995;30:252–257.

91. Valdovinos MA, Camilleri M, Thomforde GM, Frie C. Reduced accuracy of 14C-D-xylose breath test for detecting bacterial overgrowth in gastrointestinal motility disorders. *Scand J Gastroenterol.* 1993;28:963–968.

92. Rumessen JJ, Gudmand-Hoyer E, Bachmann E, Justesen T. Diagnosis of bacterial overgrowth of the small intestine. Comparison of the 14C-D-xylose breath test and jejunal cultures in 60 patients Scandinavian. *J Gastroenterol.* 1985;20:1267–1275.

93. Sellin JH, Hart R. Glucose malabsorption associated with rapid intestinal transit. *Am J Gastroenterol.* 1992;87:584–589.

94. Strocchi A, Corazza G, Ellis CJ, Gasbarrini G, Levitt MD. Detection of malabsorption of low doses of carbohydrate: accuracy of various breath H2 criteria. *Gastroenterology.* 1993;105:1404–1410.

95. Thompson DG, Binfield P, De Belder A, O'Brien J, Warren S, Wilson M. Extra intestinal influences on exhaled breath hydrogen measurements during the investigation of gastrointestinal disease. *Gut.* 1985;26:1349–1352.

96. Kerlin P, Phillips S. Differential transit of liquids and solid residue through the human ileum. *Am J Physiol.* 1983;245:G38–G43.

97. Metz G, Drasar BS, Gassull MA, Jenkins DJA, Blendis LM. Breath-hydrogen test for small-intestinal bacterial colonisation. *Lancet.* 1976;307:668–669.

98. Bond Jr JH, Levitt MD. Use of pulmonary hydrogen (H 2) measurements to quantitate carbohydrate absorption. Study of partially gastrectomized patients. *J Clin Investig.* 1972;51:1219–1225.

99. Saad RJ, Chey WD. Breath testing for small intestinal bacterial overgrowth: maximizing test accuracy. *Clin Gastroenterol Hepatol.* 2014;12:1964–1972; quiz e119–e120.

100. Pimentel M. Breath testing for small intestinal bacterial overgrowth: should we bother? *Am J Gastroenterol.* 2016;111:307–308.

101. King CE, Toskes PP. Comparison of the 1-gram [14C] xylose, 10-gram lactulose-H2, and 80-gram glucose-H2 breath tests in patients with small intestine bacterial overgrowth. *Gastroenterology.* 1986;91:1447–1451.

102. Hirakawa M, Iida M, Kohrogi N, Fujishima M. Hydrogen breath test assessment of orocecal transit time: comparison with barium meal study. *Am J Gastroenterol.* 1988;83:1361–1363.

103. Kristensen M, Hoeck HC. Abnormal flora in the small intestine. Diagnostic evaluation of the H2 breath test. *Ugeskr Laeger.* 1994;156:7530–7533.

104. Sadik R, Abrahamsson H, Stotzer PO. Gender differences in gut transit shown with a newly developed radiological procedure. *Scand J Gastroenterol.* 2003;38:36–42.

105. Riordan SM, McIver CJ, Walker BM, Duncombe VM, Bolin TD, Thomas MC. The lactulose breath hydrogen test and small intestinal bacterial overgrowth. *Am J Gastroenterol.* 1996;91:1795–1803.

106. Walters B, Vanner SJ. Detection of bacterial overgrowth in IBS using the lactulose H2 breath test: comparison with 14C-D-xylose and healthy controls. *Am J Gastroenterol.* 2005;100:1566–1570.

107. Bond Jr JH, Levitt MD, Prentiss R. Investigation of small bowel transit time in man utilizing pulmonary hydrogen (H2) measurements. *J Lab Clin Med.* 1975;85:546–555.

108. Pimentel M, Chow EJ, Lin HC. Eradication of small intestinal bacterial overgrowth reduces symptoms of irritable bowel syndrome. *Am J Gastroenterol.* 2000;95:3503–3506.

109. Pimentel M, Chow EJ, Lin HC. Normalization of lactulose breath testing correlates with symptom improvement in irritable bowel syndrome. a double-blind, randomized, placebo-controlled study. *Am J Gastroenterol.* 2003;98:412–419.

110. Pimentel M, Wallace D, Hallegua D, et al. A link between irritable bowel syndrome and fibromyalgia may be related to findings on lactulose breath testing. *Ann Rheum Dis.* 2004;63:450–452.

111. Nucera G, Gabrielli M, Lupascu A, et al. Abnormal breath tests to lactose, fructose and sorbitol in irritable bowel syndrome may be explained by small intestinal bacterial overgrowth. *Aliment Pharmacol Ther.* 2005;21:1391–1395.

112. Connolly L, Chang L. Combined orocecal scintigraphy and lactulose hydrogen breath testing demonstrate that breath testing detects orocecal transit, not small intestinal bacterial overgrowth in patients with irritable bowel syndrome. *Gastroenterology.* 2011;141:1118–1121.

113. Savage DC. Microbial ecology of the gastrointestinal tract. *Annu Rev Microbiol.* 1977;31:107–133.

114. O'Hara AM, Shanahan F. The gut flora as a forgotten organ. *EMBO Rep.* 2006;7:688–693.

115. Swidsinski A, Loening-Baucke V, Lochs H, Hale LP. Spatial organization of bacterial flora in normal and inflamed intestine: a fluorescence in situ hybridization study in mice. *World J Gastroenterol.* 2005;11:1131–1140.

116. Sekirov I, Russell SL, Antunes LCM, Finlay BB. Gut microbiota in health and disease. *Physiol Rev.* 2010;90:859–904.

117. Yang I, Nell S, Suerbaum S. Survival in hostile territory: the microbiota of the stomach. *FEMS Microbiol Rev.* 2013;37:736–761.

118. Phillips SF, Quigley EM, Kumar D, Kamath PS. Motility of the ileocolonic junction. *Gut.* 1988;29:390–406.

119. Roland BC, Ciarleglio MM, Clarke JO, et al. Low ileocecal valve pressure is significantly associated with small intestinal bacterial overgrowth (SIBO). *Dig Dis Sci.* 2014;59:1269–1277.

120. Husebye E. The pathogenesis of gastrointestinal bacterial overgrowth. *Chemotherapy.* 2005;51(suppl 1):1–22.

121. Gorbach SL, Plaut AG, Nahas L, Weinstein L, Spanknebel G, Levitan R. Studies of intestinal microflora. II. Microorganisms of the small intestine and their relations to oral and fecal flora. *Gastroenterology.* 1967;53:856–867.

122. Drasar BS, Shiner M, McLeod GM. Studies on the intestinal flora. I. The bacterial flora of the gastrointestinal tract in healthy and achlorhydric persons. *Gastroenterology.* 1969;56:71–79.

123. Drasar BS, Shiner M. Studies on the intestinal flora. II. Bacterial flora of the small intestine in patients with gastrointestinal disorders. *Gut.* 1969;10:812–819.

124. Finegold SM, Attebery HR, Sutter VL. Effect of diet on human fecal flora: comparison of Japanese and American diets. *Am J Clin Nutr.* 1974;27:1456–1469.

125. Simon GL, Gorbach SL. Intestinal flora in health and disease. *Gastroenterology.* 1984;86:174–193.

126. Hill MJ, Drasar BS. The normal colonic bacterial flora. *Gut.* 1975;16:318–323.

127. Simon GL, Gorbach SL. The human intestinal microflora. *Dig Dis Sci.* 1986;31:147S–62S.

128. Dominguez-Bello MG, Costello EK, Contreras M, et al. Delivery mode shapes the acquisition and structure of the initial microbiota across multiple body habitats in newborns. *Proc Natl Acad Sci USA.* 2010;107:11971–11975.

129. Edwards CA, Parrett AM. Intestinal flora during the first months of life: new perspectives. *Br J Nutr.* 2002;88(suppl 1):S11–S18.

130. Claesson MJ, Jeffery IB, Conde S, et al. Gut microbiota composition correlates with diet and health in the elderly. *Nature.* 2012;488:178–184.

131. Odamaki T, Kato K, Sugahara H, et al. Age-related changes in gut microbiota composition from newborn to centenarian: a cross-sectional study. *BMC Microbiol.* 2016;16:90.

132. Bäckhed F, Roswall J, Peng Y, et al. Dynamics and stabilization of the human gut microbiome during the first year of life. *Cell Host Microbe.* 2015;17:852.

133. Goodrich Julia K, Waters Jillian L, Poole Angela C, et al. Human genetics shape the gut microbiome. *Cell.* 2014;159:789–799.

134. Wang S, Charbonnier L-M, Noval Rivas M, et al. MyD88 adaptor-dependent microbial sensing by regulatory T cells promotes mucosal tolerance and enforces commensalism. *Immunity.* 2015;43:289–303.

135. David LA, Maurice CF, Carmody RN, et al. Diet rapidly and reproducibly alters the human gut microbiome. *Nature.* 2014;505:559–563.

136. Maurice Corinne F, Haiser Henry J, Turnbaugh Peter J. Xenobiotics shape the physiology and gene expression of the active human gut microbiome. *Cell.* 2013;152:39–50.

137. Cho I, Yamanishi S, Cox L, et al. Antibiotics in early life alter the murine colonic microbiome and adiposity. *Nature.* 2012;488:621–626.

138. Hsiao A, Ahmed AMS, Subramanian S, et al. Members of the human gut microbiota involved in recovery from Vibrio cholerae infection. *Nature.* 2014;515:423–426.

139. Thaiss Christoph A, Zeevi D, Levy M, et al. Transkingdom control of microbiota diurnal oscillations promotes metabolic homeostasis. *Cell.* 2014;159:514–529.

140. Fujimura KE, Demoor T, Rauch M, et al. House dust exposure mediates gut microbiome Lactobacillus enrichment and airway immune defense against allergens and virus infection. *Proc Natl Acad Sci USA.* 2014;111:805–810.

141. Wang YH, Gorvel JP, Chu YT, Wu JJ, Lei HY. *Helicobacter pylori* impairs murine dendritic cell responses to infection. *PLoS One.* 2010;5:e10844.

142. Paik CN, Choi MG, Lim CH, et al. The role of small intestinal bacterial overgrowth in postgastrectomy patients. *Neuro Gastroenterol Motil.* 2011;23:e191–e196.

143. Pyleris E, Giamarellos-Bourboulis EJ, Tzivras D, Koussoulas V, Barbatzas C, Pimentel M. The prevalence of overgrowth by aerobic bacteria in the small intestine by small bowel culture: relationship with irritable bowel syndrome. *Dig Dis Sci.* 2012;57:1321–1329.

144. Quigley EM. Small intestinal bacterial overgrowth: what it is and what it is not. *Curr Opin Gastroenterol.* 2014;30:141–146.

145. Abu-Shanab A, Quigley EM. Diagnosis of small intestinal bacterial overgrowth: the challenges persist!. *Expert Rev Gastroenterol Hepatol.* 2009;3:77–87.

146. Cole CR, Ziegler TR. Small bowel bacterial overgrowth: a negative factor in gut adaptation in pediatric SBS. *Curr Gastroenterol Rep.* 2007;9:456–462.

147. Bratten JR, Spanier J, Jones MP. Lactulose breath testing does not discriminate patients with irritable bowel syndrome from healthy controls. *Am J Gastroenterol.* 2008;103:958–963.

148. Scarpellini E, Giorgio V, Gabrielli M, et al. Prevalence of small intestinal bacterial overgrowth in children with irritable bowel syndrome: a case-control study. *J Pediatr.* 2009;155:416–420.

149. Park JS, Yu JH, Lim HC, et al. Usefulness of lactulose breath test for the prediction of small intestinal bacterial overgrowth in irritable bowel syndrome. *Korean J Gastroenterol.* 2010;56:242–248.

150. Zhao J, Zheng X, Chu H, et al. A study of the methodological and clinical validity of the combined lactulose hydrogen breath test with scintigraphic oro-cecal transit test for diagnosing small intestinal bacterial overgrowth in IBS patients. *Neuro Gastroenterol Motil.* 2014;26:794–802.

151. Rana SV, Sinha SK, Sikander A, Bhasin DK, Singh K. Study of small intestinal bacterial overgrowth in North Indian patients with irritable bowel syndrome: a case control study. *Trop Gastroenterol.* 2008;29:23–25.

152. Parodi A, Greco A, Savarino E, et al. Breath test be useful in diagnosis of IBS patients? An Italian study. In: *Gastroenterology: WB Saunders Co-Elsevier Inc 1600 John F Kennedy Boulevard, Ste 1800, Philadelphia, PA 19103-2899 USA.* May 2007:A192–A193.

153. Lombardo L, Foti M, Ruggia O, Chiecchio A. Increased incidence of small intestinal bacterial overgrowth during proton pump inhibitor therapy. *Clin Gastroenterol Hepatol.* 2010;8:504–508.

154. Sachdeva S, Rawat AK, Reddy RS, Puri AS. Small intestinal bacterial overgrowth (SIBO) in irritable bowel syndrome: frequency and predictors. *J Gastroenterol Hepatol.* 2011;26(suppl 3):135–138.

155. Lupascu A, Gabrielli M, Lauritano EC, et al. Hydrogen glucose breath test to detect small intestinal bacterial overgrowth: a prevalence case-control study in irritable bowel syndrome. *Aliment Pharmacol Ther.* 2005;22:1157–1160.

156. Posserud I, Stotzer PO, Bjornsson ES, Abrahamsson H, Simren M. Small intestinal bacterial overgrowth in patients with irritable bowel syndrome. *Gut.* 2007;56:802–808.

157. Choung RS, Ruff KC, Malhotra A, et al. Clinical predictors of small intestinal bacterial overgrowth by duodenal aspirate culture. *Aliment Pharmacol Ther.* 2011;33:1059–1067.

158. Giamarellos-Bourboulis EJ, Pyleris E, Barbatzas C, Pistiki A, Pimentel M. Small intestinal bacterial overgrowth is associated with irritable bowel syndrome and is independent of proton pump inhibitor usage. *BMC Gastroenterol.* 2016;16:67.

159. Ghoshal UC, Srivastava D, Ghoshal U, Misra A. Breath tests in the diagnosis of small intestinal bacterial overgrowth in patients with irritable bowel syndrome in comparison with quantitative upper gut aspirate culture. *Eur J Gastroenterol Hepatol.* 2014;26:753–760.

160. Shimura S, Ishimura N, Mikami H, et al. Small intestinal bacterial overgrowth in patients with refractory functional gastrointestinal disorders. *J Neurogastroenterol Motil.* 2016;22:60–68.

161. Costa MB, Azeredo Jr IL, Marciano RD, Caldeira LM, Bafutto M. Evaluation of small intestine bacterial overgrowth in patients with functional dyspepsia through H2 breath test. *Arq Gastroenterol.* 2012;49:279–283.

162. Rana SV, Sharma S, Malik A, et al. Small intestinal bacterial overgrowth and orocecal transit time in patients of inflammatory bowel disease. *Dig Dis Sci.* 2013;58:2594–2598.

163. Mishkin D, Boston FM, Blank D, Yalovsky M, Mishkin S. The glucose breath test: a diagnostic test for small bowel Stricture(s) in Crohn's disease. *Dig Dis Sci.* 2002;47:489–494.

164. Lee JM, Lee KM, Chung YY, et al. Clinical significance of the glucose breath test in patients with inflammatory bowel disease. *J Gastroenterol Hepatol.* 2015;30:990–994.

165. Rana SV, Sharma S, Kaur J, et al. Relationship of cytokines, oxidative stress and GI motility with bacterial overgrowth in ulcerative colitis patients. *J Crohn's Colitis.* 2014;8:859–865.

166. Sánchez-Montes C, Ortiz V, Bastida G, et al. Small intestinal bacterial overgrowth in inactive Crohn's disease: influence of thiopurine and biological treatment. *World J Gastroenterol.* 2014;20:13999–14003.

167. Rutgeerts P, Ghoos Y, Vantrappen G, Eyssen H. Ileal dysfunction and bacterial overgrowth in patients with Crohn's disease. *Eur J Clin Invest.* 1981;11:199–206.

168. Castiglione F, Del Vecchio Blanco G, Rispo A, et al. Orocecal transit time and bacterial overgrowth in patients with Crohn's disease. *J Clin Gastroenterol.* 2000;31:63–66.

169. Ricci JERJ, Chebli LA, Ribeiro T, et al. Small-intestinal bacterial overgrowth is associated with concurrent intestinal inflammation but not with systemic inflammation in Crohn's disease patients. *J Clin Gastroenterol.* 2018;52:530–536.

170. Klaus J, Spaniol U, Adler G, Mason RA, Reinshagen M, von Tirpitz CC. Small intestinal bacterial overgrowth mimicking acute flare as a pitfall in patients with Crohn's Disease. *BMC Gastroenterol.* 2009;9:61.

171. Rubio-Tapia A, Barton SH, Rosenblatt JE, Murray JA. Prevalence of small intestine bacterial overgrowth diagnosed by quantitative culture of intestinal aspirate in celiac disease. *J Clin Gastroenterol.* 2009;43:157–161.

172. Mooney PD, Evans KE, Sanders DS. Letter: coeliac disease and small intestinal bacterial overgrowth–is dysmotility the missing link? *Aliment Pharmacol Ther.* 2014;39:902–903.

173. Tursi A, Brandimarte G, Giorgetti G. High prevalence of small intestinal bacterial overgrowth in celiac patients with persistence of gastrointestinal symptoms after gluten withdrawal. *Am J Gastroenterol.* 2003;98:839–843.

174. George NS, Sankineni A, Parkman HP. Small intestinal bacterial overgrowth in gastroparesis. *Dig Dis Sci.* 2014;59:645–652.

175. Reddymasu SC, McCallum RW. Small intestinal bacterial overgrowth in gastroparesis: are there any predictors? *J Clin Gastroenterol.* 2010;44:e8–e13.

176. Sung HJ, Paik CN, Chung WC, Lee KM, Yang JM, Choi MG. Small intestinal bacterial overgrowth diagnosed by glucose hydrogen breath test in post-cholecystectomy patients. *J Neurogastroenterol Motil.* 2015;21:545–551.

177. Gutierrez IM, Kang KH, Calvert CE, et al. Risk factors for small bowel bacterial overgrowth and diagnostic yield of duodenal aspirates in children with intestinal failure: a retrospective review. *J Pediatr Surg.* 2012;47:1150–1154.

CHAPTER 7

Infections Associated With Irritable Bowel Syndrome

SAKTEESH V. GURUNATHAN, MD • MADHUSUDAN GROVER, MD

INTRODUCTION

Irritable bowel syndrome (IBS) is one of the most common gastrointestinal disorders in the United States and around the world. It is characterized by recurrent abdominal pain and irregular bowel habits and is defined using the Rome IV criteria (Table 7.1). The role of infections in the development of IBS, also referred to as postinfection IBS (PI-IBS), has been documented in the past but was first proposed by Chaudhary and Truelove in 1962.[1] In addition to PI-IBS, other functional gastrointestinal disorders (FGIDs) such as functional dyspepsia can also follow an episode of infectious gastroenteritis (IGE). Foodborne illness affects approximately one in six adults in the United States annually. Moreover, travel-associated diarrhea may impact up to 72 million individuals every year.[2,3] Additionally, military personnel deployed to the developing countries are particularly at an increased risk of IGE and development of PI-IBS. Studies show a wide-ranging prevalence of PI-IBS from 4% to 36%.[4] A systematic review and meta-analysis of ~21,000 patients with IGE followed up anywhere from 3 months to 10 years demonstrated that the risk of developing IBS increases fourfold after IGE as compared with unexposed individuals from the same population.[4,5] The IBS symptoms may persist for up to 8–10 years after the episode of IGE.[6] Owing to significant underreporting of IGE cases and often poor recall of the inciting IGE episode by the patient,[7] it is plausible that majority of IBS cases are postinfection in origin. In fact, mathematic modeling has predicted this to be the case.[8] Thus advancements in the understanding of PI-IBS will likely inform us about IBS in general.

Risk factors that are associated with the development of PI-IBS include female sex, younger age, psychiatric comorbidities, and severity of symptoms at the time of IGE.[4,6,10] We had limited insight about the natural history and mechanisms of PI-IBS until recently when there has been a progress in our mechanistic understanding of the clinical and molecular aspects of the disease. The available literature supports a role for epithelial, microbial, and immune factors in the pathophysiology of PI-IBS. Human studies have shown evidence of serotonergic dysfunction, impaired barrier function, and altered immune activation in the pathophysiologic condition of PI-IBS.[11] A few studies have reported altered levels of cytokines such as tumor necrosis factor (TNF)-α, interleukin IL-6, IL-8, IL-10, and IL-1β, suggesting that low-grade inflammation may play a role in the pathophysiologic condition of PI-IBS.[12]

PI-IBS usually presents as mixed (alternating diarrhea and constipation) IBS (IBS-M) or diarrhea-predominant IBS (IBS-D). As with IBS, the symptoms can be nonspecific, making it important to exclude other organic diagnoses, especially in the presence of alarm symptoms such as significant weight loss, nocturnal symptoms, and gastrointestinal bleeding.[13] A critical component of the PI-IBS management includes patient education on the role of infections in the subsequent development of chronic gastrointestinal symptoms. Patients with IBS incur significant expenditure, both direct health-related and through indirect causes such as work absenteeism. The cost is estimated to be around 25$ billion annually in the United States.[14]

TABLE 7.1
Rome IV Criteria for Diagnosis of Irritable Bowel Syndrome

Recurrent abdominal pain, on average, at least 1 day/week in the last 3 months, associated with two or more of the following criteria:
- Related to defecation
- Associated with a change in frequency of stool
- Associated with a change in form (appearance) of stool.

Criteria fulfilled for the last 3 months with symptom onset at least 6 months before diagnosis (Ref. 9)

Gastrointestinal Diseases and Their Associated Infections. https://doi.org/10.1016/B978-0-323-54843-4.00007-6
Copyright © 2019 Elsevier Inc. All rights reserved.

EPIDEMIOLOGY

Prevalence

In a meta-analysis, it was found that PI-IBS has an estimated pooled prevalence of 10% within 12 months of exposure to IGE and 14% in studies looking beyond 12 months.[4] This was similar to pooled incidence of 10% (95% confidence interval [CI], 9–85) in a previous meta-analysis.[5] The relative risk (RR) was 4 as compared with nonexposed individuals derived from the same population followed up over the same period.[4] The overall PI-IBS rate was found to be the highest with parasitic and protozoal infections (*Giardia lamblia*),[15,16] followed by bacterial (*Campylobacter jejuni, Shigella, Salmonella, and Escherichia coli* O157:H7) and viral (*Norovirus*) causes. However, within 12 months, viral infections seem to be associated with the highest prevalence, which decreases after 12 months suggesting that the PI-IBS due to viruses is a transient entity.[17] Norovirus is a major cause of food poisoning (55%), but it is a less common pathogen associated with the development of PI-IBS. Viral infections have not been associated with significant mucosal inflammation or alterations in gut microbiome, which could be the reason for the lesser incidence and shorter lasting nature of postviral IBS.

The definition of PI-IBS includes symptom onset following a clinically suspected or laboratory-proven episode of IGE. Certain pathogens have been associated with IBS state, such as *Blastocystis*[18–20] and *Brachyspira*.[21] These, however, have not been attributed to precede the onset of PI-IBS. In one study, high levels of IgG2 subclass antibodies to *Blastocystis* were found in the sera of patients with IBS, compared with healthy controls.[19] In a study of 388 patients, *Blastocystis* was recovered from 10% patients, half of whom fulfilled the Rome criteria for IBS.[18] However, in a subsequent study, no significantly higher prevalence of *Blastocystis hominis* infection was found in patients with IBS compared with healthy controls.[22] *Brachyspira* as the cause for intestinal spirochetosis was associated with higher prevalence of patients reporting IBS symptoms.[21] As with PI-IBS in general, these patients also had nonconstipation-predominant IBS.

RISK FACTORS

Gender and Age

Female sex is found to be an independent risk factor for the development of PI-IBS in many studies, with a pooled RR of 2 in a meta-analysis.[10,23–25] Some studies suggest a possibility of confounding, as females have higher prevalence of psychosocial disorders, which have also been associated with PI-IBS.[26–28] However, in a preponderance of the literature and after controlling for other risk factors, it was found that female sex is associated with higher odds of PI-IBS development.

Young age has been shown as an independent risk factor in several PI-IBS studies.[29–31] A study showed that age >60 years has a protective effect on the development of PI-IBS (RR, 0.4).[10] This is because elderly individuals have reduced immune activation and less inflammatory response to the infection. Additionally, IBS in general has higher prevalence in younger individuals. However, some of the other studies did not find a clear link between PI-IBS development and age.[28,32]

Psychological Factors

Psychological comorbidities such as anxiety, depression, somatization, hypochondriasis, adverse life events, and neuroticism at the time of infection are related to the development of PI-IBS.[4] We should also take into consideration a significant heterogeneity in studies for some of the psychosocial variables such as anxiety ($I^2 = 90\%$).[4] Another study showed that negative illness perception during IGE is associated with the development of PI-IBS.[33] Although some studies suggest that somatization and neuroticism specifically at the time of initial illness are related to the development of PI-IBS (odds ratio [OR], 4 and 3, respectively).[26,34] Gwee et al.[26] showed that the scores obtained from psychometric analysis from patients with PI-IBS remained stable even 3 months after IGE and thus can influence disease presentation .

Genetic Factors

A study done on the Walkerton outbreak cohort identified single nucleotide variants in the genes *CDH1, TLR9, and IL6* as risk factors, independent of other clinical factors, for the development of PI-IBS.[35] Toll-like receptor 9 (*TLR9*) serves as a receptor for unmethylated CpG dinucleotides, a marker of bacterial DNA, and their inflammation, while *CDH1* codes for E-cadherin, a tight junction protein in the intestinal epithelium that modulates the permeability. However, when controlled for all the single nucleotide polymorphisms studied, these did not withstand statistical significance. A study by Swan et al. showed[36] that genetic polymorphisms in TNFSF15 and TNF-α are associated with IBS-D and PI-IBS .

Role of Antibiotics

Prolonged use of antibiotics during IGE can be a predisposition for PI-IBS development.[28,37,38] One study showed that the use of more than five antibiotics after an episode of IGE has a twofold increased risk of PI-IBS compared with not receiving any antibiotics.[29] Based on seven studies, antibiotic use at the time of IGE is associated with increased risk of developing PI-IBS.[25,29,38-41] Prolonged use of antibiotics could be a marker of disease severity, which has been associated with PI-IBS, and can perhaps confound the association of antibiotic use with PI-IBS development. Additionally, some of the studies highlighting antibiotic use as a risk factor are based on a small proportion of patients with IGE treated with antibiotics.[28,38]

Smoking

Two studies found that smoking does not increase the risk of PI-IBS.[29,39] However, in a third study, it was found to be significantly associated with the development of PI-IBS (OR, 5).[42] Smoking might have an indirect effect, as it is a marker of neuroticism ,[43] which is known to be a risk factor for PI-IBS.[26,44]

Enteritis-Associated Factors

In several studies, clinical symptoms such as abdominal pain, diarrhea for >7 days, bloody stools, abdominal cramps, and weight loss (of ≥4.5 kg) were found to be associated with the development of PI-IBS.[24,38-40] But in a few other studies, fever and weight loss were not found to be significantly associated with PI-IBS.[23,30,31] A meta-analysis found that 9 out of 15 studies showed abdominal pain as one of the significant risk factors in the development of PI-IBS (OR, 3; 95% CI, 1-8).[17,24,40,45] Based on eight studies, diarrhea for more than 7 days was found to be positively associated to PI-IBS (OR, 3; 95% CI, 1-5).[10,24,31,32,38-40,46] Four studies showed that bloody stool was associated with increased odds in the development of PI-IBS (OR, 2; 95% CI, 1-3).[24,38-40] A study done for 3 months following viral gastroenteritis showed that in univariate logistic regression, emesis, duration of abdominal pain, duration of fever, weight loss, and mucus in stool were found to be associated with increased risk with the development of IBS.[17] However, in multiple logistic regression, it was found that only emesis is a significant positive predictor of IBS (OR, 10).[17] In summary, several clinical markers of IGE severity have been associated with the subsequent development of PI-IBS. This may reflect greater pathogen injury or amplified host response during IGE to cause molecular changes that predict downstream development of chronic gastrointestinal dysfunction seen in PI-IBS.

PATHOPHYSIOLOGY

Immune Activation

Studies showing altered population of immune cells in patients with PI-IBS suggest a role for immune dysregulation in PI-IBS.

Enterochromaffin Cell Hyperplasia

Enterochromaffin cells are found in the mucosa lining the digestive tract. These cells form an integral part of the enteric nervous system, as they modulate the neuronal signaling by secreting the neurotransmitter serotonin (also called 5-hydroxytryptamine [5-HT]), which also regulates the secretion and motility in the gut. In a study done on patients following *C. jejuni* enteritis, patients with persistent loose stools had an increased number of enterochromaffin cells, CD3, and intraepithelial lymphocytes in their rectal biopsies. While the number of serotonin-containing enterochromaffin cells were increased both initially and at 12 weeks, peptide YY–positive enteroendocrine L cell count was elevated initially but returned back to normal at 12 weeks.[47] Persistent enterochromaffin cell hyperplasia was also seen in another study done on patients with IBS 3 months following *C. jejuni* enteritis.[27] The putative role of serotonergic dysregulation was also seen in a mouse model study of *Citrobacter rodentium*, a model of enteropathogenic *E. coli* infection, but with contrasting results. There was evidence of reduced levels of 5-HT and somatostatin-positive enteroendocrine cells 10 days following infection, which returned to baseline at 30 days. This was accompanied by changes in inducible nitric oxide synthase immunoreactivity and the changes were not seen in an immunodeficient mouse.[48] Postprandial serotonin levels were found to be elevated in patients with PI-IBS.[47,49,50]

Inflammatory Cytokines

Counts of intraepithelial lymphocytes and T lymphocytes (CD3, CD4, CD8) were found to be increased on serial rectal biopsies obtained from patients who had *C. jejuni* enteritis. The elevated levels of these cells could last for several months after infection[27,47] and have been considered as independent predictors of PI-IBS.[27] IL-1β is an important proinflammatory cytokine that is released by lymphocytes and macrophages. There is an increased expression of IL-1β messenger RNA in the terminal ileum and rectosigmoid colon in patients with post-*Shigella* IBS as compared with disease controls.[32,51] TNF-α, IL-6, and IL-8 are the other proinflammatory mediators whose levels were found to be elevated in PI-IBS.[52] There is also an evidence of psychological stress being associated with increased levels of IL-6 and IL-1β, which reflects the complex interaction between central and peripheral factors.[53,54]

Mast Cell Activation

Mast cells play a prominent role in the immune response and mucosal injury, and their cell counts were found to be elevated in patients with post-*Shigella* IBS.[32] Another study revealed that while mast cell numbers remain the same, there is an increase in activated mast cells, mast cell area, and tryptase concentration among patients with PI-IBS.[55] Proximity of mast cells to the enteric nerves has been related to the intensity of abdominal pain in patients with IBS (not specified as PI-IBS).[56]

Impaired Barrier Function

The intestinal barrier is made up of immunologic and nonimmunologic components such as mucous coat, epithelial tight junctions, and antimicrobial metabolites secreted by the enteric flora.[57,58] An increase in the intestinal permeability allows luminal antigens to enter the mucosa and in turn incite an inflammatory response.[57] In a study where patients with post-*Campylobacter* IBS are compared with the controls, the in vivo permeability assessed by lactulose/mannitol (L/M) excretion ratio was increased immediately after infection and at 12 weeks.[47] In the Walkerton study, it was shown that L/M ratio was increased significantly in the PI-IBS group compared with the control group, and among the PI-IBS group, the patients who had increased intestinal permeability also had concurrent increase in the stool frequency.[59]

MOLECULAR CHANGES ASSOCIATED WITH PATHOGENS CAUSING POSTINFECTION IRRITABLE BOWEL SYNDROME

Campylobacter jejuni

C. jejuni is one of the most common causes of foodborne illness and has been repeatedly associated with the development of PI-IBS. The primary reservoir of the organism is poultry and the transmission mainly takes place through consumption of raw or undercooked meat.[60] The important virulent factors are the flagella, adhesion and binding factors, toxins such as cytolethal distending toxin (CDT), microtubule- and/or microfilament-dependent epithelial cell invasion, and chemokine induction (IL-8).[61] In rat models, CDT has been associated with chronic altered bowel patterns, chronic rectal inflammation, and chronic reduction of interstitial cells of Cajal, the pacemaker cells in the gut, which can be reversed with antibiotic treatment.[62] Extraintestinal sequelae include the Guillain-Barré syndrome and reactive arthritis (especially in human leukocyte antigen-B27–predisposed individuals). Molecular mimicry between neuronal GM-1 and GD-1a gangliosides and *C. jejuni* lipooligosaccharide is the basis for the axonal degeneration in Guillain-Barré syndrome.[61] It has been found that the bacterial IGE might be a factor of initiation or exacerbation of inflammatory bowel disease (IBD) (Crohn disease > ulcerative colitis) as well.[37]

Shigella

Shigella is one of the common pathogens that is associated with bacterial dysentery. In a study done on patients with shigellosis, it was found that the duration of diarrhea during acute illness is an independent risk factor.[31] Increased density of neuron-specific enolase, increase in 5-HT-immunoreactive (ir) nerve clustering adjacent to mast cells, and increases in levels of ileal mast cells, substance P, 5-HT–containing enterochromaffin cells, peptide YY–containing L cells, intraepithelial lymphocytes, CD3 lymphocytes, CD8 lymphocytes, mast cells, and CD68-ir macrophages were also seen.[32,63]

Norovirus

Norwalk-like viruses accounts for more than half of the foodborne illness in the United States.[64] It is a shorter lasting illness than bacterial enteritis. Individuals with FUT-2 gene are susceptible to norovirus gastroenteritis but those without the H type 1 oligosaccharide ligand are resistant to infection, as that seems to affect the binding.[65] Under light microscopy, partial villous flattening, villous broadening, and disorganization of intestinal epithelial cells can be noticed. Under electron microscopy, infiltration of lamina propria by mononuclear cells, increase in numbers of multivesiculate bodies, widening of intercellular spaces, and attenuated activity of brush border enzymes are seen.[66,67] The above changes undergo recovery in 2 weeks, which may explain the short-lasting nature of postviral IBS.

Giardia

Giardia has been shown to cause several pathophysiologic effects such as caspase-dependent enterocyte apoptosis, disruption of epithelial tight junction, villous atrophy, activation of signal transduction pathways, anion hypersecretion, intestinal hypermotility, intestinal fluid accumulation, loss of intestinal brush border surface area, increased disaccharidase activity, and increase in the villus/crypt ratios.[68–71] In a study done 6 years after the exposure, it was found that 39% of cases exposed to giardiasis had IBS compared with the control group (12%).[15] However, chronic giardiasis or postinfection lactose intolerance can cause symptoms that mimic PI-IBS and results from studies that do not exclude them need to be interpreted with caution.

Blastocystis

B. hominis is a common intestinal inhabitant in humans. It is known to colonize the large intestine and is found in both symptomatic and asymptomatic individuals. However, when present in high numbers, it has been associated with abdominal pain, diarrhea, and other nonspecific abdominal symptoms.[72,73] The mechanisms involved in intestinal infection are adhesion and binding, lysis, and the presence of toxin.[74] Although *Blastocystis* is known to increase IL-8 gene expression in human colonic epithelial cells in vitro and to cause barrier disruption and degradation of intestinal IgA,[75,76] it is not determined whether it causes IBS via a direct mechanism or its presence in patients with IBS reflects a favorable luminal environment for the parasite to thrive.

Brachyspira

Brachyspira species such as *Brachyspira aalborgi*, *Brachyspira pilosicoli*, and *Brachyspira hominis* are known to cause human intestinal spirochetosis.[77,78] Although the mechanism by which it causes enteric illness is unclear, it is known to colonize the epithelial cells of the colon by characteristic apical attachment. A study showed that *B. pilosicoli* was associated with inflammatory changes in the human colon.[79] The study by Walker et al.[21] found that brachyspira infection was associated with a threefold increased higher odds of presence of IBS .

CLINICAL FEATURES

The most predominant phenotype associated with PI-IBS is IBS-M, followed by IBS-D, and rarely IBS-constipation. The predominant symptoms being increased frequency of bowel movements, presence of looser stools, and increased urgency. Neal et al.[10] showed that a significant number of people complain of mucus in stool and abdominal bloating as well . Presence of abdominal discomfort and pain is required to classify a patient as having PI-IBS; however, a subset of patients complain of altered bowel function without significant issues with abdominal discomfort. These patients may fulfill the criteria for postinfection functional diarrhea. Psychosocial comorbidities such as fatigue and depression are commonly present in patients with IBS.[80]

Diagnosis

The diagnosis of PI-IBS is made by using symptom-based Rome criteria (Table 7.1). Hence, a proper assessment of the patient's history is warranted. The patient should not meet the diagnostic criteria of IBS prior to the episode of acute IGE.[81] The episode of acute IGE is characterized either by a positive stool culture result or by the presence of two or more of the following clinical features: diarrhea, fever, and vomiting.[82] To exclude other organic causes, a complete physical assessment and an initial set of investigations such as complete blood count, inflammatory markers such as C-reactive protein, and celiac serologic testing should be considered. Stool examination for ova and parasites is recommended, especially in cases following protozoal or parasitic infections. Stool culture and polymerase chain reaction results for ongoing bacterial or viral IGE is often negative and is not warranted. Endoscopic tests may be relevant for patients with a family history of colonic cancer or other alarm symptoms such as intestinal bleeding and weight loss.[83] The risk of missing an organic cause is rare when the symptom-based Rome IV criteria are met, the basic testing result is negative, and the alarm symptoms are not present.[84]

For refractory diarrhea the following tests are recommended: screening for 48-h stool volume and fat, electrolytes, and laxatives; jejunal aspirates for small intestinal bacterial overgrowth; and colonic biopsies for microscopic colitis.[84] Patients who have complaints of postprandial abdominal bloating should be considered for hydrogen or lactose breath test to rule out small intestinal bacterial overgrowth and lactose intolerance, respectively.[84]

In an animal model, antibodies to *CdtB* cross-react with antibodies to vinculin in the host gut leading to an IBS-like phenotype.[85] A study that compared the patients who have IBS-D, IBD, and celiac disease showed that anti-*CdtB* and antivinculin titers were significantly higher in the IBS-D group ($P<.001$).[85] Although it is less specific in distinguishing IBS from celiac disease, it is useful in differentiating IBS from IBD.[85] Another study done at Mexico concluded that these tests (anti-*CdtB* and antivinculin) can be used as a first-line investigation to confirm IBS-D and IBS-M.[86,87] However, the difference between PI-IBS (71.4%) and non–PI-IBS (41.7%) was not statistically significant, making these a nonspecific marker for IBS-D but not a biomarker for PI-IBS.

Differential Diagnosis

IBD: IBD and IBS can share several clinical symptoms. IBD is also characterized by extraintestinal manifestations such as musculoskeletal symptoms, fatigue, and ophthalmologic symptoms.[88] IBD is more associated with complications such as fulminant colitis, toxic megacolon, perforation, stricture, and fistulas. Although IBS is much more common, the incidence and prevalence of IBD is increasing over time.[89]

Celiac disease: A study showed that there was significant association between IGE and the subsequent development of celiac disease with an OR of 2.[90] Other studies showed that 3%–4% of the patients with IBS had concurrent celiac disease.[91,92] Hence, it is beneficial to test for celiac disease in the workup of IBS, especially IBS-D.[92]

Nonceliac gluten sensitivity (NCGS): NCGS is more common than celiac disease but the diagnosis is difficult to make.[93] It is partly due to the nonspecific nature of the symptoms. The carbohydrate component of the antigen fructan is said to mediate the abdominal symptoms in NCGS.[94] Gluten-free diet significantly improves the abdominal symptoms.

Lactose intolerance: Most of the symptoms experienced in patients with IBS may be due to clinically undiagnosed lactose intolerance.[95] It is more prevalent in the Mediterranean population. Hence, testing for lactose intolerance and adherence to lactose-free diet in those who were tested positive are recommended, as they have been shown to resolve symptoms in more than 50% of the cases.[96] However, a study done on patients in northern England that tested for lactose intolerance in 24 PI-IBS cases found that lactose intolerance is not claimed to be the cause of their IBS symptoms.[97] Hence, avoidance of dairy products in the management of PI-IBS without any evidence of lactose intolerance is not recommended.[97]

Tropical sprue: Tropical sprue is one of the notable causes of postinfection malabsorption and the symptoms can mimic PI-IBS. Tropical sprue responds well to antibiotic treatment. Some have postulated an overlap in the clinical features between tropical sprue and PI-IBS.[98,99]

Bile acid malabsorption: Bile acid malabsorption has been reported following IGE.[100] Overproduction of bile acids or impaired reabsorption in the terminal ileum can promote excessive delivery into the colon, which can result in secretory diarrhea. Up to one-third of patients with IBS-D or functional diarrhea have evidence of bile acid malabsorption. The actual prevalence of bile acid malabsorption in PI-IBS is unknown. Bile acid diarrhea usually responds well to bile acid sequestering agents.[101,102]

Microscopic colitis: Microscopic colitis is a rare cause of chronic diarrhea. It usually presents with prolonged watery diarrhea and normal radiologic and gross endoscopic findings.[103] However, colonic biopsy is the method of diagnosis for this.[104] The pathogenesis can be due to an inflammatory response that follows an inciting luminal antigen, gluten, or drugs.[105] There is at least one case report of lymphocytic colitis following an episode of *C. jejuni* IGE.[106]

MANAGEMENT

The management of PI-IBS is similar to that of IBS in general. Lifestyle and dietary modification is the key treatment in most of the FGIDs, including IBS. The medications are usually tailored according to the predominant symptom and are reviewed in detail elsewhere.[107]

Opiates

Loperamide is a peripherally acting μ-receptor agonist prescribed to improve the stool frequency. Many studies have shown that opiates have a favorable profile in delaying the rapid intestinal transit.[108,109] However, it is less effective in controlling abdominal pain.[110] In fact, the main side effects of opiates are bloating and abdominal discomfort. Caution should be adopted for risk of constipation considering the IBS-M phenotype in most patients with PI-IBS.

Antispasmodics

Meta-analyses demonstrate the efficacy of anticholinergics like cimetropium bromide, pinaverium bromide, octylonium bromide, trimebutine, and mebeverine on improving the pain aspect of the disease.[111,112] The advantage of anticholinergics is that they can be used on an as-needed basis during episodes of pain.[111] Peppermint oil is another agent in this category that has been found to be effective in managing the pain.

Prednisolone

Prednisolone, 30 mg, once a day for 3 weeks was not found to be effective over placebo in reducing the symptoms of PI-IBS.[113] The enterochromaffin cell counts remained the same, although there was a significant reduction in T-lymphocyte counts in the lamina propria, which is presumed to be an anti-inflammatory effect. However, it was not associated with any improvement in abdominal pain and diarrhea.[113]

Mesalazine

A study showed that mesalazine is effective for both patients with PI-IBS and patients with non–PI-IBS. It significantly reduced stool frequency and abdominal pain and improved stool consistency.[114] However, a statistical difference between PI-IBS and non–PI-IBS could not be found. Another study showed that although mesalazine was not effective in overall IBS-D population when compared with placebo, the PI-IBS subgroup saw an improvement in bowel symptoms.[115] However, a pilot study of 17 patients with PI-IBS[116] and another study of IBS-D[117] showed negative results. An adequately powered double-blind and placebo-controlled study in PI-IBS is needed to examine the effects of mesalazine.

Rifaximin

There are two double-blinded, placebo-controlled trials, TARGET 1 and TARGET 2, that showed that rifaximin, when compared with placebo, had a statistically significant effect (40.8% vs. 31.2%, $P = .01$ in TARGET 1; 40.6% vs. 32.2%, $P = .03$ in TARGET 2; 40.7% vs. 31.7%, $P < .001$ in the two studies combined) in reducing the symptoms in patients with IBS.[118] The effect is assessed by global relief of symptoms, bloating, abdominal pain, and stool consistency and the number needed to treat was close to 10. It is approved for treatment of IBS-D and can be used for selected cases with PI-IBS; however, it has not been studied specifically for patients with PI-IBS.

Psychotropics

Various classes of psychotropics have been tested in IBS. However, none of these trials have been in the PI-IBS population. These are extensively reviewed elsewhere.[119]

Psychological Treatment

Cognitive behavioral therapy and gut-directed hypnotherapy have been most widely studied in IBS. Drossman et al.[120] showed cognitive behavioral therapy is as effective as psychotropics for management of women with moderate to severe IBS . Studies show that the combination of medication and psychotherapy has superior outcomes in both short term and long term, improved healthcare, and is cost-effective.[121,122] Whitehead[123] reviewed 11 studies, which include 5 controlled trials, and found that hypnotherapy has positive outcomes on IBS symptoms even for those who are not satisfied with the medical therapy . None of the psychotherapies have been tested in the PI-IBS group.

REFERENCES

1. Chaudhary NA, Truelove SC. The irritable colon syndrome. A study of the clinical features, predisposing causes, and prognosis in 130 cases. *Q J Med.* 1962;31:307–322.
2. Kendall ME, Crim S, Fullerton K, et al. Travel-associated enteric infections diagnosed after return to the United States, foodborne diseases active surveillance network (FoodNet), 2004–2009. *Clin Infect Dis.* 2012;54(suppl 5):S480–S487.
3. LaRocque RC, Rao SR, Lee J, et al. Global TravEpiNet: a national consortium of clinics providing care to international travelers–analysis of demographic characteristics, travel destinations, and pretravel healthcare of high-risk US international travelers, 2009–2011. *Clin Infect Dis.* 2012;54(4):455–462.
4. Klem F, Wadhwa A, Prokop LJ, et al. Prevalence, risk factors, and outcomes of irritable bowel syndrome after infectious enteritis: a systematic review and meta-analysis. *Gastroenterology.* 2017;152(5):1042–1054.e1.
5. Thabane M, Kottachchi DT, Marshall JK. Systematic review and meta-analysis: the incidence and prognosis of post-infectious irritable bowel syndrome. *Aliment Pharmacol Ther.* 2007;26(4):535–544.
6. Marshall JK, Thabane M, Garg AX, Clark WF, Moayyedi P, Collins SM. Eight year prognosis of postinfectious irritable bowel syndrome following waterborne bacterial dysentery. *Gut.* 2010;59(5):605–611.
7. Majowicz SE, Edge VL, Fazil A, et al. Estimating the under-reporting rate for infectious gastrointestinal illness in Ontario. *Can J Public Health.* 2005;96(3):178–181.
8. Shah ED, Riddle MS, Chang C, Pimentel M. Estimating the contribution of acute gastroenteritis to the overall prevalence of irritable bowel syndrome. *J Neurogastroenterol Motil.* 2012;18(2):200–204.
9. Lacy BE, Mearin F, Chang L, et al. Bowel disorders. *Gastroenterology.* 2016;150(6):1393–1407. e5.
10. Neal KR, Hebden J, Spiller R. Prevalence of gastrointestinal symptoms six months after bacterial gastroenteritis and risk factors for development of the irritable bowel syndrome: postal survey of patients. *BMJ.* 1997;314(7083):779–782.
11. Thabane M, Marshall JK. Post-infectious irritable bowel syndrome. *World J Gastroenterol.* 2009;15(29):3591–3596.
12. Grover M, Camilleri M, Smith K, Linden DR, Farrugia G. On the fiftieth anniversary. Postinfectious irritable bowel syndrome: mechanisms related to pathogens. *Neuro Gastroenterol Motil.* 2014;26(2):156–167.
13. Vanner SJ, Depew WT, Paterson WG, et al. Predictive value of the Rome criteria for diagnosing the irritable bowel syndrome. *Am J Gastroenterol.* 1999;94(10):2912–2917.
14. Fullerton S. Functional digestive disorders (FDD) in the year 2000–economic impact. Supplement: = Acta chirurgica Supplement *Eur J Surg.* 1998:62–64. 582.
15. Hanevik K, Wensaas K-A, Rortveit G, Eide GE, Mørch K, Langeland N. Irritable bowel syndrome and chronic fatigue 6 Years after Giardia infection: a controlled prospective cohort study. *Clin Infect Dis.* 2014;59(10):1394–1400.

16. Wensaas K-A, Langeland N, Hanevik K, Mørch K, Eide GE, Rortveit G. Irritable bowel syndrome and chronic fatigue 3 years after acute giardiasis: historic cohort study. *Gut.* 2012;61(2):214–219.

17. Marshall JK, Thabane M, Borgaonkar MR, James C. Postinfectious irritable bowel syndrome after a food-borne outbreak of acute gastroenteritis attributed to a viral pathogen. *Clin Gastroenterol Hepatol.* 2007;5(4):457–460.

18. Giacometti A, Cirioni O, Fiorentini A, Fortuna M, Scalise G. Irritable bowel syndrome in patients with Blastocystis hominis infection. *Eur J Clin Microbiol Infect Dis.* 1999;18(6):436–439.

19. Hussain R, Jaferi W, Zuberi S, et al. Significantly increased IgG2 subclass antibody levels to Blastocystis hominis in patients with irritable bowel syndrome. *Am J Trop Med Hyg.* 1997;56(3):301–306.

20. Yakoob J, Jafri W, Jafri N, et al. Irritable bowel syndrome: in search of an etiology: role of Blastocystis hominis. *Am J Trop Med Hyg.* 2004;70(4):383–385.

21. Walker MM, Talley NJ, Inganas L, et al. Colonic spirochetosis is associated with colonic eosinophilia and irritable bowel syndrome in a general population in Sweden. *Hum Pathol.* 2015;46(2):277–283.

22. Tungtrongchitr A, Manatsathit S, Kositchaiwat C, et al. Blastocystis hominis infection in irritable bowel syndrome patients. *Southeast Asian J Trop Med Public Health.* 2004;35(3):705–710.

23. Moss-Morris R, Spence M. To "lump" or to "split" the functional somatic syndromes: can infectious and emotional risk factors differentiate between the onset of chronic fatigue syndrome and irritable bowel syndrome? *Psychosom Med.* 2006;68(3):463–469.

24. Marshall JK, Thabane M, Garg AX, Clark WF, Salvadori M, Collins SM. Incidence and epidemiology of irritable bowel syndrome after a large waterborne outbreak of bacterial dysentery. *Gastroenterology.* 2006;131(2):445–450; quiz 660.

25. Spence MJ, Moss-Morris R. The cognitive behavioural model of irritable bowel syndrome: a prospective investigation of patients with gastroenteritis. *Gut.* 2007;56(8):1066–1071.

26. Gwee K, Leong Y, Graham C, et al. The role of psychological and biological factors in postinfective gut dysfunction. *Gut.* 1999;44(3):400–406.

27. Dunlop SP, Jenkins D, Neal KR, Spiller RC. Relative importance of enterochromaffin cell hyperplasia, anxiety, and depression in postinfectious IBS. *Gastroenterology.* 2003;125(6):1651–1659.

28. Mearin F, Perez-Oliveras M, Perello A, et al. Dyspepsia and irritable bowel syndrome after a Salmonella gastroenteritis outbreak: one-year follow-up cohort study. *Gastroenterology.* 2005;129(1):98–104.

29. Ruigómez A, García Rodríguez LA, Panés J. Risk of irritable bowel syndrome after an episode of bacterial gastroenteritis in general practice: influence of comorbidities. *Clin Gastroenterol Hepatol.* 2007;5(4):465–469.

30. Nair P, Okhuysen PC, Jiang ZD, et al. Persistent abdominal symptoms in US adults after short-term stay in Mexico. *J Trav Med.* 2014;21(3):153–158.

31. Ji S, Park H, Lee D, Song YK, Choi JP, Lee S-I. Post-infectious irritable bowel syndrome in patients with Shigella infection. *J Gastroenterol Hepatol.* 2005;20(3):381–386.

32. Wang LH, Fang XC, Pan GZ. Bacillary dysentery as a causative factor of irritable bowel syndrome and its pathogenesis. *Gut.* 2004;53(8):1096–1101.

33. Parry SD, Corbett S, James P, Barton JR, Welfare MR. Illness perceptions in people with acute bacterial gastroenteritis. *J Health Psychol.* 2003;8(6):693–704.

34. Gwee KA, Graham JC, McKendrick MW, et al. Psychometric scores and persistence of irritable bowel after infectious diarrhoea. *Lancet.* 1996;347(8995):150–153.

35. Villani AC, Lemire M, Thabane M, et al. Genetic risk factors for post-infectious irritable bowel syndrome following a waterborne outbreak of gastroenteritis. *Gastroenterology.* 2010;138(4):1502–1513.

36. Swan C, Duroudier NP, Campbell E, et al. Identifying and testing candidate genetic polymorphisms in the irritable bowel syndrome (IBS): association with TNFSF15 and TNFalpha. *Gut.* 2013;62(7):985–994.

37. Garcia Rodriguez LA, Ruigomez A, Panes J. Acute gastroenteritis is followed by an increased risk of inflammatory bowel disease. *Gastroenterology.* 2006;130(6):1588–1594.

38. Thabane M, Simunovic M, Akhtar-Danesh N, et al. An outbreak of acute bacterial gastroenteritis is associated with an increased incidence of irritable bowel syndrome in children. *Am J Gastroenterol.* 2010;105(4):933–939.

39. Pitzurra R, Fried M, Rogler G, et al. Irritable bowel syndrome among a cohort of European travelers to resource-limited destinations. *J Travel Med.* 2011;18(4):250–256.

40. Nielsen HL, Engberg J, Ejlertsen T, Nielsen H. Psychometric scores and persistence of irritable bowel after Campylobacter concisus infection. *Scand J Gastroenterol.* 2014;49(5):545–551.

41. Törnblom H, Holmvall P, Svenungsson B, Lindberg G. Gastrointestinal symptoms after infectious diarrhea: a five-year follow-pp in a Swedish cohort of adults. *Clin Gastroenterol Hepatol.* 2007;5(4):461–464.

42. Parry SD, Barton JR, Welfare MR. Factors associated with the development of post-infectious functional gastrointestinal diseases: does smoking play a role? *Eur J Gastroenterol Hepatol.* 2005;17(10):1071–1075.

43. Munafo MR, Zetteler JI, Clark TG. Personality and smoking status: a meta-analysis. *Nicotine Tob Res.* 2007;9(3):405–413.

44. Spiller R, Garsed K. Postinfectious irritable bowel syndrome. *Gastroenterology.* 2009;136(6):1979–1988.

45. Kowalcyk BK, Smeets HM, Succop PA, De Wit NJ, Havelaar AH. Relative risk of irritable bowel syndrome following acute gastroenteritis and associated risk factors. *Epidemiol Infect.* 2014;142(6):1259–1268.

46. Koh S-J, Lee DH, Lee SH, et al. Incidence and risk factors of irritable bowel syndrome in community subjects with culture-proven bacterial gastroenteritis. *Korean J Gastroenterol.* 2012;60(1):13–18.

47. Spiller RC, Jenkins D, Thornley JP, et al. Increased rectal mucosal enteroendocrine cells, T lymphocytes, and increased gut permeability following acute Campylobacter enteritis and in post-dysenteric irritable bowel syndrome. *Gut*. 2000;47(6):804–811.

48. O'Hara JR, Skinn AC, MacNaughton WK, Sherman PM, Sharkey KA. Consequences of Citrobacter rodentium infection on enteroendocrine cells and the enteric nervous system in the mouse colon. *Cell Microbiol*. 2006;8(4):646–660.

49. Dunlop SP, Jenkins D, Spiller RC. Distinctive clinical, psychological, and histological features of postinfective irritable bowel syndrome. *Am J Gastroenterol*. 2003;98(7):1578–1583.

50. Dunlop SP, Coleman NS, Blackshaw E, et al. Abnormalities of 5-hydroxytryptamine metabolism in irritable bowel syndrome. *Clin Gastroenterol Hepatol*. 2005;3(4):349–357.

51. Gwee KA, Collins SM, Read NW, et al. Increased rectal mucosal expression of interleukin 1beta in recently acquired post-infectious irritable bowel syndrome. *Gut*. 2003;52(4):523–526.

52. Dinan TG, Quigley EM, Ahmed SM, et al. Hypothalamic-pituitary-gut axis dysregulation in irritable bowel syndrome: plasma cytokines as a potential biomarker? *Gastroenterology*. 2006;130(2):304–311.

53. Brydon L, Edwards S, Jia H, et al. Psychological stress activates interleukin-1beta gene expression in human mononuclear cells. *Brain Behav Immun*. 2005;19(6):540–546.

54. Dinan TG, Clarke G, Quigley EM, et al. Enhanced cholinergic-mediated increase in the pro-inflammatory cytokine IL-6 in irritable bowel syndrome: role of muscarinic receptors. *Am J Gastroenterol*. 2008;103(10):2570–2576.

55. Han W, Wang Z, Lu X, Guo C. Protease activated receptor 4 status of mast cells in post infectious irritable bowel syndrome. *Neuro Gastroenterol Motil*. 2012;24(2):113–119.e82.

56. Barbara G, Stanghellini V, De Giorgio R, et al. Activated mast cells in proximity to colonic nerves correlate with abdominal pain in irritable bowel syndrome. *Gastroenterology*. 2004;126(3):693–702.

57. Hollander D. Permeability in Crohn's disease: altered barrier functions in healthy relatives? *Gastroenterology*. 1993;104(6):1848–1851.

58. Walker RI, Owen RL. Intestinal barriers to bacteria and their toxins. *Annu Rev Med*. 1990;41:393–400.

59. Marshall JK, Thabane M, Garg AX, Clark W, Meddings J, Collins SM. Intestinal permeability in patients with irritable bowel syndrome after a waterborne outbreak of acute gastroenteritis in Walkerton, Ontario. *Aliment Pharmacol Ther*. 2004;20(11–12):1317–1322.

60. Schnee AE, Petri Jr WA. Campylobacter jejuni and associated immune mechanisms: short-term effects and long-term implications for infants in low-income countries. *Curr Opin Infect Dis*. 2017;30(3):322–328.

61. Dasti JI, Tareen AM, Lugert R, Zautner AE, Groß U. Campylobacter jejuni: a brief overview on pathogenicity-associated factors and disease-mediating mechanisms. *Int J Medical Microbiol*. 2010;300(4):205–211.

62. Pokkunuri V, Pimentel M, Morales W, et al. Role of Cytolethal distending toxin in altered stool form and bowel phenotypes in a rat model of post-infectious irritable bowel syndrome. *J Neurogastroenterol Motil*. 2012;18(4):434–442.

63. Kim HS, Lim JH, Park H, Lee SI. Increased immunoendocrine cells in intestinal mucosa of postinfectious irritable bowel syndrome patients 3 Years after acute Shigella infection - an observation in a small case control study. *Yonsei Med J*. 2010;51(1):45–51.

64. Scallan E, Hoekstra RM, Angulo FJ, et al. Foodborne illness acquired in the United States–major pathogens. *Emerg Infect Dis*. 2011;17(1):7–15.

65. Lindesmith L, Moe C, Marionneau S, et al. Human susceptibility and resistance to Norwalk virus infection. *Nat Med*. 2003;9(5):548–553.

66. Agus SG, Dolin R, Wyatt RG, Tousimis AJ, Northrup RS. Acute infectious nonbacterial gastroenteritis: intestinal histopathology. Histologic and enzymatic alterations during illness produced by the Norwalk agent in man. *Ann Intern Med*. 1973;79(1):18–25.

67. Levy AG, Widerlite L, Schwartz CJ, et al. Jejunal adenylate cyclase activity in human subjects during viral gastroenteritis. *Gastroenterology*. 1976;70(3):321–325.

68. Mohammed SR, Faubert GM. Purification of a fraction of Giardia lamblia trophozoite extract associated with disaccharidase deficiencies in immune Mongolian gerbils (*Meriones unguiculatus*). *Parasite*. 1995;2(1):31–39.

69. Koh WH, Geurden T, Paget T, et al. Giardia duodenalis assemblage-specific induction of apoptosis and tight junction disruption in human intestinal epithelial cells: effects of mixed infections. *J Parasitol*. 2013;99(2):353–358.

70. Scott KG, Yu LC, Buret AG. Role of CD8+ and CD4+ T lymphocytes in jejunal mucosal injury during murine giardiasis. *Infect Immun*. 2004;72(6):3536–3542.

71. Cotton JA, Beatty JK, Buret AG. Host parasite interactions and pathophysiology in Giardia infections. *Int J Parasitol*. 2011;41(9):925–933.

72. Ricci N, Toma P, Furlani M, Caselli M, Gullini S. Blastocystis hominis: a neglected cause of diarrhoea? *Lancet*. 1984;323(8383):966.

73. Phillips BP, Zierdt CH. Blastocystis hominis: pathogenic potential in human patients and in gnotobiotes. *Exp Parasitol*. 1976;39(3):358–364.

74. Zierdt CH. Blastocystis hominis–past and future. *Clin Microbiol Rev*. 1991;4(1):61–79.

75. Puthia MK, Lu J, Tan KS. Blastocystis ratti contains cysteine proteases that mediate interleukin-8 response from human intestinal epithelial cells in an NF-kappaB-dependent manner. *Eukaryot Cell*. 2008;7(3):435–443.

76. Puthia MK, Sio SW, Lu J, Tan KS. Blastocystis ratti induces contact-independent apoptosis, F-actin rearrangement, and barrier function disruption in IEC-6 cells. *Infect Immun*. 2006;74(7):4114–4123.

77. Westerman LJ, de Boer RF, Roelfsema JH, et al. Brachyspira species and gastroenteritis in humans. *J Clin Microbiol.* 2013;51(7):2411–2413.

78. Hovind-Hougen K, Birch-Andersen A, Henrik-Nielsen R, et al. Intestinal spirochetosis: morphological characterization and cultivation of the spirochete Brachyspira aalborgi gen. nov., sp. nov. *J Clin Microbiol.* 1982;16(6):1127–1136.

79. Westerman LJ, Stel HV, Schipper MEI, et al. Development of a real-time PCR for identification of Brachyspira species in human colonic biopsies. *PLoS One.* 2012;7(12):e52281.

80. Piche T, Saint-Paul MC, Dainese R, et al. Mast cells and cellularity of the colonic mucosa correlated with fatigue and depression in irritable bowel syndrome. *Gut.* 2008;57(4):468–473.

81. Ericsson CD, Hatz C, DuPont AW. Postinfectious irritable bowel syndrome. *Clin Infect Dis.* 2008;46(4):594–599.

82. DuPont AW. Postinfectious irritable bowel syndrome. *Clin Infect Dis.* 2008;46(4):594–599.

83. Longstreth GF, Thompson WG, Chey WD, Houghton LA, Mearin F, Spiller RC. Functional bowel disorders. *Gastroenterology.* 2006;130(5):1480–1491.

84. Drossman DA, Camilleri M, Mayer EA, Whitehead WE. AGA technical review on irritable bowel syndrome. *Gastroenterology.* 2002;123(6):2108–31.

85. Pimentel M, Morales W, Rezaie A, et al. Development and validation of a biomarker for diarrhea-predominant irritable bowel syndrome in human subjects. *PLoS One.* 2015;10(5):e0126438.

86. Carmona-Sánchez R. Are the anti-CdtB and anti-vinculin antibodies really ready for use in patients with diarrhea in Mexico? Regarding microscopic colitis. *Rev Gastroenterol México.* 2017;82(2):196–197.

87. Schmulson M, Balbuena R, Corona de Law C. Clinical experience with the use of anti-CdtB and anti-vinculin antibodies in patients with diarrhea in Mexico. *Rev Gastroenterol México.* 2016;81(4):236–239.

88. Monsen U, Sorstad J, Hellers G, Johansson C. Extracolonic diagnoses in ulcerative colitis: an epidemiological study. *Am J Gastroenterol.* 1990;85(6):711–716.

89. Molodecky NA, Soon IS, Rabi DM, et al. Increasing incidence and prevalence of the inflammatory bowel diseases with time, based on systematic review. *Gastroenterology.* 2012;142(1):46–54.e42.

90. Riddle MS, Murray JA, Porter CK. The incidence and risk of celiac disease in a healthy US adult population. *Am J Gastroenterol.* 2012;107(8):1248–1255.

91. Sanders DS, Carter MJ, Hurlstone DP, et al. Association of adult coeliac disease with irritable bowel syndrome: a case-control study in patients fulfilling ROME II criteria referred to secondary care. *Lancet.* 2001;358(9292):1504–1508.

92. Wahnschaffe U, Ullrich R, Riecken EO, Schulzke JD. Celiac disease-like abnormalities in a subgroup of patients with irritable bowel syndrome. *Gastroenterology.* 2001;121(6):1329–1338.

93. Levy J, Bernstein L, Silber N. Celiac disease: an immune dysregulation syndrome. *Curr Probl Pediatr Adolesc Health Care.* 2014;44(11):324–327.

94. Carroccio A, Mansueto P, D'Alcamo A, Iacono G. Non-celiac wheat sensitivity as an allergic condition: personal experience and narrative review. *Am J Gastroenterol.* 2013;108(12):1845–1852; quiz 53.

95. Bohmer CJ, Tuynman HA. The clinical relevance of lactose malabsorption in irritable bowel syndrome. *Eur J Gastroenterol Hepatol.* 1996;8(10):1013–1016.

96. Lisker R, Solomons NW, Perez Briceno R, Ramirez Mata M. Lactase and placebo in the management of the irritable bowel syndrome: a double-blind, cross-over study. *Am J Gastroenterol.* 1989;84(7):756–762.

97. Parry SD, Barton JR, Welfare MR. Is lactose intolerance implicated in the development of post-infectious irritable bowel syndrome or functional diarrhoea in previously asymptomatic people? *Eur J Gastroenterol Hepatol.* 2002;14(11):1225–1230.

98. Ramakrishna BS, Venkataraman S, Mukhopadhya A. Tropical malabsorption. *Postgrad Med.* 2006;82(974):779–787.

99. Ghoshal UC, Gwee KA. Post-infectious IBS, tropical sprue and small intestinal bacterial overgrowth: the missing link. *Nat Rev Gastroenterol Hepatol.* 2017;14(7):435–441.

100. Niaz SK, Sandrasegaran K, Renny FH, Jones BJ. Postinfective diarrhoea and bile acid malabsorption. *J R Coll Physicians Lond.* 1997;31(1):53–56.

101. Sinha L, Liston R, Testa HJ, Moriarty KJ. Idiopathic bile acid malabsorption: qualitative and quantitative clinical features and response to cholestyramine. *Aliment Pharmacol Ther.* 1998;12(9):839–844.

102. Williams AJ, Merrick MV, Eastwood MA. Idiopathic bile acid malabsorption–a review of clinical presentation, diagnosis, and response to treatment. *Gut.* 1991;32(9):1004–1006.

103. Mills LR, Schuman BM, Thompson WO. Lymphocytic colitis. A definable clinical and histological diagnosis. *Dig Dis Sci.* 1993;38(6):1147–1151.

104. Schiller LR. Diagnosis and management of microscopic colitis syndrome. *J Clin Gastroenterol.* 2004;38(5 suppl 1):S27–S30.

105. Zins BJ, Sandborn WJ, Tremaine WJ. Collagenous and lymphocytic colitis: subject review and therapeutic alternatives. *Am J Gastroenterol.* 1995;90(9):1394–1400.

106. Perk G, A Z, C P, E R. Lymphocytic colitis: a clue to an infectious trigger. *Scand J Gastroenterol.* 1999;34(1):110–112.

107. Camilleri M. Pharmacology of the new treatments for lower gastrointestinal motility disorders and irritable bowel syndrome. *Clin Pharmacol Ther.* 2012;91(1):44–59.

108. Cann PA, Read NW, Holdsworth CD, Barends D. Role of loperamide and placebo in management of irritable bowel syndrome (IBS). *Dig Dis Sci.* 1984;29(3):239–247.

109. Efskind PS, Bernklev T, Vatn MH. A double-blind placebo-controlled trial with loperamide in irritable bowel syndrome. *Scand J Gastroenterol.* 1996;31(5):463–468.

110. Hovdenak N. Loperamide treatment of the irritable bowel syndrome. *Scand J Gastroenterol Suppl.* 1987;130:81–84.

111. Poynard T, Regimbeau C, Benhamou Y. Meta-analysis of smooth muscle relaxants in the treatment of irritable bowel syndrome. *Aliment Pharmacol Ther.* 2001;15(3):355–361.

112. Ford AC, Talley NJ, Spiegel BM, et al. Effect of fibre, antispasmodics, and peppermint oil in the treatment of irritable bowel syndrome: systematic review and meta-analysis. *BMJ.* 2008;337:a2313.

113. Dunlop SP, Jenkins D, Neal KR, et al. Randomized, double-blind, placebo-controlled trial of prednisolone in post-infectious irritable bowel syndrome. *Aliment Pharmacol Ther.* 2003;18(1):77–84.

114. Bafutto M, Almeida JR, Leite NV, Oliveira EC, Gabriel-Neto S, Rezende-Filho J. Treatment of postinfectious irritable bowel syndrome and noninfective irritable bowel syndrome with mesalazine. *Arq Gastroenterol.* 2011;48(1):36–40.

115. Lam C, Tan W, Leighton M, et al. A mechanistic multicentre, parallel group, randomised placebo-controlled trial of mesalazine for the treatment of IBS with diarrhoea (IBS-D). *Gut.* 2016;65(1):91–99.

116. Tuteja AK, Fang JC, Al-Suqi M, Stoddard GJ, Hale DC. Double-blind placebo-controlled study of mesalamine in post-infective irritable bowel syndrome–a pilot study. *Scand J Gastroenterol.* 2012;47(10):1159–1164.

117. Barbara G, Cremon C, Annese V, et al. Randomised controlled trial of mesalazine in IBS. *Gut.* 2016;65(1):82–90.

118. Pimentel M, Lembo A, Chey WD, et al. Rifaximin therapy for patients with irritable bowel syndrome without constipation. *N Engl J Med.* 2011;364(1):22–32.

119. Grover M, Drossman DA. Psychotropic agents in functional gastrointestinal disorders. *Curr Opin Pharmacol.* 2008;8(6):715–723.

120. Drossman DA, Toner BB, Whitehead WE, et al. Cognitive-behavioral therapy versus education and desipramine versus placebo for moderate to severe functional bowel disorders. *Gastroenterology.* 2003;125(1):19–31.

121. Creed F, Fernandes L, Guthrie E, et al. The cost-effectiveness of psychotherapy and paroxetine for severe irritable bowel syndrome. *Gastroenterology.* 2003;124(2):303–317.

122. Svedlund J, Sjodin I, Ottosson JO, Dotevall G. Controlled study of psychotherapy in irritable bowel syndrome. *Lancet.* 1983;2(8350):589–592.

123. Whitehead WE. Hypnosis for irritable bowel syndrome: the empirical evidence of therapeutic effects. *Int J Clin Exp Hypn.* 2006;54(1):7–20.

CHAPTER 8

Appendicitis and Infections of the Appendix

MOJGAN HOSSEINI, MD • LAURA W. LAMPS, MD

INTRODUCTION

The presence of the organ that we now know as the vermiform appendix was probably first noticed by the Egyptians around 300 BC. Centuries later, around the year 1500, the appendix was sketched by Leonardo Da Vinci, who used the term "orecchio" to describe what he likened to an ear projecting from the cecum. The organ was formally described by the anatomist da Capri in 1521, and again by Vesalius in 1543. The first report of acute appendicitis was published by the German surgeon Lorenz Heister, followed by the first documented appendectomy, which was performed by Claudius Amyand in England in 1735.[1,2]

Appendectomies are one of the most commonly performed surgical procedures. The pathologic spectrum of an acutely inflamed appendix includes a wide range of infectious and noninfectious etiologies, some with overlapping morphologic features that may require extensive diagnostic evaluation and clinicopathologic correlation to differentiate. The appendix may be the sole site of involvement in certain disorders, or it may be involved in a more widespread gastrointestinal or systemic inflammatory process.

MORPHOLOGIC PATTERNS OF APPENDICITIS

Acute "nonspecific" appendicitis (AA) is the most common abdominal surgical emergency, with a peak incidence in the second and third decades of life. However, it can occur at any age, from infancy to late adulthood. AA typically presents with periumbilical pain that is colicky in nature, with gradual onset and increasing severity. Nausea, vomiting, anorexia, fever, and malaise are variably present, and diarrhea or constipation may occur as well. The pain typically localizes to the right lower quadrant within 6–18 h, and guarding and rebound tenderness may develop.[3,4]

The pathogenesis of AA remains controversial, and there are likely multiple etiologic factors. Obstruction, by a fecalith, adhesions, or foreign material, has been the most popular theory. Advocates theorize that the obstruction and increase in intraluminal pressure interfere with vascular flow to the appendiceal mucosa, leading to ischemia, ulceration, and infection.[3,5] Others argue that obstruction is not the cause, but rather the result, of appendicitis.[6] Other theories point to a compromise of the serosal vasculature, mucosal ulceration due to various infections, and constipation due to a low fiber diet with slow fecal transit time as other possible etiologies.[7–9]

Both the gross and histologic features of acute nonspecific AA are variable, and the gross and microscopic findings may not correlate in terms of extent of inflammation. Macroscopic changes begin with dilatation of the serosal vessels, and progress to hyperemia, fibrinopurulent exudate, and frank gangrenous necrosis.[3] Histologically, acute suppurative appendicitis is characterized by neutrophilic infiltration of the muscularis propria (Fig. 8.1). Lesser degrees of inflammation (i.e., inflammation limited to the mucosa or superficial submucosa) may represent the earliest phase of acute suppurative appendicitis, but may also be seen in infections or secondary to fecaliths.[3,4,10]

The role of enteric bacteria in the development of AA has been the subject of much debate, and a wide variety of organisms, both anaerobic and aerobic, have been isolated.[11,12] *Bacteroides fragilis* has been the most commonly identified, but its role as a causative factor has never been established.[13,14]

Granulomatous Appendicitis

Granulomatous appendicitis is rare, seen in less than 1%–2% of cases.[15] Historically, it was considered to represent isolated Crohn's disease in the ileocecal valve region; however, as only approximately 5%–10% of patients with isolated granulomatous appendicitis will

Gastrointestinal Diseases and Their Associated Infections. https://doi.org/10.1016/B978-0-323-54843-4.00008-8
Copyright © 2019 Elsevier Inc. All rights reserved.

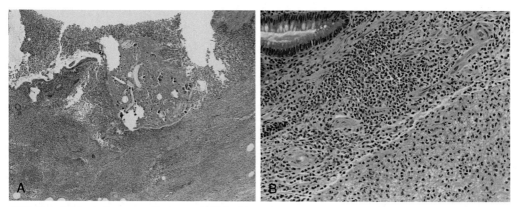

FIG. 8.1 **(A)** Acute "non-specific appendicitis" with surface mucosal erosion and acute inflammation involving the mucosa, submucosa, and muscularis propria. Fecal material is seen at the surface. **(B)** Purulent/neutrophilic inflammation within appendiceal wall.

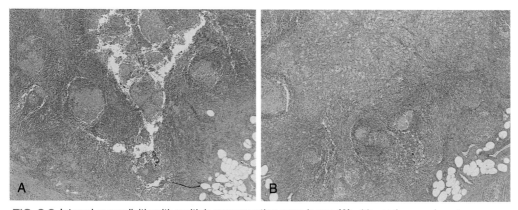

FIG. 8.2 Interval appendicitis with multiple noncaseating granulomas **(A)** with xanthogranulomatous inflammation **(B)** Periodic acid–Schiff (PAS) stain.

develop Crohn's disease in the future, other underlying etiologies are now recognized as more important causes of granulomatous appendicitis.[16,17]

Etiologies such as sarcoidosis, foreign body reaction, and mycobacterial, fungal, and parasitic infections have been increasingly implicated as causes of granulomatous appendicitis.[16–21] In recent years, infections by *Yersinia* species and subacute/recurrent or interval appendicitis have emerged as the most common causes.[18,22] The presence of large numbers of confluent granulomas is suggestive of an infectious process, especially if necrosis and central abscess formation are present.[19] Interval appendicitis refers to ruptured acute appendicitis that has been treated with antibiotics and drainage for a period of time prior to a delayed appendectomy. About 60% of interval appendectomies show a granulomatous appendicitis, and they often show a xanthogranulomatous reaction

as well (Fig. 8.2). A Crohn's-like reaction, including transmural lymphoid aggregates and fibrosis, is seen in a minority of cases.[22]

Chronic Appendicitis

Chronic appendicitis is both a poorly defined term and a controversial diagnosis. Clinically, patients may suffer from chronic, ongoing symptoms, which can be due to recurrent bouts of acute appendicitis prior to resection, adhesions, fecaliths, peri-appendiceal abscesses, or true chronic infections, such as *Mycobacterium tuberculosis*. However, there are no specific histologic criteria that correlate with the clinical scenario of a patient with prolonged symptoms. For this reason, the term "primary chronic appendicitis" should be avoided.[3] However, the surgical pathologist occasionally encounters an appendix with destructive, predominantly mononuclear or plasmacytic inflammation and scarring, in a

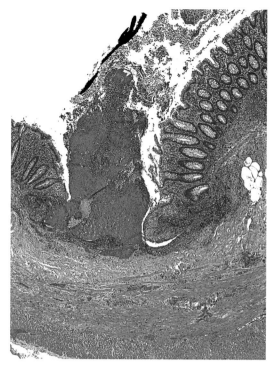

FIG. 8.3 PCR-proven *Campylobacter jejuni* acute appendicitis, featuring mucosal erosion with a neutrophilic infiltrate in mucosa and submucosa.

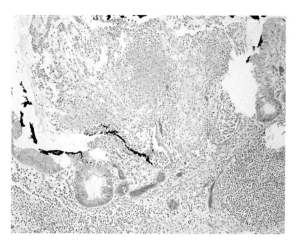

FIG. 8.4 Involvement of the appendix in a case of *C. difficile* colitis.

patient with recurrent or prolonged symptoms. In these cases, "chronic ongoing appendicitis" may be used in the absence of Crohn's disease, interval appendectomy, identifiable infections, or other chronic diseases.

APPENDICITIS DUE TO SPECIFIC INFECTIOUS ENTITIES

Bacterial Infections

Bacterial infections occasionally cause appendicitis in isolation, but often are associated with infection involving the surrounding bowel. In many cases, the infection is only diagnosed after appendectomy, and finding the infection in the appendix may indicate more widespread disease.

Campylobacter species. *Campylobacter* species, particularly *C. jejuni*, have been isolated from appendectomy specimens using molecular, microbiological, immunohistochemical, and electron microscopic methods. Morphologic findings are those of early, nonspecific AA, with inflammatory changes that are typically limited to the mucosa, without transmural inflammation or periappendicitis (Fig. 8.3).[23,24]

Clostridium difficile. Appendicitis related to *C. difficile* infection has historically been a rare event, with only a few cases reported in the literature. However, in recent years, due to the increase in the incidence of *C. difficile* colitis, more cases of *C. difficile* appendicitis have also been reported.[25,26] Appendiceal involvement usually develops in the setting of colonic infection, and isolated appendiceal *C. difficile* infection is extremely rare.[25,27,28] The appendices show typical feature of *C. difficile* pseudomembranous colitis with volcano or mushroom-like mucosal neutrophilic eruptions, and dilated and necrotic crypts giving rise to the pseudomembrane composed of fibrin, mucin, and neutrophils (Fig. 8.4). Grossly, the overall appearance may be that of phlegmonous or gangrenous appendicitis.[25,27] Recognition of a possible *C. difficile* infection in the appendix is important, so that appropriate treatment can be instituted.

Yersinia enterocolitica and pseudotuberculosis. Yersinia is the most common cause of bacterial enteritis in Western and Northern Europe, and the incidence is also increasing in North America and Australia. *Y. enterocolitica* (YE) and *Y. pseudotuberculosis* (YP) are the two species that are implicated in human gastrointestinal disease. Both are Gram-negative coccobacilli that prefer cold temperatures, and are transmitted orally through consumption of contaminated food, including meat, dairy products, chocolate, poultry, produce, and through contaminated water.[18,29–33]

As noted earlier, *Yersinia* causes granulomatous appendicitis, with or without associated enterocolitis or mesenteric lymphadenitis.[18,29] The involved appendix has a thickened, edematous wall with nodular inflammatory masses centered on Peyer's patches. Aphthoid and

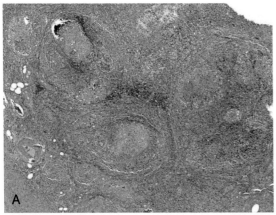

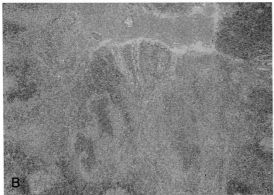

FIG. 8.5 **(A)** Granulomatous appendicitis due to *Yersinia enterocolitica* infection featuring granulomas with prominent lymphoid cuffs. **(B)** *Yersinia pseudotuberculosis* with necrotizing granulomatous inflammation.

linear ulcers may be seen, and perforation is common. Both suppurative and granulomatous patterns of inflammation may be seen with either YE or YP, and a mixture of the two is common.[18,34–36] Epithelioid granulomas with prominent lymphoid cuffs are very characteristic of Yersinia infection (Fig. 8.5). Some patients with *Yersinia* infection and signs and symptoms of appendicitis actually have inflammation of the terminal ileum and mesenteric nodes that clinically mimics appendicitis (the so-called pseudoappendicular syndrome).[29,31,35,37,38]

Yersinia can be quite challenging to diagnose in tissue sections. Special stains are not helpful, because the organisms are small, usually present in low numbers, and difficult to distinguish from other nonpathogenic colonic flora. Bacterial culture is challenging as well, as *Yersinia* are fastidious organisms that require specific conditions for successful culture. PCR analysis performed from the tissue block or from stool may be very helpful for diagnosis.[18,39,40]

Uncomplicated *Yersinia* infection in immunocompetent patients tends to be self-limited, and usually resolves spontaneously. Immunocompromised patients, or those at high risk of disseminated infection due to high body iron content, such as those on desferrioxamine therapy or those with hereditary hemochromatosis, may require antibiotic therapy.[41–43]

The primary differential diagnoses for *Yersinia* infection include Crohn's disease and other infections, particularly *Salmonella* and mycobacterial infection. PCR from stool or tissue can help distinguish between Yersinia and other infections, as can acid-fast stains in the case of mycobacterial infection. Distinction between *Yersinia* and Crohn's disease can be especially problematic. The presence of other features of chronicity (e.g., pyloric metaplasia and neural hyperplasia) and involvement of other segments of the gastrointestinal (GI) tract favor Crohn's disease.[18,19]

Other enteric pathogens. *Salmonella* has only rarely been isolated from an acutely inflamed appendix, and the clinical presentation and histologic findings are identical to acute nonspecific appendicitis.[44,45] In the rare instance that *Salmonella* is isolated from the appendix, patients require antibiotic treatment following appendectomy as they tend to remain febrile without treatment.[46] AA has also rarely been reported in association with *Shigella* infection and dysentery.[47,48] Stool culture with matrix-assisted laser desorption/ionization time-of-flight mass spectrometry (MALDI-TOF) or PCR performed on tissue or stool is the preferred method of detection for these organisms.[46,49]

Tuberculosis. Tuberculosis is a common global disease with a worldwide estimated incidence of 10.4 million new cases in 2015 according to the most recent WHO "Global Tuberculosis Report, 2016." HIV patients accounted for 1.2 million (11%) of all TB cases in 2015.[50,51] Although the ileocecum is involved in over 40% of cases of abdominal tuberculosis, the appendix is only rarely involved (~1% of cases).[52–54] Despite its proximity to the ileocecum, appendiceal involvement is usually related to mycobacterial infection of the ileocecum, genitourinary system, or peritoneal cavity. Only 20% of intestinal tuberculosis is associated with pulmonary TB.[52,53]

Patients may present with typical signs and symptoms of AA, or with milder, more chronic and nonspecific symptoms including intermittent right iliac fossa pain.[53] When confronted with a case of granulomatous appendicitis, tuberculosis should be considered in individuals from endemic areas, as well as in immunocompromised patients in both endemic and nonendemic

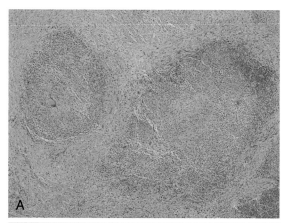

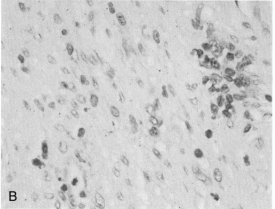

FIG. 8.6 **(A)** Tuberculous appendicitis with caseating granulomas in the wall of the appendix. **(B)** Acid-Fast Bacilli (AFB) stain shows rare mycobacteria.

countries.[52] Patients typically require long-term antitubercular therapy after appendectomy.[55,56]

The appendix is usually macroscopically inflamed, with mural thickening, serosal adhesions, and abdominal lymphadenitis.[52–54] Appendiceal histology shows lymphoid hyperplasia with associated caseating granulomas (Fig. 8.6).[54] Mucosal ulceration may be present. Organisms may be rare and undetectable by special stains for acid-fast bacilli, and culture and molecular assays may be needed for diagnosis.

Atypical mycobacteria (particularly *Mycobacterium avium-intracellulare* [MAI]) are also a rare cause of appendicitis. It is almost exclusively seen in immunocompromised patients. The diffuse histiocytic infiltrate characteristic of other gastrointestinal MAI infections can be seen, and mycobacterial pseudotumors have been reported in acquired immune deficiency syndrome (AIDS) patients.[57,58]

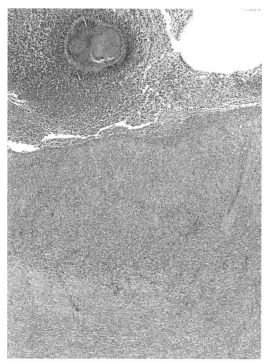

FIG. 8.7 Appendicitis due to Actinomyces, with surface ulceration and a sulfur granule with associated acute inflammation.

Actinomyces

Actinomyces israelii is a filamentous anaerobic Grampositive bacterium that is part of the normal bacterial flora of the oral cavity and upper gastrointestinal tract. The appendix, followed by the right colon, is the most common intraabdominal organ involved in actinomycosis. It occasionally causes chronic granulomatous appendicitis. Patients present with abdominal pain, weight loss, and fever and, occasionally, a palpable mass that may mimic malignancy.[59–62] The correct diagnosis is usually dependent upon microscopic examination of the appendectomy specimen.

Grossly affected appendices are enlarged and indurated, with serosal adhesions. The enlargement is due to the presence of transmural inflammation, lymphoid hyperplasia, and marked mural fibrosis. Palisading histiocytes, giant cells, and granulomas are often admixed with neutrophilic inflammation. Mucosal ulceration and architectural distortion as well as small sinus tracts and mural abscesses may be seen.[59–61]

The organism itself produces typical actinomycotic (sulfur) granules (Fig. 8.7), consisting of irregular round clusters of bacteria rimmed by eosinophilic

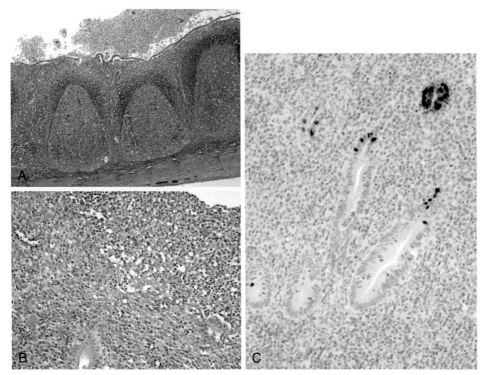

FIG. 8.8 Adenovirus appendiceal infection with lymphoid hyperplasia **(A)** and viral inclusions (smudge cells) within detached epithelial cells **(B)**. Viral inclusions are highlighted by adenovirus immunostain **(C)**.

club-like projections of proteinaceous material (Splendore-Hoeppli material). The filamentous, Gram-positive organisms can be highlighted with Gram, Grocott methenamine silver (GMS), and Warthin–Starry stains. Histologic differentiation must be made between commensal actinomyces present at the luminal surface of the appendix with no inflammatory response, versus invasive actinomycosis, which is characterized by invasion of the appendiceal wall with an associated inflammatory response. After appendectomy and/or abscess drainage, long-term antibiotic therapy is necessary due to limited drug penetration into the fibrous tissue and increased risk of recurrence.[59–63]

Spirochetosis

Spirochetosis is typically seen in the large bowel in immunosuppressed (particularly HIV positive) patients, and it is rarely seen in the appendix.[64–68] Appendiceal spirochetosis appears to be an incidental finding in most reported cases, and not the causative agent of the patient's symptoms.[66,69] Most patients present with diarrhea and have nonspecific endoscopic findings in the colon, such as edema or erosion. Histologically, the organisms are seen as a prominent brush border on hematoxylin and eosin staining and can be further highlighted with Warthin–Starry, GMS, periodic acid–Schiff (PAS), and/or immunostains for *Treponema pallidum* organisms.

Rickettsia. Rickettsial infections are extremely rare causes of AA. When this does occur, it is usually associated with Rocky Mountain spotted fever, in which the presenting symptoms of fever, nausea, vomiting, and diarrhea prompt an abdominal examination, and thus consideration of appendicitis or cholecystitis.[70–72] Organisms have been isolated from endothelial cell in the appendix in patients with symptomatic AA.

Appendectomy is not curative as rickettsial diseases are systemic infections, and thus antibiotic therapy is required.[70–73]

APPENDICITIS DUE TO VIRAL INFECTIONS

Adenovirus. Adenovirus is one of the more common viral infections of the appendix. It is associated with ileal and ileocecal intussusception, particularly in children, because the prominent lymphoid hyperplasia interferes with gut motility. Most patients do not have symptoms of appendicitis, and the adenovirus is found in segmental resection specimens for intussusception.

Morphological changes are subtle, and include lymphoid hyperplasia with overlying disorderly proliferation and degeneration of the surface epithelium (Fig. 8.8). Viral inclusions are exclusively intranuclear and are typically found in the superficial epithelium in areas of degenerative changes.[74,75] The most common adenovirus inclusions, known as smudge cells, have enlarged, basophilic nuclei without a clear nuclear membrane. Homogenous, eosinophilic inclusions surrounded by halos with distinct nuclear membranes (Cowdry A-type) are less common.[75–77] In the appendix, viral inclusions are noted in only one third of the cases on routine stains in patients with intussusception. As a result, other detection methodologies such as immunohistochemistry, PCR, and in situ hybridization are recommended.[74–77] Positive serologies or fecal identification of the virus does not necessarily represent current infection, because viral shedding and increased serologic titers may persist for months after the initial infection.[74]

Cytomegalovirus (CMV). CMV is very common, and approximately 60% of the US population, across multiple ethnicities, has evidence of infection. The prevalence increases with age to about 90% in individuals who are 80 or more years old.[78] Thus, it is not surprising that CMV is the most common GI pathogen in immunosuppressed patients, including HIV positive patients, organ transplant recipients, and those on ongoing immunosuppression for inflammatory bowel disease. It is found in the appendices of HIV patients with increasing frequency.[79–81] It is also detected in 21% of pediatric appendectomies.[82] Primary CMV infection in the immunocompetent individual is typically asymptomatic or presents with a mononucleosis-like syndrome.[83] In HIV patients, the presentation is often prolonged, with weeks of fever, diarrhea, and abdominal pain that eventually may localize to the right lower quadrant. Appendiceal perforation is common. Because CMV is almost always a systemic infection, antiviral treatment is required after appendectomy, particularly in the immunocompromised.

Appendectomy specimens show ulcerated appendiceal mucosa with a transmural mixed inflammatory infiltrate, including neutrophils, histiocytes, plasma cells, and lymphocytes. CMV inclusions can be intranuclear or intracytoplasmic. The characteristic "owl's

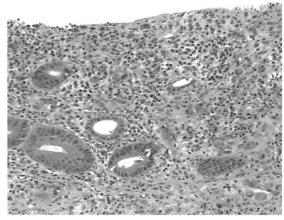

FIG. 8.9 CMV appendicitis showing typical owl's eye nuclear inclusions as well as basophilic granular cytoplasmic inclusions. (Courtesy Dr. Joseph Misdraji.)

eye" CMV inclusions can be seen in the nuclei of epithelial, endothelial, histiocytic, or stromal cells, and smudgy granular basophilic inclusions may be seen in the cytoplasm (Fig. 8.9).[79,80] Immunohistochemistry, PCR assays, in situ hybridization, and CMV serological studies/antigen tests can aid in diagnosis. Isolation of CMV in culture does not imply active disease because the virus may be excreted for months to years after a primary infection.[84,85]

Epstein–Barr Virus

AA can develop during infectious mononucleosis due to systemic infection by the Epstein–Barr virus (EBV). Changes in the appendiceal lymphoid tissue mimic those occurring in the lymph nodes.[86] EBV has also been detected by PCR in up to 5% of appendiceal specimens from children with AA, although the clinical significance of this remains unclear.[82] Multiple serologic tests are available for diagnosis, such as Viral capsid antigen (VCA) IgM and IgG, Early antigen (EA) IgG, EBV nuclear antigen (EBNA), Monospot test, and viral titer determination by PCR.

Measles. Involvement of the appendix in measles infection has been reported, and appendicitis can happen during either the prodromal or fully developed stage.[87,88] The classic feature of measles infection in the appendix is that of Warthin–Finkeldey giant cells, which are also found in hyperplastic lymphoid tissue elsewhere in the body during measles infection.[87,88] If necessary, diagnosis can be confirmed by serologic testing for measles IgG and IgM or PCR testing.[89]

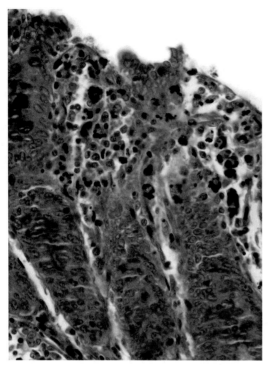

FIG. 8.10 Histoplasma are seen within macrophages in the appendix of an immunocompromised baby. (H&E/Methamine silver stain).

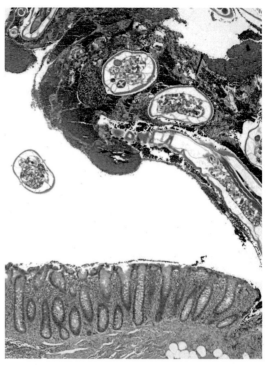

FIG. 8.11 *Enterobius vermicularis* (pinworm) present in the appendiceal lumen. Internal organs and lateral ala of *Enterobius* are visible.

APPENDICITIS DUE TO FUNGAL INFECTIONS

Fungal appendicitis is very rare, and is typically part of systemic infection in severely immunocompromised patients. Mucormycosis has been reported as the cause of right lower quadrant inflammatory masses involving the appendix, ileum, and cecum.[90,91] *Histoplasma* may also involve the appendix as part of a generalized infection of the gastrointestinal tract, usually in immunocompromised patients (Fig. 8.10).[92] Appendicitis due to *Candida* and *Aspergillus* has also been rarely reported.[93]

APPENDICITIS DUE TO PARASITIC INFECTIONS

Enterobius vermicularis (pinworm). Enterobius (*Oxyuris vermicularis* in the older literature) is one of the most common human parasites, with a reported gastrointestinal tract infection rate of 4%–28% worldwide, and an especially high prevalence among children ages 5–10 years.[94–97] The infective eggs are found in dust and soil, and transmission is considered to be fecal-oral. The worms live and reproduce in the ileum, cecum,

proximal colon, and appendix; the female worm migrates to the anus to deposit her eggs, and then dies. The perianal eggs and worms produce the characteristic symptoms of pruritis ani, which typically leads to perianal scratching and resultant insomnia. Many infections are asymptomatic, however.

The relationship between the presence of pinworms in the appendiceal lumen, symptoms of AA, and a possible causative role in AA remains controversial. As both worms and ova may cause obstruction of the appendiceal lumen, similar to fecaliths, a similar obstructive mechanism for the development of AA has been postulated.[94–96,98] Although actual invasion of the appendiceal mucosa by *Enterobius* has been documented, it is rare, and even invasive worms typically incite no or very little inflammatory response. Granulomas and necrosis may occur as a reaction to degenerating worms or ova. The worms are white or ivory, 2–5 mm long, with pointed ends; the posterior end is curved. They may be seen with the naked eye. Morphologically, pinworms have prominent lateral alae with easily visible internal organs (Fig. 8.11). *Enterobius* eggs are oval, with one flat side and a bilayered refractile shell.[94–96,98]

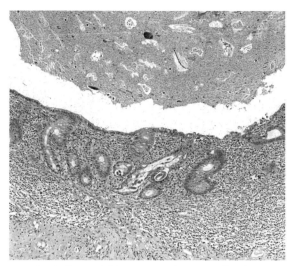

FIG. 8.12 *Strongyloides* are seen the appendiceal crypts with associated eosinophilic inflammation. (Courtesy Dr. Dennis Baroni-Cruz.)

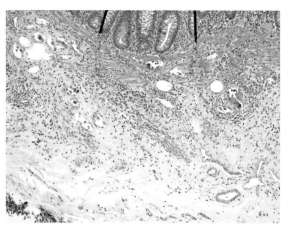

FIG. 8.13 Calcified schistosome eggs with associated fibrosis and giant cell reaction.

Strongyloides stercoralis. *Strongyloides stercoralis* is a common nematode that is endemic in tropical climates, including the southeastern United States, Brazil, Thailand, and certain areas of Japan. It is also common in urban areas with large immigrant populations, and in mental institutions.[99-101] Infection is acquired from contaminated soil. Risk factors include Human T-cell leukemia virus type 1 (*HTLV-1*) infection and chronic illnesses including alcoholism.[102] Patients with AIDS do not seem to be particularly susceptible, although rare cases have been reported.[102-104]

Strongyloides stercoralis is a rare cause of appendicitis, and its clinical presentation is similar to nonspecific AA. Additional findings that may be encountered include mesenteric adenopathy, rash, urticaria, peripheral eosinophilia and leukocytosis, and concomitant pulmonary symptoms. Affected appendices typically show a marked transmural eosinophilic infiltrate; granulomas are variably present, and larvae may be found within them (Fig. 8.12). Adult worms characteristically have sharply pointed tails that are often curved. Stool examination and serologic studies may be helpful for diagnosis.[100,101]

Schistosomiasis

Schistosomes, most commonly *S. haematobium*, only rarely cause appendicitis even in endemic areas. Presentation is similar to nonspecific AA, although some cases are associated with inflammatory masses. Histologically, appendices show transmural eosinophilic inflammation with a granulomatous reaction to the ova (Fig. 8.13). Older infections may show hyalinized, fibrotic granulomas with calcification of ova. Patients may require antischistosomal therapy postappendectomy.[105-108]

Entamoeba histolytica. *Entamoeba histolytica* is occasionally found in the lumen of the appendix, usually representing extension from right colon infection.[97,99,108-112] There is typically no accompanying inflammation, and this parasite is rarely associated with clinical signs of AA.

Amoebic trophozoites have distinct cell membranes with foamy cytoplasm, round and eccentrically located nuclei with peripheral margination of chromatin, and a central karyosome. The presence of ingested red blood cells is essentially pathognomonic of *Entamoeba histolytica* and helps to distinguish it from other amoebae. Distinction of trophozoites from macrophages within inflammatory exudates may be difficult. Amoebae are trichrome and periodic acid–Schiff positive, and macrophages can be highlighted by immunostains for CD163 or CD68. *Entamoeba histolytica* can also be detected through stool examination for cysts and trophozoites, stool culture, serologic tests, and PCR assays.[113]

Balantidium coli

Balantidium coli is the largest and the only ciliate protozoan that infects humans, who are typically accidental hosts after fecal/oral exposure. *B. coli* has a worldwide distribution, and pigs are the reservoir hosts. Human Balanitis is very rare, and directly correlates with the density of the pig population in a given community.[114] Appendicitis due to *B. coli* is exceedingly rare, and usually secondary to severe colonic infection.[115–117] The organisms are large, round to oval bodies with a large, dark macronucleus and a prominent brush border covered in cilia. Trophozoites can be detected in stool or in urine in patients with genitourinary involvement.[118,119]

Toxoplasma. Toxoplasma infection are extremely common throughout the world. It is acquired through ingestion of contaminated food or water, undercooked meat, or accidental ingestion from the environment, most commonly from contact with cat feces.[120–122] Infections during pregnancy are particularly harmful due to development of congenital toxoplasmosis in the fetus with high risk of developmental abnormalities and stillborn. Clinically, acute appendicitis due to Toxoplasma is exceedingly rare.[123] Morphological features include florid follicular hyperplasia with prominent monocytoid B cells and tingible body macrophages. Granulomas are unusual. Organisms can occasionally be highlighted with Giemsa stain. Diagnostic tests include serologic testing and PCR.[124]

Cryptosporidium parvum

Cryptosporidium is the most common human coccidian intestinal parasite, and is acquired through ingestion of water contaminated with oocytes or spores. Cryptosporidial infections of the appendix are very rare, and have been reported primarily in immunocompromised patients.[125–127] Histologic features include surface epithelial apoptosis and nuclear disarray, along with a mild intraepithelial lymphocytosis. The organism appears as small blue beads or globules at the brush border.[128,129] Stool ova and parasite studies with special stains (modified acid-fast or safranin) may be useful, along with molecular studies.[130]

Echinococcus

Echinococcosis (hydatid disease) is a worldwide zoonotic infection caused by cestodes (tapeworms) of the genus Echinococcus.[131] Rare cases of AA in association with intraluminal or intraabdominal cystic echinococcosis have been reported.[132–134] Echinococcosis is transmitted by the fecal-oral route, through ingestion of food and water contaminated with the feces of carnivorous hosts such as dogs (definitive host) or herbivorous hosts such as sheep and cattle (intermediate hosts).[135] Features include intraluminal organisms with the characteristic germinal layer, protoscoleces and hooklets, in addition to appendiceal wall necrosis and an eosinophilic inflammatory infiltrate.[134] Serologic tests may be very useful in confirming infection.[136]

Trichuris sp. (Whipworms)

Trichuris is a colorectal helminth with a worldwide distribution, particularly in the tropics and parts of Asia. Infection is most commonly seen in children, and is transmitted by ingestion of infective ova through contaminated food or water. The cecum is the primary site of infection (sometimes with the involvement of ileum), followed by the rectum. Appendicitis and peritonitis have been rarely reported.[137,138] Most patients are asymptomatic, although infection in children can lead to malnutrition and growth restriction, and rarely trichuriasis can mimic Crohn's disease.[139,140] The worms are about 4 cm in size and can be seen with the naked eye. Laboratory diagnosis is established by examination of stool for ova and parasites, revealing the distinctive ovoid eggs with bilateral mucus plugs.

Ascaris sp. (Roundworms)

Ascaris is the largest roundworm and the most common human helminthic infection. Prevalence is highest in tropical and subtropical climates, and is associated with poverty and poor sanitation. Ingestion of fertilized eggs leads to infection, most of which are asymptomatic; however, chronic infection in children can cause malnutrition and growth restriction.[141,142]

Rare cases of appendiceal involvement with perforation and peritonitis have been reported.[143,144] Microscopic examination of the stool for eggs can be helpful, and larva can sometimes be identified in sputum or in gastric aspirates. Adult worms occasionally pass through the rectum or oronasal openings as well.[142]

IMPORTANT NONINFECTIOUS ENTITIES IN THE DIFFERENTIAL DIAGNOSIS

Chronic Idiopathic Inflammatory Bowel Disease

Isolated involvement of the appendix is only rarely reported, in less than 2% of Crohn's cases. When the appendix is involved in chronic idiopathic inflammatory bowel disease, it is most often associated with ileocecal Crohn's disease, and can be seen in up to 50% patients with ileocecal involvement.[145,146] Morphologic features include active inflammation, transmural lymphoid aggregates, and mural fibrosis with or without granulomas, and thus Crohn's disease of the appendix may be encountered in the differential diagnosis of granulomatous appendicitis. Inflammation of the appendiceal orifice and the appendix proper can be seen in association with ulcerative colitis as well (Fig. 8.14).[147–150]

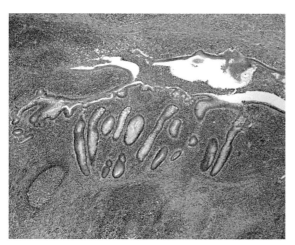

FIG. 8.14 Mucosal ulceration, architectural distortion, and basal plasmacytosis in an appendix involved by ulcerative colitis.

Appendiceal Involvement in Collagen-Vascular Disorders

Vasculitis in the appendix has been reported in the context of Henoch–Schonlein purpura, rheumatoid arthritis, lupus, and enterocolic lymphocytic phlebitis, among others.[151] Although there are rare reports of isolated appendiceal vasculitis, involvement is almost always present as a component of systemic disease, with involvement of other visceral and mesenteric vessels.[151]

REFERENCES

1. Golden RL, Reginald H. Fitz, appendicitis, and the Osler connection–a discursive review. *Surgery.* 1995;118(3):504–509.
2. Thomas Jr CG. Experiences with early operative interference in cases of disease of the vermiform appendix by Charles McBurney, M.D., visiting surgeon to the Roosevelt Hospital, New York city. *Rev Surg.* 1969;26(3):153–166.
3. Carr NJ. The pathology of acute appendicitis. *Ann Diagn Pathol.* 2000;4(1):46–58.
4. Williams RAMP. *Inflammatory Disorders of the Appendix.* London: Chapman and Hall Medical Press; 1994.
5. Wangensteen OH, Bowers WF. Significance of the obstructive factor in the genesis of acute appendicitis. *Arch Surg.* 1937;34:496.
6. Arnbjornsson E, Bengmark S. Role of obstruction in the pathogenesis of acute appendicitis. *Am J Surg.* 1984;147:390–392.
7. Arnbjornsson E. Acute appendicitis and dietary fiber. *Arch Surg.* 1983;118(7):868–870.
8. Arnbjornsson E. Acute appendicitis related to faecal stasis. *Ann Chir Gynaecol.* 1985;74(2):90–93.
9. Sisson RG, Ahlvin RC, Harlow MC. Superficial mucosal ulceration and the pathogenesis of acute appendicitis. *Am J Surg.* 1971;122(3):378–380.
10. Gray Jr GF, Wackym PA. Surgical pathology of the vermiform appendix. *Pathol Annu.* 1986;21(Pt 2):111–144.
11. Jindal N, Kaur GD, Arora S. Rajiv. Bacteriology of acute appendicitis with special reference to anaerobes. *Indian J Pathol Microbiol.* 1994;37(3):299–305.
12. Roberts JP. Quantitative bacterial flora of acute appendicitis. *Arch Dis Child.* 1988;63(5):536–540.
13. Pieper R, Kager L, Weintraub A, Lindberg AA, Nord CE. The role of Bacteroides fragilis in the pathogenesis of acute appendicitis. *Acta Chirurgica Scandinavica.* 1982;148(1):39–44.
14. Elhag KM, Alwan MH, Al-Adnani MS, Sherif RA. Bacteroides fragilis is a silent pathogen in acute appendicitis. *J Med Microbiol.* 1986;21(3):245–249.
15. Higgins MJ, Walsh M, Kennedy SM, Hyland JM, McDermott E, O'Higgins NJ. Granulomatous appendicitis revisited: report of a case. *Dig Surg.* 2001;18(3):245–248.
16. Dudley Jr TH, Dean PJ. Idiopathic granulomatous appendicitis, or Crohn's disease of the appendix revisited. *Hum Pathol.* 1993;24(6):595–601.
17. Huang JC, Appelman HD. Another look at chronic appendicitis resembling Crohn's disease. *Mod Pathol.* 1996;9(10):975–981.
18. Lamps LW, Madhusudhan KT, Greenson JK, et al. The role of Yersinia enterocolitica and Yersinia pseudotuberculosis in granulomatous appendicitis: a histologic and molecular study. *Am J Surg Pathol.* 2001;25(4):508–515.
19. Bronner MP. Granulomatous appendicitis and the appendix in idiopathic inflammatory bowel disease. *Semin Diagn Pathol.* 2004;21(2):98–107.
20. Clarke H, Pollett W, Chittal S, Ra M. Sarcoidosis with involvement of the appendix. *Arch Intern Med.* 1983;143(8):1603–1604.
21. Veress B, Alafuzoff I, Juliusson G. Granulomatous peritonitis and appendicitis of food starch origin. *Gut.* 1991;32(6):718–720.
22. Guo G, Greenson JK. Histopathology of interval (delayed) appendectomy specimens: strong association with granulomatous and xanthogranulomatous appendicitis. *Am J Surg Pathol.* 2003;27(8):1147–1151.
23. van Spreeuwel JP, Lindeman J, Bax R, Elbers HJ, Sybrandy R, Meijer CJ. Campylobacter-associated appendicitis: prevalence and clinicopathologic features. *Pathol Annu.* 1987;22(Pt 1):55–65.
24. Campbell LK, Havens JM, Scott MA, Lamps LW. Molecular detection of Campylobacter jejuni in archival cases of acute appendicitis. *Mod Pathol.* 2006;19(8):1042–1046.
25. Coyne JD, Dervan PA, Haboubi NY. Involvement of the appendix in pseudomembranous colitis. *J Clin Pathol.* 1997;50(1):70–71.
26. Brown TA, Rajappannair L, Dalton AB, Bandi R, Myers JP, Kefalas CH. Acute appendicitis in the setting of *Clostridium difficile* colitis: case report and review of the literature. *Clin Gastroenterol Hepatol.* 2007;5(8):969–971.

27. Martirosian G, Bulanda M, Wojcik-Stojek B, et al. Acute appendicitis: the role of enterotoxigenic strains of Bacteroides fragilis and *Clostridium difficile*. *Med Sci Mon Int Med J Exp Clin Res*. 2001;7(3):382–386.

28. Hackford AW, Tally FP, Reinhold RB, Barza M, Gorbach SL. Prospective study comparing imipenem-cilastatin with clindamycin and gentamicin for the treatment of serious surgical infections. *Arch Surg*. 1988;123(3):322–326.

29. Naktin J, Beavis KG. Yersinia enterocolitica and Yersinia pseudotuberculosis. *Clin Lab Med*. 1999;19(3):523–536, vi.

30. Saebo A, Lassen J. Acute and chronic gastrointestinal manifestations associated with Yersinia enterocolitica infection. A Norwegian 10-year follow-up study on 458 hospitalized patients. *Ann Surg*. 1992;215(3):250–255.

31. Baert F, Peetermans W, Knockaert D. Yersiniosis: the clinical spectrum. *Acta Clinica Belgica*. 1994;49(2):76–85.

32. Bennion RS, Thompson Jr JE, Gil J, Schmit PJ. The role of Yersinia enterocolitica in appendicitis in the southwestern United States. *Am Surg*. 1991;57(12):766–768.

33. Rosner BM, Werber D, Hohle M, Stark K. Clinical aspects and self-reported symptoms of sequelae of Yersinia enterocolitica infections in a population-based study, Germany 2009–2010. *BMC Infect Dis*. 2013;13:236.

34. Gleason TH, Patterson SD. The pathology of Yersinia enterocolitica ileocolitis. *Am J Surg Pathol*. 1982;6(4):347–355.

35. El-Maraghi NR, Mair NS. The histopathology of enteric infection with Yersinia pseudotuberculosis. *Am J Clin Pathol*. 1979;71(6):631–639.

36. Lamps LW. Yersinia enterocolitica and Yersinia pseudotuberculosis. In: Lamps L, ed. *Surgical Pathology of the Gastrointestinal System: Bacterial, Fungal, Viral, and Parasitic Infections*. New York: Springer-Verlag; 2010.

37. Attwood SE, Mealy K, Cafferkey MT, et al. Yersinia infection and acute abdominal pain. *Lancet (Lond Engl)*. 1987;1(8532):529–533.

38. Van Noyen R, Selderslaghs R, Bekaert J, Wauters G, Vandepitte J. Causative role of Yersinia and other enteric pathogens in the appendicular syndrome. *Eur J Clin Microbiol Infect Dis*. 1991;10(9):735–741.

39. Dekker JP, Frank KM. Salmonella, Shigella, and yersinia. *Clin Lab Med*. 2015;35(2):225–246.

40. Buss SN, Leber A, Chapin K, et al. Multicenter evaluation of the BioFire FilmArray gastrointestinal panel for etiologic diagnosis of infectious gastroenteritis. *J Clin Microbiol*. 2015;53(3):915–925.

41. Gayraud M, Scavizzi MR, Mollaret HH, Guillevin L, Hornstein MJ. Antibiotic treatment of Yersinia enterocolitica septicemia: a retrospective review of 43 cases. *Clin Infect Dis*. 1993;17(3):405–410.

42. Pham JN, Bell SM, Lanzarone JY. Biotype and antibiotic sensitivity of 100 clinical isolates of Yersinia enterocolitica. *J Antimicrob Chemother*. 1991;28(1):13–18.

43. Pham JN, Bell SM, Martin L, Carniel E. The beta-lactamases and beta-lactam antibiotic susceptibility of Yersinia enterocolitica. *J Antimicrob Chemother*. 2000;46(6):951–957.

44. Kazlow PG, Freed J, Rosh JR, et al. *Salmonella typhimurium* appendicitis. *J Pediatr Gastroenterol Nutr*. 1991;13(1):101–103.

45. Golakai VK, Makunike R. Perforation of terminal ileum and appendix in typhoid enteritis: report of two cases. *East Afr Med J*. 1997;74(12):796–799.

46. CDC. *Salmonella*; 2017. https://www.cdc.gov/salmonella/general/.

47. Lending RE, Buchsbaum HW, Hyland RN. Shigellosis complicated by acute appendicitis. *South Med J*. 1986;79(8):1046–1047.

48. Nussinovitch M, Shapiro RP, Cohen AH, Varsano I. Shigellosis complicated by perforated appendix. *Pediatr Infect Dis J*. 1993;12(4):352–353.

49. CDC. *Shigella – Shigellosis*; 2017. https://www.cdc.gov/shigella/index.html.

50. Maharjan S. An uncommon case of chronic tubercular appendicitis. *Case Rep Pathol*. 2015;2015:534838.

51. WHO. *Global Tuberculosis Report 2016*. Geneva, Switzerland: World Health Organization; 2016. http://www.who.int/tb/publications/global_report/en/.

52. Horvath KD, Whelan RL. Intestinal tuberculosis: return of an old disease. *Am J Gastroenterol*. 1998;93(5):692–696.

53. Singh MK, Arunabh KVK. Tuberculosis of the appendix–a report of 17 cases and a suggested aetiopathological classification. *Postgrad Med*. 1987;63(744):855–857.

54. Mittal VK, Khanna SK, Gupta NM, Aikat M. Isolated tuberculosis of appendix. *Am Surg*. 1975;41(3):172–174.

55. Agarwal P, Sharma D, Agarwal A, et al. Tuberculous appendicitis in India. *Trop Doct*. 2004;34(1):36–38.

56. Chong VH, Telisinghe PU, Yapp SK, Chong CF. Tuberculous appendix: a review of clinical presentations and outcomes. *Singap Med J*. 2011;52(2):90–93.

57. Livingston RA, Siberry GK, Paidas CN, Eiden JJ. Appendicitis due to *Mycobacterium avium* complex in an adolescent infected with the human immunodeficiency virus. *Clin Infect Dis*. 1995;20(6):1579–1580.

58. Basilio-de-Oliveira C, Eyer-Silva WA, Valle HA, Rodrigues AL, Pinheiro Pimentel AL, Morais-De-Sa CA. Mycobacterial spindle cell pseudotumor of the appendix vermiformis in a patient with aids. *Braz J Infect Dis*. 2001;5(2):98–100.

59. Ferrari TC, Couto CA, Murta-Oliveira C, Conceicao SA, Silva RG. Actinomycosis of the colon: a rare form of presentation. *Scand J Gastroenterol*. 2000;35(1):108–109.

60. Mueller MC, Ihrler S, Degenhart C, Bogner JR. Abdominal actinomycosis. *Infection*. 2008;36(2):191.

61. Schmidt P, Koltai JL, Weltzien A. Actinomycosis of the appendix in childhood. *Pediatr Surg Int*. 1999;15(1):63–65.

62. Ridha A, Oguejiofor N, Al-Abayechi S, Njoku E. Intraabdominal actinomycosis mimicking malignant abdominal disease. *Case Rep Infect Dis*. 2017;2017:1972023.

63. Ng N, Ng G, Davis BR, Meier DE. Actinomyces appendicitis: diagnostic dilemma–malignancy or infection? *Am Surg*. 2014;80(1):E33–E35.

64. Tateishi Y, Takahashi M, Horiguchi S, et al. Clinicopathologic study of intestinal spirochetosis in Japan with

special reference to human immunodeficiency virus infection status and species types: analysis of 5265 consecutive colorectal biopsies. *BMC Infect Dis.* 2015;15:13.

65. Ogata S, Shimizu K, Nakanishi K. Human intestinal spirochetosis: right-side preference in the large intestine. *Ann Diagn Pathol.* 2015;19(6):414–417.

66. Henrik-Nielsen R, Lundbeck FA, Teglbjaerg PS, Ginnerup P, Hovind-Hougen K. Intestinal spirochetosis of the vermiform appendix. *Gastroenterology.* 1985;88(4):971–977.

67. Umeda S, Serizawa H, Kobayashi T, et al. Clinical significance of human intestinal spirochetosis: a retrospective study. *Nihon Shokakibyo Gakkai zasshi.* 2017;114(2):230–237.

68. Ogata S, Shimizu K, Oda T, Tominaga S, Nakanishi K. Immunohistochemical detection of human intestinal spirochetosis. *Hum Pathol.* 2016;58:128–133.

69. Westerman LJ, Schipper ME, Stel HV, Bonten MJ, Kusters JG. Appendiceal spirochaetosis in children. *Gut Pathog.* 2013;5(1):40.

70. Tseng BY, Yang HH, Liou JH, Chen LK, Hsu YH. Immunohistochemical study of scrub typhus: a report of two cases. *Kaohsiung J Med Sci.* 2008;24(2):92–98.

71. Walker DH, Lesesne HR, Varma VA, Thacker WC. Rocky Mountain spotted fever mimicking acute cholecystitis. *Arch Intern Med.* 1985;145(12):2194–2196.

72. Randall MB, Walker DH. Rocky Mountain spotted fever. Gastrointestinal and pancreatic lesions and rickettsial infection. *Arch Pathol Lab Med.* 1984;108(12):963–967.

73. Horney LF, Walker DH. Meningoencephalitis as a major manifestation of Rocky Mountain spotted fever. *South Med J.* 1988;81(7):915–918.

74. Reif RM. Viral appendicitis. *Hum Pathol.* 1981;12(2):193–196.

75. Yunis EJ, Atchison RW, Michaels RH, DeCicco FA. Adenovirus and ileocecal intussusception. *Lab Investig J Tech Methods Pathol.* 1975;33(4):347–351.

76. Porter HJ, Padfield CJ, Peres LC, Hirschowitz L, Berry PJ. Adenovirus and intranuclear inclusions in appendices in intussusception. *J Clin Pathol.* 1993;46(2):154–158.

77. Montgomery EA, Popek EJ. Intussusception, adenovirus, and children: a brief reaffirmation. *Hum Pathol.* 1994;25(2):169–174.

78. Staras SA, Dollard SC, Radford KW, Flanders WD, Pass RF, Cannon MJ. Seroprevalence of cytomegalovirus infection in the United States, 1988-1994. *Clin Infect Dis.* 2006;43(9):1143–1151.

79. Neumayer LA, Makar R, Ampel NM, Zukoski CF. Cytomegalovirus appendicitis in a patient with human immunodeficiency virus infection. Case report and review of the literature. *Arch Surg.* 1993;128(4):467–468.

80. Valerdiz-Casasola S, Pardo-Mindan FJ. Cytomegalovirus infection of the appendix in patient with the acquired immunodeficiency syndrome. *Gastroenterology.* 1991;101(1):247–249.

81. Baroco AL, Oldfield EC. Gastrointestinal cytomegalovirus disease in the immunocompromised patient. *Curr Gastroenterol Rep.* 2008;10(4):409–416.

82. Katzoli P, Sakellaris G, Ergazaki M, Charissis G, Spandidos DA, Sourvinos G. Detection of herpes viruses in children with acute appendicitis. *J Clin Virol.* 2009;44(4):282–286.

83. Kotton H. *Cytomegalovirus and Human Herpesvirus Types 6–8. Harrison's Principles of Internal Medicine.* New York, NY: McGraw-Hill; 2015.

84. Chetty R, Roskell DE. Cytomegalovirus infection in the gastrointestinal tract. *J Clin Pathol.* 1994;47(11):968–972.

85. Kotton CN. CMV: prevention, diagnosis and therapy. *Am J Transplant.* 2013;13(suppl 3):24–40; quiz 40.

86. Lopez-Navidad A, Domingo P, Cadafalch J, Farrerons J, Allende L, Bordes R. Acute appendicitis complicating infectious mononucleosis: case report and review. *Rev Infect Dis.* 1990;12(2):297–302.

87. Paik SY, Oh JT, Choi YJ, Kwon KW, Yang WI. Measles-related appendicitis. *Arch Pathol Lab Med.* 2002;126(1):82–84.

88. Galloway WH. Appendicitis in the course of measles. *Br Med J.* 1953;2(4851):1412–1414.

89. CDC. Measles. https://www.cdc.gov/measles/lab-tools/index.html.

90. ter Borg F, Kuijper EJ, van der Lelie H. Fatal mucormycosis presenting as an appendiceal mass with metastatic spread to the liver during chemotherapy-induced granulocytopenia. *Scand J Infect Dis.* 1990;22(4):499–501.

91. Baig WW, Ravindra Prabhu A, Natraj KS, Mathew M. Combined mucormycosis and candidiasis of the cecum presenting as a right iliac fossa mass in a patient with chronic kidney disease. *Trav Med Infect Dis.* 2008;6(3):145–147.

92. Lamps LW, Molina CP, West AB, Haggitt RC, Scott MA. The pathologic spectrum of gastrointestinal and hepatic histoplasmosis. *Am J Clin Pathol.* 2000;113(1):64–72.

93. Larbcharoensub N, Boonsakan P, Kanoksil W, et al. Fungal appendicitis: a case series and review of the literature. *Southeast Asian J Trop Med Publ Health.* 2013;44(4):681–689.

94. Sinniah B, Leopairut J, Neafie RC, Connor DH, Voge M. Enterobiasis: a histopathological study of 259 patients. *Ann Trop Med Parasitol.* 1991;85(6):625–635.

95. Arca MJ, Gates RL, Groner JI, Hammond S, Caniano DA. Clinical manifestations of appendiceal pinworms in children: an institutional experience and a review of the literature. *Pediatr Surg Int.* 2004;20(5):372–375.

96. Wiebe BM. Appendicitis and Enterobius vermicularis. *Scand J Gastroenterol.* 1991;26(3):336–338.

97. Yildirim S, Nursal TZ, Tarim A, Kayaselcuk F, Noyan T. A rare cause of acute appendicitis: parasitic infection. *Scand J Infect Dis.* 2005;37(10):757–759.

98. Mogensen K, Pahle E, Kowalski K. Enterobius vermicularis and acute appendicitis. *Acta Chirurgica Scandinavica.* 1985;151(8):705–707.

99. Nadler S, Cappell MS, Bhatt B, Matano S, Kure K. Appendiceal infection by Entamoeba histolytica and Strongyloides stercoralis presenting like acute appendicitis. *Dig Dis Sci.* 1990;35(5):603–608.

100. Shakir AA, Youngberg G, Alvarez S. Strongyloides infestation as a cause of acute appendicitis. *J Tenn Med Assoc.* 1986;79(9):543–544.

101. Noodleman JS. Eosinophilic appendicitis. Demonstration of Strongyloides stercoralis as a causative agent. *Arch Pathol Lab Med.* 1981;105(3):148–149.

102. Schar F, Trostdorf U, Giardina F, et al. Strongyloides stercoralis: global distribution and risk factors. *PLoS Neglected Trop Dis.* 2013;7(7):e2288.

103. Komenaka IK, Wu GC, Lazar EL, Cohen JA. Strongyloides appendicitis: unusual etiology in two siblings with chronic abdominal pain. *J Pediatr Surg.* 2003;38(9):E8–E10.

104. Felekouras E, Kontos M, Kyriakou V, et al. Strongyloides stercoralis infection as a cause of acute granulomatous appendicitis in an HIV-positive patient in Athens, Greece. *Scand J Infect Dis.* 2002;34(11):856–857.

105. Adebamowo CA, Akang EE, Ladipo JK, Ajao OG. Schistosomiasis of the appendix. *Br J Surg.* 1991;78(10):1219–1221.

106. Satti MB, Tamimi DM, Al Sohaibani MO, Al Quorain A. Appendicular schistosomiasis: a cause of clinical acute appendicitis? *J Clin Pathol.* 1987;40(4):424–428.

107. Badmos KB, Komolafe AO, Rotimi O. Schistosomiasis presenting as acute appendicitis. *East Afr Med J.* 2006;83(10):528–532.

108. Doudier B, Parola P, Dales JP, Linzberger N, Brouqui P, Delmont J. Schistosomiasis as an unusual cause of appendicitis. *Clin Microbiol Infect.* 2004;10(2):89–91.

109. Rivasi F, Pampiglione S. Appendicitis associated with presence of Schistosoma haematobium eggs: an unusual pathology for Europe. Report of three cases. *APMIS.* 2006;114(1):72–76.

110. Ramdial PK, Madiba TE, Kharwa S, Clarke B, Zulu B. Isolated amoebic appendicitis. *Virchows Arch.* 2002;441(1):63–68.

111. Gotohda N, Itano S, Okada Y, et al. Acute appendicitis caused by amebiasis. *J Gastroenterol.* 2000;35(11):861–863.

112. Singh NG, Mannan AA, Kahvic M. Acute amebic appendicitis: report of a rare case. *Indian J Pathol Microbiol.* 2010;53(4):767–768.

113. Eslick G. Infectious causes of appendicitis. In: Mollering R, ed. *Diseases of the Gastrointestinal Tract and Associated Infections.* Saunders; 2010:995–1017.

114. Solaymani-Mohammadi S, Rezaian M, Anwar MA. Human balantidiasis in Iran: an unresolved enigma? *Trends Parasitol.* 2005;21(4):160–161.

115. Gonzalez Sanchez O. [Acute appendicitis caused by Balantidium coli]. *Rev Cubana Med Trop.* 1978;30(1):9–13.

116. Dodd LG. Balantidium coli infestation as a cause of acute appendicitis. *J Infect Dis.* 1991;163(6):1392.

117. Dorfman S, Rangel O, Bravo LG. Balantidiasis: report of a fatal case with appendicular and pulmonary involvement. *Trans R Soc Trop Med Hyg.* 1984;78(6):833–834.

118. Schuster FL, Ramirez-Avila L. Current world status of Balantidium coli. *Clin Microbiol Rev.* 2008;21(4):626–638.

119. Garcia-Laverde A, de Bonilla L. Clinical trials with metronidazole in human balantidiasis. *Am J Trop Med Hyg.* 1975;24(5):781–783.

120. Dubey JP, Jones JL. Toxoplasma gondii infection in humans and animals in the United States. *Int J Parasitol.* 2008;38(11):1257–1278.

121. Paquet C, Yudin MH. Toxoplasmosis in pregnancy: prevention, screening, and treatment. *J Obstet Gynaecol Can.* 2013;35(1):78–81.

122. Stansfeld AG. The histological diagnosis of toxoplasmic lymphadenitis. *J Clin Pathol.* 1961;14(6):565–573.

123. Ojo OS, Udeh SC, Odesanmi WO. Review of the histopathological findings in appendices removed for acute appendicitis in Nigerians. *J R Coll Surg Edinb.* 1991;36(4):245–248.

124. Liu Q, Wang ZD, Huang SY, Zhu XQ. Diagnosis of toxoplasmosis and typing of Toxoplasma gondii. *Parasites Vectors.* 2015;8:292.

125. Oberhuber G, Lauer E, Stolte M, Borchard F. Cryptosporidiosis of the appendix vermiformis: a case report. *Zeitschrift fur Gastroenterologie.* 1991;29(11):606–608.

126. Ramsden K, Freeth M. Cryptosporidial infection presenting as an acute appendicitis. *Histopathology.* 1989;14(2):209–211.

127. Buch K, Nguyen S, Divino CM, Weber K, Morotti RA. Cryptosporidiosis presenting as acute appendicitis: a case report. *Am Surg.* 2005;71(6):537–538.

128. Chen XM, Keithly JS, Paya CV, LaRusso NF. Cryptosporidiosis. *N Engl J Med.* 2002;346(22):1723–1731.

129. Bouzid M, Hunter PR, Chalmers RM, Tyler KM. Cryptosporidium pathogenicity and virulence. *Clin Microbiol Rev.* 2013;26(1):115–134.

130. Checkley W, White Jr AC, Jaganath D, et al. A review of the global burden, novel diagnostics, therapeutics, and vaccine targets for cryptosporidium. *Lancet Infect Dis.* 2015;15(1):85–94.

131. Thompson RC. Biology and systematics of Echinococcus. *Adv Parasitol.* 2017;95:65–109.

132. Vaizey CJ, Sanne I, Gilbert JM. Periappendiceal hydatidosis: an unusual cause of right iliac fossa pain. *Br J Surg.* 1994;81(9):1371–1372.

133. Mondal K, Mandal R. Acute appendicitis caused by an echinococcal Brood capsule unmasks an asymptomatic hepatic hydatid cyst. *ACG Case Rep J.* 2017;4:e74.

134. Hajizadeh M, Ahmadpour E, Sadat ATE, Spotin A. Hydatidosis as a cause of acute appendicitis: a case report. *Asian Pac J Trop Dis.* 2013;3(1):71–73.

135. Eckert J, Deplazes P. Biological, epidemiological, and clinical aspects of echinococcosis, a zoonosis of increasing concern. *Clin Microbiol Rev.* 2004;17(1):107–135.

136. Tamarozzi F, Covini I, Mariconti M, et al. Comparison of the diagnostic accuracy of three rapid tests for the Serodiagnosis of hepatic cystic echinococcosis in humans. *PLoS Neglected Trop Dis.* 2016;10(2):e0004444.

137. Dorfman S, Cardozo J, Dorfman D, Del Villar A. The role of parasites in acute appendicitis of pediatric patients. *Invest Clin.* 2003;44(4):337–340.

138. Haines DO, Buckley JJ, Pester FR. A cryptic infection of an appendix with the whipworm, Trichuris trichiura in Britain. *J Helminthol.* 1968;42(3):289–294.

139. Cook GC. The clinical significance of gastrointestinal helminths–a review. *Trans R Soc Trop Med Hyg.* 1986;80(5):675–685.

140. CDC. Trichuriasis. https://www.cdc.gov/dpdx/trichuriasis/index.html.

141. Khuroo MS. Ascariasis. *Gastroenterol Clin N Am.* 1996;25(3):553–577.

142. CDC. Ascariasis. https://www.cdc.gov/dpdx/ascariasis/index.html.

143. Sinha SN, Sinha BN. Appendicular perforation due to *Ascaris lumbricoides. J Indian Med Assoc.* 1974;63(12):396–397.

144. Gahukamble DB, Gahukamble L. Granulomatous peritonitis due to *Ascaris lumbricoides. Ann Trop Paediatr.* 1987;7(2):142–144.

145. Vanek VW, Spirtos G, Awad M, Badjatia N, Bernat D. Isolated Crohn's disease of the appendix. Two case reports and a review of the literature. *Arch Surg.* 1988;123(1):85–87.

146. Machado NO, Chopra PJ, Hamdani AA. Crohn's disease of the appendix with enterocutaneous fistula post-appendicectomy: an approach to management. *N Am J Med Sci.* 2010;2(3):158–161.

147. Anzai H, Hata K, Kishikawa J, et al. Appendiceal orifice inflammation is associated with proximal extension of disease in patients with ulcerative colitis. *Colorectal Dis.* 2016;18(8):O278–O282.

148. D'Haens G, Geboes K, Peeters M, Baert F, Ectors N, Rutgeerts P. Patchy cecal inflammation associated with distal ulcerative colitis: a prospective endoscopic study. *Am J Gastroenterol.* 1997;92(8):1275–1279.

149. Matsumoto T, Nakamura S, Shimizu M, Iida M. Significance of appendiceal involvement in patients with ulcerative colitis. *Gastrointest Endosc.* 2002;55(2):180–185.

150. Mutinga ML, Odze RD, Wang HH, Hornick JL, Farraye FA. The clinical significance of right-sided colonic inflammation in patients with left-sided chronic ulcerative colitis. *Inflamm Bowel Dis.* 2004;10(3):215–219.

151. Richards T, Strabac M, Ludeman L. Vasculitic appendicitis. *J R Soc Med.* 2004;97(9):439–440.

CHAPTER 9

Infectious Organisms Associated With Colorectal Cancer

MIN YOUNG PARK, MD, BMUSSTUDIES •
GUY D. ESLICK, DRPH, PHD, FACE, FFPH

Colorectal cancer (CRC) is the third most common malignancy diagnosed worldwide[1] and more than half of all incidence rates occur in developed countries. It is the third leading cause of cancer-related mortality in both men and women, and also one of the major catalysts for morbidity in those who suffer from the disease. Efforts have been made to enhance our understanding of the pathogenesis of CRC as a multistep process from years of interplay between genetic and environmental factors. Approximately 20%–25% of all CRCs originate from familial basis, and as many as 5% of colon cancers have an identifiable single gene modification.[2] Some of the most notable single gene syndromes include familial adenomatous polyposis (FAP), hereditary nonpolyposis colorectal cancer or Lynch syndrome, and Gardner syndrome. Thus far, accumulating evidence has regarded lifestyle high in red meat consumption, low fiber diet, and tobacco smoking as some of the recognizable epigenetic parameters potentially contributing to the occurrence of CRC (Fig. 9.1). In the past decades, infectious agents including human papilloma virus (HPV), hepatitis virus B, C, and *Helicobacter pylori* have become to be acknowledged as the primary carcinogens for cervical cancer, liver cancer, and gastric cancer, respectively. Consequently, there has been increasing number of studies to elucidate a potential relationship between various pathogens and CRC. Although infectious agents are still not included in the long list of risk factors for colorectal tumorigenesis, the current literature evidence appears to support this causal link. This article aims to review proposed mechanisms and assess the current literature evidence for the involvement of microbes as carcinogens for CRC.

The pathogenesis of CRC is a slow, sequential process that involves acquisition of premalignant lesions and transformation into cancerous cells due to multiple molecular alterations over a course of years or even up to decades. A number of molecular pathways have been implicated in the occurrence of both familial and sporadic forms of CRC including chromosomal instability and the CpG island hypermethylation.[3] The human gastrointestinal tract is a habitat for over 100 trillion bacteria from more than 500 different species.[4] This microbial community is essential for mucosal immune system and nutrient absorption.[5] Considering the pivotal role of gut microbiota in maintaining functional homeostasis and other beneficial effects, the exact mechanism of bacterial commensals in induction of colorectal oncogenesis has been difficult to elucidate. A combination of mutagenic toxins from the bacteria and cytotoxic damage from immune response is likely to produce a synergistic effect for the initiation of chronic inflammation (Fig. 9.2). Activation of cyclooxygenase-2 (COX-2) is considered to be responsible for chronic inflammation through downstream signaling pathways that inhibit apoptosis, increase angiogenesis, reduce the production of antitumorigenic cytokines, and disseminate tumor cells to colonic epithelial cells. COX-2 has been shown to be highly expressed in individuals with clinically diagnosed CRC in comparison with healthy controls.[5–10] The importance of the enzyme was further emphasized in chemoprotective effects of both nonspecific and specific COX-2 inhibitor against colorectal tumorigenesis although higher cardiovascular risk was observed in the latter agents.[12–18] Furthermore, overexpression of COX-2 was correlated to higher propensity for the development of CRC in mouse models, whereby various mutant models of tumor suppressor gene adenomatous *Polyposis coli* (*APC*) had decreased CRC incidence after deletion of COX-2 gene.[19–22] Once initiated, chronic inflammation cascades p53 mutations and disrupts the symbiotic relationship in gut microbiota. The incidence rates of adenomas and adenocarcinomas decreased significantly in T-cell receptor β (TCRβ)/p53 knockout and *Apc*^{min} mice models (representative model of human FAP) raised in germ-free condition, respectively.[22–25] Emerging evidence has indicated a selective pool of bacteria, and viruses can

Copyright © 2019 Elsevier Inc. All rights reserved.

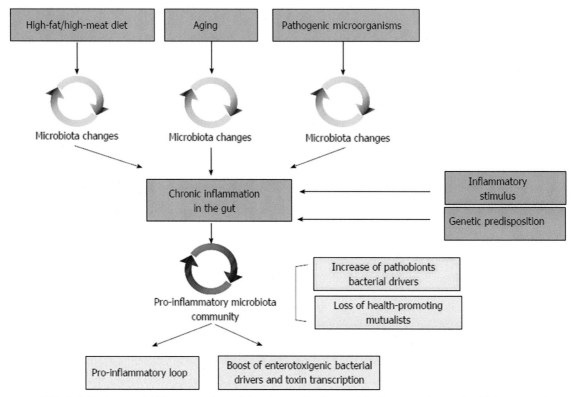

FIG. 9.1 Environmental triggers, such as diet, aging, and pathogen infections, can force microbiota changings that, in a genetically susceptible host, can drive to chronic inflammation in the gut. Inflammation shifts the gut microbiota toward a proinflammatory configuration, supporting colorectal cancer (CRC) drivers as pathobionts at the expense of health-promoting CRC-protective microbiota components. As a consequence, a proinflammatory loop is established in the gut, directly supporting CRC onset and favoring colonization by toxigenic bacterial drivers directly involved in CRC promotion. (From Candela M, Turroni S, Biagi E, et al. Inflammation and colorectal cancer, when microbiota-host mutualism breaks. *World J Gastroenterol*. 2014;20(4):908–922.)

produce mutagenic toxins for direct modulation of colonic epithelial cells leading to neoplasia or activate the immune system to generative reactive species causing genomic or chromosomal instability.

STREPTOCOCCUS BOVIS

Streptococcus bovis is a Gram-positive, nonenterococcal bacterium that is well recognized as one of the gastrointestinal commensals found in approximately 11%–16% of asymptomatic individuals.[28] The bacterium initially underwent a nomenclature change from *S. bovis* into *S. gallolyticus* after its pathogenic potential for CRC was acknowledged in a study by Osawa and colleagues.[29] Schlegel et al. proposed another taxonomic change after three subspecies were recognized for their

differences in molecular characteristics as *S. gallolyticus* subsp *gallolyticus* (I), *S. infantarius* subsp *infantarius* and *S. infantarius* subsp *coli* (both II/1), and *S. gallolyticus* subsp *pastuerianus* (II/2).[30] The relationship between *S. bovis* and CRC was first proposed in a case report during the 1950s when bacteremia and infective endocarditis have already been acknowledged as serious clinical manifestations of opportunistic infection from this organism.[31,32] The prevalence of *S. bovis* in CRC cases has previously been shown to range from 10% to 80% in relation to those with diagnosis of endocarditis.[33–37] A recent meta-analysis indicated increased odds ratios of 7.48 (95% CI 3.10–18.06) for CRC in patients with *S. bovis* septicemia and 14.5 (95% CI 5.66–37.35) in *S. bovis* infective endocarditis.[38] In contrast, the association between *S. bovis* and CRC could

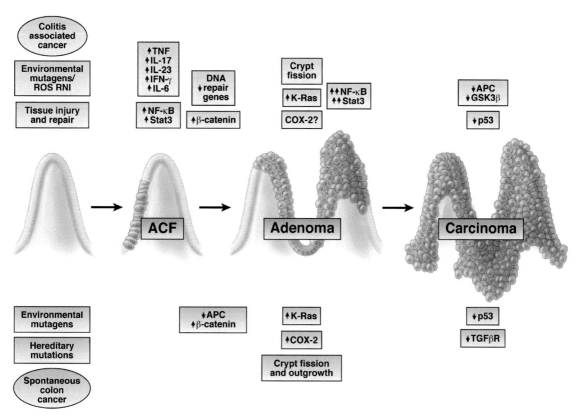

FIG. 9.2 Mechanisms of colorectal cancer (CRC) and colitis-associated cancer (CAC) development. CRC is caused by accumulation of mutations in oncogenes and tumor suppressor genes; some of these lead to aberrant activation of β-catenin signaling. Mutations in adenomatous polyposis coli (APC), β-catenin, or other components of this pathway mediate the transition of single preneoplastic cells to aberrant crypt foci (ACF) and then to adenoma and colorectal carcinoma. Chronic inflammation, which leads to CAC, is characterized by production of proinflammatory cytokines that can induce mutations in oncogenes and tumor suppressor genes (APC, p53, K-ras) and genomic instability via various mechanisms. Persistent inflammation facilitates tumor promotion by activating proliferation and antiapoptotic properties of premalignant cells, as well as tumor progression and metastasis. There is considerable overlap in mechanisms of CRC and CAC pathogenesis. GSK-β, glycogen synthase kinase-β; RNI, reactive nitrogen intermediates; TGF, transforming growth factor. (From Terzić J, Grivennikov S, Karin E, Karin M. Inflammation and colon cancer. *Gastroenterology*. 2010;138(6):2101–2114.e5, with permission.)

not be clearly defined based on inconsistent results obtained from fecal antigen studies.[38–42] Collated evidence from studies using culturing techniques has also not been convincing due to variability in molecular biology techniques and logistical obstacles arising from these.[42–46] A number of serological studies have shown higher antibody titer with immunoglobulin G (IgG) in individuals with *S. bovis* colonization compared with controls, but the findings were not statistically significant due to small sample size.[45,47] Studies with more sensitive biochemical tests[34,43] have indicated clinically confirmed *S. bovis* septicemia and/or endocarditis can increase likelihood of CRC in affected patients or being diagnosed with the cancer at a younger age of less than 65 years of age once initial infection has resolved.[48] Among subspecies of *S. bovis* (or *S. gallolyticus*), *S. bovis* (I) has been suggested as the main driving force in initiating oncologic process of colorectal neoplasia.[49–51] Isolates from *S. bovis* (I) showed greater capacity for biofilm formation through adhesion of pilus protein from the bacterium to collagen types I and IV found in heart muscles, which eventually leads to a higher incidence rate of endocarditis.[34,52–56] Once colonized, S. bovis (I) induces cyclo-oxygenase 2 pathway to create a proinflammatory environment suitable for cancer cells to proliferate.[43,57,58] Nevertheless, transition of data from experimental and epidemiological studies into the actual clinical practice for understanding the relationship between S. bovis and CRC remains questionable, as a recent 17-year longitudinal cohort study did not detect any advanced colonic lesion in patients with S. bovis.[42] Future research directions should be aimed at understanding whether S. bovis plays a pivotal part in the etiology of CRC or maintaining a procarcinogenic status through its virulent factors. Clinical practice should also ideally be altered, whereby confirmed S. bovis cases in CRC patients to be more closely monitored with possible options of treating the bacterial infection for improved oncological outcome.

HELICOBACTER PYLORI

Helicobacter pylori is a Gram-negative bacterium and was classified as a group 1 human carcinogen in association with gastric cancer by International Agency for Research on Cancer (IARC) in 1994.[59] The pathogen has an extensive influence on causality of multiple premalignant lesions and chronic inflammatory conditions including chronic gastritis, gastric/duodenal ulcer, and intestinal metaplasia. Due to its infection found in around half of the adult population in many countries,[60,61] its linkages with other intestinal pathologies and colorectal carcinogenicity have been investigated. Considering the organism is difficult to culture, polymerase chain reaction and the C-urea breath test have been accepted as alternative detection methods. A recent meta-analysis conducted by Wu et al. has demonstrated increased odds ratios of H. pylori infection for both colorectal cancer and colorectal adenoma, 1.39 (95% CI 1.18–1.64) and 1.66 (95% CI 1.39–1.97), respectively.[62] However, there was significant heterogeneity between included studies and evidence for publication bias. Furthermore, two prospective studies included in the meta-analysis have shown that there was no increased risk for acquisition of CRC from H. pylori infection. Findings from these studies were conflicting in comparison with retrospective case–control, pilot, and cross-sectional studies. There are two main proposed mechanisms of CRC carcinogenesis in relation to H. pylori infection out of some of the other suggested hypotheses. Chronic inflammation in intestinal epithelial cells is induced by interaction of cytotoxin-associated gene (CagA) with SHP-2, which promotes interleukin-8 (IL-8) secretion and eventually

unregulated cell growth.[63] Furthermore, hosts infected with CagA positive H. pylori have been shown to acquire hypergastrinemia. Increased gastrin level from H. pylori infection is another suggested mechanism due to its possible involvement as a growth factor in tumor angiogenesis and trophic effects in intestinal mucosa.[64–66] However, the role of H. pylori in oncogenesis of CRC remains inconclusive, which is largely attributed to conflicted findings from more recent[67–69] studies in comparison with preceded concept of positive association between H. pylori and CRC.

ESCHERICHIA COLI

Escherichia coli (E. coli) are rod-shaped, Gram-negative bacteria found as commensal flora in human gastrointestinal tract. They are aero-anaerobic and one of the most cultivatable organisms in stool cultures. E. coli are categorized into four phylogenetic groups depending on their virulence factors (A, B1, B2, and D).[70–72] Among these subtypes, E. coli groups B2 and D have been shown to be more enteropathogenic, associated with Crohn's disease[73–75] and also cause extraintestinal diseases. In particular, some strains from phylogroup B2 have been implicated in CRC tumorigenesis after a number of studies have shown mucosal E. coli to be more prevalent in colonic tissue samples from patients with CRC, but not in controls.[76–78] One of the cyclomodulin (CM)-encoding E. coli strains, commonly known as pks island, encodes colibactin. This is a polypeptide with high genotoxic potentials for inducing carcinogenesis through cellular senescence that causes DNA damage, but not necessarily with intestinal inflammation, as seen in both in vitro and in vivo studies. These findings have provided a glimpse into the mechanism of the linkage between E. coli and colorectal neoplasia. Further studies are needed to verify the capability of these toxins in changing genetic configuration of cancer-free samples and their subsequent long-term effects.

ENTEROCOCCUS FAECALIS

Enterococcus faecalis is a part of Gram-positive coccus and facultative anaerobes that are commonly found as one of the human intestinal commensals. Along with other enterococci, E. faecalis can generate oxygen-free radicals in a genetically susceptible host to induce chronic inflammation that is suitable for the development of CRC, as shown in interleukin-10 (IL-10) knockout mice models.[79,80] These byproducts interact with lipophilic membrane of colonic epithelial cells to produce oxidized fatty acids that can lead to genomic stress[81] and chromosomal instability in mammalian cells.[82] Also known as a 'macrophage-induced bystander effect',[83] this cellular mechanism of producing extracellular superoxides is recognized as the main driving force in colorectal tumorigenic process in vitro and in vivo studies.[82,84] However, findings from laboratory studies have not been reproducible in clinical practice after a prospective cohort study by Winter and colleagues had contrasting findings between the initial and 1-year follow-up results.[85] This study initially showed that 40% of stool samples obtained from patients with CRC had free oxygen radical-producing E. faecalis, but microbiota composition of the same patients changed drastically in a follow-up collection of samples 1 year later.

BACTEROIDES FRAGILIS

Bacteroides fragilis is a Gram-negative, rod-shaped anaerobe that comprises a small portion of the normal microbial symbiont in human gastrointestinal tract. There are two subtypes—nontoxigenic and enterotoxigenic (ETBF), which is responsible for inflammatory diarrheal diseases[86] including CRC.[87] B. fragilis toxin (BFT) is the primary culprit in inducing DNA damage and promoting proinflammatory cytokines in colonic epithelial cells through specific receptor binding.[86,87] In particular, the role of IL-17 has been highlighted in relation to regulatory T cells, which have paradoxically been shown to reduce the likelihood of intestinal neoplasia from chronic inflammation.[88] Although a number of laboratory studies in mouse models have supported the orchestration of the bacterium in colorectal oncogenesis, there have been only two studies where the results were translational in humans.[89,90] The most recent study conducted by Boleij and his colleagues demonstrated higher detection rate of BFT in colorectal cancer cases (75%) with no prior history of antibiotic treatment than in controls (67%). Considering the impact of B. fragilis on colonic epithelial cells in experiments, further clinical studies with long-term data are warranted to affirm their association.

FUSOBACTERIUM NUCLEATUM

Fusobacterium nucleatum is an obligate, Gram-negative microorganism. It commonly forms a part of commensal flora of the human oral cavity along with a number of other anaerobes. In spite of being one of the most abundant microbiomes in human body, it is implicated in a wide spectrum of diseases—most notably in periodontal diseases, intrauterine infection, appendicitis, inflammatory bowel disease, and liver abscess.[91] There has been increasing evidence for the pathogenicity of F. nucleatum in colorectal tumorigenesis after a number of laboratory studies have demonstrated its overpopulation in patient samples compared with healthy controls and also in mice models.[92–101] The adhesive nature of the bacterium may allow horizontal gene transfer from coexisting microbiota. There are two notable virulence factors including FadA and Fap2. FadA has been shown to activate B-catenin signaling pathway to promote tumor cell progression and also invade epithelial and/or endothelial cell layers to generate proinflammatory cytokines.[102] Fap2 creates a suitable microenvironment for the development of CRC through interaction with immune cell activities.[103] In reference to the aforementioned potential mechanisms, detection methods for F. nucleatum and tissue preparation are largely variable between studies. These differences in turn showed contrasting results, whereby one study showed impressive 87.13%[97] detection rate of the bacterium in CRC patients as opposed to other studies showing inconsistent rates.[98,99,105–106] Long-term data with prospective study designs are needed to ascertain the actual clinical impact of the microorganism in the context of CRC progression.

HUMAN PAPILLOMA VIRUS

HPV is a double-stranded DNA virus with over 100 genotypes, and 40 of these have been identified to infect basal layer of epithelial cells through microscopic abrasions.[107] These subtypes can be largely classified into two groups based on their risk potential for causing cervical cancer. Subtypes including HPV-6 and 11 are primarily responsible for benign lesions including anogenital warts and laryngeal papillomatosis.[108] HPV-16 and 18 are acknowledged as carcinogens for cervical, anal, head, and neck squamous cell carcinomas through years of extensive research.[109] Other HPV subtypes have also been linked to cancers in oropharyngeal[110] and anogenital tract.[111] E6 and 7 oncoproteins have been implicated in colorectal tumorigenesis through interference with p53 tumor suppressor and inactivation of retinoblastoma protein (pRb) to promote uncontrolled cell growth, respectively.[112,113] Considering the etiological role of p53 in numerous malignancies, including colorectal cancer,[114,115] HPV has been hypothesized to be involved in CRC. However, consensus regarding the association has been debatable due to continuation of inconsistent results beginning from differences in early case reports and studies.[117–123] Improvements in analytical methods and sample preparation techniques initially appeared to produce analogous findings to verify contribution of the virus in oncogenesis of CRC.[124–129] A meta-analysis by Baandrup et al. showed a positive association between HPV and CRC with a pooled prevalence 11.2% of viral infection in 2630 adenocarcinoma samples, but a wide range from 0% to 80%.[129] There was a significant heterogeneity between the studies included for quantitative analysis and geographical variation. Another meta-analysis with focus on Iranian patients has also revealed higher HPV in colorectal cancer samples. However, the authors have indicated a potential pitfall of establishing involvement of the viral infection in carcinogenesis based on DNA presence alone. A causal role of HPV has continued to be uncertain in studies published by researchers from a number of western countries even after the meta-analysis. Vuitton and colleagues showed HPV 16 and 18 could not be extracted after performing a real-time PCR (qPCR) and genotyping assay in 210 clinically confirmed cases of colorectal malignancy in France.[130] The finding from this case–control study advocates other negative reports that have been published close to date.[128,132–138] In spite of mounting data, there still seems to be insufficient evidence for reaching a consensus with regards to the association of HPV and CRC.

JOHN CUNNINGHAM VIRUS

John Cunningham virus (JCV) is one of the most prevalent viruses in humans that is often acquired in childhood or during adolescent years. It is a nonenveloped small double-stranded DNA (dsDNA) virus with affinity for replication and infection in a limited number of species. Increased susceptibility for CRC from JCV infection was first reported in a study showing a 10-fold higher viral load in patient samples by a semiquantitative polymerase chain reaction (PCR) method.[139] Subsequent studies have examined this association using either the same or different detection methods including nested-PCR, in situ hybridization (ISH), or immunoassays with focus on a role of T-cell antigen (Ag) in colorectal neoplasia. A study with 100 CRC samples and 100 healthy controls showed an impressive JCV DNA detection rate of 90% in those with the diagnosis of the cancer using nested-PCR.[140] In comparison, a study by Rollison and colleagues using immunoassay on collected blood samples did not show any positive correlation between the virus and CRC. T-Ag takes up over a half of the JCV genome and is primarily responsible for mediating transcriptional activities in host cells.[141] Its etiological potential for CRC has been eluded to be through interaction with β-catenin that essentially facilitates oncogenic process in downstream effect.[143–145] With the exception of two large cohort studies,[145,146] those with relatively small sample size showed comparatively higher likelihood of association between CRC and chronic JCV infection.

HUMAN HERPESVIRUS

Epstein–Barr virus is a DNA virus, also called human herpesvirus 4 (HHV-4), of the Gamma-herpesvirinae family and known to have infected approximately over 95% of human population worldwide.[147] The virus is implicated in a wide spectrum of conditions including infectious mononucleosis in the context of acute viral infection. At its latency, Epstein Barr Virus (EBV) can also be a primary driving factor in etiology of Burkitt lymphoma, Hodgkin disease, nasopharyngeal, gastric cancers, and other malignancies. Due to its clinical significance and prevalence, the potential role of the virus in oncogenesis of CRC has been investigated. An early study by Yuen et al. indicated that none of the 36 colorectal adenocarcinoma samples detected EBV using either ISH or an Epstein–Barr encoded RNA (EBER) probe.[148] This negative finding was consistent in following studies that utilized other various techniques such as immunohistochemistry and/or PCR amplification.[150–152] Even in a group of inflammatory bowel disease (IBD) patients with CRC, EBV DNA could not be found with ISH.[152] In contrast, three Chinese studies and one Syrian study have indicated involvement of EBV in the development of CRC using similar methods.[154–156] Furthermore, the Syrian study specified Fascin protein to be closely associated with upregulation of colorectal neoplastic process based on their finding and previous studies showing abundant expression of the protein in other malignancies. The exact role of the virus in CRC cannot be clearly defined on the basis of conflicting evidence that exist to date.

Cytomegalovirus (CMV) is also known as human herpesvirus 5 (HHV-5) and usually remains subclinical once a host acquires this ubiquitous viral infection. However, it can transform into a deadly pathogen especially in immunocompromised individuals. The identification of CMV nucleic acids and proteins in glioblastoma[156] has sparked interest in elucidating potential contribution of the virus in the causality of CRC. Oncogenic properties of CMV to modulate cell transcription have been emphasized in relation to IE1-72 protein, which causes p53 inhibition through interruption on p53 binding site.[157,158] In the context of colorectal tumorigenesis, the mechanistic role of CMV is yet to be defined. One of the early studies by Huang et al. reported CMV genomic sequences in four of the seven adenocarcinoma cases using cRNA-DNA hybridization. Nevertheless, results obtained from studies in following years have been contrary with each other[160–163] despite application of the same analytical method such as immunohistochemistry[163,164] or examination of the same type of tissue samples.[165,166] A study using nested-PCR between CRC and adenoma control samples showed no correlation between CMV and colorectal malignancy.[167] This observation contradicted the positive finding from a study published a few years later that also used nested-PCR on CRC and matched healthy control samples.[168] Considering the differences in currently available data, further studies are required to validate the involvement of CMV in inducing CRC and its influence on long-term survival.

SUMMARY

The clinical impacts of viral and bacterial agents in the etiology of sporadic CRC still remain to be confirmed due to a range of factors. The complexity of colorectal tumorigenesis, geographical variations in incidence rates of CRC, and shortcomings of detection methods used in small-scale studies have provided limited insight into clarifying the association between infectious agents and CRC. Culturing has been the choice of investigation for isolating these microorganisms from tissue or blood samples of CRC patients, which were both time consuming and allowed analysis of a small sample size. In addition, fecal analysis of bacterial composition may not be reflective of the commensal flora found in individual gastrointestinal tract. One of the significant limitations under these circumstances is inability to replicate these findings in larger populations. Advances in molecular technology and next generation sequencing[170–174] have shown promises in addressing the aforementioned confounding factors with regards to differences in individual microbial composition and/or susceptibility to viral infection. These techniques can be applied in large prospective cohorts recruited from both affected patients and healthy controls to collect data. They may also help in elucidating signaling pathways other than those mediated by COX-2 and to determine particular viral or bacterial species with higher virulent factors for the development of CRC. More widespread and consistent usage of these constantly improving techniques in prospectively designed studies with adequate sample size will enable better understanding of this growing field of research.

REFERENCES

1. Cancer IAfRo. *Cancer Fact Sheets: Colorectum*; 2012. Available from: http://globocan.iarc.fr/Pages/fact_sheets_cancer.aspx.
2. Arnold CN, Goel A, Blum HE, Boland CR. Molecular pathogenesis of colorectal cancer. *Cancer.* 2005;104(10):2035–2047.
3. Bosman F, Yan P. Molecular pathology of colorectal cancer. *Pol J Pathol.* 2014;65(4):257–266.
4. Hooper L, Gordon J. Commensal host-bacterial relationships in the gut. *Science.* 2001;292:1115–1118.
5. Fujimura KE, Slusher NA, Cabana MD, Lynch SV. Role of the gut microbiota in defining human health. *Expert Rev Anti Infect Ther.* 2010;8(4):435.
6. Eberhart CE, Coffey RJ, Radhika A, Giardiello FM, Ferrenbach S, Dubois RN. Up-regulation of cyclooxygenase 2 gene expression in human colorectal adenomas and adenocarcinomas. *Gastroenterology.* 1994; 107(4):1183–1188.
7. Hao X, Bishop AE, Wallace M, et al. Early expression of cyclo-oxygenase-2 during sporadic colorectal carcinogenesis. *J Pathol.* 1999;187(3):295–301.
8. Masunaga R, Kohno H, Dhar DK, et al. Cyclooxygenase-2 expression correlates with tumor neovascularization and prognosis in human colorectal carcinoma patients. *Clin Cancer Res.* 2000;6(10):4064–4068.
9. Sano H, Kawahito Y, Wilder RL, et al. Expression of cyclooxygenase-1 and -2 in human colorectal cancer. *Cancer Res.* 1995;55(17):3785–3789.
10. Sheehan KM, Sheahan K, O'Donoghue DP, et al. The relationship between cyclooxygenase-2 expression and colorectal cancer. *J Am Med Assoc.* 1999;282(13):1254–1257.
11. Zhang H, Sun X-F. Overexpression of cyclooxygenase-2 correlates with advanced stages of colorectal cancer. *Am J Gastroenterol.* 2002;97:1037.
12. Arber N, Eagle CJ, Spicak J, et al. Celecoxib for the prevention of colorectal adenomatous polyps. *N Engl J Med.* 2006;355(9):885–895.
13. Brown W, Skinner S, Malcontenti-Wilson C, Vogiagis D, O'Brien P. Non-steroidal anti-inflammatory drugs with activity against either cyclooxygenase 1 or cyclooxygenase 2 inhibit colorectal cancer in a DMH rodent model by inducing apoptosis and inhibiting cell proliferation. *Gut.* 2001;48(5):660.
14. Chan AT, Ogino S, Fuchs CS. Aspirin use and survival after diagnosis of colorectal cancer. *J Am Med Assoc.* 2009;302(6):649–658.
15. Gupta RA, DuBois RN. Colorectal cancer prevention and treatment by inhibition of cyclooxygenase-2. *Nat Rev Canc.* 2001;1:11.
16. Half E, Arber N. Colon cancer: preventive agents and the present status of chemoprevention. *Expet Opin Pharmacother.* 2009;10(2):211–219.
17. Kumar N, Drabu S, Mondal SC. NSAID's and selectively COX-2 inhibitors as potential chemoprotective agents against cancer. *Arab J Chem.* 2013;6(1):1–23.

18. Lanas A. Nonsteroidal antiinflammatory drugs and cyclooxygenase inhibition in the gastrointestinal tract: a trip from peptic ulcer to colon cancer. *Am J Med Sci.* 2009;338(2):96–106.

19. Al-Salihi MA, Terrece Pearman A, Doan T, et al. Transgenic expression of cyclooxygenase-2 in mouse intestine epithelium is insufficient to initiate tumorigenesis but promotes tumor progression. *Cancer Lett.* 2008;273(2):225–232.

20. Chulada PC, Thompson MB, Mahler JF, et al. Genetic disruption of *Ptgs-1*, as well as of *Ptgs-2*, reduces intestinal tumorigenesis in *Min* mice. *Cancer Res.* 2000;60(17):4705–4708.

21. Oshima M, Dinchuk JE, Kargman SL, et al. Suppression of intestinal polyposis in Apc delta716 knockout mice by inhibition of cyclooxygenase 2 (COX-2). *Cell.* 1996;87(5):803.

22. Dove WF, Clipson L, Gould KA, et al. Intestinal neoplasia in the ApcMin mouse: independence from the microbial and natural killer (beige locus) status. *Cancer Res.* 1997;57(5):812.

23. Ivanov II, Frutos RL, Manel N, et al. Specific microbiota direct the differentiation of IL-17-producing T-helper cells in the mucosa of the small intestine. *Cell Host Microbe.* 2008;4(4):337–349.

24. Kado S, Uchida K, Funabashi H, et al. Intestinal microflora are necessary for development of spontaneous adenocarcinoma of the large intestine in T-cell receptor beta chain and p53 double-knockout mice. *Cancer Res.* 2001;61(6):2395.

25. Mazmanian SK, Round JL, Kasper DL. A microbial symbiosis factor prevents intestinal inflammatory disease. *Nature.* 2008;453(7195):620+.

26. Terzić J, Grivennikov S, Karin E, Karin M. Inflammation and colon cancer. *Gastroenterology.* 2010;138(6):2101–2114.e5.

27. Candela M, Turroni S, Biagi E, et al. Inflammation and colorectal cancer, when microbiota-host mutualism breaks. *World J Gastroenterol.* 2014;20(4):908–922.

28. Noble CJ. Carriage of group D streptococci in the human bowel. *J Clin Pathol.* 1978;31:1182–1186.

29. Osawa R, Fujusawa T, Sly L. *Streptococcus gallolyticus* sp. nov.; gallate degrading organisms formerly assigned to *Streptococcus bovis*. *Syst Appl Microbiol.* 1995;18:74–78.

30. Schlegel L, Grimont F, Ageron E, Grimont PAD, Bouvet A. Reappraisal of the taxonomy of the *Streptococcus bovis/Streptococcus equinus* complex and related species: description of *Streptococcus gallolyticus* subsp. *gallolyticus* subsp. nov., *S. gallolyticus* subsp. *macedonicus* subsp. nov. and *S. gallolyticus* subsp. *pasteurianus* subsp. nov. *Int J Syst Evol Microbiol.* 2003;53:631–645.

31. McCoy W, Mason 3rd JM. Enterococcal endocarditis associated with carcinoma of the sigmoid: report of a case. *J Med Assoc State Ala.* 1951;21:162–166.

32. Bisno A. Streptococcal infection. In: *Harrison's Principles of Internal Medicine*. 12th ed. New York: McGraw-Hill; 1991:563–569.

33. Alazmi W, Bustamante M, O'Loughlin C, Gonzalez J, Raskin JB. The association of *Streptococcus bovis* bacteremia and gastrointestinal diseases: a retrospective analysis. *Dig Dis Sci.* 2006;51(4):732–736.

34. Boleij A, Roelofs R, Danne C, et al. Selective antibody response to *Streptococcus gallolyticus* pilus proteins in colorectal cancer patients. *Cancer Prev Res.* 2012;5(2):260–265.

35. Gold JS, Bayar S, Salem RR. Association of *Streptococcus bovis* bacteremia with colonic neoplasia and extracolonic malignancy. *Arch Surg.* 2004;139(7):760–765.

36. Klein RS, Recco RA, Catalano MT, Edberg SC. Association of *Streptococcus bovis* with carcinoma of the colon. *N Engl J Med.* 1977;297(15):800–802.

37. Lazarovitch T, Shango M, Levine M, et al. The relationship between the new taxonomy of *Streptococcus bovis* and its clonality to colon cancer, endocarditis, and biliary disease. *Infection.* 2013;41(2):329–337.

38. Krishnan S, Eslick GD. *Streptococcus bovis* infection and colorectal neoplasia: a meta-analysis. *Colorectal Dis.* 2014;16:672–680.

39. Potter MA, Cunliffe NA, Smith M, Miles RS, Flapan AD, Dunlop MG. A prospective controlled study of the association of *Streptococcal bovis* with colorectal carcinoma. *J Clin Pathol.* 1998;51:473–474.

40. Dubrow R, Edberg S, Wikfors E, Callan D, Troncale F, Vender R, et al. Faecal carriage of *Streptococcus bovis* and colorectal adenomas. *Gastroenterology.* 1991;101:721–725.

41. Chirouze C, Patry I, Duval X, Baty V, Tattevin P, Aparico T, et al. *Streptococcus bovis/Streptococcus equinus* complex fecal carriage, colorectal carcinoma, and infective endocarditis: a new appraisal of a complex connection. *Eur J Clin Microbiol Infect Dis.* 2013;32(9):1171–1176.

42. Boltin D, Goldberg E, Bugaevsky O, Kelner E, Dickman R. Colonic carriage of *Streptococcus bovis* and colorectal neoplasia: a prospective 17-year longitudinal case-control study. *Eur J Gastroenterol Hepatol.* 2015;28:1449–1453.

43. Abdulamir AS, Hafidh RR, Bakar FA. Molecular detection, quantification, and isolation of *Streptococcus gallolyticus* bacteria colonising colorectal tumours: inflammation-driven potential of carcinogenesis via IL-1, COX-2, and IL-8. *Mol Canc.* 2010;9(249):1–18.

44. Norfleet RG, Mitchell PD. *Streptococcus bovis* does not selectively colonize colorectal cancer and polyps. *J Clin Gastroenterol.* 1993;17(1):25–28.

45. Tjalsma H, Scholler-Guinard M, Lasonder E, Ruers TJ, Willems HL, Swinkels DW. Profiling the humoral immune response in colon cancer patients: diagnostic antigens from *Streptococcus bovis*. *Int J Canc.* 2006;119(9):2127–2135.

46. Tsai C-E, Chiu C-T, Rayner CK, et al. Associated factors in *Streptococcus bovis* bacteremia and colorectal cancer. *Kaohsiung J Med Sci.* 2016;32(4):196–200.

47. Darjee R, Gibb AP. Serological investigation into the association between *Streptococcus bovis* and colorectal cancer. *J Clin Pathol.* 1993;47(12):1116–1119.

48. Butt J, Romero-Hernandez B, Perez-Gomez B, et al. Association of *Streptococcus gallolyticus* subspecies *gallolyticus* with colorectal cancer: serological evidence. *Int J Canc.* 2016;138(7):1670–1679.

49. Boleij A, van Gelder MMHJ, Swinkels DW, Tjalsma H. Clinical importance of *Streptococcus gallolyticus* infection among colorectal cancer patients: systematic review and meta-analysis. *Clin Infect Dis.* 2011;53(9): 870–878.

50. Corredoira J, Grau I, Garcia-Rodriguez JF, et al. The clinical epidemiology and malignancies associated with *Streptococcus bovis* biotypes in 506 cases of bloodstream infections. *J Infect.* 2015;71(3):317–325.

51. Ruoff K, Miller S, Garner C, Ferraro M, Calderwood S. Bacteremia with *Streptococcus bovis* and *Streptococcus salivarius*: clinical correlates of more accurate identification of isolates. *J Clin Microbiol.* 1989;27(2):305–308.

52. Boleij A, Muytjens CMJ, Bukhari SI, et al. Novel clues on the specific association of *Streptococcus gallolyticus* subsp. gallolyticus with colorectal cancer. *J Infect Dis.* 2011;203(8):1101–1109.

53. Danne C, Entenza JM, Mallet A, et al. Molecular characterization of a *Streptococcus gallolyticus* genomic island encoding a pilus involved in endocarditis. *J Infect Dis.* 2011;204(12):1960–1970.

54. Martins M, Aymeric L, du Merle L, et al. *Streptococcus gallolyticus* Pil3 pilus is required for adhesion to colonic mucus and for colonization of mouse distal colon. *J Infect Dis.* 2015;212(10):1646–1655.

55. Rusinok C, Couve E, Da Cunha V, et al. Genome sequence of *Streptococcus gallolyticus*: insights into its adaptation to the bovine rumen and its ability to cause endocarditis. *J Bacteriol.* 2010;192(8):2266–2276.

56. Sillanpää J, Nallapareddy SR, Singh KV, Ferraro MJ, Murray BE. Adherence characteristics of endocarditis-derived *Streptococcus gallolyticus* ssp. gallolyticus (*Streptococcus bovis* biotype I) isolates to host extracellular matrix proteins. *FEMS (Fed Eur Microbiol Soc) Microbiol Lett.* 2008;289(1):104–109.

57. Biarc J, Nguyen IS, Pini A, et al. Carcinogenic properties of proteins with pro-inflammatory activity from *Streptococcus infantarius* (formerly *S. bovis*). *Carcinogenesis.* 2004;25(8):1477–1484.

58. Ellmerich S, Schöller M, Duranton B, et al. Promotion of intestinal carcinogenesis by *Streptococcus bovis*. *Carcinogenesis.* 2000;21(4):753–756.

59. IARC. Schistosomes, liver flukes and *Helicobacter pylori*. *IARC Monogr Eval Carcinog Risks Hum.* 1994;61. Lyon.

60. Group TES. An international association between *Helicobacter pylori* infection and gastric cancer. *Lancet.* 1993;341(8857):1359–1362.

61. Parkin DM. The global health burden of infection-associated cancers in the year 2002. *Int J Canc.* 2006;118: 3030–3044.

62. Wu Q, Yang ZP, Xu P, Gao LC, Fan DM. Association between *Helicobacter pylori* infection and the risk of colorectal neoplasia: a systematic review and meta-analysis. *Colorectal Dis.* 2013;15:e352–e364.

63. Robinson K, Argent RH, Atherton JC. The inflammatory and immune response to *Helicobacter pylori* infection. *Best Pract Res Clin Gastroenterol.* 2007;21(2):237–259.

64. Hartwich A, Konturek SJ, Pierzchalski P, Zuchowicz M, Labza H. *Helicobacter pylori* infection, gastrin, cyclooxygenase-2, and apoptosis in colorectal cancer. *Int J Colorectal Dis.* 2001;16:202–210.

65. Georgopoulos SD, Polymeros D, Triantafyllou K, et al. Hypergastrinemia is associated with increased risk of distal colon adenomas. *Digestion.* 2006;74:42–46.

66. Thorburn CM, Friedman GD, Dickinson CJ, Vogelman JH, Orentreich N, Parsonnet J. Gastrin and colorectal cancer: a prospective study. *Gastroenterology.* 1998;115(2):275–280.

67. Blase JL, Campbell PT, Gapstur SM, et al. Prediagnostic *Helicobacter pylori* antibodies and colorectal cancer risk in an elderly, caucasian population. *Helicobacter.* 2016;21(6):488–492.

68. Epplein M, Pawlita M, Michel A, Peek RM, Cai Q, Blot WJ. *Helicobacter pylori* protein-specific antibodies and risk of colorectal cancer. *Cancer Epidemiol Biomark Prev.* 2013;22.

69. Fernández de Larrea-Baz N, Michel A, Romero B, et al. *Helicobacter pylori* antibody reactivities and colorectal cancer risk in a case-control study in Spain. *Front Microbiol.* 2017;8:888.

70. Clermont O, Bonacorsi S, Bingen E. Rapid and simple determination of the *Escherichia coli* phylogenetic group. *Appl Environ Microbiol.* 2000;66(10):4555–4558.

71. Herzer PJ, Inouye S, Inouye M, Whittam TS. Phylogenetic distribution of branched RNA-linked multicopy single-stranded DNA among natural isolates of *Escherichia coli*. *J Bacteriol.* 1990;172(11):6175–6181.

72. Picard B, Garcia JS, Gouriou S, et al. The link between phylogeny and virulence in *Escherichia coli* extraintestinal infection. *Infect Immun.* 1999;67(2):546–553.

73. Martin HM, Campbell BJ, Hart CA, et al. Enhanced *Escherichia coli* adherence and invasion in crohn's disease and colon cancer. *Gastroenterology.* 2004;127: 80–93.

74. Darfeuille-Michaud A, Neut C, Barnich N, et al. Presence of adherent *Escherichia coli* strains in ileal mucosa of patients with Crohn's disease. *Gastroenterology.* 1998;115(6):1405–1413.

75. Darfeuille-Michaud A, Boudeau J, Bulois P, et al. High prevalence of adherent-invasive *Escherichia coli* associated with ileal mucosa in Crohn's disease. *Gastroenterology.* 2004;127(2):412–421.

76. Arthur JC, Perez-Chanona E, Muhlbauer M, et al. Intestinal inflammation targets cancer-inducing activity of the microbiota. *Science.* 2012;338(6103):120–123.

77. Buc E, Dubois D, Sauvanet P, Raisch J, Bonnet R. High prevalence of mucosa-associated *E. coli* producing cyclomodulin and genotoxin in colon cancer. *PLoS One.* 2013;8:e56964.

78. Bonnet M, Buc E, Sauvanet P, et al. Colonization of the human gut by *E. coli* and colorectal cancer risk. *Clin Cancer Res.* 2013;20(4):859–867.

79. Balish E, Warner T. *Enterococcus faecalis* induces inflammatory bowel disease in interleukin-10 knockout mice. *Am J Pathol.* 2002;160(6):2253–2257.

80. Kim SC, Tonkonogy SL, Albright CA, et al. Variable phenotypes of enterocolitis in interleukin 10-deficient mice monoassociated with two different commensal bacteria. *Gastroenterology.* 2005;128(4):891–906.

81. Blair IA. Lipid hydroperoxide-mediated DNA damage. *Exp Gerontol.* 2001;36(9):1473–1481.

82. Huycke MM, Abrams V, Moore DR. *Enterococcus faecalis* produces extracellular superoxide and hydrogen peroxide that damages colonic epithelial cell DNA. *Carcinogenesis.* 2002;23(3):529–536.

83. Wang X, Allen TD, May RJ, Lightfoot S, Houchen CW, Huycke MM. *Enterococcus faecalis* induces aneuploidy and tetraploidy in colonic epithelial cells through a bystander effect. *Cancer Res.* 2008;68(23):9909–9917.

84. Huycke MM, Moore DR. In vivo production of hydroxyl radical by *Enterococcus faecalis* colonizing the intestinal tract using aromatic hydroxylation. *Free Radic Biol Med.* 2002;33(6):818–826.

85. Winters MD, Schlinke TL, Joyce WA, Glore SR, Huycke MM. Prospective case-cohort study of intestinal colonization with enterococci that produce extracellular superoxide and the risk for colorectal adenomas or cancer. *Am J Gastroenterol.* 1998;93(12):2491–2500.

86. Sears CL. Enterotoxigenic *Bacteroides fragilis*: a rogue among symbiotes. *Clin Microbiol Rev.* 2009;22(2):349–369.

87. Goodwin AC, Shields CED, Wu S, et al. Polyamine catabolism contributes to enterotoxigenic *Bacteroides fragilis*-induced colon tumorigenesis. *Proc Natl Acad Sci USA.* 2011;108(37):15354–15359.

88. Geis AL, Fan H, Wu X, et al. Regulatory T-cell response to enterotoxigenic *Bacteroides fragilis* colonisation triggers IL17-dependent colon carcinogenesis. *Cancer Discov.* 2015;5(10):1098–1109.

89. Boleij A, Hechenbleikner EM, Goodwin AC, Badani R, Sears CL. The *Bacteroides fragilis* toxin gene is prevalent in the colon mucosa of colorectal cancer patients. *Clin Infect Dis.* 2015;60(2):208–215.

90. Toprak NU, Yagci A, Gulluoglu BM, et al. A possible role of *Bacteroides fragilis* enterotoxin in the aetiology of colorectal cancer. *Clin Microbiol Infect.* 2006;12(8):782–786.

91. Han Y. *Fusobacterium nucleatum*: a commensal-turned pathogen. *Curr Opin Microbiol.* 2015;23:141–147.

92. Castellarin M, Warren R, Freeman J, et al. *Fusobacterium nucleatum* infection is prevalent in human colorectal carcinoma. *Genome Res.* 2012;22:299–306.

93. Kostic A, Gevers D, Pedamallu C, et al. Genomic analysis identifies association of *Fusobacterium* with colorectal carcinoma. *Genome Res.* 2012;22:292–298.

94. McCoy A, Araújo-Pérez F, Azcárate-Peril A, Yeh J, Sandler R, Keku T. *Fusobacterium* is associated with colorectal adenomas. *PLoS One.* 2013;8:e53653.

95. Warren R, Freeman D, Plesance S, et al. Co-occurence of anaerobic bacteria in colorectal carcinomas. *Microbiome.* 2013;1(16):1–12.

96. Zeller G, Tap J, Voigt A, et al. Potential of fecal microbiota for early-stage detection of colorectal cancer. *Mol Syst Biol.* 2014;41(1):1–10.

97. Mima K, Sukawa Y, Nishihara R, et al. *Fusobacterium nucleatum* and T Cells in colorectal carcinoma. *JAMA Oncol.* 2015;1(5):653–661.

98. Ito K, Kanno S, Nosho K, et al. Association of *Fusobacterium nucleatum* with clinical and molecular features in colorectal serrated pathway. *Int J Canc.* 2015;137(6):1258–1268.

99. Tahara T, Yamamoto E, Suzuki H, et al. *Fusobacterium* in colonic flora and molecular features of colorectal carcinoma. *Cancer Res.* 2014;74:1311–1318.

100. Yang Y, Weng W, Peng J, et al. *Fusobacterium nucleatum* increases proliferation of colorectal cancer cells and tumor development in mice by activating toll-like receptor 4 signaling to nuclear factor-κB, and upregulating expression of MicroRNA-21. *Gastroenterology.* 2017;152(4):851–866.

101. Wong S, Kwong T, Chow T, et al. Quantitation of faecal *Fusobacterium* improves faecal immunochemical test in detecting advanced colorectal neoplasia. *Gut.* 2017;66(8):1441–1448.

102. Rubinstein M, Wang X, Liu W, Hao Y, Cai G, Han Y. *Fusobacterium nucleatum* promotes colorectal carcinogenesis by modulating E-cadherin/β-catenin signaling via its FadA adhesin. *Cell Host Microbe.* 2013;14(2):195–206.

103. Gur C, Ibrahim Y, Isaacson B, et al. Binding of the Fap2 protein of *Fusobacterium nucleatum* to human inhibitory receptor TIGIT protects tumors from immune cell attack. *Immunity.* 2015;42(2):344–355.

104. Mima K, Cao Y, Chan AT, et al. *Fusobacterium nucleatum* in colorectal carcinoma tissue according to tumor location. *Clin Transl Gastroenterol.* 2016;7:e200.

105. Nosho K, Sukawa Y, Adachi Y, et al. Association of *Fusobacterium nucleatum* with immunity and molecular alterations in colorectal cancer. *World J Gastroenterol.* 2016;22(2):557–566.

106. Suehiro Y, Sakai K, Nishioka M, et al. Highly sensitive stool DNA testing of *Fusobacterium nucleatum* as a marker for detection of colorectal tumours in a Japanese population. *Ann Clin Biochem.* 2017;54(1):86–91.

107. Schiffman M, Castle PE. Human papillomavirus: epidemiology and public health. *Arch Pathol Lab Med.* 2003;127(8):930–934.

108. Wiley D, Masongsong E. Human papillomavirus: the burden of infection. *Obstet Gynecol Surv.* 2006;61(6):S3–S14.

109. Muñoz N. Human papillomavirus and cancer: the epidemiological evidence. *J Clin Virol.* 2000;19(1):1–5.

110. Mehanna H, Beech T, Nicholson T, et al. Prevalence of human papillomavirus in oropharyngeal and nonoropharyngeal head and neck cancer—systematic review and meta-analysis of trends by time and region. *Head Neck.* 2013;35(5):747–755.

111. Steenbergen RDM, de Wilde J, Wilting SM, Brink AATP, Snijders PJF, Meijer CJLM. HPV-mediated transformation of the anogenital tract. *J Clin Virol.* 2005;32:25–33.

112. Lizano M, Berumen J, García-Carrancá A. HPV-related carcinogenesis: basic concepts, viral types and variants. *Arch Med Res.* 2009;40(6):428–434.

113. Buitrago-Pérez Á, Garaulet G, Vázquez-Carballo A, Paramio JM, García-Escudero R. Molecular signature of HPV-induced carcinogenesis: pRb, p53 and gene expression profiling. *Curr Genom.* 2009;10(1):26–34.

114. Slattery ML, Curtin K, Schaffer D, Anderson K, Samowitz W. Associations between family history of colorectal cancer and genetic alterations in tumors. *Int J Canc.* 2002;97(6):823–827.

115. Ricciardi R, Ghabreau L, Yasmeen A, Darnel AD, Akil N, Moustafa A-E. Role of E6/E7 onco-proteins of high-risk human papillomaviruses in human colorectal carcinogenesis. *Cell Cycle.* 2009;8(12):1964–1965.

116. Boguszakova L, Hirsch I, Brichacek B, et al. Absence of cytomegalovirus, Epstein-Barr virus, and papillomavirus DNA from adenoma and adenocarcinoma of the colon. *Acta Virol.* 1988;32(3):303–308.

117. Cheng J, Sheu L, Lin J, Meng C. Detection of human papillomavirus DNA in colorectal adenomas. *Arch Surg.* 1995;130(1):73–76.

118. Kirgan D, Manalo P, Hall M, McGregor B. Association of human papillomavirus and colon neoplasms. *Arch Surg.* 1990;125(7):862–865.

119. Koulos J, Symmans F, Chumas J, Nuovo G. Human papillomavirus detection in adenocarcinoma of the anus. *Mod Pathol.* 1991;4(1):58–61.

120. McGregor B, Byrne P, Kirgan D, Albright J, Manalo P, Hall M. Confirmation of the association of human papillomavirus with human colon cancer. *Am J Surg.* 1993;166(6):738–742.

121. Shah KV, Daniel RW, Simons JW, Vogelstein B. Investigation of colon cancers for human papillomavirus genomic sequences by polymerase chain reaction. *J Surg Oncol.* 1992;51(1):5–7.

122. Shroyer KR, Kim JG, Manos M, Greer CE, Pearlman NW, Franklin WA. Papillomavirus found in anorectal squamous carcinoma, not in colon adenocarcinoma. *Arch Surg.* 1992;127(6):741–744.

123. Bodaghi S, Yamanegi K, Xiao S-Y, Da Costa M, Palefsky JM, Zheng Z-M. Colorectal papillomavirus infection in patients with colorectal cancer. *Clin Cancer Res.* 2005;11(8):2862–2867.

124. Buyru N, Tezol A, Dalay N. Coexistence of K-ras mutations and HPV infection in colon cancer. *BMC Canc.* 2006;6(1):115.

125. Damin DC, Caetano MB, Rosito MA, et al. Evidence for an association of human papillomavirus infection and colorectal cancer. *Eur J Surg Oncol.* 2007;33(5):569–574.

126. Lee YM, Leu SY, Chiang H, Fung CP, Liu WT. Human papillomavirus type 18 in colorectal cancer. *J Microbiol Immunol Infect.* 2001;34(2):87–91.

127. Pérez LO, Abba MC, Laguens RM, Golijow CD. Analysis of adenocarcinoma of the colon and rectum: detection of human papillomavirus (HPV) DNA by polymerase chain reaction. *Colorectal Dis.* 2005;7(5):492–495.

128. Yavuzer D, Karadayi N, Salepci T, Baloglu H, Dabak R, Bayaramicli OU. Investigation of human papillomavirus DNA in colorectal carcinomas and adenomas. *Med Oncol.* 2011;28(1):127–132.

129. Baandrup L, Thomsen LT, Olesen TB, Andersen KK, Norrild B, Kjaer SK. The prevalence of human papillomavirus in colorectal adenomas and adenocarcinomas: a systematic review and meta-analysis. *Eur J Canc.* 2014;50(8):1446–1461.

130. Vuitton L, Jaillet C, Jacquin E, et al. Human papillomaviruses in colorectal cancers: a case-control study in western patients. *Dig Liver Dis.* 2017;49(4):446–450.

131. Aghakhani A, Hamkar R, Ramezani A, et al. Lack of human papillomavirus DNA in colon adenocarcinoma and adenoma. *J Canc Res Therapeut.* 2014;10(3):531–534.

132. Gornick M, Castellsague X, Sanchez G, et al. Human papillomavirus is not associated with colorectal cancer in a large international study. *Cancer Causes Control.* 2010;21:737.

133. Karpinski P, Myszka A, Ramsey D, Kielan W, Sasiadek MM. Detection of viral DNA sequences in sporadic colorectal cancers in relation to CpG island methylation and methylator phenotype. *Tumor Biol.* 2011;32(4):653–659.

134. Khabaz MN. HPV and the development of colorectal cancer. *Global J Health Sci.* 2017;9(4):251–256.

135. Meshkat M, Tayyebi Meibodi N, Sepahi S, Fadaee N, Salehpour M, Meshkat Z. The frequency of human papillomaviruses in colorectal cancer samples in Mashhad, northeastern Iran. *Turk J Med Sci.* 2014;44:501–503.

136. Ranjbar R, Saberfar E, Shamsaie A, Ghasemian E. The aetiological role of human papillomavirus in colorectal carcinoma: an iranian population-based case control study. *Asian Pac J Cancer Prev.* 2014;15(4):1521–1525.

137. Taherian H, Tafvizi F, Fard ZT, Abdirad A. Lack of association between human papillomavirus infection and colorectal cancer. *Przegląd Gastroenterol.* 2014;9(5):280–284.

138. Yantiss RK, Goodarzi M, Zhou XK, et al. Clinical, pathologic, and molecular features of early-onset colorectal carcinoma. *Am J Surg Pathol.* 2009;33(4):572–582.

139. Laghi L, Randolph AE, Chauhan DP, et al. JC virus DNA is present in the mucosa of the human colon and in colorectal cancers. *Proc Natl Acad Sci USA.* 1999;96(13):7484–7489.

140. Coelho TR, Gaspar R, Figueiredo P, Mendonça C, Lazo PA, Almeida L. Human JC polyomavirus in normal colorectal mucosa, hyperplastic polyps, sporadic adenomas, and adenocarcinomas in Portugal. *J Med Virol.* 2013;85(12):2119–2127.

141. Raj GV, Gallia GL, Chang CF, Khalili K. T-antigen-dependent transcriptional initiation and its role in the regulation of human neurotropic JC virus late gene expression. *J Gen Virol.* 1998;79(9):2147–2155.

142. Enam S, Del Valle L, Lara C, et al. Association of human polyomavirus JCV with colon cancer. Evidence for interaction of viral T-antigen and β-catenin. *Cancer Res.* 2002;62(23):7093–7101.

143. Niv Y, Ajay G, Richard B. JC virus and colorectal cancer: a possible trigger in the chromosomal instability pathways. *Curr Opin Gastroenterol.* 2005;21(1):85–89.

144. Goel A, Li MS, Nagasaka T, et al. Association of JC virus T-antigen expression with the methylator phenotype in sporadic colorectal cancers. *Gastroenterology.* 2006;130(7):1950–1961.

145. Lundstig A, Stattin P, Persson K, et al. No excess risk for colorectal cancer among subjects seropositive for the JC polyomavirus. *Int J Canc.* 2007;121(5):1098–1102.

146. Rollison DE, Helzlsouer KJ, Lee J-H, et al. Prospective study of JC virus seroreactivity and the development of colorectal cancers and adenomas. *Cancer Epidemiol Biomark Prev.* 2009;18(5):1515–1523.

147. Jenson H. Epstein-Barr virus. *Pediatr Rev.* 2011;32(9):375–385.

148. Yuen ST, Chung LP, Leung SY, Luk IS, Chan SY, Ho J. In situ detection of Epstein-Barr virus in gastric and colorectal adenocarcinomas. *Am J Surg Pathol.* 1994;18(11):1158–1163.

149. Grinstein S, Preciado MV, Gattuso P, et al. Demonstration of Epstein-Barr virus in carcinomas of various sites. *Cancer Res.* 2002;62(17):4876–4878.

150. Mehrabani-Khasraghi S, Ameli M, Khalily F. Demonstration of herpes simplex virus, cytomegalovirus, and Epstein-Barr virus in colorectal cancer. *Iran Biomed J.* 2016;20(5):302–306.

151. Tafvizi F, Fard ZT, Assareh R. Original paper
Epstein-Barr virus DNA in colorectal carcinoma in Iranian patients. *Pol J Pathol.* 2015;66(2):154–160.

152. Wong N, Herbst H, Herrmann K, et al. Epstein–Barr virus infection in colorectal neoplasms associated with inflammatory bowel disease: detection of the virus in lymphomas but not in adenocarcinomas. *J Pathol.* 2003;201(2):312–318.

153. Al-Antary N, Farghaly H, Aboulkassim T, Yasmeen A, Akil N. Al Moustafa A-E. Epstein–Barr virus and its association with Fascin expression in colorectal cancers in the Syrian population: a tissue microarray study. *Hum Vaccines Immunother.* 2017;13(7):1573–1578.

154. Liu H-X, Ding Y-Q, Li X, Yao K-T. Investigation of Epstein-Barr virus in Chinese colorectal tumors. *World J Gastroenterol.* 2003;9(11):2464–2468.

155. Liu H-X, Ding Y-Q, Sun Y-O, et al. Detection of Epstein-Barr virus in human colorectal cancer by in situ hybridazition. *Di Yi Jun Yi Da Xue Xue Bao.* 2002;22(10):915–917.

156. Lawler SE. Cytomegalovirus and glioblastoma; controversies and opportunities. *J Neuro Oncol.* 2015;123(3):465–471.

157. Cobbs CS, Harkins L, Samanta M, et al. Human cytomegalovirus infection and expression in human malignant glioma. *Cancer Res.* 2002;62(12):3347–3350.

158. Hwang E-S, Zhang Z, Cai H, et al. Human cytomegalovirus IE1-72 protein interacts with p53 and inhibits p53-dependent transactivation by a mechanism different from that of IE2-86 protein. *J Virol.* 2009;83(23):12388–12398.

159. Akintola-Ogunremi O, Luo Q, He T-C, Wang HL. Is cytomegalovirus associated with human colorectal tumorigenesis? *Am J Clin Pathol.* 2005;123(2):244–249.

160. Avni A, Haikin H, Feuchtwanger MM, et al. Antibody pattern to human cytomegalovirus in patients with adenocarcinoma of the colon. *Intervirology.* 1981;16(4):244–249.

161. Knösel T, Schewe C, Dietel M, Schlag PM, Petersen I. Cytomegalovirus associated with progression and metastasis of colorectal cancer? *Pathol Res Pract.* 2004;200(4):322.

162. Roche JK, Cheung KS, Huang IB, Lang DJ. Cytomegalovirus: detection in human colonic and circulating mononuclear cells in association with gastrointestinal disease. *Int J Canc.* 1981;27(5):659–667.

163. Harkins L, Volk AL, Samanta M, et al. Specific localisation of human cytomegalovirus nucleic acids and proteins in human colorectal cancer. *Lancet.* 2002;360(9345):1557–1563.

164. Mariguela VC, Chacha SGF, Cunha AA, Troncon LEA, Zucoloto S, Figueiredo LTM. Cytomegalovirus in colorectal cancer and idiopathic ulcerative colitis. *Rev do Inst Med Trop São Paulo.* 2008;50:83–87.

165. Dimberg J, Hong TT, Skarstedt M, Lofgren S, Zar N, Matussek A. Detection of cytomegalovirus DNA in colorectal tissue from Swedish and Vietnamese patients with colorectal cancer. *Anticancer Res.* 2013;33(11):4947–4950.

166. Rüger R, Fleckenstein B. Cytomegalovirus DNA in colorectal carcinoma tissues. *Klin Wochenschr.* 1985;63(9):405–408.

167. Bender C, Zipeto D, Bidoia C, et al. Analysis of colorectal cancers for human cytomegalovirus presence. *Infect Agents Canc.* 2009;4(1):6.

168. Tafvizi F, Fard ZT. Detection of human cytomegalovirus in patients with colorectal cancer by nested-PCR. *Asian Pac J Cancer Prev.* 2014;15:1453–1457.

169. Ahn J, Sinha R, Pei Z, et al. Human gut microbiome and risk for colorectal cancer. *J Natl Cancer Inst.* 2013;105(24):1907–1911.

170. Weir TL, Manter DK, Sheflin AM, Barnett BA, Heuberger AL, Ryan EP. Stool microbiome and metabolome differences between colorectal cancer patients and healthy adults. *PLoS One.* 2013;8(8):e70803.

171. Zackular JP, Rogers MAM, Ruffin tMT, Schloss PD. The human gut microbiome as a screening tool for colorectal cancer. *Cancer Prev Res.* 2014;7(11):1112–1121.

172. Mira-Pascual L, Cabrera-Rubio R, Ocon S, et al. Microbial mucosal colonic shifts associated with the development of colorectal cancer reveal the presence of different bacterial and archaeal biomarkers. *J Gastroenterol.* 2015;50(2):167–179.

173. Vogtmann E, Hua X, Zeller G, et al. Colorectal cancer and the human gut microbiome: reproducibility with whole-genome shotgun sequencing. *PLoS One.* 2016;11(5):e0155362.

CHAPTER 10

Infections and Pancreatic Cancer

DOMINIQUE S. MICHAUD, SCD

INTRODUCTION

Pancreatic cancer is the third leading cause of cancer deaths in the United States,[1] where an estimated 53,670 men and women were diagnosed with pancreatic cancer and 43,090 individuals died of this disease in 2017.[1] Incidence of pancreatic cancer has remained relatively constant over the past four decades, with a slight 1% increase among whites in the past decade.[2] Over the past decade, pancreatic cancer death rates have increased by 0.3% per year in white men, remained stable in white women, and decreased by 0.5% per year in black men and women.[1] Globally, pancreatic cancer incidence rates are higher in more developed countries[2a]; the majority of new cases are diagnosed in Asia (42%), followed by Europe (30%) and North America (14%).

Age-adjusted incidence rates for pancreatic cancer in the United States are slightly higher for men than women (14 per 100,000 for men vs. 11 per 100,000 for women), and African-American men have the highest pancreatic cancer incidence rates (15.4 per 100,000), whereas Asians have the lowest rates (9.7 per 100,000 for both sexes).[2] Pancreatic cancer is the most rapidly fatal cancer; in the United States, the 5-year survival rate is 8% .[1]

KNOWN RISK FACTORS OF PANCREATIC CANCER

Although a number of risk factors have been linked to pancreatic cancer, only about one-third of pancreatic cancer cases can be attributed to these factors,[3] leaving two-thirds of these cancers with unknown cause. Consistency in findings across numerous observational studies, especially large prospective cohort studies with long follow-up periods, has provided convincing evidence for a number of risk factors, including tobacco smoke, long-standing diabetes, obesity, family history, AB blood type, and heavy alcohol consumption.[4]

Cigarette smoke accounts for the largest number of pancreatic cancers worldwide; the estimated population attributable risk for smoking ranges between 11% and 32%, depending on the prevalence of exposure in the country.[3,4] Current smokers have an approximately twofold higher risk of pancreatic cancer than never smokers.[5–9] In addition, the risk of pancreatic cancer increases with the number of cigarettes smoked.[10] Smoking cigars has also been associated with elevated pancreatic cancer risk, but smoking pipes does not appear to increase the risk of pancreatic cancer.[10]

Although it is well documented that type 2 diabetes can develop as a consequence of pancreatic cancer and is often identified close to cancer diagnosis, there has been substantial controversy over the role of diabetes as a cause of pancreatic cancer. To begin to address the causality question, observational studies have examined the relation among glucose levels, insulin levels, and types 2 diabetes decades before pancreatic cancer diagnosis. Elevated glucose levels in the blood of subjects obtained five or more years prior to pancreatic cancer diagnosis have been strongly associated with a higher risk of pancreatic cancer.[11,12] Insulin levels and insulin resistance have also been associated with higher pancreatic cancer risk in two prospective studies.[11,13] Similarly, risk for pancreatic cancer remains elevated over 20 years after diagnosis of diabetes type 2, providing support that diabetes plays a causal role in carcinogenesis.[14–16] For example, the risk of pancreatic cancer is higher when diabetes type 2 is diagnosed within 1 year of the cancer diagnosis (relative risk [RR] = 5.38; 95% confidence interval [CI], 3.49–8.30) than when diabetes is diagnosed 10 or more years earlier (RR = 1.51; 95% CI, 1.16–1.96[15]).

Obesity has only recently been widely accepted as a risk factor for pancreatic cancer, given the consistent results obtained from prospective cohort studies. In the largest meta-analysis conducted (including 23 prospective studies and 9504 pancreatic cancer cases), a 10% increase in risk was reported for each 5-unit increase in BMI (RR, 1.10; 95% CI, 1.07–1.14).[17] A similar magnitude between obesity and pancreatic cancer was

Gastrointestinal Diseases and Their Associated Infections. https://doi.org/10.1016/B978-0-323-54843-4.00010-6
Copyright © 2019 Elsevier Inc. All rights reserved.

reported in another pooled analysis; however, the association was not linear, as the increase in risk was more dramatic among very obese patients (RR, 1.55; 95% CI, 1.16–2.07, comparing BMI >35 to BMI <25 kg/m^2).[18] Associations with obesity and pancreatic cancer are similar in men and women, but appear to be stronger among never smokers.[17]

Family history of pancreatic cancer only explains a small fraction of pancreatic cases (<5%)[4]; even though individuals with a first-degree relative with pancreatic cancer have a moderately higher risk than those without a family history (RR, 1.76; 95% CI, 1.19–2.61),[19] familial pancreatic cancer is relatively uncommon (and thus explains little of the overall cases). Germline mutations in BRCA2, CDKN2A, STK11, PRSS1, SPINK1, PRSS2, and CTRC genes and DNA mismatch repair have been associated with pancreatic cancer risk,[20] similarly explaining only a small percentage of all cases.

Genome-wide association studies (GWASs) have uncovered new areas of genetic susceptibility for pancreatic cancer.[21,22] Of particular interest, because of its role in immunity,[23] is the region in the ABO gene (rs687289 at 9q34.2) that was identified as being strongly associated with the risk of pancreatic cancer in three GWAS analyses (PanScan III: ABO; OR, 1.27; 95% CI, 1.20–1.35; $P = 1.6 \times 10^{-16}$).[21,22,24] These findings are consistent with studies that examined the role of blood groups directly, including suggestions for these associations as early as 1960.[25] Individuals with blood group A (hazard ratio [HR], 1.32; 95% CI, 1.02–1.72), AB (HR, 1.51; 95% CI, 1.02–2.23), or B (HR, 1.72; 95% CI, 1.25–2.38) had a higher risk of pancreatic cancer than those with blood group O.[26] It has been estimated that as much as 17% of the pancreatic cancer cases can be attributed to inheriting a non-O blood group (blood group A, B, or AB).[26]

Several large pooled analyses on alcohol intake and pancreatic cancer have consistently reported elevated risks at higher levels of alcohol intake (six or more drinks per day), while risk does not appear to be consistently elevated at lower levels of alcohol consumption.[27–29]

Many of the known risk factors of pancreatic cancer, described earlier, are thought to modify risk by causing mutations (e.g., family history, tobacco smoke), altering hormonal pathways that can impact oxidative stress and tumor growth (e.g., obesity and diabetes),[30] or possibly through inflammatory pathways (e.g., obesity, tobacco smoke). In the next section, factors more directly associated with inflammation are discussed.

OBSERVATIONAL STUDIES LINKING INFLAMMATION AND INFECTIOUS CONDITIONS TO PANCREATIC CANCER

Chronic Pancreatitis and the Role of Inflammation

Associations between chronic pancreatitis and pancreatic cancer risk have been very strong, providing compelling evidence that chronic local inflammation in the pancreas can lead to carcinogenesis. The most convincing evidence that chronic pancreatitis plays a causal role in pancreatic cancer comes from studies on patients with hereditary pancreatitis, as these patients have extremely high rates of pancreatic cancer (compared with the general population). Moreover, symptoms of pancreatitis in patients with hereditary pancreatitis occur at a mean age of 10 years[31] and pancreatic cancer develops at younger ages than those in the general population. In a national series study of 200 patients with hereditary pancreatitis, the average age at cancer onset was 55 years, and the incidence rate for pancreatic cancer in this group of patients was remarkably higher than the incidence rate in the general population (standardized incidence ratio [SIR] = 87; 95% CI, 42–113).[32] Other hereditary pancreatitis studies have also reported elevated SIRs.[33,34] In addition, smoking among subjects with hereditary pancreatitis is associated with substantially earlier age at onset (50 years for ever smokers vs. 70 years for never smokers),[35] adding to the evidence that both these factors contribute to cancer onset.

Studies examining the temporal relationship between chronic pancreatitis and the diagnosis of pancreatic cancer have noted decreasing rates of cancer as the lag period increases,[36] suggesting that pancreatitis may also be a consequence of the cancer. Nevertheless, the risk remains elevated, albeit attenuated, with long latency periods. A 5.8-fold increase in risk of pancreatic cancer was estimated from six studies that excluded pancreatic cancer cases diagnosed within 2 years from chronic pancreatitis diagnosis (95% CI, 2.1–15.9).[36] With a 10-year lag, the largest cohort study based on registry data reported an RR of 2.2 (95% CI, 0.9–4.4; the association was not quite statistically significant because of the smaller numbers in this analysis).[37] Elevated local inflammation of the pancreas, present in both hereditary and chronic pancreatitis, is likely creating a microenvironment in the pancreas that can be conducive to tumor development. Indeed, induction of pancreatitis in pancreatic cancer mouse models has been shown to cause dramatic acceleration of pancreatic carcinoma.[38]

Peptic Ulcers and Role of *Helicobacter pylori* Infection

A number of observational studies have examined the associations between peptic ulcers and pancreatic cancer. Positive associations have been observed for gastric ulcers and pancreatic cancer in prospective cohort studies, with detailed information on the type of peptic ulcers.[39,40] In one study the risk of pancreatic cancer was almost threefold higher in subjects who had a gastric ulcer 10–19 years prior to the pancreatic cancer diagnosis (RR, 2.89; 95% CI, 1.26–6.64).[39] In contrast, no association was noted for a history of duodenal ulcers in the same population.[39] Similar findings were reported in a second prospective cohort study gastric, but not duodenal, ulcers were associated with a twofold higher risk of pancreatic cancer in patients who had a gastric ulcer and underwent gastric resection 20 years prior to the diagnosis of pancreatic cancer.[40] Gastric ulcers are associated with low acid production, whereas duodenal ulcers are associated with hyperacidity; consequently, nitrosamine levels are higher in individuals with gastric ulcers and may explain the association with pancreatic cancer risk.[40] Low acidity, however, also allows for the colonization of bacteria that may not usually colonize the stomach, which may lead to dysbiosis in the stomach and changes to the gut microbiota.

Reported associations between *H. pylori* and pancreatic cancer risk have been conflicting. The first case-control study on this topic, published 20 years ago, reported a positive association between *H. pylori* and pancreatic cancer risk (OR = 2.1; 95% CI, 1.09–4.05)[41] and initiated the motivation to research the potential role of this bacteria in pancreatic cancer. In a large prospective cohort study of male smokers, men with *H. pylori* antibodies or CagA-positive strains had about a twofold higher risk of pancreatic cancer than those who were seronegative for those antibodies (OR, 1.87; 95% CI, 1.05–3.34 and OR, 2.01; 95% CI, 1.09–3.70, respectively).[42] However, findings from subsequent observational studies with large pancreatic cancer cases did not reproduce findings from the first two studies.[43–46] Results from meta-analyses conducted on this association are inconsistent and largely influenced by the quality of studies included.[47–49]

Although there does not appear to be an association between *H. pylori* and pancreatic cancer overall, an interesting trend has emerged, suggesting that the direction of the association depends on the strain of *H. pylori* (i.e., CagA-positive or negative). In a meta-analysis separating out results for CagA-positive and CagA-negative strains, an inverse association was noted for CagA-positive strains (OR, 0.78; 95% CI, 0.67–0.91 in six studies), whereas a positive association was found for CagA-negative strains (OR, 1.30; 95% CI, 1.02–1.65 in five studies).[49] The authors of this meta-analysis suggest that the lack of overall association for *H. pylori* may be due to differences in strain prevalence in different studies and argue that CagA-positive strains may be protective of pancreatic cancer by reducing acidity in the stomach.[49] This explanation, however, is inconsistent with the observations noted on the association between gastric ulcers and pancreatic cancer (as gastric ulcers are associated with hypoacidity). Of interest, periodontal disease has been linked to peptic ulcer disease, independent of *H. pylori*,[50] suggesting other bacteria may be involved in the pathogenesis of ulcer disease. The complex results and lack of consistency for *H. pylori* and pancreatic cancer highlight the need for research to include a microbiome approach that is more comprehensive.

Periodontal Diseases and the Role of Periodontal Pathogens

Periodontal disease is an inflammatory disease of the gums that can lead to gum recession, soft tissue damage, bone loss, and tooth loss (severe periodontitis).[51] A number of keystone pathogenic bacteria have been linked to the severity of periodontitis, but it is also clear that periodontal disease is a complex polymicrobial disease that involves the immune response.[52] In addition, as with many chronic diseases, periodontal disease has multiple risk factors, including smoking, socioeconomic status, and type 2 diabetes.[51] Positive associations between periodontal disease and pancreatic cancer risk have been reported in four prospective cohort studies.[53–56] In the first study to report an association between periodontitis and pancreatic cancer, individuals with periodontitis at baseline had a higher risk of fatal pancreatic cancer than those with a healthy periodontium (RR, 1.77; 95% CI, 0.85–1.85), after controlling for age and sex.[53] Unfortunately, cigarette smoking was not adjusted for in this cohort, as it was an exploratory analysis.[53] In a prospective study of male health professionals, men who reported having periodontal disease at baseline had a 64% higher risk of pancreatic cancer than those reporting no periodontal disease, after adjusting for age, smoking, diabetes, and body mass index.[54] In the same study, a twofold increase in pancreatic cancer risk was observed among never smokers (RR, 2.09; 95% CI, 1.18–3.71). Similar positive associations were reported in three additional cohort studies, with detailed data on periodontitis,[55–57] but smoking was not adjusted in one of these studies.[57]

In contrast to reports on periodontal disease and pancreatic cancer, findings on tooth loss (a marker of severe periodontitis) and pancreatic cancer have been inconsistent.[58]

Efforts to better understand the link between periodontal disease and pancreatic cancer have included examination of oral bacteria in relation to pancreatic cancer risk. *Porphyromonas gingivalis*, a keystone periodontal disease pathogen, has been extensively studied for its unique ability to evade immune response.[59] The association between antibodies to periodontal pathogens and the risk of pancreatic cancer was first examined in a large European cohort using stored blood samples from over 385,000 men and women at baseline (i.e., prior to cancer diagnosis).[60] In this study, a greater than twofold increase in risk of pancreatic cancer was observed among those with high levels of antibodies to a pathogenic strain of *P. gingivalis* (OR, 2.38; 95% CI, 1.16–4.90, comparing >200 ng/mL with <200 ng/mL) after adjusting for known risk factors, including smoking.[60] In the NHANES III (Third National Health and Nutrition Examination Survey) cohort study, elevated levels of antibodies to *P. gingivalis* (>69.1 enzyme-linked immunosorbent assay units of IgG (EU) compared with <69.1 EU) were associated with a threefold increase risk of orodigestive cancer mortality (RR, 3.03; 95% CI, 0.99–9.31). A separate examination of *P. gingivalis* with pancreatic cancer mortality could not be conducted in that study because of insufficient case numbers.[55] In a third cohort study, DNA of oral bacteria were measured directly in saliva using 16S RNA genes (samples had been obtained and stored at study recruitment prior to cancer diagnosis) to examine their relation to pancreatic cancer risk; a 1.6-fold increased risk was reported for *P. gingivalis* and a twofold increase risk was observed for *Aggregatibacter actinomycetemcomitans*, another periodontal pathogen.[61] These findings are highly consistent with the results on periodontal disease.

Microbiota and Pancreatic Cancer

Only a few studies have measured bacteria directly in the pancreatic tissue or in fluids near the pancreas. Two studies reported the presence of numerous and diverse bacterial colonization on pancreatic and biliary stents; large interindividual differences in bacterial profiles were observed, but *Streptococcus* species were commonly identified (in both studies) and often present with *Veillonella* species.[62,63] Other studies have only measured specific bacterial DNA in the pancreatic tissue (tumor and surrounding tissue), namely, for *Helicobacter* species[64] and *Fusobacterium* species.[65] *Fusobacterium* species was identified in 8.8% of pancreatic cancer tissues (283

tissues tested), and while it was not related to clinical or molecular features, it was associated with higher mortality.[65] *Helicobacter* species was common in pancreatic cancer patients (75% of patients tested positive in the tumor and/or surrounding tissues) and was also commonly identified in patients with chronic pancreatitis (60%), but *Helicobacter* was not identified in the pancreatic tissue of patients with benign conditions.[64]

A study reported the presence of a large number of bacterial populations in fluid collected from the bile duct, pancreas, and jejunum of pancreatic cancer patients undergoing pancreaticoduodenectomy, using 16S RNA genes.[66] Bacteria present in fluids obtained from the pancreatic ducts and the common bile duct included *Prevotella*, *Haemophilus*, *Aggregatibacter*, and *Fusobacterium*.[66] Microbial communities in the pancreas, bile, and jejunal fluids were similar within individuals, but differed between individuals.[66] Similar observations were made in a study examining bacterial DNA from 16S RNA genes obtained from fresh pancreatic and duodenum tissue[67]; bacterial profiles were much more similar within individuals across different tissue types (including duodenum, pancreatic duct, pancreatic tissue) than they were across different individuals. The bacterial profiles also differed in cancer versus noncancer patients in this cross-sectional study.[67] At this time, it is not clear if the relative abundance in bacteria obtained from pancreatic tissue changes as a result of the cancer (and associated systemic immune changes) or if they contribute to the disease in a causal way.

Several studies have looked at the involvement of bacteria in biliary and pancreatic diseases and have observed a high number of bacterial taxa present in the calcified pancreatic duct epithelium and in pancreatic abscesses.[68–72] Anaerobic bacterial taxa have been found at a variable rate in pancreatitis; the results depend on the process of bacterial identification.[68–70] Previous studies have also reported the presence of bacteria in bile.[73,74] In a study of six patients with gallstones, 16S RNA gene sequencing identified highly relative abundances of *Escherichia*, *Klebsiella*, and *Pyramidobacter* in the bile, and the bacterial profile of the bile was very similar to that in the duodenum of the same patients.[74]

A study published in *Science*[75] reported high abundance of *Fusobacterium nucleatum* in the tumor tissue of patients with colorectal cancer and also found very similar bacterial profiles in metastatic tumors (to the liver). This study is of interest, as it suggests that bacteria may be directly involved in the progression of cancer and might open up new therapeutic opportunities. More research is needed to determine if this may also apply to pancreatic cancer.

BIOLOGICAL PATHWAYS LINKING BACTERIAL INFECTIOUS AGENTS TO PANCREATIC CANCER

Experimental data has provided important clues into how bacteria can directly impact cancer development.[76] Extensive research on *H. pylori* has provided insights into how it activates the inflammatory response, induces oxidative stress and DNA damage, and increases cell proliferation.[77] Moreover, research on virulence factors of *H. pylori* has clarified pathways to carcinogenesis.[78] Understanding the mechanisms through which *H. pylori* can lead to stomach cancer contributed to the classification of this bacterium as a Class I carcinogen by the International Agency for Research on Cancer in 1994.

New research has focused on oral bacteria, especially *F. nucleatum* and *P. gingivalis*. Interest in *F. nucleatum* increased substantially after two papers published in 2012 reported the presence of this bacterium in colon cancer tissue.[79,80] Research on *F. nucleatum* has provided clues on how this bacterium may cause cancer; immune suppression appears to be central to the ability of *F. nucleatum* in inducing carcinogenesis.[81] For example, through the production of the protein Fap2, *F. nucleatum* can inhibit antitumor immunity by natural killer cells,[82] providing evidence for its ability to modulate the tumor-immune microenvironment. Other carcinogenic pathways include promotion of cell proliferation by FadA adhesin (produced by *F. nucleatum*).[83]

Studies on pancreatic cancer mouse model have shown that experimental pancreatitis dramatically accelerates tumor initiation and progression of pancreatic ductal adenocarcinoma.[84–91] *P. gingivalis* has been shown to promote low-grade chronic inflammation by modulating the innate and adaptive immune response[92] and has been extensively studied to understand mechanisms that may explain its strong link with heart disease.[93] Importantly, *P. gingivalis* has been shown to evade the immune response by modification of its lipid A, the biological core of bacterial lipopolysaccharide, universally recognized by the TLR4-MD2 (toll-like receptor 4/myeloid differentiation factor 2) complex.[94–96] TLR4 is overexpressed in human pancreatic cancer and inhibition of this receptor has protective effects on pancreatic cancer progression and invasiveness[97]; understanding if certain bacteria, such as *P. gingivalis*, can impact these key immune pathways and enhance cancer progression will be critical to understand whether they play a causal role. In addition, *P. gingivalis* has been shown to alter dendritic cell maturation[98,99] and promote expansion of myeloid-derived suppressor cells,[100] providing further support for its active role in immune evasion and suppression.

Mechanistic studies demonstrating the ability of *F. nucleatum* and *P. gingivalis* to suppress the host immune response provide support for a potential role in carcinogenesis.[76] Research on these two bacteria and cancer is at its infancy and much more work is needed to elucidate their role in cancer progression. More importantly, however, these pathogens are not likely to be the only two important bacteria; research suggests that their activities and pathogenic properties may be linked to a much more complex microbiome environment.[101] Examining how the microbiome impacts the innate immunity and causes inflammation is becoming an important field in cancer research.

VIRAL INFECTIONS

There is ample evidence demonstrating that viruses cause cancer; in fact, some of these associations were established over 50 years ago.[102,103] Hepatitis B virus (HBV) and hepatocellular carcinoma is one of the strongest virus–cancer associations. HBV can integrate into the DNA, possibly causing direct DNA mutations,[104] but it also causes substantial inflammation of the liver, leading to fibrosis and hyperproliferation of cells in the liver.[105] In contrast, the association between HBV and pancreatic cancer was not examined until recently and remains somewhat controversial. The first study suggesting a link between HBV infection and pancreatic cancer was published in 2008[106]; in this case-control study, a statistically significant twofold increase in risk was observed in individuals who demonstrated past HBV infection (antibody for HBV core antigen positive). Following this study, a number of other observational studies have reported on the association between HBV and pancreatic cancer. While results are somewhat inconsistent, the overall trend suggests that a positive association exists between chronic HBV carriers (meta-analysis summary: RR = 1.39; 95% CI, 1.22–1.59) and those with past HBV exposure (meta-analysis summary: RR = 1.41; 95% CI, 1.06–1.87).[107] The associations are consistent in case-control and cohort studies.[107] Two studies also reported that active HBV infection may be associated with a greater risk than past or chronic HBV infection (summary RR = 3.83; 95% CI, 1.76–8.36).[107] Further research is needed to confirm these findings in larger cohort studies, including confirming the observation made in a cohort study that individuals with chronic HBV infection have a very high rate of pancreatic cancer before the age of 50 years.[108]

MICROBIOME AND DIAGNOSTIC/MANAGEMENT OF PANCREATIC CANCER

The role of the microbiome in the diagnosis and management of pancreatic cancer remains understudied but will undoubtedly gain more attention in the near future. A number of experimental studies conducted at other cancer sites suggest that there may be new opportunities for early detection or targeted therapy with microbiome research. In mouse models, infection with *F. nucleatum* or *P. gingivalis* was shown to promote tumor progression in the oral cavity,[109] and similarly, *F. nucleatum* infection was shown to increase colorectal tumor growth.[110] In a study, antimicrobial treatment reduced *Fusobacterium* load in mouse with xenografts of human primary colorectal adenocarcinoma positive for *Fusobacterium*.[75] In addition, the antimicrobial treatment was shown to reduce cancer cell proliferation and overall tumor growth.[75] In pancreatic cancer, patients with tumors positive for *Fusobacterium* species were found to have worse prognosis than patients with tumors negative for *Fusobacterium* $(P = .02)$,[65] suggesting that these tumors may be similar to colorectal cancers (with respect to the role of bacterial infections).

Taken together, these experimental and observational studies provide strong and compelling evidence that bacteria play a role in gastrointestinal cancers, including pancreatic cancer. The next decade of research should shed light on if, and how, the microbiome can be modulated to improve prevention and treatment of this devastating cancer.

SUMMARY

There is increasing evidence that bacterial infections play a role in pancreatic carcinogenesis; studies to date support a role for oral bacteria in pancreatic carcinogenesis. Biological mechanisms of interest include inflammatory pathways, both systemic and local, as well as altered immune response. Viruses, such as HBV, may also play a role in this cancer. However, substantial research remains to be carried out to understand the pathways and whether bacteria, or viruses, are causing cancer, or are acting as opportunistic microbiota. Experimental and observational studies are urgently needed to address these critical questions and to determine whether microbiome may provide new opportunities to reduce pancreatic cancer incidence or mortality.

REFERENCES

1. ACS. *Cancer Facts & Figures 2017*. Atlanta: American Cancer Society, Inc; 2017.
2. Surveillance, Epidemiology, and End Results (SEER) Program. *SEER*Stat Database: Incidence - SEER 9 Regs Research Data, Nov 2013 Sub (1973-2011) <Katrina/Rita Population Adjustment> - Linked to County Attributes - Total U.S., 1969-2012 Counties, National Cancer Institute, DCCPS, Surveillance Research Program, Surveillance Systems Branch, Released April 2014*. National Cancer Institute, DCCPS, Surveillance Research Program; 2014. www.seer.cancer.gov. www.seer.cancer.gov/seerstat.
2a. Ferlay J, Soerjomataram I, Dikshit R, Eser S, Mathers C, Rebelo M, et al. Cancer incidence and mortality worldwide: sources, methods and major patterns in GLOBOCAN 2012. *Int J Cancer*. 2015;136(5):E359–86.
3. Parkin DM. 1. The fraction of cancer attributable to lifestyle and environmental factors in the UK in 2010. *Br J Cancer*. 2011;105(suppl 2):S2–S5.
4. Maisonneuve P, Lowenfels AB. Risk factors for pancreatic cancer: a summary review of meta-analytical studies. *Int J Epidemiol*. 2015;44(1):186–198.
5. Bosetti C, Lucenteforte E, Silverman DT, et al. Cigarette smoking and pancreatic cancer: an analysis from the international pancreatic cancer case-control consortium (Panc4). *Ann Oncol*. 2012;23(7):1880–1888.
6. Lynch SM, Vrieling A, Lubin JH, et al. Cigarette smoking and pancreatic cancer: a pooled analysis from the pancreatic cancer cohort consortium. *Am J Epidemiol*. 2009;170(4):403–413.
7. Heinen MM, Verhage BA, Goldbohm RA, van den Brandt PA. Active and passive smoking and the risk of pancreatic cancer in The Netherlands Cohort Study. *Cancer Epidemiol Biomark Prev*. 2010;19(6):1612–1622.
8. Vrieling A, Bueno-de-Mesquita HB, Boshuizen HC, et al. Cigarette smoking, environmental tobacco smoke exposure and pancreatic cancer risk in the European Prospective Investigation into Cancer and Nutrition. International journal of cancer. *J Int Cancer*. 2010;126(10):2394–2403.
9. Fuchs CS, Colditz GA, Stampfer MJ, et al. A prospective study of cigarette smoking and the risk of pancreatic cancer. *Arch Intern Med*. 1996;156(19):2255–2260.
10. Bertuccio P, La Vecchia C, Silverman DT, et al. Cigar and pipe smoking, smokeless tobacco use and pancreatic cancer: an analysis from the International Pancreatic Cancer Case-Control Consortium (PanC4). *Ann Oncol*. 2011;22(6):1420–1426.
11. Stolzenberg-Solomon RZ, Graubard BI, Chari S, et al. Insulin, glucose, insulin resistance, and pancreatic cancer in male smokers. *JAMA*. 2005;294(22):2872–2878.
12. Gapstur SM, Gann PH, Lowe W, Liu K, Colangelo L, Dyer A. Abnormal glucose metabolism and pancreatic cancer mortality. *JAMA*. 2000;283(19):2552–2558.
13. Wolpin BM, Bao Y, Qian ZR, et al. Hyperglycemia, insulin resistance, impaired pancreatic beta-cell function, and risk of pancreatic cancer. *J Natl Cancer Inst*. 2013;105(14):1027–1035.

14. Huxley R, Ansary-Moghaddam A, Berrington de Gonzalez A, Barzi F, Woodward M. Type-II diabetes and pancreatic cancer: a meta-analysis of 36 studies. *Br J Cancer.* 2005;92(11):2076–2083.
15. Bosetti C, Rosato V, Li D, et al. Diabetes, antidiabetic medications, and pancreatic cancer risk: an analysis from the International Pancreatic Cancer Case-Control Consortium. *Ann Oncol.* 2014;25(10):2065–2072.
16. Ben Q, Cai Q, Li Z, et al. The relationship between new-onset diabetes mellitus and pancreatic cancer risk: a case-control study. *Eur J Cancer.* 2011;47(2):248–254.
17. Aune D, Greenwood DC, Chan DS, et al. Body mass index, abdominal fatness and pancreatic cancer risk: a systematic review and non-linear dose-response meta-analysis of prospective studies. *Ann Oncol.* 2012;23(4):843–852.
18. Arslan AA, Helzlsouer KJ, Kooperberg C, et al. Anthropometric measures, body mass index, and pancreatic cancer: a pooled analysis from the Pancreatic Cancer Cohort Consortium (PanScan). *Arch Intern Med.* 2010;170(9):791–802.
19. Jacobs EJ, Chanock SJ, Fuchs CS, et al. Family history of cancer and risk of pancreatic cancer: a pooled analysis from the Pancreatic Cancer Cohort Consortium (PanScan). *Int J Cancer.* 2010;127(6):1421–1428.
20. Landi S. Genetic predisposition and environmental risk factors to pancreatic cancer: a review of the literature. *Mutat Res.* 2009;681(2–3):299–307.
21. Amundadottir L, Kraft P, Stolzenberg-Solomon RZ, et al. Genome-wide association study identifies variants in the ABO locus associated with susceptibility to pancreatic cancer. *Nat Genet.* 2009;41(9):986–990.
22. Wolpin BM, Rizzato C, Kraft P, et al. Genome-wide association study identifies multiple susceptibility loci for pancreatic cancer. *Nat Genet.* 2014;46(9):994–1000.
23. Cooling L. Blood groups in infection and host susceptibility. *Clin Microbiol Rev.* 2015;28(3):801–870.
24. Petersen GM, Amundadottir L, Fuchs CS, et al. A genome-wide association study identifies pancreatic cancer susceptibility loci on chromosomes 13q22.1, 1q32.1 and 5p15.33. *Nat Genet.* 2010;42(3):224–228.
25. Aird I, Lee DR, Roberts JA. ABO blood groups and cancer of oesophagus, cancer of pancreas, and pituitary adenoma. *Br Med J.* 1960;1(5180):1163–1166.
26. Wolpin BM, Chan AT, Hartge P, et al. ABO blood group and the risk of pancreatic cancer. *J Natl Cancer Inst.* March 18, 2009;101(6):424–431.
27. Michaud DS, Vrieling A, Jiao L, et al. Alcohol intake and pancreatic cancer: a pooled analysis from the pancreatic cancer cohort consortium (PanScan). *Cancer Causes Control.* 2010;21(8):1213–1225.
28. Genkinger JM, Spiegelman D, Anderson KE, et al. Alcohol intake and pancreatic cancer risk: a pooled analysis of fourteen cohort studies. *Cancer Epidemiol Biomark Prev.* 2009;18(3):765–776.
29. Lucenteforte E, La Vecchia C, Silverman D, et al. Alcohol consumption and pancreatic cancer: a pooled analysis in the international pancreatic cancer case-control consortium (PanC4). *Ann Oncol.* 2012;23(2):374–382.
30. Giovannucci E, Michaud D. The role of obesity and related metabolic disturbances in cancers of the colon, prostate, and pancreas. *Gastroenterology.* 2007;132(6):2208–2225.
31. Rebours V, Boutron-Ruault MC, Schnee M, et al. The natural history of hereditary pancreatitis: a national series. *Gut.* 2009;58(1):97–103.
32. Rebours V, Boutron-Ruault MC, Schnee M, et al. Risk of pancreatic adenocarcinoma in patients with hereditary pancreatitis: a national exhaustive series. *Am J Gastroenterol.* 2008;103(1):111–119.
33. Lowenfels AB, Maisonneuve P, DiMagno EP, et al. Hereditary pancreatitis and the risk of pancreatic cancer. International hereditary pancreatitis study group. *J Natl Cancer Inst.* 1997;89(6):442–446.
34. Howes N, Lerch MM, Greenhalf W, et al. Clinical and genetic characteristics of hereditary pancreatitis in Europe. *Clin Gastroenterol Hepatol.* 2004;2(3):252–261.
35. Lowenfels AB, Maisonneuve P, Whitcomb DC, Lerch MM, DiMagno EP. Cigarette smoking as a risk factor for pancreatic cancer in patients with hereditary pancreatitis. *JAMA.* 2001;286(2):169–170.
36. Raimondi S, Lowenfels AB, Morselli-Labate AM, Maisonneuve P, Pezzilli R. Pancreatic cancer in chronic pancreatitis; aetiology, incidence, and early detection. *Best Pract Res Clin Gastroenterol.* 2010;24(3):349–358.
37. Karlson BM, Ekbom A, Josefsson S, McLaughlin JK, Fraumeni Jr JF, Nyren O. The risk of pancreatic cancer following pancreatitis: an association due to confounding? *Gastroenterology.* 1997;113(2):587–592.
38. Murtaugh LC. Pathogenesis of pancreatic cancer: lessons from animal models. *Toxicol Pathol.* 2014;42(1):217–228.
39. Bao Y, Spiegelman D, Li R, Giovannucci E, Fuchs CS, Michaud DS. History of peptic ulcer disease and pancreatic cancer risk in men. *Gastroenterology.* 2010;138(2):541–549.
40. Luo J, Nordenvall C, Nyren O, Adami HO, Permert J, Ye W. The risk of pancreatic cancer in patients with gastric or duodenal ulcer disease. International journal of cancer. *J Int Cancer.* 2007;120(2):368–372.
41. Raderer M, Wrba F, Kornek G, et al. Association between *Helicobacter pylori* infection and pancreatic cancer. *Oncology.* 1998;55(1):16–19.
42. Stolzenberg-Solomon RZ, Blaser MJ, Limburg PJ, et al. *Helicobacter pylori* seropositivity as a risk factor for pancreatic cancer. *J Natl Cancer Inst.* 2001;93(12):937–941.
43. de Martel C, Llosa AE, Friedman GD, et al. *Helicobacter pylori* infection and development of pancreatic cancer. *Cancer Epidemiol Biomark Prev.* 2008;17(5):1188–1194.
44. Lindkvist B, Johansen D, Borgstrom A, Manjer J. A prospective study of *Helicobacter pylori* in relation to the risk for pancreatic cancer. *BMC Cancer.* 2008;8:321.
45. Risch HA, Yu H, Lu L, Kidd MS. ABO blood group, *Helicobacter pylori* seropositivity, and risk of pancreatic cancer: a case-control study. *J Natl Cancer Inst.* 2010;102(7):502–505.

46. Yu G, Murphy G, Michel A, et al. Seropositivity to *Helicobacter pylori* and risk of pancreatic cancer. *Cancer Epidemiol Biomark Prev.* 2013;22(12):2416–2419.

47. Wang Y, Zhang FC, Wang YJ. *Helicobacter pylori* and pancreatic cancer risk: a meta- analysis based on 2,049 cases and 2,861 controls. *Asian Pac J Cancer Prev.* 2014;15(11):4449–4454.

48. Xiao M, Wang Y, Gao Y. Association between *Helicobacter pylori* infection and pancreatic cancer development: a meta-analysis. *PLoS One.* 2013;8(9):e75559.

49. Schulte A, Pandeya N, Fawcett J, et al. Association between *Helicobacter pylori* and pancreatic cancer risk: a meta-analysis. *Cancer Causes Control.* 2015;26(7):1027–1035.

50. Boylan MR, Khalili H, Huang ES, et al. A prospective study of periodontal disease and risk of gastric and duodenal ulcer in male health professionals. *Clin Transl Gastroenterol.* 2014;5:e49.

51. Papapanou PN. Periodontal diseases: epidemiology. *Ann Periodontol.* 1996;1(1):1–36.

52. Hajishengallis G. Periodontitis: from microbial immune subversion to systemic inflammation. *Nat Rev Immunol.* 2015;15(1):30–44.

53. Hujoel PP, Drangsholt M, Spiekerman C, Weiss NS. An exploration of the periodontitis-cancer association. *Ann Epidemiol.* 2003;13(5):312–316.

54. Michaud DS, Joshipura K, Giovannucci E, Fuchs CS. A prospective study of periodontal disease and pancreatic cancer in US male health professionals. *J Natl Cancer Inst.* 2007;99(2):171–175.

55. Ahn J, Segers S, Hayes RB. Periodontal disease, Porphyromonas gingivalis serum antibody levels and orodigestive cancer mortality. *Carcinogenesis.* 2012;33(5):1055–1058.

56. Arora M, Weuve J, Fall K, Pedersen NL, Mucci LA. An exploration of shared genetic risk factors between periodontal disease and cancers: a prospective co-twin study. *Am J Epidemiol.* 2010;171(2):253–259.

57. Chang JS, Tsai CR, Chen LT, Shan YS. Investigating the association between periodontal disease and risk of pancreatic cancer. *Pancreas.* 2016;45(1):134–141.

58. Michaud DS, Fu Z, Shi J, Chung M. Periodontal disease, tooth loss, and cancer risk. *Epidemiol Rev.* 2017;39(1):49–58.

59. Tribble GD, Kerr JE, Wang BY. Genetic diversity in the oral pathogen Porphyromonas gingivalis: molecular mechanisms and biological consequences. *Future Microbiol.* 2013;8:607–620.

60. Michaud DS, Izard J, Wilhelm-Benartzi CS, et al. Plasma antibodies to oral bacteria and risk of pancreatic cancer in a large European prospective cohort study. *Gut.* 2013;62(12):1764–1770.

61. Fan X, Alekseyenko AV, Wu J, et al. Human oral microbiome and prospective risk for pancreatic cancer: a population-based nested case-control study. *Gut.* 2018;67(1):120–127.

62. Schneider J, Schenk P, Obermeier A, et al. Microbial colonization of pancreatic duct stents: a prospective analysis. *Pancreas.* 2015;44(5):786–790.

63. Scheithauer BK, Wos-Oxley ML, Ferslev B, Jablonowski H, Pieper DH. Characterization of the complex bacterial communities colonizing biliary stents reveals a host-dependent diversity. *ISME J.* 2009;3(7):797–807.

64. Nilsson HO, Stenram U, Ihse I, Wadstrom T. Helicobacter species ribosomal DNA in the pancreas, stomach and duodenum of pancreatic cancer patients. *World J Gastroenterol.* 2006;12(19):3038–3043.

65. Mitsuhashi K, Nosho K, Sukawa Y, et al. Association of Fusobacterium species in pancreatic cancer tissues with molecular features and prognosis. *Oncotarget.* 2015;6(9):7209–7220.

66. Rogers MB, Aveson V, Firek B, et al. Disturbances of the perioperative microbiome across multiple body sites in patients undergoing pancreaticoduodenectomy. *Pancreas.* 2017;46(2):260–267.

67. Del Castillo E, Meier R, Chung M, et al. The Microbiomes of Pancreatic and Duodenum Tissue Overlap and are Highly Subject Specific but Differ between Pancreatic Cancer and Non-Cancer Subjects. *Cancer Epidemiol Biomarkers Prev.* October 29, 2018. https://doi.org/10.1158/1055-9965.EPI-18-0542.

68. Swidsinski A, Schlien P, Pernthaler A, et al. Bacterial biofilm within diseased pancreatic and biliary tracts. *Gut.* 2005;54(3):388–395.

69. Schmid SW, Uhl W, Friess H, Malfertheiner P, Buchler MW. The role of infection in acute pancreatitis. *Gut.* 1999;45(2):311–316.

70. Brook I, Frazier EH. Microbiological analysis of pancreatic abscess. *Clin Infect Dis.* 1996;22(2):384–385.

71. Hill MC, Dach JL, Barkin J, Isikoff MB, Morse B. The role of percutaneous aspiration in the diagnosis of pancreatic abscess. *Am J Roentgenol.* 1983;141(5):1035–1038.

72. Tsui NC, Zhao E, Li Z, et al. Microbiological findings in secondary infection of severe acute pancreatitis: a retrospective clinical study. *Pancreas.* 2009;38(5):499–502.

73. Wu T, Zhang Z, Liu B, et al. Gut microbiota dysbiosis and bacterial community assembly associated with cholesterol gallstones in large-scale study. *BMC Genomics.* 2013;14:669.

74. Ye F, Shen H, Li Z, et al. Influence of the biliary system on biliary bacteria revealed by bacterial communities of the human biliary and upper digestive tracts. *PLoS One.* 2016;11(3):e0150519.

75. Bullman S, Pedamallu CS, Sicinska E, et al. Analysis of Fusobacterium persistence and antibiotic response in colorectal cancer. *Science.* 2017;358(6369):1443–1448.

76. Gagnaire A, Nadel B, Raoult D, Neefjes J, Gorvel JP. Collateral damage: insights into bacterial mechanisms that predispose host cells to cancer. *Nat Rev Microbiol.* 2017;15(2):109–128.

77. Salama NR, Hartung ML, Muller A. Life in the human stomach: persistence strategies of the bacterial pathogen *Helicobacter pylori*. *Nat Rev Microbiol.* 2013;11(6):385–399.

78. Hatakeyama M. *Helicobacter pylori* CagA and gastric cancer: a paradigm for hit-and-run carcinogenesis. *Cell Host Microbe.* 2014;15(3):306–316.

79. Kostic AD, Gevers D, Pedamallu CS, et al. Genomic analysis identifies association of Fusobacterium with colorectal carcinoma. *Genome Res.* 2012;22(2):292–298.
80. Castellarin M, Warren RL, Freeman JD, et al. Fusobacterium nucleatum infection is prevalent in human colorectal carcinoma. *Genome Res.* 2012;22(2):299–306.
81. Bashir A, Miskeen AY, Bhat A, Fazili KM, Ganai BA. Fusobacterium nucleatum: an emerging bug in colorectal tumorigenesis. *Eur J Cancer Prev.* 2015;24(5):373–385.
82. Gur C, Ibrahim Y, Isaacson B, et al. Binding of the Fap2 protein of Fusobacterium nucleatum to human inhibitory receptor TIGIT protects tumors from immune cell attack. *Immunity.* 2015;42(2):344–355.
83. Rubinstein MR, Wang X, Liu W, Hao Y, Cai G, Han YW. Fusobacterium nucleatum promotes colorectal carcinogenesis by modulating E-cadherin/beta-catenin signaling via its FadA adhesin. *Cell Host Microbe.* 2013;14(2):195–206.
84. Daniluk J, Liu Y, Deng D, et al. An NF-kappaB pathway-mediated positive feedback loop amplifies Ras activity to pathological levels in mice. *J Clin Investig.* 2012;122(4):1519–1528.
85. De La OJP, Murtaugh LC. Notch and Kras in pancreatic cancer: at the crossroads of mutation, differentiation and signaling. *Cell Cycle (Georgetown, Tex).* 2009;8(12):1860–1864.
86. Carriere C, Young AL, Gunn JR, Longnecker DS, Korc M. Acute pancreatitis markedly accelerates pancreatic cancer progression in mice expressing oncogenic Kras. *Biochem Biophys Res Commun.* 2009;382(3):561–565.
87. Ji B, Tsou L, Wang H, et al. Ras activity levels control the development of pancreatic diseases. *Gastroenterology.* 2009;137(3):1072–1082, 1082.e1071–e1076.
88. Guerra C, Schuhmacher AJ, Canamero M, et al. Chronic pancreatitis is essential for induction of pancreatic ductal adenocarcinoma by K-Ras oncogenes in adult mice. *Cancer Cell.* 2007;11(3):291–302.
89. Khasawneh J, Schulz MD, Walch A, et al. Inflammation and mitochondrial fatty acid beta-oxidation link obesity to early tumor promotion. *Proc Natl Acad Sci USA.* 2009;106(9):3354–3359.
90. Morris JP, Cano DA, Sekine S, Wang SC, Hebrok M. Beta-catenin blocks Kras-dependent reprogramming of acini into pancreatic cancer precursor lesions in mice. *J Clin Investig.* 2010;120(2):508–520.
91. Philip B, Roland CL, Daniluk J, et al. A high-fat diet activates oncogenic Kras and COX2 to induce development of pancreatic ductal adenocarcinoma in mice. *Gastroenterology.* 2013;145(6):1449–1458.
92. Kramer CD, Genco CA. Microbiota, immune subversion, and chronic inflammation. *Front Immunol.* 2017;8:255.
93. Gibson 3rd FC, Yumoto H, Takahashi Y, Chou HH, Genco CA. Innate immune signaling and Porphyromonas gingivalis-accelerated atherosclerosis. *J Dental Res.* 2006;85(2):106–121.
94. Akira S, Takeda K, Kaisho T. Toll-like receptors: critical proteins linking innate and acquired immunity. *Nat Immunol.* 2001;2(8):675–680.
95. Miller SI, Ernst RK, Bader MW. LPS, TLR4 and infectious disease diversity. *Nat Rev Microbiol.* 2005;3(1):36–46.
96. Reife RA, Coats SR, Al-Qutub M, et al. Porphyromonas gingivalis lipopolysaccharide lipid A heterogeneity: differential activities of tetra- and penta-acylated lipid A structures on E-selectin expression and TLR4 recognition. *Cell Microbiol.* 2006;8(5):857–868.
97. Vaz J, Andersson R. Intervention on toll-like receptors in pancreatic cancer. *World J Gastroenterol.* 2014;20(19):5808–5817.
98. Miles B, Scisci E, Carrion J, Sabino GJ, Genco CA, Cutler CW. Noncanonical dendritic cell differentiation and survival driven by a bacteremic pathogen. *J Leukoc Biol.* 2013;94(2):281–289.
99. Miles B, Zakhary I, El-Awady A, et al. Secondary lymphoid organ homing phenotype of human myeloid dendritic cells disrupted by an intracellular oral pathogen. *Infect Immun.* 2014;82(1):101–111.
100. Su L, Xu Q, Zhang P, Michalek SM, Katz J. Phenotype and function of myeloid-derived suppressor cells induced by Porphyromonas gingivalis infection. *Infect Immun.* 2017;85(8).
101. Dejea CM, Sears CL. Do biofilms confer a pro-carcinogenic state? *Gut Microbes.* 2016;7(1):54–57.
102. Marx JL. How DNA viruses may cause cancer. *Science.* 1989;243(4894 Pt 1):1012–1013.
103. Evans AS, Mueller NE. Viruses and cancer. Causal associations. *Ann Epidemiol.* 1990;1(1):71–92.
104. Brechot C, Pourcel C, Louise A, Rain B, Tiollais P. Presence of integrated hepatitis B virus DNA sequences in cellular DNA of human hepatocellular carcinoma. *Nature.* 1980;286(5772):533–535.
105. Kremsdorf D, Soussan P, Paterlini-Brechot P, Brechot C. Hepatitis B virus-related hepatocellular carcinoma: paradigms for viral-related human carcinogenesis. *Oncogene.* 2006;25(27):3823–3833.
106. Hassan MM, Li D, El-Deeb AS, et al. Association between hepatitis B virus and pancreatic cancer. *J Clin Oncol.* 2008;26(28):4557–4562.
107. Luo G, Hao NB, Hu CJ, et al. HBV infection increases the risk of pancreatic cancer: a meta-analysis. *Cancer Causes Control.* 2013;24(3):529–537.
108. Iloeje UH, Yang HI, Jen CL, et al. Risk of pancreatic cancer in chronic hepatitis B virus infection: data from the REVEAL-HBV cohort study. *Liver Int.* 2010;30(3):423–429.
109. Binder Gallimidi A, Fischman S, Revach B, et al. Periodontal pathogens Porphyromonas gingivalis and Fusobacterium nucleatum promote tumor progression in an oral-specific chemical carcinogenesis model. *Oncotarget.* 2015;6(26):22613–22623.
110. Kostic AD, Chun E, Robertson L, et al. Fusobacterium nucleatum potentiates intestinal tumorigenesis and modulates the tumor-immune microenvironment. *Cell Host Microbe.* 2013;14(2):207–215.

CHAPTER 11

Viral Gastroenteritis

NICOLA ANNE PAGE, PHD, MPH, MSC (MED), BSC (AGRIC) (HONS), BSC (AGRIC) •
SANDRAMA NADAN, PHD, MSC, BSC (HONS), BSC •
JANET MANS, PHD, MSC, BSC (HONS), BSC

INTRODUCTION

Gastroenteritis is defined as inflammation of the stomach and intestines that may result in a wide range of symptoms from asymptomatic infections through mild complaints to life-threatening conditions that lead to death. Vulnerable populations at increased risk of fatal outcomes include children, immune-compromised patients, and the elderly. The Global Burden of Diseases study estimated that in 2015 there were 2.39 billion episodes of diarrhea globally, which resulted in 1.31 million deaths.[1] In children, an estimated 957.5 million episodes occurred with 499,000 mortality outcomes.[1] Between 2005 and 2015, mortality due to diarrhea declined by 20.8% overall and by 34.3% in children.[1] However, the incidence of diarrhea has not decreased in similarly large increments with only a 5.9% overall reduction and a 10.4% reduction in children.[1]

Diarrhea can be caused by various infectious (viruses, bacteria, and parasites) and noninfectious (food poisoning, chronic diseases, food allergies, and antibiotics) sources. Various pathogens and conditions present with similar clinical signs including watery nonbloody diarrhea, vomiting, and fever. Although a laboratory diagnosis is essential in differentiating enteric pathogens, most diarrheal episodes do not require a diagnosis to begin treatment and rehydration therapies can be initiated immediately. In this chapter, we concentrate on the viruses associated with diarrheal diseases. The terms gastroenteritis and diarrhea are used interchangeably.

Viruses tended to be implicated as a cause of diarrhea when no other bacterial or parasitic pathogen could be found. That meant that our knowledge of diarrhea-associated viruses was based solely on our ability to detect them. Enteric virus detection methods began with fine filters that removed bacteria and parasites but not viral particles, moved onto growth in cell cultures and detection using electron microscopes and antibodies to the genome age with molecular detection by polymerase chain reaction (PCR) and Sanger sequencing.[2] Detection methods have continued to evolve and currently include sequence independent next generation sequencing methodologies and direct sequencing of viral genomes from clinical specimens.

Establishing a causal relationship between a diarrheal disease and a virus is a complex process, and the difficulty in establishing causality was recognized early as the 19th century. During this time, Koch laid out a set of guidelines that enabled the classification of microorganisms as pathogens. A microbe fulfilling the following criteria was deemed a pathogen: (1) the microbe could be detected in cases with the disease outcome from infected tissues or clinical specimens, (2) the microbe was not associated with any other disease or asymptomatic infection and, (3) the microbe could be isolated, grown in pure culture, and induce the same disease in healthy individuals.[2,3] Trying to assign causality using Koch's guidelines proves problematic for enteric viruses on a few fronts: (1) enteric viruses can cause asymptomatic infections,[4–7] (2) enteric viruses can be shed for prolonged periods,[8,9] and (3) enteric viruses may be difficult to grow in culture.[10]

Postulates for virus causality have been revised to reflect changes in our understanding of virus biology and evolving detection methods.[2,3,11] For enteric viruses, the challenges that remain include an inability to demonstrate pathogenicity in human cell lines, limited case–control studies to establish disease association, no or limited viral antigens to screen sera for immune responses, numerous coinfections with multiple pathogens capable of producing the disease outcome and the broad viral genetic diversity.[11,12]

Viruses that are known to cause diarrheal diseases include rotavirus (RV), norovirus (NoV), sapovirus (SaV), adenovirus (AdV), and astrovirus (AstV). Other viruses that have demonstrated some association with

Gastrointestinal Diseases and Their Associated Infections. https://doi.org/10.1016/B978-0-323-54843-4.00011-8
Copyright © 2019 Elsevier Inc. All rights reserved.

diarrhea are Aichi virus, torovirus, and picobirnaviruses.[13] New viruses detected in the gastrointestinal tract by next generation sequencing with an unknown association with diarrhea include novel astroviruses, Saffold virus, Cosavirus, Klassevirus/Salivirus, novel polyomaviruses, Bufavirus, Tusavirus, and Recovirus.[13] This chapter will focus on the epidemiology, diagnosis, and management of the five most common enteric viruses associated with diarrhea.

ENTERIC VIRUSES

Rotavirus

Rotaviruses are classified within the virus family *Reoviridae*. The genome consists of 11 individual segments of double-stranded (ds) RNA (18 500 bp in total) enclosed by three protein layers: the core, inner capsid, and outer capsid (Fig. 11.1A). The proteins of the inner and outer capsid layers include epitopes that aid in the classification of RV strains. Epitopes on the inner capsid

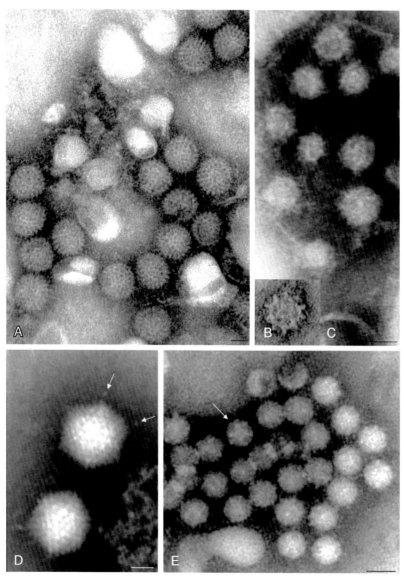

FIG. 11.1 Negatively-stained, pathogenic virions with characteristic morphologies of: (a) Reoviridae, Sedovirinae, Rotavirus; (b and c) Caliciviridae, Norovirus; inset: Vesivirus; (d) Adenoviridae, Mastadenovirus — arrows indicate the ends of pentameric fibres; (e) Asteroviridae, Astrovirus — arrow highlights a particle with taxonomically relevant starry appearance. Scale bars = 30 nm. (Reproduced with permission of Monica Birkhead, NICD).

protein (VP6) allow classification of RVs into eight species (termed RVA–RVH). Epidemiological studies have shown that group A RVs are commonly associated with human disease.[14]

The outer capsid proteins, VP7 and VP4, are able to independently elicit an immune response and were important epitopes during vaccine development.[15] These proteins specify the G and P genotypes, respectively, and to date 35G and 50P genotypes have been described.[16,17] The G types, G1-4, G8, G9, and G12, and P types, P[8], P[6], and P[4], are considered to predominate in human infections.[18,19] The remaining nine genes are classified according to nucleotide sequence identities, and all new types are established by the Rotavirus Classification Working Group (RCWG).[16,17]

Epidemiology

Rotavirus is a childhood diarrheal disease with most children experiencing an infection by 3 years of age, even in high-income countries with access to clean water, proper sewerage, and good standards of healthcare.[20] Globally, RV is the leading cause of diarrhea and related mortality in children <5 years. Etiology studies investigating both moderate-to-severe diarrhea in a case–control study design (Global Enteric Multisite Study; GEMS) and community-acquired diarrhea in a cohort study design (MAL-ED) identified RV as the most important diarrheal pathogen in children <2 years of age.[21–23]

Rotavirus is typically detected in 40% of hospitalized diarrhea cases although the percentage varies depending on location, time of year, healthcare setting, age of patients, and socioeconomic strata.[20,24] The RV prevalence in hospitalized diarrhea patients <5 years is typically double the prevalence in outpatients with an additional 3% of RV cases detected in healthy controls.[25] Rotavirus has been estimated to be fatal in roughly 28% of RV positive diarrhea cases in children <5 years.[25] In global terms, RV mortality in children <5 years was estimated at 527,000 (465,000–591,000) in 2000 although by 2013, the estimate had declined to 215,000 (197,000–233,000).[26]

The greatest number of deaths and disproportionate burden occurs in sub-Saharan Africa.[26] Children living in Africa are exposed to RV at an earlier age than children in Europe or Asia.[20,24] Furthermore, poor caregiver knowledge about dehydration danger signs, failure to seek medical care, failure to implement oral rehydration therapy (ORT) at home or at the health center, poor implementation of the World Health Organization (WHO) Integrated Management of Childhood

Illnesses (IMCI) guidelines, and a lack of zinc provision are some of the factors that contribute to mortality.[27]

In high- and middle-income countries with temperate climates, RVs have a distinct winter seasonality.[15,28] In contrast, in low-income countries in Africa and Asia, seasonality is less pronounced and RVs circulate throughout the year.[28] A study by Patel and colleagues[29] showed that the level of country development was a better predictor of RV seasonality than latitude or geography with poorer countries displaying limited seasonal variation compared to richer countries with a more marked seasonality. Another modeling study found that high birth and transmission rates contributed to the lack of seasonality in low-income countries.[30] Generally, RVs are detected more frequently during the cooler, drier months of the year.

Pathogenesis

Rotavirus infects the mature enterocytes on the small intestinal villi tips resulting in the shortening and atrophy of the villi.[14,15] Rotavirus causes diarrhea by destroying the epithelium that leads to malabsorptive diarrhea, reducing the blood supply within the villi, the NSP4 viral enterotoxin action, and activation of the enteric nervous system.[14,15] Rotavirus can escape the gut and RV nucleic acid, antigen, and infectious particles have been detected in serum and other bodily fluids including cerebrospinal fluid and throat swabs.[31,32]

Natural RV infections do not provide complete protection against a subsequent infection or associated mild disease.[33] Reinfection in the first few years of life appears to be common, although infants usually experience a milder illness during subsequent RV infections.[34,35] Although RV cases are rare in adults, RV is readily transmitted within households from symptomatic children and cause asymptomatic or mildly symptomatic infections in adults.[36]

Norovirus

Norovirus is a member of the *Caliciviridae* family of single-stranded (ss), positive sense RNA viruses. The ~7.5 kb genome encodes three open reading frames (ORFs). ORF1 encodes a polyprotein that is proteolytically cleaved into six nonstructural proteins, whereas ORF2 and ORF3 encode the major (VP1) and minor (VP2) capsid proteins, respectively (Fig. 11.1B and C). Noroviruses are genetically and antigenically diverse with six genogroups (G) defined, of which GI, GII, and GIV infect humans. Genogroups are further subdivided into >30 genotypes based on the relatedness of the RNA-dependent RNA polymerase (RdRp) and complete capsid gene.[37] Standard nomenclature requires both the RdRp and capsid genotypes be indicated if available, with the polymerase type denoted by P, for example, GII.P16/GII.4.[38]

Noroviruses evolve rapidly by a combination of genetic drift and recombination. Despite the number of genotypes, the genogroup II, genotype 4 (GII.4) strains predominate globally.[39] Mutations in the protruding domain of VP1 modulate the virus' ability to interact with host attachment factors, the histo-blood group antigens (HBGAs), and to escape from host immune response (herd immunity).[40] Intra- and inter-genotype recombination between NoV strains is common. The recombination breakpoint is located around the ORF1/ORF2 junction.[41] Many recombinant strains have been described and some polymerase genotypes (e.g., GII. Pg) are frequently detected in combination with different capsid genotypes.[42]

Epidemiology

Norovirus is estimated to cause 18% (95% confidence interval (CI) 17–20) of gastroenteritis in all ages worldwide. Higher NoV prevalence is observed in the community (24%, 95% CI 28–30) compared to hospitalized individuals (17%, 95% CI 17–20).[43] The global economic burden of NoV is projected at $4.2 billion per year in direct health system costs and at $60.3 billion per year in societal costs, mostly due to lost productivity.[44] As the introduction of universal RV vaccination, NoV has replaced RV as the leading cause of hospitalizations in children with gastroenteritis in some settings.[45,46] Norovirus is a primary cause of foodborne illness and was estimated to cause 125 million cases of foodborne illness and 35,000 related deaths in 2010.[47] A recent review of waterborne gastroenteritis outbreaks identified NoV as a major pathogen, affecting >16,000 consumers over 14 years.[48]

A recent study evaluated NoV infections in healthcare workers and food handlers in outbreak settings.[49] They found that 59.1% of employees' stool specimens tested positive for NoV and >70% were infected asymptomatically. There was no significant difference in the duration or level of shedding between symptomatic and asymptomatic individuals. However, in nosocomial outbreaks, it has been shown that symptomatic individuals are more likely to transmit NoV, probably due to efficient spread via vomiting and diarrhea.[50] Infected individuals could be a potential source of secondary NoV transmission and strict hygiene practices should be enforced for all employees or sick persons.

Norovirus infections occur throughout the year, however in the northern hemisphere, outbreaks peak in the winter months.[51] In other parts of the world, a summer seasonality or no distinct seasonality is observed.[52]

Pathogenesis

Norovirus uses human HBGAs as attachment factors to facilitate infection.[53] The expression of HBGAs gastrointestinal tract cells and secretions is regulated by the fucosyltransferase 2 (FUT2) enzyme. Individuals with two inactive *FUT2* alleles, do not express certain HBGAs on their intestinal epithelium or in secretions and are termed nonsecretors.[54] Norovirus genotypes differ in their ability to bind to different HBGAs and nonsecretors in general are less susceptible to NoV infections than secretors.[53] The mutated *FUT2* alleles occur in approximately 20%–30% of individuals of African and European descent.[54]

Although the primary site of NoV replication has not been determined, cellular changes were noted in jejunal tissue including broadening and blunting of the villi and infiltration of mononuclear cells in the lamina propria.[37] Reduced gastric motility is also noted; considered to be associated with vomiting and nausea.[37] Asymptomatic NoV infections are common with factors that determine symptomatic versus asymptomatic presentation unclear, although frequent exposure to the virus may lead to asymptomatic reinfections due to acquired immunity.[55]

Sapovirus

Sapoviruses are also members of the *Caliciviridae* family. Although similar to NoV in composition and size, they differ in the 7.1–7.7 kb genome that only has two open reading frames (ORF-1 and ORF-2).[56] The first reading frame encodes a large polyprotein containing nonstructural proteins and the major capsid protein, VP1, while ORF-2 encodes the minor capsid protein, VP2.[57] Currently, SaVs are classified into 15 genogroups based on the major capsid protein VP1.[56] Human SaV strains are typically found in four genogroups (GI, GII, GIV, GV).[56] Similarly to NoV, SaV strains display large genetic diversity.

Epidemiology

Sapoviruses are associated with both sporadic cases and epidemic outbreaks of acute diarrhea in all age groups.[57] In the United Kingdom, SaVs were detected in 3.8%–8.8% of all diarrhea cases while in Japan, SaVs were detected in 9.3%–12.7% of patients with diarrhea.[57] Sapoviruses have been identified in daycare centers, schools, and colleges, hospitals, nursing homes, food venues, and cruise ship outbreaks.[57]

Sapovirus infections may be more common in children <5 years than previously considered. The reanalysis of MAL-ED specimens using molecular assays showed that SaVs were the second most common pathogen detected in community-acquired diarrhea and were associated with dehydration and vomiting symptoms.[58] In addition, SaV was identified as one of the top 10 pathogens associated with moderate-to-severe diarrhea in all three age groups in the reanalysis of GEMS specimens.[21] A recent review described SaV in children <5 years in 5.4%–12.7% of diarrhea cases.[57]

Pathogenesis

Different from NoV, SaV infections have not been linked to HBGA phenotypes, and no human genetic factors have been identified for susceptibility or resistance to SaV.[57] However, for growth in cell culture, porcine SaVs require bile salts and bind to sialic acid cellular receptors on glycoproteins attached via O-linked glycosylation.[59,60] Recent studies have identified SaV in both fecal and nasopharyngeal swabs at high viral concentrations and in patients with acute hepatitis of unknown etiology.[61,62] Further studies are required to elucidate these findings.

Adenovirus

Adenoviruses, belonging to the *Adenoviridae* family, are nonenveloped, icosahedral viruses with a 30–38 kb linear ds DNA genome.[63] Viral particles are composed of 11 structural proteins with three proteins (hexon, penton, and fiber) making up the capsid (Fig. 11.1D).[63] The hexon and fiber (terminal knob) proteins have epitopes that define adenovirus group and type species.[63] Although 75 types of human AdV (HAdV) have been identified, 51 serotypes were classified based on traditional serotyping methods such as hemagglutination and serum neutralization assays. The remaining 24 types have been defined by genomics and molecular analysis.[64-68] The 75 HAdV types are classified into seven species (A–G) based on their immunological, biological, and biochemical characteristics.[67-69]

Adenoviruses cause disease in humans and various animal species including simian, bovine, equine, ovine, canine, and opossum hosts.[63] In human infections, they produce a wide range of syndromes including respiratory diseases, conjunctivitis, hepatitis, hemorrhagic cystitis, and acute diarrhea.[63] Human AdV species F (types 40 and 41) and A (types 12, 18, 31, and 61) have been associated with diarrhea although all HAdV species can be detected in stool specimens.[63] The detection of HAdV in stool makes it difficult to assign causality to diarrheal episodes especially as details regarding accompanying respiratory, ocular, or urinary symptoms are not captured. Therefore, the true numbers of diarrhea cases attributed to "enteric" HAdV in the overall burden is probably an underestimation.

Epidemiology

Human AdV type 40/41 was detected in 1.8%–4.5% of all moderate-to-severe diarrhea cases in the original GEMS etiology and population-based burden of pediatric diarrheal disease in sub-Saharan Africa and south Asia.[23] The study used an HAdV-specific as well as a HAdV type 40/41-specific enzyme immunoassay (EIA) to screen stool specimens of cases and age-matched community controls. Retesting of 11,400 stool specimens from 5700 cases and controls using a more sensitive quantitative PCR (qPCR) revealed HAdV type 40/41 in 1.5%–22.4% of moderate-to-severe diarrhea cases.[21]

A similar screening approach (HAdV-specific EIA) was performed for the pathogen-specific burden of community diarrhea in developing countries (MAL-ED) study.[22] Human AdV was detected 1.1%–3.9% of diarrhea cases. Preliminary data from the reanalysis of the specimens using qPCR showed that HAdV type 40/41 was the second most common pathogen in children 0–11 months (after RV) and fifth most common pathogen in children 12–24 months.[58] Etiology studies in both hospitalized and community-acquired diarrhea showed the importance of species F HAdV in diarrhea burden in children <5 years.[21-23,58]

Pathogenesis

Adenoviruses infect the epithelial cells of the intestines and different HAdV species have been detected in different parts of the bowels.[70] HAdV species A was commonly detected in the duodenum and jejunum (range 10^1–10^3 virus copies per million cells) while species E (range 10^2–10^7) and F (range 10^2–10^9) were detected in the colon.[70] Species C was detected in the terminal ileum, primarily within the lymphoid cells in the lamina propria, and in the jejunum and colon (range 10^1–10^3).[70] Cell cytotoxicity leading to tissue damage may occur due to three activities: production of viral proteins, infiltration of cellular inflammatory substances, or the effect of cytokines triggered by the viral infection.[63]

Astrovirus

Astrovirus are part of the *Astroviridae* family with a nonenveloped icosahedral structure and 6.8–7.3 kb ss RNA genome.[71] The polyadenylated genome encodes three ORFs: ORF1a encodes a serine protease and a putative VPg protein, ORF1b encodes the RdRp, and ORF2 encodes the structural proteins (Fig. 11.1E).[71] Eight classic genotypes of human AstVs (HAstV), HAstV type 1 (HAstV-1) to HAstV-8, have been identified based on ORF2 sequences.[71] Recombinant strains typically display the identities of two different classic HAstVs in a single genome in ORF1b and ORF2.[72] Novel genotypes (AstV-MLB, AstV-VA and AstV-HMO), usually associated with extraintestinal infections, have also been detected and characterized based on unique nucleotide sequences.[62,73]

Epidemiology

Surveillance studies detected HAstV in ~11% of diarrhea cases in children <5 years with a prevalence of 7% reported in urban and 23% in rural areas.[71] Other epidemiology studies reported HAstV prevalence at 0.6%–3.9% in Vietnam (hospitalized patients and outpatients <15 years), 1.9% in the former Soviet Union (outpatients <5 years), 4.8% in Ghana (outpatients <5 years), 6.3% in Gabon (outpatients <5 years), 6.9% in Bulgaria (hospitalized patients <3 years), 3.1%–4.9% in the United States (hospitalized patients and outpatients <5 years), and 1.5%–29.7% in Venezuela (hospitalized patients and outpatients <6 years).[73] In the MAL-ED study, HAstVs were detected in 2.7% of cases 0–11 months and in 4.2% of cases 12–24 months using EIA-based methods.[22] For GEMS reanalysis using molecular assays, HAstV was detected in 0.2%–5.5% of moderate-to-severe diarrhea cases in children 0–11 months and 0.9%–5.5% in children 12–23 months.[21] Astroviruses were detected in 0.5%–20.7% of children without diarrhea in Brazil.[74]

Astrovirus infections occur throughout the year, with a slight increase in the cooler seasons. When seasonality is observed, it is usually during winter months in temperate regions and rainy seasons in tropical climates.[71,75]

The severity of HAstV infections may be genotype related although further research is needed to confirm the observation.[76] Classic HAstV-1 is the prevalent genotype worldwide and novel AstVs have been reported at varied prevalence.[73] Overall, a decrease in classic HAstVs has been observed with replacement by novel or recombinant strains.[71,73]

Pathogenesis

Astrovirus infects the epithelial cells in the lower regions of the villi, entering the cells via a clathrin-mediated cytosis.[77] Astroviruses cause diarrhea in unconventional manner as no inflammation or cell death is observed but the tight junctions between cells are disrupted allowing an influx of water that results in diarrhea.[76] The increased intestinal permeability disrupts water and nutrient absorption and may also allow extraintestinal dissemination via the lumen, the serosa, and the bloodstream.[76]

Human AstVs have been associated with nondiarrheal diseases such as celiac disease[78] and neurotropic conditions in immune-compromised individuals.[79] A novel strain, HAstV-VA1/HMO-C-UK1, was identified separately from two patients with unexplained fatal encephalitis[80,81] and recombinant HAstVs have been detected in stool specimens of patients with nonpolio acute flaccid paralysis.[72]

A retrospective study that screened stool specimens from pediatric oncology patients detected classic and novel AstVs at higher prevalence as compared with NoV and SaV. Furthermore, these AstVs were associated with prolonged virus shedding.[82] Astroviruses have also been linked to medical conditions such as intussusception,[83] necrotizing enterocolitis,[84] hand–foot and mouth disease,[85] and even death due to persistent diarrhea.[86]

Other Enteric Viruses

The use of molecular methods has improved diarrhea enteric pathogen attribution to levels of 89.3% in GEMS and 64.9% in the MAL-ED study.[21,58] However, there still remains a proportion of diarrhea without an assigned pathogen. Aichivirus was first associated with an oyster-associated outbreak of gastroenteritis in Japan and has subsequently been detected in Europe and Asia. However, most studies report Aichivirus prevalence less than 4%.[87,88] Torovirus were suspected of an association with pediatric diarrhea as they were related to animal viruses that caused diarrhea and were detected in more diarrheic children than controls.[89,90] However, since the late 1990 studies, no additional prevalence or case–control studies have been conducted. The contribution of torovirus to the diarrhea burden remains unanswered.

Sequence-independent amplification techniques and unbiased next generation sequencing have been used to detect novel viruses in stool specimens.[13] Human bocavirus, first detected in 2005 using sequencing methods, was initially associated with respiratory tract infections (HBoV1).[91] Subsequent HBoV strains (HBoV2-4) were detected in stool specimens and their role in diarrhea was investigated.[92,93] A recent systematic review and meta-analysis suggests that HBoV is not associated with diarrheal disease; detected at similar

TABLE 11.1
Clinical Presentation of Enteric Viruses Associated With Diarrhea

Virus	Incubation Period[a] (in days; 95% CI)	Fever[c]	Stool Frequency[c]	Vomiting[c]	Dehydration[c]	Duration (in days)
Rotavirus	2.0 (1.4–2.4)	+++	+++	+++	+++	4–7[e,f]
Norovirus GII	1.2 (1.2–1.3)			+++	+++	1.8–4[f,g]
Norovirus GI	1.1 (1.1–1.2)			++[d]		
Sapovirus	1.7 (1.5–1.8)			+++	++	3–6[f,h]
Adenovirus type 40/41	3–10[b]				+++	5–12[f]
Astrovirus	4.5 (3.9–5.2)					1–4[f]

[a]Data from Lee et al.[95]
[b]Data from Kotloff et al.[96]
[c]Data from Platts-Mills et al.[58]; odds ratio of >1.5 = +++; odds ratio of <1.5 = ++.
[d]Data from Kirby et al.[97]
[e]Data from Mohan et al.[98]
[f]Data from Eckardt and Baumgart.[99]
[g]Data from Devasia et al.[100]
[h]Data from Liu et al.[101]

prevalence in cases and controls. However, exclusion of HBoV1 in the analysis shows an association between HBoV2 and acute gastroenteritis.[94]

Viruses detected in gastroenteritis cases with unknown disease pathogenesis include Saffold virus, Cosavirus, Klassevirus/Salivirus, novel polyomaviruses, Bufavirus, Tusavirus, and Recovirus.[13] Most of these new viruses demonstrate limited association with disease in case–control studies and/or are detected at low incidence.[13] Additional surveillance of diarrhea cases including a broad range of severity as well as healthy controls and alternative syndromes (acute flaccid paralysis, encephalitis/meningitis, fever of unknown origin) should be considered to elucidate the role played by these viruses in diarrhea or other syndromes.

Clinical Presentation of Enteric Viruses

The incubation period of enteric viruses associated with diarrhea varies from 1 to 10 days (Table 11.1). The clinical presentation of enteric virus gastroenteritis is nonspecific and includes watery nonbloody diarrhea of varying frequency and duration, vomiting, fever, and dehydration (Table 11.1). In some cases, vomiting may be present without diarrhea, especially in the case of norovirus infections.[97] Additional symptoms may also include nausea, stomach cramps, headache, myalgia, chills, anorexia, and fatigue.[71,97] Laboratory screening is often required to correctly identify the causal virus as a diagnosis based on clinical presentation alone is difficult.

Rotavirus disease is considered the most severe of all viral gastroenteritis infections, associated with severe dehydration, acidosis at admission, and diarrhea-associated mortality.[26,102,103] Rotavirus disease severity increases in young children (<5 months) or immunocompromised patients.[103,104] Norovirus has been reported to cause disease severity similar to RV although less dehydration was noted.[102] Vulnerable individuals including young children, the elderly, and immune-compromised individuals with NoV experience more severe illness of extended duration and associated mortality.[52,105]

A milder clinical presentation is considered to be associated with SaV and HAstV infections[106–108] However, complications such as dehydration and disseminated disease associated with HAstV can develop in patients with underlying gastrointestinal disease, poor nutritional status, and mixed infections.[109,110] Enteric AdV infections are also considered milder than RV or NoV although the diarrhea symptoms are described as persistent or prolonged (8–12 days).[96,111]

Diagnosis of Enteric Virus Infections

A laboratory diagnosis is not required for the symptomatic treatment of diarrhea and routine testing of diarrhea cases, especially in resource-constrained settings, is not recommended by the WHO. However, the 2017 Infectious Diseases Society of America (IDSA) Infectious Diarrhea guidelines recommend that among individuals with gastroenteritis, children younger than 5 years of age, the elderly, people who are immuno-compromised, and those with bloody diarrhea, severe abdominal pain or tenderness, or signs of sepsis should be tested for diarrheal pathogens.[112]

Circumstances where a diagnosis may be sought include diarrheal surveillance programs, during an outbreak of diarrhea or when an increase in diarrhea cases is noted, to monitor the impact of rotavirus vaccine introduction, complicated or prolonged diarrhea cases, or diarrhea cases where administration of antibiotics is being considered. Individuals should be tested within 48–72 h after onset of symptoms and the best specimen for virus testing is whole stool, although rectal swabs or vomitus could be used in some cases where stool specimen cannot be obtained.[113]

Norovirus infections can be diagnosed on clinical and epidemiological characteristics if no specimens are available (Kaplan criteria developed in 1982 during a large waterborne outbreak of gastroenteritis).[114] The criteria are (1) a mean incubation period of 24–48 h; (2) a mean duration of illness of between 12 and 60 h; (3) >50% of patients with vomiting; and (4) no bacterial pathogens detected in the stool specimens.[114] The criteria are highly specific in foodborne outbreak scenarios, and may be less useful during hospital outbreaks where the duration of symptoms could exceed 60 h.[113]

Enzyme immunoassays

Enzyme immunoassays (EIA) detect the virus antigen (Ag) in patient stool specimens and are easier to implement than electron microscopy or cell culture. The gold standard for RV diagnosis is detection of the inner capsid antigen (VP6) in stool and many commercial EIA kits are available. Antigen detection correlates well with clinical disease despite EIA being less sensitive than molecular methods.

Astrovirus EIA kits detect the capsid protein (ORF2) of classic HAstVs at 10^5–10^6 viral particles per gram of stool.[115] Although the EIA assays generally correlated with RT-PCR detection, they are less sensitive than molecular methods.[116] Commercial EIA kits are available for virus-specific or group-specific HAdV detection and target the hexon protein.[63] However, recent epidemiological studies showed that HAdV 40/41 incidence was five times greater when molecular methods were used compared to EIA.[21] Although EIA use may be suitable in resource constrained settings for HAdV detection, molecular testing should be considered to improve diagnostic proficiency.

For NoV, EIAs are highly specific but lack sensitivity as the assays fail to detect many strains due to the high antigenic diversity. Rapid NoV tests are less specific and sensitive than quantitative RT-PCR, but may be useful in settings where molecular technology is not available and very rapid results are needed. Sapoviruses can be detected using enzyme immunoassays but these assays are not commercially available and are rarely used.[57] This is mainly due to difficulty in generating antibodies that can detect a wide variety of genetically diverse strains and the higher sensitivity offered by molecular methods.

Molecular detection

Real-time or quantitative reverse transcription (qRT)—PCR can be used to detect all enteric viruses in stool specimens. However, positive results must be considered with the clinical symptoms as enteric viruses can cause asymptomatic infections or be shed for prolonged periods[73,117] and multiple enteric pathogens are often detected in diarrhea cases.[21,58]

Recent studies using molecular detection methods have determined the cycle threshold (Ct) values that correlate with clinically relevant RV infections and range from Ct = 17.2 (in EIA-positive specimens in India)[117] to Ct = 26.7 (in EIA-positive specimens in Malawi).[4] Although the appropriate Ct value could be determined for specific diagnostic settings, the GEMS reanalysis showed that RV was generally associated with diarrhea whenever it was detected (Ct = 35).[21] However, RV qRT-PCR results should still be evaluated in association with clinical background.

The current gold standard for NoV detection is qRT-PCR, and various commercial kits are available in monoplex as well as multiplex (GI + GII) formats. In addition, a variety of viral gastroenteritis multiplex assays that utilize different technologies/chemistries have been developed.[113] Most of the panels provide comprehensive qualitative results, but as mixed infections are common, interpretation of the data can be problematic due to a lack of quantitative information.

Quantitative RT-PCR is the method of choice for detection of SaV due to the sensitivity and specificity. Multiple primers and probes that target the RdRp, the RdRp-VP1 junction, or the VP1 regions have been used in SaV diagnostics. However, assays targeting the RdRp-VP1 junction appear to have the highest detection rates and assays targeting the VP1 gene may be used for assigning genotype.[57]

Adenoviruses contain three capsid proteins (hexon, fibre, and penton) that can be used to differentiate strains diagnostically. The species-specific epitopes are located on the hexon gene, and are hypervariable regions designated loop 1 and 2 (L1 and L2).[69] Most detection assays target one of these regions while typing relies on sequencing and phylogenetic analysis of L2.[69] Although the fiber protein has also been used for classification, it cannot differentiate all HAdV species and is therefore not frequently utilized.[69]

Although AstV-specific RT-PCR assays are rapid, sensitive, and specific, they cannot distinguish between infectious and noninfectious viral particles.[118] However, HAstVs have been detected more often in specimens by RT-PCR than by EIA.[116] Accurate HAstV load quantification is an important step to determine whether the degree of viral replication contributes to the clinical outcome of the infection.[73]

Transmission and Prevention

Viruses associated with diarrhea are primarily transmitted via the fecal–oral route and spread via direct person-to-person contact or food- and waterborne exposure. Enteric viruses are shed at high concentrations in feces, are highly stable in the environment, and have a very low infectious dose.[14,119,120] Enteric viruses can, therefore, cause extensive outbreaks in confined situations where large numbers of individuals share the same space, for example, cruise ships, military camps, and daycare centers. In addition, nosocomial spread and fomites have been implicated as modes of enteric virus transmission.[121]

Norovirus is also frequently implicated in nosocomial outbreaks with significant economic implications for affected healthcare institutions. Shellfish, specifically oysters,[122] and fresh produce such as berries[123] and salads[124] have often been linked NoV outbreaks. Shellfish water catchments are regularly contaminated by sewage discharges,[125] and polluted irrigation water has been linked to contaminated leafy greens and berries.[126] Global foodborne NoV outbreaks from single source involving multiple countries have been described.[127]

The interruption of transmission is most important in preventing the spread of enteric viruses.[119] Universal hygiene procedures must be enforced in hospitals, daycare centers, and other institutions where person-to-person transmissions are likely to occur. Food handlers must be aware of the dangers posed by their personal diarrheal disease infections.[71]

Management

The WHO recommends an immediate assessment of dehydration followed by therapy aimed at preventing dehydration using a standard oral rehydration solution (ORS).[128] Intravenous fluids (Ringer's Lactate or saline) should be administered if oral rehydration fails, if the patient is severely dehydrated or in shock. Early feeding after rehydration of children with diarrhea is recommended and should include breast milk or formula and age appropriate foods such as complex carbohydrates, lean meats, yoghurt, fruits, and vegetables.

There are no licensed antivirals to treat NoV infections, but efforts are underway to develop specific antivirals including compounds that block NoV/HBGA interactions and the nonstructural proteins such as the protease and RdRp.[129] The new human intestinal enteroid NoV cell culture system[130] will likely have a dramatic impact on the progress in identifying and evaluating norovirus antivirals.

Good progress was demonstrated in a patient with HAstV-associated encephalitis following intravenous immunoglobulin and interferon treatment.[131] Exogenous IFN-β was able to reduce the HAstV infection ability and barrier permeability.[132] In addition, features of the HAstV protein structure have been identified as potential options for medical interventions such as inhibitors or adaptation of existing antivirals against the AstV proteases.[133]

Enteric virus vaccines

The burden of diarrheal disease and the failure of improved sanitation or access to clean water to reduce RV incidence led to the development of vaccines. Two oral RV vaccines (Rotarix, GlaxoSmithKline Biologicals and RotaTeq, Merck & Co) available globally, have been shown to be safe and effective.[134,135] The introduction of rotavirus vaccines has played a role in reducing the numbers of diarrhea cases by 10%, the number of diarrhea-related deaths by 34% and the number of rotavirus-related deaths by 44%.[134]

Developing country manufacturers are producing similar oral RV vaccine products and currently the Lanzhou Lamb vaccine (LLR) in China, Rotavin-M1 in Vietnam, Rotavac and Rotasiil in India are licensed locally.[134] In addition, a neonatal strain RV3BB is in development in Australia, and a subunit vaccine has undergone Phase II trials in South Africa.[134,136]

The immune response following norovirus infection in humans are not well understood. Early studies indicated that infection only induced short-term immunity,[137] but more recent modeling studies based on the literature and age-specific incidence data from the United Kingdom suggest that immunity may range from 4 to 9 years.[138] Studies have shown that there is cross-protection within genogroups but not between genogroups suggesting that a successful vaccine would have to contain both GI and GII, the most commonly identified genogroups in humans.[139]

The main challenge in norovirus vaccine development is to generate a cost-effective vaccine that induces broadly protective neutralizing antibodies that will protect against heterologous and newly emerging norovirus strains as well as provide long-lasting immunity. Modeling studies have suggested that pediatric vaccination would have the largest impact to prevent norovirus disease and death compared to vaccination in the elderly.[140] Although there are some promising vaccine candidates, future studies have to determine whether these will be effective in the pediatric, elderly, and otherwise immune-compromised populations, which are at greatest risk for severe norovirus infection.

Different types of norovirus vaccines are in various stages of development, including virus-like particle (VLP)-based vaccines, oral adenovirus-vectored vaccines, and P-particle vaccines, which consist of the protruding domain of the norovirus major capsid protein.[139] The Takeda VLP-based vaccine, a combination of GI.1 and GII.4-derived VLPs, can prevent norovirus illness and to some extent infection by intranasal or intramuscular administration.[141] Another approach is dual rotavirus/norovirus vaccines that combine the rotavirus VP6 protein with norovirus GI.3 and GII.4 VLPs. This vaccine candidate was shown to be immunogenic in preclinical animal studies.[142]

A NoV-AstV-HEV trivalent vaccine has shown a significant antibody response in mice compared to a mixed vaccine of the three separate viral antigens.[143] An engineered antibody, PL-2, has demonstrated neutralization of the HAstV capsid by blocking the virus attachment to cells.[144]

Conclusions

Enteric viruses continue to play an important role in diarrheal disease burden, especially in the first year of life and, therefore, require continued research. Although much work has been done, gaps still exist for pathogenesis in human infections, mechanisms of disease, immunity, and correlates of protection. The molecular surveillance results from the GEMS and MAL-ED studies as well as the reverse genetics system for RV, the new human intestinal enteroid NoV cell culture system and next generation or whole genome sequencing of enteric virus populations, and the human microbiome will provide new tools and insights into how enteric viruses interact with human hosts.

DISCLOSURE STATEMENT

Disclosure of any relationship with a commercial company that has a direct financial interest in subject matter or materials discussed in article or with a company making a competing product.
Nicola Page has received personal fees from GlaxoSmithKline, Merck, and Aspen Pharma.

REFERENCES

1. Global Burden of Diseases Diarrhoeal Diseases Collaborators. Estimates of global, regional, and national morbidity, mortality, and aetiologies of diarrhoeal diseases: a systematic analysis for the Global Burden of Disease Study 2015. *Lancet Infect Dis.* 2017;17: 909–948.
2. Fredericks DN, Relman DA. Sequence-based identification of microbial pathogens: a reconsideration of Koch's postulate. *Clin Microbiol Rev.* 1996;9:18–33.
3. River TM. Viruses and Koch's postulate. *J Bacteriol.* 1937;33:1–12.
4. Bennett A, Bar-Zeev N, Jere KC, et al. Determination of a viral load threshold to distinguish symptomatic versus asymptomatic rotavirus infection in a high-disease-burden African population. *J Clin Microbiol.* 2015;53: 1951–1954.
5. Robilotti E, Deresinski S, Pinsky BA. Norovirus. *Clin Microbiol Rev.* 2015;28:134–164.
6. Dey RS, Ghosh S, Chawla-Sarkar M, et al. Circulation of a novel pattern of infections by enteric adenovirus serotype 41 among children below 5 years of age in Kolkata, India. *J Clin Microbiol.* 2011;49:500–505.
7. Méndez-Toss M, Griffin DD, Calva J, et al. Prevalence and genetic diversity of human astroviruses in Mexican children with symptomatic and asymptomatic infections. *J Clin Microbiol.* 2004;42:151–157.
8. Ye S, Whiley DM, Ware RS, Kirkwood CD, Lambert SB, Grimwood K. Multivalent rotavirus vaccine and wild-type rotavirus strain shedding in Australian infants: a birth cohort study [published online ahead of print Nov 15 2017]. *Clin Infect Dis.* 2017. https://doi.org/10.1093/cid/cix1022.
9. Newman KL, Moe CL, Kirby AE, Flanders WD, Parkos CA, Leon JS. Norovirus in symptomatic and asymptomatic individuals: cytokines and viral shedding. *Clin Exp Immunol.* 2016;184:347–357.
10. Papafragkou E, Hewitt J, Park GW, Greening G, Vinjé J. Challenges of culturing human norovirus in three-dimensional organoid intestinal cell culture models. *PLoS One.* 2013;8(6):e63485. https://doi.org/10.1371/journal.pone.0063485.
11. Heubner RJ. Criteria for etiologic association of prevalent viruses with prevalent diseases; the virologist's dilemma. *Ann N Y Acad Sci.* 1957;67:430–438.
12. Li L, Delwart E. From orphan virus to pathogen: the path to the clinical lab. *Curr Opin Virol.* 2011;1:282–288.
13. Oude Munnink BB, van der Hoek L. Viruses causing gastroenteritis: the known, the new and those beyond. *Viruses.* 2016;8(2):e42. https://doi.org/10.3390/v8020042.
14. Desselberger U. Rotaviruses. *Virus Res.* 2014;190:75–96.
15. Estes MK, Kapikian AZ. Rotavirus. In: Knipe DM, Howley PM, eds. *Fields Virology.* 5th ed. Philadelphia, PA: Lippincott Williams & Wilkins; 2007:1917–1974.
16. Matthijnssens J, Ciarlet M, McDonald SM, et al. Uniformity of rotavirus strain nomenclature proposed by the Rotavirus Classification Working Group (RCWG). *Arch Virol.* 2011;156:1397–1413.

17. Rotavirus Classification Working Group: RCWG. *List of Accepted Genotypes*. KU Leuven; 2017. https://rega.kuleuven.be/cev/viralmetagenomics/virus-classification/rcwg. Updated July 24.

18. Bányai K, László B, Duque J, et al. Systematic review of regional and temporal trends in global rotavirus strain diversity in the pre rotavirus vaccine era: insights for understanding the impact of rotavirus vaccination programs. *Vaccine*. 2012;30:A122–A130.

19. Dóró R, László B, Martella V, et al. Review of global rotavirus strain prevalence data from six years post vaccine licensure surveillance: is there evidence of strain selection from vaccine pressure? *Infect Genet Evol*. 2014;28:446–461.

20. Steele AD, Madhi SA, Cunliffe NA, et al. Incidence of rotavirus gastroenteritis by age in Africa, Asia and European children: relevance for timing of rotavirus vaccination. *Hum Vaccines Immunother*. 2016;12:2406–2412.

21. Liu J, Platts-Mills JA, Juma J, et al. Use of quantitative molecular diagnostic methods to identify causes of diarrhoea in children: a reanalysis of the GEMS case-control study. *Lancet*. 2016;388:1291–1301.

22. Platts-Mills JA, Babji S, Bodhidatta L, et al. Pathogen-specific burdens of community diarrhoea in developing countries: a multisite birth cohort study (MAL-ED). *Lancet Glob Health*. 2015;3(9):e564–e575. https://doi.org/10.1016/S2214-109X(15)00151-5.

23. Kotloff KL, Nataro JP, Blackwelder WC, et al. Burden and aetiology of diarrhoeal disease in infants and young children in developing countries (the Global Enteric Multicenter Study, GEMS): a prospective, case-control study. *Lancet*. 2013;382:209–222.

24. World Health Organization. Rotavirus vaccines. WHO position paper – January 2013. *Wkly Epidemiol Rec*. 2013;88:49–64.

25. Clark A, Black R, Tate J, et al. Estimating global, regional and national rotavirus deaths in children aged <5 years: current approaches, new analyses and proposed improvements. *PLoS One*. 2017;12(9):e0183392. https://doi.org/10.1371/journal.pone.0183392.

26. Tate JE, Burton AH, Boschi-Pinto C. UD Parashar. Global, regional, and national estimates of rotavirus mortality in children <5 years of age, 2000–2013. *Clin Infect Dis*. 2016;62:S96–S105.

27. Nasrin D, Wu Y, Blackwelder WC, et al. Health care seeking for childhood diarrhea in developing countries: evidence from seven sites in Africa and Asia. *Am J Trop Med Hyg*. 2013;89(suppl 1):3–12.

28. Cook SM, Glass RI, LeBaron CW, Ho MS. Global seasonality of rotavirus infections. *Bull World Health Organ*. 1990;68:171–177.

29. Patel MM, Pitzer VE, Alonso WJ, et al. Global seasonality of rotavirus disease. *Pediatr Infect Dis J*. 2013;32(4):e134–e147. https://doi.org/10.1097/INF.0b013e31827d3b68.

30. Pitzer VE, Viboud C, Lopman BA, Patel MM, Parashar UD, Grenfell BT. Influence of birth rates and transmission rates on the global seasonality of rotavirus incidence. *J R Soc Interface*. 2011;8:1584–1593.

31. Ushijima H, Xin K, Nishimura S, Morikawa S, Abe T. Detection and sequencing of rotavirus VP7 gene from human materials (stools, sera, cerebrospinal fluids, and throat swabs) by reverse transcription and PCR. *J Clin Microbiol*. 1994;32:2893–2897.

32. Blutt SE, Matson DO, Crawford SE, et al. Rotavirus antigenemia in children is associated with viremia. *PLoS Med*. 2007;4(4):e121. https://doi.org/10.1371/journal.pmed.0040121.

33. Lewnard JA, Lopman BA, Parashar UD, et al. Naturally acquired immunity against rotavirus infection and gastroenteritis in children: paired reanalyses of birth cohort studies. *J Infect Dis*. 2017;216:317–326.

34. Gladstone BP, Ramani S, Mukhopadhya I, et al. Protective effect of natural rotavirus infection in an Indian birth cohort. *N Engl J Med*. 2011;365:337–346.

35. Velázquez FR, Matson DO, Calva JJ, et al. Rotavirus infection in infants as protection against subsequent infections. *N Engl J Med*. 1996;335:1022–1028.

36. Lopman BA, Vicuña Y, Salazar F, et al. Household transmission of rotavirus in a community with rotavirus vaccination in Quininde, Ecuador. *PLoS One*. 2013;8(7):e67763. https://doi.org/10.1371/journal.pone.0067763.

37. Green K. Caliciviridae: the noroviruses. In: Knipe DM, Howley PM, eds. *Fields Virology*. 6th ed. Philadelphia, PA: Lippincott Williams & Wilkins; 2013:582–608.

38. Kroneman A, Vega E, Vennema H, et al. Proposal for a unified norovirus nomenclature and genotyping. *Arch Virol*. 2013;158:2059–2068.

39. Siebenga JJ, Vennema H, Zheng DP, et al. Norovirus illness is a global problem: emergence and spread of norovirus GII.4 variants, 2001-2007. *J Infect Dis*. 2009;200:802–812.

40. Lindesmith LC, Donaldson EF, Lobue AD, et al. Mechanisms of GII.4 norovirus persistence in human populations. *PLoS Med*. 2008;5(2):e31. https://doi.org/10.1371/journal.pmed.0050031.

41. Bull RA, Tanaka MM, White PA. Norovirus recombination. *J Gen Virol*. 2007;88:3347–3359.

42. Mans J, Murray TY, Nadan S, Netshikweta R, Page NA, Taylor MB. Norovirus diversity in children with gastroenteritis in South Africa from 2009 to 2013: GII.4 variants and recombinant strains predominate. *Epidemiol Infect*. 2016;144:907–916.

43. Ahmed SM, Hall AJ, Robinson AE, et al. Global prevalence of norovirus in cases of gastroenteritis: a systematic review and meta-analysis. *Lancet Infect Dis*. 2014;14:725–730.

44. Bartsch SM, Lopman BA, Ozawa S, Hall AJ, Lee BY. Global economic burden of norovirus gastroenteritis. *PLoS One*. 2016;11(4):e0151219. https://doi.org/10.1371/journal.pone.0151219.

45. Bucardo F, Reyes Y, Svensson L, Nordgren J. Predominance of norovirus and sapovirus in Nicaragua after implementation of universal rotavirus vaccination. *PLoS One*. 2014;9(5):e98201. https://doi.org/10.1371/journal.pone.0098201.

46. Payne DC, Vinje J, Szilagyi PG, et al. Norovirus and medically attended gastroenteritis in U.S. children. *N Engl J Med*. 2013;368:1121–1130.

47. Havelaar AH, Kirk MD, Torgerson PR, et al. World Health Organization global estimates and regional comparisons of the burden of foodborne disease in 2010. *PLoS Med.* 2015;12(12):e1001923. https://doi.org/10.1371/journal. pmed.1001923.

48. Moreira NA, Bondelind M. Safe drinking water and waterborne outbreaks. *J Water Health.* 2017;15:83–96.

49. Sabria A, Pinto RM, Bosch A, et al. Norovirus shedding among food and healthcare workers exposed to the virus in outbreak settings. *J Clin Virol.* 2016;82:119–125.

50. Sukhrie FH, Teunis P, Vennema H, et al. Nosocomial transmission of norovirus is mainly caused by symptomatic cases. *Clin Infect Dis.* 2012;54:931–937.

51. Glass RI, Parashar UD, Estes MK. Norovirus gastroenteritis. *N Engl J Med.* 2009;361:1776–1785.

52. Page NA, Groome MJ, Nadan S, et al. Norovirus epidemiology in South African children <5 years hospitalised for diarrhoeal illness between 2009 and 2013. *Epidemiol Infect.* 2017;145(9):1942–1952.

53. Nordgren J, Sharma S, Kambhampati A, Lopman N, Svensson L. Innate resistance and susceptibility to norovirus infection. *PLoS Pathog.* 2016;12(4):e1005385. https://doi.org/10.1371/journal.ppat.1005385.

54. Ferrer-Admetlla A, Sikora M, Laayouni H, et al. A natural history of FUT2 polymorphism in humans. *Mol Biol Evol.* 2009;26:1993–2003.

55. Lopman B, Steele AD, Kirkwood CD, Parashar UD. The vast and varied global burden of norovirus: prospects for prevention and control. *PLoS Med.* 2016;13(4):e1001999. https://doi.org/10.1371/journal.pmed.1001999.

56. Oka T, Lu Z, Phan T, Delwart EL, Saif LJ, Wang Q. Genetic characterization and classification of human and animal sapoviruses. *PLoS One.* 2016;11(5):e0156373. https://doi.org/10.1371/journal.pone.0156373.

57. Oka T, Wang Q, Katayama K, Saif LJ. Comprehensive review of human sapoviruses. *Clin Microbiol Rev.* 2015;28:32–53.

58. Platts-Mills JA, Liu J, Rogawski ET, et al. Use of quantitative molecular diagnostic methods to assess the aetiology, burden, and clinical characteristics of diarrhoea in children in low-resource settings: a reanalysis of the MAL-ED cohort study, Lancet Glob Health. 2018. pii: S2214-109X(18)30349-8. https://doi.org/10.1016/S2214-109X(18)30349-8.

59. Hosmillo M, Sorgeloos F, Hiraide R, Lu J, Goodfellow I, Cho KO. Porcine sapovirus replication is restricted by the type I interferon response in cell culture. *J Gen Virol.* 2015;96:74–84.

60. Kim DS, Hosmillo M, Alfajaro MM, et al. Both α2,3- and α2,6-linked sialic acids on O-linked glycoproteins act as functional receptors for porcine sapovirus. *PLoS Pathog.* 2014;10(6):e1004172. https://doi.org/10.1371/journal. ppat.1004172.

61. Neres Silva T, Dábilla N, Souza Fiaccadori F, et al. Sapovirus in fecal and nasopharyngeal swab samples of children with symptoms of acute gastroenteritis [published online ahead of print Nov 14 2017]. *Pediatr Infect Dis J.* 2017. https://doi.org/10.1097/INF.0000000000001833.

62. Gonzales-Gustavson E, Timoneda N, Fernandez-Cassi X, et al. Identification of sapovirus GV.2, astrovirus VA3 and novel anelloviruses in serum from patients with acute hepatitis of unknown aetiology. *PLoS One.* 2017;12(10):e0185911. https://doi.org/10.1371/journal. pone.0185911.

63. Ruuskanen O, Metcalf JP, Meurman O, Akusjärvi. Adenoviruses. In: Richman DD, Whitley RJ, Hayden FG, eds. *Clinical Virology.* 3rd ed. Washington, DC: ASM Press; 2009:559–579.

64. Hage E, Dhingra A, Liebert UG, Bergs S, Ganzenmueller T, Heim A. Three novel, multiple recombinant types of species of human mastadenovirus D (HAdV-D 73, 74 & 75) isolated from diarrhoeal faeces of immunocompromised patients [published online ahead of print Nov 2 2017]. *J Gen Virol.* 2017. https://doi.org/10.1099/ jgv.0.000968.

65. Ismail AM, Lee JS, Dyer DW, Seto D, Rajaiya J, Chodosh J. Selection pressure in the human adenovirus fiber knob drives cell specificity in epidemic keratoconjunctivitis. *J Virol.* 2016;90:9598–9607.

66. Hage E, Gerd Liebert U, Bergs S, Ganzenmueller T, Heim A. Human mastadenovirus type 70: a novel, multiple recombinant species D mastadenovirus isolated from diarrhoeal faeces of a haematopoietic stem cell transplantation recipient. *J Gen Virol.* 2015;96:2734–2742.

67. Ghebremedhin B. Human adenovirus: viral pathogen with increasing importance. *Eur J Microbiol Immunol.* 2014;4:26–33.

68. Singh G, Robinson CM, Dehghan S, et al. Homologous recombination in E3 genes of human adenovirus species D. *J Virol.* 2013;87:12481–12488.

69. Madisch I, Harste G, Pommer H, Heim A. Phylogenetic analysis of the main neutralization and hemagglutination determinants of all human adenovirus prototypes as a basis for molecular classification and taxonomy. *J Virol.* 2005;79:15265–15276.

70. Kosulin K, Geiger E, Vécsei A, et al. Persistence and reactivation of human adenoviruses in the gastrointestinal tract. *Clin Microbiol Infect.* 2016;22:381.e1–381.e8. https://doi.org/10.1016/j.cmi.2015.12.013.

71. Bosch A, Pintó RM, Guix S. Human astroviruses. *Clin Microbiol Rev.* 2014;27:1048–1074.

72. Shaukat S, Angez M, Alam MM, et al. Identification and characterization of unrecognized viruses in stool samples of non-polio acute flaccid paralysis children by simplified VIDISCA. *Virol J.* 2014;11:146. https://doi. org/10.1186/1743-422X-11-146.

73. Vu DL, Bosch A, Pintó RM, Guix S. Epidemiology of classic and novel human astrovirus: gastroenteritis and beyond. *Viruses.* 2017;9(2):e33. https://doi.org/10.3390/ v9020033.

74. Resque HR, Munford V, Castilho JG, Schmich H, Caruzo TAR, Rácz ML. Molecular characterization of astrovirus in stool samples from children in Sao Paulo, Brazil. *Mem Inst Oswaldo Cruz.* 2007;102: 969–974.

75. Zaraket H, Abou-El-Hassan H, Kreidieh K, et al. Characterization of astrovirus-associated gastroenteritis in hospitalized children under five years of age. *Infect Genet Evol.* 2017;53:94–99.

76. Johnson C, Hargest V, Cortez V, Meliopoulos VA, Schultz-Cherry S. Astrovirus pathogenesis. *Viruses.* 2017;9(1):22. https://doi.org/10.3390/v9010022.

77. Méndez E, Muñoz-Yañez C, Sánchez-San MC, et al. Characterization of human astrovirus cell entry. *J Virol.* 2014;88:2452–2460.

78. Smits SL, van Leeuwen M, van der Eijk AA, et al. Human astrovirus infection in a patient with new-onset celiac disease. *J Clin Microbiol.* 2010;48:3416–3418.

79. Kennedy PG, Quan P-L, Lipkin WI. Viral encephalitis of unknown cause: current perspective and recent advances. *Viruses.* 2017;9(6):138. https://doi.org/10.3390/v9060138.

80. Naccache SN, Peggs KS, Mattes FM, et al. Diagnosis of neuroinvasive astrovirus infection in an immunocompromised adult with encephalitis by unbiased next-generation sequencing. *Clin Infect Dis.* 2015;60:919–923.

81. Brown JR, Morfopoulou S, Hubb J, et al. Astrovirus VA1/HMO-C: an increasingly recognized neurotropic pathogen in immunocompromised patients. *Clin Infect Dis.* 2015;15(60):881–888.

82. Cortez V, Freiden P, Gu Z, Adderson E, Hayden R, Schultz-Cherry S. Persistent infections with diverse co-circulating astroviruses in pediatric oncology patients, Memphis, Tennessee, USA. *Emerg Infect Dis.* 2017;23:288–290.

83. Aminu M, Ameh E, Geyer A, Esona M, Taylor M, Steele A. Role of astrovirus in intussusception in Nigerian infants. *J Trop Pediatr.* 2009;55:192–194.

84. Chappé C, Minjolle S, Dabadie A, Morel L, Colimon R, Pladys P. Astrovirus and digestive disorders in neonatal units. *Acta Paediatr.* 2012;101(5):e208–e212. https://doi.org/10.1111/j.1651-2227.2011.02569.

85. Linsuwanon P, Poovorawan Y, Li L, Deng X, Vongpunsawad S, Delwart E. The fecal virome of children with hand, foot, and mouth disease that tested PCR negative for pathogenic enteroviruses. *PLoS One.* 2015;10(8):e0135573. https://doi.org/10.1371/journal.pone.0135573.

86. Unicomb LE, Banu NN, Azim T, et al. Astrovirus infection in association with acute, persistent and nosocomial diarrhea in Bangladesh. *Pediatr Infect Dis J.* 1998;17:611–614.

87. Nielsen AC, Gyhrs ML, Nielsen LP, Pedersen C, Böttiger B. Gastroenteritis and the novel picornaviruses aichi virus, cosavirus, saffold virus, and salivirus in young children. *J Clin Virol.* 2013;5:239–242.

88. Rueter G, Boros A. Pankovics. Kobuvirus – a comprehensive review. *Rev Med Virol.* 2011;21:32–41.

89. Jamieson FB, Wang EE, Bain C, Good J, Duckmanton L, Petric M. Human torovirus: a new nosocomial gastrointestinal pathogen. *J Infect Dis.* 1998;178:1263–1269.

90. Koopmans MP, Goosen ES, Lima AA, et al. Association of torovirus with acute and persistent diarrhea in children. *Pediatr Infect Dis J.* 1997;16:504–507.

91. Allander T, Tammi MT, Eriksson M, Bjerkner A, Tiveljung-Lindell A, Andersson B. Cloning of a human parvovirus by molecular screening of respiratory tract samples. *Proc Natl Acad Sci U S A.* 2005;102:12891–12896.

92. Arthur JL, Higgins GD, Davidson GP, Givney RC, Ratcliff RM. A novel bocavirus associated with acute gastroenteritis in Australian children. *PLoS Pathog.* 2009;5(4):e1000391. https://doi.org/10.1371/journal.ppat.1000391.

93. Kapoor A, Simmonds P, Slikas E, et al. Human bocaviruses are highly diverse, dispersed, recombination prone, and prevalent in enteric infections. *J Infect Dis.* 2010;201:1633–1643.

94. De R, Liu L, Qian Y, et al. Risk of acute gastroenteritis associated with human bocavirus infection in children: a systematic review and meta-analysis. *PLoS One.* 2017;12(9):e0184833. https://doi.org/10.1371/journal.pone.0184833.

95. Lee RM, Lessler J, Lee RA, et al. Incubation periods of viral gastroenteritis: a systematic review. *BMC Infect Dis.* 2013;13:446. https://doi.org/10.1186/1471-2334-13-446.

96. Kotloff KL, Losonsky GA, Morris Jr JG, Wasserman SS, Singh-Naz N, Levine MM. Enteric adenovirus infection and childhood diarrhea: an epidemiologic study in three clinical settings. *Pediatrics.* 1989;84:219–225.

97. Kirby AE, Streby A, Moe CL. Vomiting as a symptom and transmission risk in norovirus illness: evidence from human challenge studies. *PLoS One.* 2016;11(4):e0143759. https://doi.org/10.1371/journal.pone.0143759.

98. Mohan VR, Karthikeyan R, Babji S, et al. Rotavirus infection and disease in a multisite birth cohort: results from the MAL-ED study. *J Infect Dis.* 2017;216:305–316.

99. Eckardt AJ, Baumgart DC. Viral gastroenteritis in adults. *Recent Pat Anti-Infect Drug Discov.* 2011;6:54–63.

100. Devasia T, Lopman B, Leon J, Handel A. Association of host, agent and environment characteristics and the duration of incubation and symptomatic periods of norovirus gastroenteritis. *Epidemiol Infect.* August 2015;143(11):2308–2314.

101. Liu X, Jahuira H, Gilman RH, et al. Etiological role and repeated infections of sapovirus among children aged less than 2 years in a cohort study in a peri-urban community of Peru. *J Clin Microbiol.* 2016;54:1598–1604.

102. Riera-Montes M, O'Ryan M, Verstraeten T. Norovirus and rotavirus disease severity in children: systematic review and meta-analysis [published online ahead of print Nov 11 2017]. *Pediatr Infect Dis J.* 2017. https://doi.org/10.1097/INF.0000000000001824.

103. Mathew A, Rao PS, Sowmyanarayanan TV, Kang G. Severity of rotavirus gastroenteritis in an Indian population: report from a 3 year surveillance study. *Vaccine.* 2014;32(suppl 1):A45–A48.

104. Bruijning-Verhagen P, Nipshagen MD, de Graaf H, Bonten MJM. Rotavirus disease course among immunocompromised patients; 5-year observations from a tertiary care medical centre. *J Infect.* 2017;75:448–454.

105. Teunis PF, Sukhrie FH, Vennema H, Bogerman J, Beersma MF, Koopmans MP. Shedding of norovirus in symptomatic and asymptomatic infections. *Epidemiol Infect.* 2015;143:1710–1717.

106. Sakai Y, Nakata S, Honma S, Tatsumi M, Numata-Kinoshita K, Chiba S. Clinical severity of Norwalk virus and Sapporo virus gastroenteritis in children in Hokkaido, Japan. *Pediatr Infect Dis J.* 2001;20:849–853.

107. Naficy AB, Rao MR, Holmes JL, et al. Astrovirus diarrhea in Egyptian children. *J Infect Dis.* 2000;182:685–690.

108. Marie-Cardine A, Gourlain K, Mouterde O, et al. Epidemiology of acute viral gastroenteritis in children hospitalized in Rouen, France. *Clin Infect Dis.* 2002;34:1170–1178.

109. Liste MB, Natera I, Suarez JA, Pujol FH, Liprandi F, Ludert JE. Enteric virus infections and diarrhea in healthy and human immunodeficiency virus-infected children. *J Clin Microbiol.* 2000;38:2873–2877.

110. Moser LA, Schultz-Cherry S. Pathogenesis of astrovirus infection. *Viral Immunol.* 2005;18:4–10.

111. Uhnoo I, Olding-Stenkvist E, Kreuger A. Clinical features of acute gastroenteritis associated with rotavirus, enteric adenoviruses, and bacteria. *Arch Dis Child.* 1986;61:732–738.

112. Shane AL, Mody RK, Crump JA, et al. 2017 infectious diseases society of America clinical practice guidelines for the diagnosis and management of infectious diarrhea. *Clin Infect Dis.* 2017;65:1963–1973.

113. Vinje J. Advances in laboratory methods for detection and typing of norovirus. *J Clin Microbiol.* 2015;53:373–381.

114. Kaplan JE, Goodman RA, Schonberger LB, Lippy EC, Gary GW. Gastroenteritis due to Norwalk virus: an outbreak associated with a municipal water system. *J Infect Dis.* 1982;146:190–197.

115. Méndez E, Arias CF. Astroviruses. In: Knipe DM, Howley PM, eds. *Fields Virology.* 6th ed. Philadelphia, PA: Lippincott Williams & Wilkins Lippincott; 2013:609–628.

116. Mitchell DK, Monroe SS, Jiang X, Matson DO, Glass RI, Pickering LK. Virologic features of an astrovirus diarrhea outbreak in a day care center revealed by reverse transcriptase-polymerase chain reaction. *J Infect Dis.* 1995;172:1437–1444.

117. Mukhopadhya I, Sarkar R, Menon VK, et al. Rotavirus shedding in symptomatic and asymptomatic children using reverse transcription-quantitative PCR. *J Med Virol.* 2013;85:1661–1668.

118. Grimm AC, Cashdollar JL, Williams FP, Fout GS. Development of an astrovirus RT-PCR detection assay for use with conventional, real-time, and integrated cell culture/RT-PCR. *Can J Microbiol.* 2004;50:269–278.

119. Jarchow-Macdonald AA, Halley S, Chandler D, Gunson R, Shepherd SJ, Parcell BJ. First report of an astrovirus type 5 gastroenteritis outbreak in a residential elderly care home identified by sequencing. *J Clin Virol.* 2015;73:115–119.

120. Teunis PF, Moe CL, Liu P, et al. Norwalk virus: how infectious is it? *J Med Virol.* 2008;80:1468–1476.

121. Gallimore CI, Taylor C, Gennery AR, et al. Use of a heminested reverse transcriptase PCR assay for detection of astrovirus in environmental swabs from an outbreak of gastroenteritis in a pediatric primary immunodeficiency unit. *J Clin Microbiol.* 2005;43:3890–3894.

122. Hassard F, Sharp JH, Taft H, et al. Critical review on the public health impact of norovirus contamination in shellfish and the environment: a UK perspective. *Food Environ Virol.* 2017;9:123–141.

123. Tavoschi L, Severi E, Niskanen T, et al. Food-borne diseases associated with frozen berries consumption: a historical perspective, European Union, 1983 to 2013. *Euro Surveill.* 2015;20(29):21193.

124. Callejón RM, Rodríguez-Naranjo MI, Ubeda C, Hornedo-Ortega R, Garcia-Parrilla MC, Troncoso AM. Reported foodborne outbreaks due to fresh produce in the United States and European Union: trends and causes. *Foodb Pathog Dis.* 2015;12:32–38.

125. Campos CJA, Kershaw S, Morgan OC, Lees DN. Risk factors for norovirus contamination of shellfish water catchments in England and Wales. *Int J Food Microbiol.* 2017;241:318–324.

126. Kokkinos P, Kozyra I, Lazic S, et al. Virological quality of irrigation water in leafy green vegetables and berry fruits production chains. *Food Environ Virol.* 2017;9:72–78.

127. Verhoef L, Kouyos RD, Vennema H, et al. An integrated approach to identifying international foodborne norovirus outbreaks. *Emerg Infect Dis.* 2011;17:412–418.

128. World Health Organization. *The Treatment of Diarrhoea: A Manual for Physicians and Other Senior Health Workers.* 4th ed. Geneva: WHO; 2005.

129. Rocha-Pereira J, Neyts J, Jochmans D. Norovirus: targets and tools in antiviral drug discovery. *Biochem Pharmacol.* 2014;91:1–11.

130. Ettayebi K, Crawford SE, Murakami K, et al. Replication of human noroviruses in stem cell-derived human enteroids. *Science.* 2016;353:1387–1393.

131. Frémond M-L, Perot P, Muth E, et al. Next-generation sequencing for diagnosis and tailored therapy: a case report of astrovirus-associated progressive encephalitis. *J Pediatric Infect Dis Soc.* 2015;4(3):e53–e57. https://doi.org/10.1093/jpids/piv040.

132. Marvin SA. The immune response to astrovirus infection. *Viruses.* 2016;9(1):e1. https://doi.org/10.3390/v9010001.

133. Speroni S, Rohayem J, Nenci S, et al. Structural and biochemical analysis of human pathogenic astrovirus serine protease at 2.0 Å resolution. *J Mol Biol.* 2009;387:1137–1152.

134. O'Ryan M. Rotavirus vaccines: a story of success with challenges ahead. *F1000Res.* 2017;6:e1517. https://doi.org/10.12688/f1000research.11912.1.

135. Lamberti LM, Ashraf S, Fischer Walker CL, Black RE. A systematic review of the effect of rotavirus vaccination on diarrhoea outcomes among children younger than 5 years. *Pediatr Infect Dis J.* 2016;35:992–998.

136. Groome MJ, Koen A, Fix A, et al. Safety and immuno-genicity of a parenteral P2-VP8-P[8] subunit rotavirus vaccine in toddlers and infants in South Africa: a ran-domised, double-blind, placebo-controlled trial. *Lancet Infect Dis*. 2017;17:843–853.

137. Parrino TA, Schreiber DS, Trier JS, Kapikian AZ, Blacklow NR. Clinical immunity in acute gastroenteritis caused by Norwalk agent. *N Engl J Med*. 1977;297:86–89.

138. Simmons K, Gambhir M, Leon J, Lopman B. Duration of immunity to norovirus gastroenteritis. *Emerg Infect Dis*. 2013;19:1260–1267.

139. Cortes-Penfield NW, Ramani S, Estes MK, Atmar RL. Prospects and challenges in the development of a noro-virus vaccine. *Clin Therapeut*. 2017;39:1537–1549.

140. Steele MK, Remais JV, Gambhir M, et al. Targeting pedi-atric versus elderly populations for norovirus vaccines: a model-based analysis of mass vaccination options. *Epidemics*. 2016;17:42–49.

141. Bernstein DI, Atmar RL, Lyon GM, et al. Norovirus vaccine against experimental human GII.4 virus ill-ness: a challenge study in healthy adults. *J Infect Dis*. 2015;211:870–878.

142. Blazevic V, Lappalainen S, Nurminen K, Huhti L, Vesikari T. Norovirus VLPs and rotavirus VP6 protein as combined vaccine for childhood gastroenteritis. *Vaccine*. 2011;29:8126–8133.

143. Xia M, Wei C, Wang L, et al. A trivalent vaccine candi-date against hepatitis E virus, norovirus, and astrovirus. *Vaccine*. 2016;34:905–913.

144. Bogdanoff WA, Campos J, Perez EI, Yin L, Alexander DL, DuBois RM. Structure of a human astrovirus capsid-antibody complex and mechanistic insights into virus neutralization. *J Virol*. 2017;91(2):e01859–16. https://doi.org/10.1128/JVI.01859-16.

CHAPTER 12

Bacterial Gastroenteritis

KAREN HELENA KEDDY, MBBCH, DTM&HBSC (MED), MMED, FCPATH (SA), PHD • ANTHONY M. SMITH, PHD

The burden of disease estimates have recognized that globally, the morbidity and mortality associated with enteric pathogens, including bacteria, may have been seriously underestimated, particularly in children aged less than 5 years.[1] Globally, the burden of diarrhea from all pathogens has been estimated at over 2 billion episodes, with over 1.3 million deaths and 71 million disability-adjusted life-years (DALYs) associated.[2] Infections may be associated with food- or waterborne diseases, resulting in large-scale outbreaks or epidemics, or maintained through person-to-person spread. The greatest disease burden is in developing countries, where endemic diarrhea is a common, but often ignored, challenge. Postinfectious sequelae are associated with a number of these pathogens and add to the DALYs.

Gastroenteritis is frequently underdiagnosed, leading to misapprehension on the importance of various gastrointestinal pathogens. However, global attempts to describe the burden of the disease have suggested that certain pathogens may contribute more than previously anticipated to disease burdens, particularly in the developing world and in vulnerable populations.[1,3,4] These data are critical in health planning and prevention of morbidity and mortality, and modern molecular diagnostic techniques have made a significant difference to our understanding of the epidemiology of bacterial gastroenteritis.

Molecular diagnosis of gastrointestinal bacterial pathogens involves detection of specific gene sequences on the genome of bacteria. Some gene sequences are unique to either a particular species of bacterium or a particular virulence phenotype of a bacterium, so detection of specific gene sequences can diagnose the presence of a particular bacterial pathogen. Molecular diagnosis of gastrointestinal pathogens are preferably (and most commonly) performed on a bacterial culture. Molecular diagnosis can also be performed directly on clinical specimens, such as stool. However, clinical specimens (particularly stool) can be very complex, so care must be taken to choose a suitable specimen processing method in order to extract DNA of good integrity, quality, and quantity. Currently, the most preferred and commonly documented molecular diagnostic method is the polymerase chain reaction (PCR), both conventional PCR and real-time PCR. PCR assays are often "multiplex" where multiple gene sequences are targeted, resulting in the diagnosis of multiple bacterial species and multiple bacterial phenotypes.

Should laboratory expertise not be available to design and implement in-house molecular diagnostic testing based on published data, then there are various commercial kits available as an alternative. Commercial kits are mostly based on the principle of real-time PCR; examples of commercial kits include TaqMan Array Card Systems, Fast Track Diagnostics kits, Seegene Allplex/Seeplex panels, BioFire FilmArray panels, and Luminex panels.[5–12] Commercial kits target a range of pathogens including bacteria, viruses, and parasites. In particular, a typical TaqMan Array Card System can target 19 enteropathogens including bacteria, viruses, and parasites,[9] while a Bacterial Gastroenteritis Fast Track Diagnostics kit will target *Salmonella* species, *Shigella* species/enteroinvasive *Escherichia coli* (EIEC), *Campylobacter* species, Shiga toxin–producing *E. coli* (STEC), *C. difficile*, and *Yersinia enterocolitica*.

CAMPYLOBACTER

Campylobacter is the commonest foodborne bacterial pathogen in many parts of the world[1,13] and is the most common cause in high-income countries.[14] It is a zoonotic pathogen frequently associated with birds and domesticated animals.[13] It is a motile, gram-negative rod that was previously called *Vibrio fetus*[15] because of its motility and "comma" shape.

Epidemiology

The World Health Organization estimates that campylobacteriosis is responsible for 166 million (95% uncertainty interval [UI], 92–300 million) illnesses annually, of which approximately 60% are foodborne.[1] Waterborne diseases have been associated with large outbreaks of gastroenteritis due to water

Gastrointestinal Diseases and Their Associated Infections. https://doi.org/10.1016/B978-0-323-54843-4.00012-X
Copyright © 2019 Elsevier Inc. All rights reserved.

contamination.[16–18] Source attribution studies in Canada have suggested that chicken is the most commonly associated meat (up to 70% of attributable cases), while exposure to cattle manure, through water contamination, ranked second (from 14% to 19% of attributablecases).[16]Humanimmunodeficiencyvirus(HIV)-associated infections have also been described.[19–21]

Pathogenicity

After ingestion, *Campylobacter* passes through the gastric acid barrier of the stomach; hence, increased gastric pH may increase the risk of infection.[22] An enterotoxin, cytolethal distending toxin, has been associated with *Campylobacter* and causes apoptosis of eukaryotic cells,[23] but it does not appear necessary for the pathogenesis of diarrhea, as toxin-negative strains can also cause disease.[22] The organisms can bind to the enteric epithelium via surface adhesion,[24] although *Campylobacter* flagella appear to have a role in the adhesion as well.[25] Invasion of the gut mucosa is supported by the finding of red blood cells in stool examination.[26]

Clinical Presentation

Campylobacter diarrhea is typically self-limiting and nonfatal, although symptoms can be severe, including diarrhea (which may be bloody), nausea, asthenia, headache, anorexia, fever, and abdominal pain.[14,15] The infectious dose is typically low: studies in adult volunteers showed between 50 and 500 organisms were sufficient to cause disease, and the development of illness was not clearly related to the infectious dose.[26] The incubation period is around 3 days, but ranges between 1 and 7 days, and illness is usually self-limiting with recovery within 6 days.[22] Mortality is rare and typically associated with comorbidity, including older age, HIV infection, and invasive disease.[27,28] Postinfectious sequelae contribute significantly to the DALYs and include Guillain-Barré syndrome (GBS), specifically in association with the Penner serotype 19[29] (see later discussion) and reactive arthritis.[15]

Diagnosis

Campylobacter is fastidious and its diagnosis requires specialized laboratory equipment and media, including microaerophilic conditions and selective agar or filtration techniques.[22] Owing to these challenges, many laboratories have moved toward molecular diagnosis. As *Campylobacter jejuni* and *Campylobacter coli* account for the majority of human campylobacteriosis, most molecular diagnostics target these two species. Numerous PCR-based methods have been described to target different *Campylobacter* species, including *C. jejuni* and

C. coli.[30–34] Among the more commonly used methods to diagnose *C. jejuni* and *C. coli*, one method is multiplex real-time PCR, described by Best and coworkers,[30] that targets the *mapA* gene specific for *C. jejuni* and the *ceuE* gene specific for *C. coli*. For a universal detection of all *Campylobacter* species, PCR assays have been described, which target gene sequences unique to all *Campylobacter* species, such as regions of the 16S ribosomal RNA gene.[35]

Antimicrobial resistance testing is recommended because of increasing resistance in these pathogens and should be undertaken according to the internationally standardized protocols.[36]

Management

Although the disease is typically self-limiting in healthy adults, in selected cases, antimicrobial treatment is a necessity in some patients, including those patients with high fever, immunosuppressed patients, patients presenting with dysentery, and extremes of age. *Campylobacter* is intrinsically resistant to β-lactam antibiotics, including cephalosporins, and previously, erythromycin was the treatment of choice.[22] Alternatives would include tetracycline or ciprofloxacin.[22] Increasing incidence of antimicrobial resistance is a cause for concern: there have been increasing reports of resistance to the fluoroquinolones, in association with increased use in animal husbandry and particularly the poultry industry.[37] Azithromycin has been used for treatment more recently, although resistance is increasingly being reported.[38–40] Long-term sequelae need to be managed on a cause-specific basis, including life support for severe cases of GBS and anti-inflammatory drugs for reactive arthritis.

DIARRHEAGENIC *ESCHERICHIA COLI*

E. coli are primarily harmless commensals of the human intestine, belonging to the family Enterobacteriaceae. They are gram-negative, non–spore forming, flagellated bacilli. Certain highly adapted *E. coli* strains are capable of causing diarrheagenic infection.[41] Diarrheagenic *E. coli* (DEC) are divided into six main categories, each with a distinct pathogenic mechanism: STEC (which includes the enterohemorrhagic *E. coli*), enterotoxigenic *E. coli* (ETEC), enteropathogenic *E. coli* (EPEC), EIEC, enteroaggregative *E. coli* (EAggEC), and diffusely adherent *E. coli* (DAEC) (Table 12.1).

Epidemiology

Water is the commonest vehicle for the transmission of DEC, excluding STEC, particularly in developing

TABLE 12.1
Clinical Presentation and Selected Virulence Characteristics of Diarrheagenic *Escherichia coli*

Diarrheagenic *E. coli*	Abbreviation	Clinical Presentation	Virulence Genes	Toxins
Shiga toxigenic (enterohemorrhagic) *E. coli*	STEC (EHEC)	Diarrhea associated with colitis/hemorrhagic colitis, hemolytic uremic syndrome, thrombocytopenic purpura	stx_1, stx_2, *eae*, *bfp*	Shiga toxin (Stx) 1 Stx2
Enterotoxigenic *E. coli*	ETEC	Watery diarrhea with cramps, fever that is low grade or absent	*elt*, *etx*	Heat-labile toxin (LT), heat-stable toxin (ST)
Enteropathogenic *E. coli*	EPEC	Watery diarrhea accompanied by fever and vomiting, may occasionally be associated with prolonged enteritis	*eae*, *bfp*	
Enteroinvasive *E. coli*	EIEC	Acute watery diarrhea with abdominal cramps and fever, stools may become bloody and mucoid (resembling shigellosis)	*ipaH*	
Enteroaggregative *E. coli*	EAggEC	May cause acute, bloody, or persistent diarrhea	*aggR*	
Diffusely adherent *E. coli*	DAEC	Role in diarrhea not fully elucidated; it has been associated with outbreaks but may also be a "passenger" in diarrhea because of other causes.		

countries. STEC has been associated with major outbreaks, accounting for 2.5 million illnesses (UI, 1.6–5.4 million),[1] which may be waterborne, whereas foodborne infections account for 48%.[1] STEC outbreaks tend to occur in association with certain serotypes, including, but not limited to, STEC O157, O111, O26. Other serotypes have also been implicated and may cause sporadic disease.[42] STEC causes hemorrhagic colitis and hemolytic uremic syndrome (HUS), a triad of uremia, thrombocytopenia and microangiopathic anemia, secondary to the production of Shiga toxin. Both EPEC and ETEC have been associated with diarrhea and infants under 5 years of age,[43] accounting for 81 million (UI, 40–171 million) and 241 million (UI, 161–377 million) illnesses, respectively.[1] In addition, ETEC is the commonest pathogen identified in traveler's diarrhea.[44,45] EAggEC and DAEC have been associated with diarrhea in both children and HIV-infected patients and have been described in outbreaks.[46–56] A large outbreak of EAggEC, associated with Shiga toxin production in Germany, that spread to neighboring countries as well as North America served as an alert to the potential of DEC virulence genes to transfer between pathotypes, with devastating consequences.[57]

Pathogenicity

Depending on the pathotype, DEC cause diarrhea through different mechanisms (Table 12.1). Both STEC and EPEC attach to the gut epithelium via attaching to and effacement of the epithelial cells, with the bundle forming pilus (bfp) assisting in the attachment. STEC additionally contains Shiga toxin, an AB subunit toxin that binds to the kidney glomerulus and causes disruption of intracellular protein manufacture, resulting in renal failure and HUS.[58] ETEC heat-labile toxin (ETEC-LT) is similar to cholera toxin, and the mechanism of action also relies on the formation of cyclic AMP, causing the active efflux of sodium ions from the epithelial cells and resulting in osmotic water loss. The heat-stable toxin of ETEC (ETEC-ST) causes osmotic water loss through a different mechanism. EAggEC adhere to the gut epithelium and to each other to form a "stacked brick" appearance, resulting in diarrhea that is partially chemically medicated. DAEC adhere diffusely to the epithelium and their role in diarrhea is not fully elucidated.[58]

Clinical Presentation

Clinical features associated with the different DEC pathotypes are listed in Table 12.1.[58] Infections typically start within 24–48 h of exposure to the implicated source, but may be longer (up to 2 weeks) for STEC. Although the infectious dose has been calculated at 10^5 organisms, it has been shown that in STEC infections, this may be as low as 10–100 organisms.[58] Postinfectious sequelae are primarily associated with STEC, where mortality is high and patients may go on to develop permanent renal failure.[58]

Diagnosis

Phenotypic diagnosis depends on culturing and the use of selective media. *E. coli* grow easily in culture, but normal commensals must be differentiated from pathogenic strains. MacConkey agar with sorbitol may assist in the diagnosis of non–sorbitol-fermenting STEC O157 strains, but it will not assist in the identification of other STEC serotypes. Serotyping has assisted in differentiating between *E. coli* strains, particularly in outbreaks, and certain serotypes may be associated with specific pathotypes.[58] Serotyping (against O somatic and H flagellar antigens) is done following the methods developed by the Orskovs.[59] Older methods of cell culture have largely been superseded by molecular methods.

Numerous molecular methods have been described to target gene sequences coding for virulence determinants associated with different categories of DEC[60–64] (Fig. 12.1). In particular, PCR-based diagnosis of STEC is well described,[62–66] with further molecular characterization of STEC, including PCR-based tests for determination of the *E. coli* serotype (O157, O111, O26, etc.)[65,67,68] and the Shiga-toxin subtype associated with STEC,[69] to establish pathogenicity and strain relatedness.

Antimicrobial susceptibility testing may assist in those cases where antimicrobial management has become necessary and should be done according to standardized methods.[70]

Management

Although DEC infections are frequently self-limiting, antimicrobials may be necessary for severe (more than six stools per day) or prolonged diarrhea (persisting for more than 1 week), dysentery with fever, or immunocompromised status.[71] Use of antibiotics in patients presenting with suspected STEC infection must be exercised with caution, as there are concerns that antimicrobials may worsen the diarrhea.[72]

Antimicrobial options are being limited by emerging antimicrobial resistance and the older antimicrobials,

ampicillin and co-trimoxazole, may no longer be effective. Newer treatment options include azithromycin and fluoroquinolones. Fluoroquinolones, azithromycin, and rifaximin have been used in travelers for noninvasive infections.[71]

Vaccines against DEC are in different stages of development and those against ETEC are the most advanced.[73–75] Additionally, cholera vaccine has been shown to provide some protection against ETEC infection.[76] Currently, however, there are no suitable vaccines for the other DEC pathotypes.

SALMONELLA

Salmonella species include *Salmonella enterica* and *Salmonella bongori* and these gram-negative bacilli and fall within the family Enterobacteriaceae. These pathogens represent a range of organisms that may be highly host specific, such as *S. enterica* serotype Typhi (*Salmonella* Typhi), which is highly adapted to invasive human diseases, or may be less adapted and affect a wider range of hosts, such as *Salmonella* Enteritidis and *Salmonella* Typhimurium.

Epidemiology

Most nontyphoidal *Salmonella* (NTS) infections are zoonoses and these pathogens are frequently associated with foodborne infections, causing enteritis, although animal exposures are well described.[77] NTS may cause systemic infections, particularly in HIV-infected individuals, with extremes of age, in the presence of malaria coinfection, and in patients with sickle cell disease.[78] *Salmonella* Typhi and *Salmonella* Paratyphi A and Paratyphi B cause invasive enteric fever and are predominantly acquired by exposure to contaminated water, but they may also be acquired by contaminated foods or rarely by direct person-to-person spread, and they are rarely associated with diarrhea. The global burden of noninvasive NTS infections is 153 million (UI, 64–382 million), of which 52% are foodborne. By comparison, the burden of typhoid fever is 21 million (UI, 7–44 million) and paratyphoid fever, due to *Salmonella* Paratyphi A, is 5 million.[1] Typhoid fever and paratyphoid fever are more common in the developing world, where they may cause major waterborne outbreaks.

Pathogenicity

Pathogenicity islands in the *Salmonella* genome function to promote host invasion and intracellular survival and to induce host immunity. *Salmonella* invade nonphagocytic and phagocytic microfold (M) cells[120] of the intestinal epithelium where they exist with

Center for Genomic Epidemiology

KmerFinder 2.0 results:

Hit	Score	z-score	Query Coverage [%]	Template Coverage [%]	Depth	Total Query Coverage [%]	Total Template Coverage [%]	Total Depth
Escherichia coli, Escherichia coli O26:H11, Escherichia coli O26:H11 str. 11368 get sequence	10699	512.3	95.40	95.42	0.89	95.40	95.42	0.89

SpeciesFinder-1.2 Server - Results

Species
Escherichia coli

SerotypeFinder-1.1 Server - Results

H type						
Serotype gene	%Identity	Query/HSP length	Contig	Position in contig	Predicted serotype	Accession number
fliC	99.93	1459 / 1467	YA00028237a-ECO_S6_L001_R1_001_(paired)_trimmed_(paired)_contig_121	12482..13940	H11	AY337465

O type						
Serotype gene	%Identity	Query/HSP length	Contig	Position in contig	Predicted serotype	Accession number
wzx	99.66	592 / 1263	YA00028237a-ECO_S6_L001_R1_001_(paired)_trimmed_(paired)_contig_54	11..602	O26	AF529080
wzy	100.00	577 / 1023	YA00028237a-ECO_S6_L001_R1_001_(paired)_trimmed_(paired)_contig_428	1..577	O26	AF529080

Predicted Serotype: O26:H11

Shiga-toxin genes						
Virulence factor	%Identity	Query/HSP length	Contig	Position in contig	Protein function	Accession number
stx2	100.00	1241 / 1241	YA00028237a-ECO_S6_L001_R1_001_(paired)_trimmed_(paired)_contig_100	1091..2331	O157 SF-3573-98, variant a	AB030484

MLST-1.8 Server - Typing Results

Sequence Type: *ST-21*

Locus	% Identity	HSP Length	Allele Length	Gaps	Allele
adk	100.00	536	536	0	adk-16
fumc	100.00	469	469	0	fumc-4
gyrb	100.00	460	460	0	gyrb-12
icd	100.00	518	518	0	icd-16
mdh	100.00	452	452	0	mdh-9
pura	100.00	478	478	0	pura-7
reca	100.00	510	510	0	reca-7

FIG. 12.1 Results following WGS data analysis (of a query diarrheagenic *Escherichia coli* isolate) at the CGE bioinformatics pipelines (http://cge.cbs.dtu.dk/services/); showing the identification and characterization of a Shiga toxin-producing *E. coli*.

membrane-bound *Salmonella*-containing vacuoles (SCVs), avoiding killing by preventing lysosome fusion and surviving and replicating in the SCVs. The pathogen translocates to the host cytoplasm rearranging the cytoskeleton and invades basolaterally through the epithelial lining to the Peyer patches, stimulating an immune response and inflammatory diarrhea.[79,80]

Clinical Presentation

NTS typically cause enteritis in healthy individuals, with diarrhea developing between 6 h and 3 days following exposure.[81] Common vehicles include contaminated eggs and chicken meat, although many other food stuffs have been implicated.[82,83] Patients may present with mild diarrhea, profuse watery diarrhea, or dysentery, in association with abdominal pain and fever of 38–39°C.[81] Resolution may occur within a couple of days of symptomatic infection, but in rare cases the infection may be more protracted and may require antimicrobial management, as does bloody diarrhea. Antimicrobials are mandatory for immunosuppressed patients because of the risk of invasive disease.[78]

Diagnosis

Phenotypic diagnosis depends on the subculture of stool specimens onto selective and nonselective media, followed by specific biochemical tests to confirm the species identity.[81] Serotype is defined by the O and H antigens, as for *E. coli*, following methods described by Ewing and White-Kaufmann-Le Minor.[84,85] With rapidly emerging resistance being a well-identified problem,[86,87] antimicrobial susceptibility testing using standardized protocols is a critical part of diagnosis.[70]

Molecular diagnostics for detection of *Salmonella* species have commonly targeted the pathogenic gene sequences[88–91] (Fig. 12.2). For determination of a specific *Salmonella* serotype, a gene sequence associated with a specific serotype is targeted; such gene sequences most often code for specific O and H antigens.[89,92–97] Globally, *Salmonella* Typhimurium and *Salmonella* are the two most commonly reported serotypes of NTS in humans, so PCR-based diagnostic methods are particularly well described for these two serotypes. Multilocus sequence typing (MLST) has proved to be a reliable tool to infer *Salmonella* serotype. MLST involves nucleotide sequence analysis of seven housekeeping genes; each unique allelic variant of a gene is assigned a unique number and each unique combination of alleles (allelic numbers) for the seven genes are assigned a unique sequence type (ST). Each *Salmonella* serotype has been found to be associated with a specific ST, so the ST of an isolate is predictive of its serotype. Public

Health England has adopted an MLST approach as a replacement for traditional *Salmonella* serotyping; this has even been extended to whole-genome sequencing (WGS) as a routine tool for full characterization of *Salmonella*, including in silico analysis of WGS data to determine MLST STs and to infer serotype.[98]

Management

Rapidly emerging resistance to the first-line antimicrobials ampicillin and trimethoprim-sulfamethoxazole in the 1990s has necessitated the introduction of fluoroquinolones and azithromycin as alternative drugs, but resistance to these antimicrobials is also developing.[86,87] Although there are commercially available vaccines to prevent typhoid fever, currently vaccines for NTS are still in the development and trial stages.[99]

SHIGELLA

Shigella species are members of the Enterobacteriaceae and include four species: *Shigella dysenteriae*, *Shigella boydii*, *Shigella flexneri*, and *Shigella sonnei*. They are the commonest cause of bacillary dysentery and have the potential to cause large-scale outbreaks or epidemics, because of the small numbers of organisms required for infection as well as the ease of transmission through water, food, and environmental contamination (fingers, flies, food, and feces). Global estimates based on enhanced molecular diagnostics and large cooperative studies suggest that disease burdens are much higher than previously thought, with 191 million (UI, 97–363 million) cases[1] and 55,000 (UI, 27,000–94,000) deaths occurring annually, mostly in young children.[100]

Epidemiology

Humans are the only known hosts of *Shigella*, and the largest burden of disease is in children under 5 years of age, particularly in developing countries.[4] *Shigella* is also one of the greatest contributors to diarrheal diseases in older children and adults, and two-thirds of the deaths due to shigellosis are in this age group.[2] While all *Shigella* species are capable of causing outbreaks, epidemic dysentery has been specifically associated with *S. dysenteriae* type 1, often in settings associated with conflict and refugees.[101] The pathogens may additionally become invasive in immunosuppressed patients, including HIV-infected adults and severely malnourished children.[102]

Pathogenicity

Shigella enters the epithelial cells of the large intestine, utilizing a type III secretion system (T3SS),

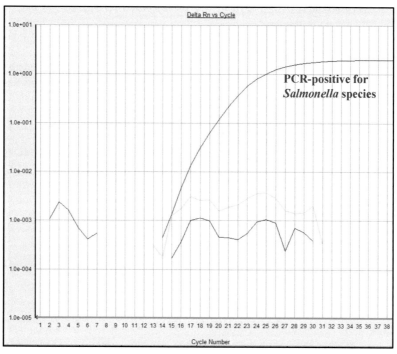

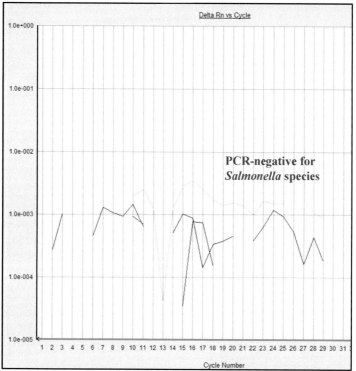

FIG. 12.2 Results for molecular diagnosis of a *Salmonella* species using real-time PCR; showing PCR-positive and PCR-negative results.

preferentially via the M cells through macropinocytosis. From the M cells, they are passed to the resident macrophages, inducing apoptosis of the host cell, destabilizing the intestinal tissue, and permitting basolateral invasion of the gut epithelial cells. The organisms multiply within the cytoplasm. Massive and rapid colonization of the epithelial cells is followed by recruitment of polymorphonuclear cells and extensive epithelial cell destruction.[103]

Clinical Presentation

The incubation period for shigellosis is 1–7 days after exposure. Clinically, patients may present with mild diarrhea to severe dysentery. Fever, cramping, and abdominal pain may be associated. Untreated, the disease in healthy individuals may last between 1 and 2 weeks. Patients presenting with S. *dysenteriae* type 1 may develop HUS, similar to those with STEC infection, because of the presence of Shiga toxin, which is highly related to the Stx1 of STEC.[104]

Diagnosis

Subculture of patients' stool specimens is necessary for phenotypic diagnosis of shigellosis. Both selective and nonselective media can be used to isolate *Shigella* colonies prior to performing specific diagnostic tests.[104] *Shigella* speciation is dependent on the use of polyvalent antisera to identify the serogroups (species), prior to *Shigella* serotyping.[104] Owing to the somewhat fastidious nature of *Shigella*, new studies have suggested that conventional methods may be inadequate[105] for diagnostics and molecular methods are becoming the method of choice for diagnosis. Antimicrobial susceptibility testing is a critical part of the diagnosis.[70]

Accurate molecular diagnosis of *Shigella* species has proved very challenging because of its close relationship with *E. coli*. Most genetic markers described for *Shigella* are not adequate to differentiate between a *Shigella* species and DEC, particularly EIEC. Nonetheless, there have been some reports claiming success in molecular (mostly PCR-based) diagnosis of *Shigella* species, where gene sequences coding for virulence factors such as invasion proteins (including the IpaH antigen) are commonly targeted.[106–109]Kim and coworkers[110] used comparative genomics to screen genome sequences of *Shigella* species to identify gene sequences unique to *Shigella*; this resulted in the design of a successful multiplex PCR that was able to both identify the genus *Shigella* and distinguish between the four species. Other studies have also reported success in using PCR-based methods to differentiate *Shigella* species and serotype some *Shigella* species.[111–114]

Management

Increasing reports of multidrug resistance in *Shigella* species[102] have limited management options to fluoroquinolones and azithromycin in many places, although resistance to these antimicrobials is emerging as well. There are currently no vaccines available for shigellosis, although a number of candidate vaccines are in an advanced state of development.[74,75]

VIBRIO CHOLERAE AND NONCHOLERA VIBRIOS

Most human infections by *Vibrio cholerae* are due to the serogroup O1, the cause of pandemic cholera. The organisms are members of the Vibrionaceae family, gram negative, motile curved bacilli, and typically halophilic and inhabit aquatic environments. The global burden of cholera is estimated at 3.2 million (UI, 2.2–4.4 million) and results in 105,000 deaths.[1] Cholera is the commonest cause of death due to diarrhea in children aged 5–14 years (13,000 deaths or 25%), with the major burden being in sub-Saharan Africa and southeast Asia.[4] Although *V. cholerae* O139 may also cause cholera, it has so far been restricted to Asia.[115]

Epidemiology

Cholera is primarily a waterborne disease, but it may be also be foodborne in about 25% of cases.[1] It is associated with large outbreaks and pandemics; the seventh pandemic started in the 1960s. Molecular evidence has shown that virtually all cholera epidemics originate from the Bay of Bengal[116] and human population movements have accounted for much of the transmission.[116,117] Most of the large outbreaks reported recently have been in Africa.[117]

Pathogenicity

The organisms bind to the gut via the toxin-coregulated pilus, which is encoded on a filamentous phage inserted into the *V. cholerae* genome, with the genes encoding the cholera toxin. *V. cholerae* O1 (and O139) produces an enterotoxin that stimulates the secretion of fluid into the intestine, leading to severe watery diarrhea. The toxin is an AB subunit toxin, with the B subunit binding to the GM1 ganglioside on the epithelial cell of the small intestine. This binding permits entry of the A subunit into the epithelial cells, enabling a cascade of events in the cytosol, initially through the activation of adenylate cyclase and the formation of cyclic AMP. Chloride ions and water molecules are secreted into the gut lumen and absorption of NaCl is ,inhibited resulting in a severe osmotic diarrhea.[115]

Clinical Presentation

The incubation period is typically 24–48 h but may be as short as 6 h. Clinical infection may range from being asymptomatic in about 70% of cases to profuse watery diarrhea, associated with "rice-water" stools in about 5% of cases. Most fluid loss occurs within the first couple of days of illness, with typical signs of decreased skin turgor, dry mucous membranes, rapid thready pulse, sunken eyeballs, and orthostatic hypotension. In the absence of adequate rehydration, patient may go into hypovolemic shock, metabolic acidosis, and hypokalemia.[115]

Diagnosis

Severe cholera, presenting with rapid dehydration and typical rice-water stools, may not require laboratory confirmation; however, diagnosis is mandatory when there is an increase in diarrheal cases in an area at risk for cholera, during an outbreak to monitor the evolution of an outbreak, and to establish the molecular epidemiologic links of an outbreak. A pragmatic approach to diagnosis has been published.[118]

Stool specimens should be collected early in the course of illness and submitted to the laboratory as soon as possible to prevent overgrowth of normal flora from the gut. *V. cholerae* will grow on nonselective media, such as blood agar, but diagnosis may be made easier through the use of highly selective agar such as thiosulfate citrate-bile salts-sucrose (TCBS) agar, on which it appears as large yellow colonies.[115] *V. cholerae* are seen as oxidase-positive large greyish colonies on blood agar. Serogrouping for serogroups O1 and O139 should be done from nonselective media to prevent autoagglutination.

Molecular diagnosis of these toxigenic *V. cholerae* are well described in the literature and typically target DNA sequences encoding two major virulence determinants associated with toxigenic *V. cholerae*, namely, the cholera toxin and the toxin-coregulated pilus. A typical PCR-based method would start with determination of the presence/absence of a *V. cholerae* species and the presence/absence of cholera toxin.[118–121] Additionally, detection of DNA sequences specific for O1/O139 antigen biosynthesis can assist with confirmation of diagnosis of *V. cholerae* serogroup O1 or O139.[120,122,123] Finally, the biotype (El Tor or classical) of *V. cholerae* O1 can be determined by further PCR assays targeting gene sequences coding for the toxin-coregulated pilus.[119,124]

Management

Rehydration is the mainstay of cholera management, and the choice of rehydration, whether to administer orally or intravenously, as well as attention to volumes required are critical for patient survival.[125] This mandates good clinical review of the patient's response to ensure that rehydration is optimized. Antimicrobials may have a secondary role, in that these do decrease the volume of diarrhea as well as the numbers of viable organisms excreted, but resistance is rapidly emerging and hence these must be used with caution.

Vaccination has been shown to be effective in the prevention of cholera outbreaks if used timely in areas under threat, such as refugee populations,[126] and the WHO keeps a stockpile of cholera vaccine for this purpose. The current vaccines are oral whole-cell vaccines containing a recombinant B subunit (WC-rBS), and adequate protective antibody levels take about 2 weeks to develop.[126]

The provision of safe water and adequate disposal of human wastes is the possible and most critical intervention to prevent disease transmission.

Noncholera Vibrios

A certain number of the noncholera vibrios may also be associated with gastroenteritis. The commonest is *Vibrio parahaemolyticus*, which is associated with diarrhea due to consumption of contaminated seafood, particularly when eaten raw. It primarily causes diarrhea, which may rarely become bloody,[127] and can be isolated from nonselective agars or TCBS, on which it appears as large green colonies.[127] Molecular epidemiologic techniques have enabled the comparison of different strains associated with outbreaks.[128]

CLOSTRIDIUM DIFFICILE

Clostridium difficile is a gram-positive, anaerobic bacillus that is spore-forming. This pathogen has now become the commonest cause of diarrheal death in all ages in the developed world ,[4] in association with antimicrobial treatment, and causes pseudomembranous colitis. Macrolides, including clindamycin, penicillins, third-generation cephalosporins and fluoroquinolones are the antibiotics most frequently associated with infection, as they suppress the normal gut flora during treatment.[129]

Epidemiology

Infection rates in symptomatic patients in low- to middle-income countries range around 16%, compared with 20%–30% in high-income countries.[130] Global disease burdens have increased 39.8% (UI, 29.6%–49.9%) between 2005 and 2015, particularly in patients over 70 years of age, in whom the increase had been greater than 60%.[4] *C. difficile* infection is primarily associated with nosocomial transmission, although outpatients, particularly if attending clinics, may also be affected.[130] Between 20% and 35% of patients will fail initial antibiotic treatment, and of these, 40%–60% will have a second recurrence.[129] Antimicrobial stewardship is a critical part of disease control and helps reduce in-hospital infection rates.[131]

Pathogenicity

C. difficile may be asymptomatic colonizers or may cause a toxin-mediated disease ranging in severity from watery diarrhea to pseudomembranous colitis and toxic megacolon. The production of the clostridial toxins A and B (TcdA and TcdB, respectively), which are large glycosylating toxins, as well as the presence and health of the normal gut flora and the health of the host, all contribute to disease.[132] TcdA is an enterotoxin and is primarily associated with diarrhea through stimulating secretion of water and salts into the gut lumen, as well as neutrophil chemotaxis and proinflammatory cytokine secretion. TcdB is cytopathic and primarily targeted in toxin neutralization tests but contributes to the pathogenesis of diarrhea and pseudomembranous colitis.[132–135]

Clinical Presentation

Exposure to *C. difficile* spores in the hospital or clinic environment is the first step toward colonization. Infection may range from asymptomatic colonization to severe diarrhea, bloody stools and pseudomembranous colitis or toxic megacolon, and fatal infection.[135] Patients with moderate diarrhea have fever and abdominal cramps, which become severe with more severe disease and the progression to ileus and toxic megacolon.[135] The risk of mortality increases with increasing age and comorbid conditions including hepatic disease, renal disease, and cardiac disease.[135]

Diagnosis

Patients may carry the organisms symptomatically, so any patient presenting with nosocomial diarrhea should have stool sent for culture for other enteric bacteria, as well as *C. difficile*. Traditionally, diagnostics depended on cell culture assay, and toxin neutralization of the *C. difficile* toxin with *Clostridium sordellii* antitoxin.[134,135] Technical demands of this test however has seen a swing to the use of kits, including enzyme immunoassays and molecular diagnostics.[135–137] *C. difficile* molecular diagnostics have been well reviewed and published.[135,137–139] The most commonly used target is the *tcdA* and/or *tcdB* genes encoding TcdA

and TcdB, respectively, located on a large pathogenicity locus; numerous PCR-based methods have been described targeting these genes.[140] Detection strategies sometimes also include the targeting of species-specific genes, for example, the *tpi* gene encoding triose phosphate isomerase.[141] A number of different techniques have been used to confirm disease outbreak, including ribotyping and MLST.[135,137]

Management

The management of an initial CDI recurrence includes repeat administration of either oral metronidazole or vancomycin for 10–14 days.[129,142] Resistance is emerging to this pathogen because of selective pressures,[142] and novel therapies include the use of probiotics and donor fecal transplants, anion resins, secondary bile acids, or antitoxin antibodies.[129] However, toxic megacolon may require surgery.[135] Due attention to antimicrobial stewardship and maintenance of optimal infection control procedures and hospital policies are important contributions toward controlling the disease. Vaccine development is in its early stages.[143]

YERSINIA ENTEROCOLITICA AND *YERSINIA PSEUDOTUBERCULOSIS*

Y. enterocolitica and *Y. pseudotuberculosis* are gram-negative bacilli and members of the family Enterobacteriaceae, most frequently acquired through contaminated foods and cause a mild, usually self-limiting, diarrhea. Not all *Y. enterocolitica* strains are pathogenic, so a distinction needs to be made between pathogenic and nonpathogenic isolates. *Y. pseudotuberculosis* may more frequently additionally go on to cause mesenteric adenitis.

Epidemiology

Y. enterocolitica infection has classically been associated with consumption of pork products[144] and is a rare cause of foodborne infection predominantly in countries with colder climates in the northern hemisphere.[1] Infection in humans is most commonly due to the serotype O:3, for which pigs are the sole reservoir.[145] Molecular studies have confirmed the association with pork, although rarely other animals may be associated.[144,146] In France, *Y. enterocolitica* isolations have outnumbered *Y. pseudotuberculosis* isolations by a factor of 15.[144]

Pathogenicity

Similar to *Salmonella* species, *Yersinia* species contain T3SS effector proteins, encoded on a 70 kb virulence plasmid, that are injected by direct cell contact through a needle-like structure into the host cell to disrupt a cellular response. Translocation of the effector proteins into the target host cell disrupts the cytoskeleton and inhibits phagocytosis, downregulates the proinflammatory cytokine response, and induces apoptosis of the target cell.[147]

Clinical Presentation

Acute infection manifests as diarrhea or, less frequently, as bloody diarrhea, particularly in children under 5 years of age, associated with low-grade fever, abdominal pain, and headache.[145] In older children and adults the infection may manifest as a pseudoappendicitis, with inflammation of mesenteric lymph nodes or the terminal ileum.[145] Infection is normally self-limiting, but significant postinfectious sequelae with an autoimmune component are well recognized. Typically, this occurs in Scandinavian patients over the age of 10 years, who carry the human leukocyte antigen B27.[145] The postinfectious sequelae include reactive arthritis, occurring between 1 and 2 weeks after initial infection; erythema nodosum; Reiter syndrome; glomerulonephritis; and uveitis.[145]

Diagnosis

Isolation requires the use of enrichment media and low-temperature incubation. The bacteria grow well on most enteric media, but selective media for *Yersinia* are also available.[145] Serotyping depends on the identification of the O antigen.[145] Low levels of bacteria may mean that the organism is not isolated from the stool, but serologic diagnosis of a preceding *Yersinia* infection in a patient presenting with reactive arthritis has been described.[148]

Molecular diagnosis of *Y. enterocolitica* has been described in the literature; however, these techniques are not as well published as those of the previously mentioned bacterial pathogens. For molecular diagnosis, the *ail* gene, encoding a virulence determinant associated with attachment/invasion of host cells, is commonly targeted to identify pathogenic *Y. enterocolitica*[149-153]; occasionally, detection strategies may also target species-specific genes (such as *foxA*) to diagnose the general presence of all types of *Y. enterocolitica*.[149]

Management

As the diarrhea is mostly self-limiting, antimicrobial therapy is not a prerequisite; however, antimicrobial therapy may be used for complicated conditions, including invasion.[154] Antimicrobial resistance appears to be less common than described in other enteric

bacteria.[155] Autoimmune manifestations would require the use of appropriate anti-inflammatory and immunosuppressive therapy.

REFERENCES

1. Kirk MD, Pires SM, Black RE, et al. World health Organization estimates of the global and regional disease burden of 22 foodborne bacterial, Protozoal, and viral diseases, 2010: a data synthesis. *PLoS Med.* 2015;12(12):e1001921.
2. Global, regional, and national age-sex specific mortality for 264 causes of death, 1980–2016: a systematic analysis for the Global Burden of Disease Study 2016. *Lancet (Lond Engl)*. 2017;390(10100):1151–1210.
3. Global, regional, and national life expectancy, all-cause mortality, and cause-specific mortality for 249 causes of death, 1980–2015: a systematic analysis for the Global Burden of Disease Study 2015. *Lancet (Lond Englg)*. 2016;388(10053):1459–1544.
4. Estimates of global, regional, and national morbidity, mortality, and aetiologies of diarrheal diseases: a systematic analysis for the Global Burden of Disease Study 2015. *Lancet Infect Dis.* 2017;17(9):909–948.
5. Piralla A, Lunghi G, Ardissino G, et al. FilmArray GI panel performance for the diagnosis of acute gastroenteritis or hemorrhagic diarrhea. *BMC Microbiol.* 2017;17(1):111.
6. Huang RS, Johnson CL, Pritchard L, Hepler R, Ton TT, Dunn JJ. Performance of the Verigene(R) enteric pathogens test, Biofire FilmArray gastrointestinal panel and Luminex xTAG(R) gastrointestinal pathogen panel for detection of common enteric pathogens. *Diagn Microbiol Infect Dis.* 2016;86(4):336–339.
7. Rintala A, Munukka E, Weintraub A, Ullberg M, Eerola E. Evaluation of a multiplex real-time PCR kit Amplidiag(R) Bacterial GE in the detection of bacterial pathogens from stool samples. *J Microbiol Methods.* 2016;128:61–65.
8. Liu J, Kabir F, Manneh J, et al. Development and assessment of molecular diagnostic tests for 15 enteropathogens causing childhood diarrhea: a multicentre study. *Lancet Infect Dis.* 2014;14(8):716–724.
9. Liu J, Gratz J, Amour C, et al. A laboratory-developed TaqMan Array Card for simultaneous detection of 19 enteropathogens. *J Clin Microbiol.* 2013;51(2):472–480.
10. Buss SN, Leber A, Chapin K, et al. Multicenter evaluation of the BioFire FilmArray gastrointestinal panel for etiologic diagnosis of infectious gastroenteritis. *J Clin Microbiol.* 2015;53(3):915–925.
11. Wessels E, Rusman LG, van Bussel MJ, Claas EC. Added value of multiplex Luminex Gastrointestinal Pathogen Panel (xTAG(R) GPP) testing in the diagnosis of infectious gastroenteritis. *Clin Microbiol Infect.* 2014;20(3):O182–O187.
12. Onori M, Coltella L, Mancinelli L, et al. Evaluation of a multiplex PCR assay for simultaneous detection of bacterial and viral enteropathogens in stool samples of paediatric patients. *Diagn Microbiol Infect Dis.* 2014;79(2):149–154.

13. Kaakoush NO, Castano-Rodriguez N, Mitchell HM, Man SM. Global epidemiology of Campylobacter infection. *Clin Microbiol Rev.* 2015;28(3):687–720.

14. Sheppard SK, Maiden MC. The evolution of Campylobacter jejuni and Campylobacter coli. *Cold Spring Harbor Perspect Biol.* 2015;7(8):a018119.

15. Moore JE, Corcoran D, Dooley JS, et al. Campylobacter. *Vet Res.* 2005;36(3):351–382.

16. Gibney KB, O'Toole J, Sinclair M, Leder K. Burden of disease attributed to waterborne transmission of selected enteric pathogens, Australia, 2010. *Am J Trop Med Hyg.* 2017;96(6):1400–1403.

17. Kuhn KG, Falkenhorst G, Emborg HD, et al. Epidemiological and serological investigation of a waterborne Campylobacter jejuni outbreak in a Danish town. *Epidemiol Infect.* 2017;145(4):701–709.

18. Ravel A, Hurst M, Petrica N, et al. Source attribution of human campylobacteriosis at the point of exposure by combining comparative exposure assessment and subtype comparison based on comparative genomic fingerprinting. *PLoS One.* 2017;12(8):e0183790.

19. Larsen IK, Gradel KO, Helms M, et al. Non-typhoidal Salmonella and Campylobacter infections among HIV-positive patients in Denmark. *Scand J Infect Dis.* 2011;43(1):3–7.

20. Manfredi R, Calza L, Chiodo F. Enteric and disseminated Campylobacter species infection during HIV disease: a persisting but significantly modified association in the HAART era. *Am J Gastroenterol.* 2002;97(2):510–511.

21. Meier PA, Dooley DP, Jorgensen JH, Sanders CC, Huang WM, Patterson JE. Development of quinolone-resistant Campylobacter fetus bacteremia in human immunodeficiency virus-infected patients. *J Infect Dis.* 1998;177(4):951–954.

22. Hu L, Kopecko DJ. Campylobacter species. In: Miliotis MD, Bier JW, eds. *International Handbook of Foodborne Pathogens.* New York: Marcel Dekker; 2003:181–198.

23. Whitehouse CA, Balbo PB, Pesci EC, Cottle DL, Mirabito PM, Pickett CL. Campylobacter jejuni cytolethal distending toxin causes a G2-phase cell cycle block. *Infect Immun.* 1998;66(5):1934–1940.

24. Kervella M, Pages JM, Pei Z, Grollier G, Blaser MJ, Fauchere JL. Isolation and characterization of two Campylobacter glycine-extracted proteins that bind to HeLa cell membranes. *Infect Immun.* 1993;61(8):3440–3448.

25. Grant CC, Konkel ME, Cieplak Jr W, Tompkins LS. Role of flagella in adherence, internalization, and translocation of Campylobacter jejuni in nonpolarized and polarized epithelial cell cultures. *Infect Immun.* 1993;61(5):1764–1771.

26. Black RE, Levine MM, Clements ML, Hughes TP, Blaser MJ. Experimental Campylobacter jejuni infection in humans. *J Infect Dis.* 1988;157(3):472–479.

27. Skirrow MB, Jones DM, Sutcliffe E, Benjamin J. Campylobacter bacteraemia in England and Wales, 1981–91. *Epidemiol Infect.* 1993;110(3):567–573.

28. Smith GS, Blaser MJ. Fatalities associated with Campylobacter jejuni infections. *JAMA.* 1985;253(19):2873–2875.

29. Kuroki S, Saida T, Nukina M, et al. Campylobacter jejuni strains from patients with Guillain-Barre syndrome belong mostly to Penner serogroup 19 and contain beta-N-acetylglucosamine residues. *Ann Neurol.* 1993;33(3):243–247.

30. Best EL, Powell EJ, Swift C, Grant KA, Frost JA. Applicability of a rapid duplex real-time PCR assay for speciation of Campylobacter jejuni and Campylobacter coli directly from culture plates. *FEMS Microbiol Lett.* 2003;229(2):237–241.

31. On SL, Jordan PJ. Evaluation of 11 PCR assays for species-level identification of Campylobacter jejuni and Campylobacter coli. *J Clin Microbiol.* 2003;41(1):330–336.

32. Gonzalez I, Grant KA, Richardson PT, Park SF, Collins MD. Specific identification of the enteropathogens Campylobacter jejuni and Campylobacter coli by using a PCR test based on the ceuE gene encoding a putative virulence determinant. *J Clin Microbiol.* 1997;35(3):759–763.

33. Leblanc-Maridor M, Beaudeau F, Seegers H, Denis M, Belloc C. Rapid identification and quantification of Campylobacter coli and Campylobacter jejuni by real-time PCR in pure cultures and in complex samples. *BMC Microbiol.* 2011;11:113.

34. Wang G, Clark CG, Taylor TM, et al. Colony multiplex PCR assay for identification and differentiation of Campylobacter jejuni, C. coli, C. lari, C. upsaliensis, and C. fetus subsp. fetus. *J Clin Microbiol.* 2002;40(12):4744–4747.

35. Lund M, Nordentoft S, Pedersen K, Madsen M. Detection of Campylobacter spp. in chicken fecal samples by real-time PCR. *J Clin Microbiol.* 2004;42(11):5125–5132.

36. Clinical Laboratory Standards Institute. *M45: Methods for Antimicrobial Dilution and Disk Susceptibility Testing of Infrequently Isolated or Fastidious Bacteria.* 3rd ed. Clinical Laboratory Standards Institute; 2015.

37. Iovine NM. Resistance mechanisms in Campylobacter jejuni. *Virulence.* 2013;4(3):230–240.

38. Mason CJ, Sornsakrin S, Seidman JC, et al. Antibiotic resistance in Campylobacter and other diarrheal pathogens isolated from US military personnel deployed to Thailand in 2002–2004: a case-control study. *Trop Dis Trav Med Vaccines.* 2017;3:13.

39. Shobo CO, Bester LA, Baijnath S, Somboro AM, Peer AK, Essack SY. Antibiotic resistance profiles of Campylobacter species in the South Africa private health care sector. *J Infect Dev Ctries.* 2016;10(11):1214–1221.

40. Szczepanska B, Andrzejewska M, Spica D, Klawe JJ. Prevalence and antimicrobial resistance of Campylobacter jejuni and Campylobacter coli isolated from children and environmental sources in urban and suburban areas. *BMC Microbiol.* 2017;17(1):80.

41. Croxen MA, Law RJ, Scholz R, Keeney KM, Wlodarska M, Finlay BB. Recent advances in understanding enteric pathogenic *Escherichia coli. Clin Microbiol Rev.* 2013;26(4):822–880.

42. Goldwater PN, Bettelheim KA. *Escherichia coli* 'O' group serology of a haemolytic uraemic syndrome (HUS) epidemic. *Scand J Infect Dis*. 2000;32(4):385–394.

43. Kotloff KL, Nataro JP, Blackwelder WC, et al. Burden and aetiology of diarrheal disease in infants and young children in developing countries (the Global Enteric Multicenter Study, GEMS): a prospective, case-control study. *Lancet (Lond Engl)*. 2013;382(9888):209–222.

44. Goldsmid JM, Leggat PA. The returned traveller with diarrhea. *Aust Fam Physician*. 2007;36(5):322–327.

45. Black RE. Epidemiology of travelers' diarrhea and relative importance of various pathogens. *Rev Infect Dis*. 1990;12(suppl 1):S73–S79.

46. Ahmed SF, Shaheen HI, Abdel-Messih IA, et al. The epidemiological and clinical characteristics of diarrhea associated with enteropathogenic, enteroaggregative and diffuse-adherent *Escherichia coli* in Egyptian children. *J Trop Pediatr*. 2014;60(5):397–400.

47. Forestier C, Meyer M, Favre-Bonte S, et al. Enteroadherent *Escherichia coli* and diarrhea in children: a prospective case-control study. *J Clin Microbiol*. 1996;34(12):2897–2903.

48. Hii JH, Guccion JG, Gilbert CL. Enteroadherent eaeA-positive *Escherichia coli* associated with chronic AIDS-related diarrhea. *Ann Intern Med*. 1996;125(6):523.

49. Lozer DM, Souza TB, Monfardini MV, et al. Genotypic and phenotypic analysis of diarrheagenic *Escherichia coli* strains isolated from Brazilian children living in low socioeconomic level communities. *BMC Infectious Diseases*. 2013;13:418.

50. Morelli R, Baldassarri L, Falbo V, Donelli G, Caprioli A. Detection of enteroadherent *Escherichia coli* associated with diarrhea in Italy. *J Med Microbiol*. 1994;41(6):399–404.

51. Oberhelman RA, Laborde D, Mera R, et al. Colonization with enteroadherent, enterotoxigenic and enterohemorrhagic *Escherichia coli* among day-care center attendees in New Orleans, Louisiana. *Pediatr Infect Dis J*. 1998;17(12):1159–1162.

52. Sullivan PB, Coles MA, Aberra G, Ljungh A. Enteropathogenic and enteroadherent-aggregative *Escherichia coli* in children with persistent diarrhea and malnutrition. *Ann Trop Paediatr*. 1994;14(2):105–110.

53. Samie A, Obi CL, Dillingham R, Pinkerton RC, Guerrant RL. Enteroaggregative *Escherichia coli* in Venda, South Africa: distribution of virulence-related genes by multiplex polymerase chain reaction in stool samples of human immunodeficiency virus (HIV)-positive and HIV-negative individuals and primary school children. *Am J Trop Med Hyg*. 2007;77(1):142–150.

54. Huang DB, Dupont HL. Enteroaggregative *Escherichia coli*: an emerging pathogen in children. *Semin Pediatr Infect Dis*. 2004;15(4):266–271.

55. Huang DB, Nataro JP, DuPont HL, et al. Enteroaggregative *Escherichia coli* is a cause of acute diarrheal illness: a meta-analysis. *Clin Infect Dis*. 2006;43(5):556–563.

56. Spencer J, Smith HR, Chart H. Characterization of enteroaggregative *Escherichia coli* isolated from outbreaks of diarrheal disease in England. *Epidemiol Infect*. 1999;123(3):413–421.

57. Bielaszewska M, Mellmann A, Zhang W, et al. Characterisation of the *Escherichia coli* strain associated with an outbreak of haemolytic uraemic syndrome in Germany, 2011: a microbiological study. *Lancet Infect Dis*. 2011;11(9):671–676.

58. Nataro JP, Kaper JB. Diarrheagenic *Escherichia coli*. *Clin Microbiol Rev*. 1998;11(1):142–201.

59. Orskov I, Orskov F, Jann B, Jann K. Serology, chemistry, and genetics of O and K antigens of *Escherichia coli*. *Bacteriol Rev*. 1977;41(3):667–710.

60. Lopez-Saucedo C, Cerna JF, Villegas-Sepulveda N, et al. Single multiplex polymerase chain reaction to detect diverse loci associated with diarrheagenic *Escherichia coli*. *Emerg Infect Dis*. 2003;9(1):127–131.

61. Schmidt H, Knop C, Franke S, Aleksic S, Heesemann J, Karch H. Development of PCR for screening of enteroaggregative *Escherichia coli*. *J Clin Microbiol*. 1995;33(3):701–705.

62. Vidal M, Kruger E, Duran C, et al. Single multiplex PCR assay to identify simultaneously the six categories of diarrheagenic *Escherichia coli* associated with enteric infections. *J Clin Microbiol*. 2005;43(10):5362–5365.

63. Cebula TA, Payne WL, Feng P. Simultaneous identification of strains of *Escherichia coli* serotype O157:H7 and their Shiga-like toxin type by mismatch amplification mutation assay-multiplex PCR. *J Clin Microbiol*. 1995;33(1):248–250.

64. Paton AW, Paton JC. Detection and characterization of Shiga toxigenic *Escherichia coli* by using multiplex PCR assays for stx1, stx2, eaeA, enterohemorrhagic *E. coli* hlyA, rfbO111, and rfbO157. *J Clin Microbiol*. 1998;36(2):598–602.

65. Jenkins C, Lawson AJ, Cheasty T, Willshaw GA. Assessment of a real-time PCR for the detection and characterization of verocytotoxigenic *Escherichia coli*. *J Med Microbiol*. 2012;61(Pt 8):1082–1085.

66. Hidaka A, Hokyo T, Arikawa K, et al. Multiplex real-time PCR for exhaustive detection of diarrheagenic *Escherichia coli*. *J Appl Microbiol*. 2009;106(2):410–420.

67. Perelle S, Dilasser F, Grout J, Fach P. Detection by 5′-nuclease PCR of Shiga-toxin producing *Escherichia coli* O26, O55, O91, O103, O111, O113, O145 and O157:H7, associated with the world's most frequent clinical cases. *Mol Cell Probes*. 2004;18(3):185–192.

68. Sanchez S, Llorente MT, Echeita MA, Herrera-Leon S. Development of three multiplex PCR assays targeting the 21 most clinically relevant serogroups associated with Shiga toxin-producing *E. coli* infection in humans. *PLoS One*. 2015;10(1):e0117660.

69. Scheutz F, Teel LD, Beutin L, et al. Multicenter evaluation of a sequence-based protocol for subtyping Shiga toxins and standardizing Stx nomenclature. *J Clin Microbiol*. 2012;50(9):2951–2963.

70. Institute CLS. *Performance Standards for Antimicrobial Susceptibility Testing; Twenty-fifth Informational Supplement* Pennsylvania, USA. ; 2015. Report No: M100-S25.

71. Zollner-Schwetz I, Krause R. Therapy of acute gastroenteritis: role of antibiotics. *Clin Microbiol Infect.* 2015;21(8):744–749.

72. Freedman SB, Xie J, Neufeld MS, Hamilton WL, Hartling L, Tarr PI. Shiga toxin–producing *Escherichia coli* infection, antibiotics, and risk of developing hemolytic uremic syndrome: a meta-analysis. *Clin Infect Dis.* 2016;62(10):1251–1258.

73. Ahmed T, Bhuiyan TR, Zaman K, Sinclair D, Qadri F. Vaccines for preventing enterotoxigenic *Escherichia coli* (ETEC) diarrhea. *Cochrane Database Syst Rev.* 2013;7:CD009029. https://doi.org/10.1002/14651858. CD009029.pub2.

74. Bohles N, Busch K, Hensel M. Vaccines against human diarrheal pathogens: current status and perspectives. *Hum Vaccin Immunother.* 2014;10(6):1522–1535.

75. Parker EP. Advances in enteric disease vaccines: from innovation to implementation. *Expert Rev Vaccines.* 2014;13(3):317–319.

76. Lundkvist J, Steffen R, Jonsson B. Cost-benefit of WC/rBS oral cholera vaccine for vaccination against ETEC-caused travelers' diarrhea. *J Travel Med.* 2009;16(1):28–34.

77. Aiken AM, Lane C, Adak GK. Risk of Salmonella infection with exposure to reptiles in England, 2004–2007. *Euro Surveill.* 2010;15(22):19581.

78. Ao TT, Feasey NA, Gordon MA, Keddy KH, Angulo FJ, Crump JA. Global burden of invasive nontyphoidal salmonella disease, 2010(1). *Emerg Infect Dis.* 2015;21(6):941–949.

79. Hurley D, McCusker MP, Fanning S, Martins M. Salmonella-host interactions - modulation of the host innate immune system. *Front Immunol.* 2014;5:481. https://doi.org/10.3389/fimmu.2014.00481. eCollection@2014.:481.

80. Dandekar T, Fieselmann A, Fischer E, Popp J, Hensel M, Noster J. Salmonella-how a metabolic generalist adopts an intracellular lifestyle during infection. *Front Cell Infect Microbiol.* 2015;4:191. https://doi.org/10.3389/fcimb.2014.00191. eCollection;%2014.:191.

81. Hanes D. Nontyphoid Salmonella. In: Miliotis MD, Bier JW, eds. *International Handbook of Foodborne Pathogens.* New York: Marcel Dekker; 2003:137–149.

82. DEK LV, Pires SM, Hald T. Using surveillance and monitoring data of different origins in a Salmonella source attribution model: a European Union example with challenges and proposed solutions. *Epidemiol Infect.* 2015;143(6):1148–1165.

83. Pires SM, Vieira AR, Hald T, Cole D. Source attribution of human salmonellosis: an overview of methods and estimates. *Foodborne Pathogens Dis.* 2014;11(9):667–676.

84. Ewing WH, Bruner DW. The use of a polyvalent antiserum for preliminary identification of Salmonella cultures. *J Bacteriol.* 1947;53(3):362.

85. Le Minor L, Veron M, Popoff M. [A proposal for Salmonella nomenclature]. *Ann Microbiol (Paris).* 1982;133(2):245–254.

86. Crump JA, Medalla FM, Joyce KW, et al. Antimicrobial resistance among invasive nontyphoidal *Salmonella enterica* isolates in the United States: national antimicrobial resistance monitoring system, 1996 to 2007. *Antimicrob Agents Chemother.* 2011;55(3):1148–1154.

87. Cloeckaert A, Schwarz S. Molecular characterization, spread and evolution of multidrug resistance in *Salmonella enterica* typhimurium DT104. *Vet Res.* 2001;32(3–4):301–310.

88. Rahn K, De Grandis SA, Clarke RC, et al. Amplification of an invA gene sequence of *Salmonella typhimurium* by polymerase chain reaction as a specific method of detection of Salmonella. *Mol Cell Probes.* 1992;6(4):271–279.

89. Pui CF, Wong WC, Chai LC, et al. Multiplex PCR for the concurrent detection and differentiation of Salmonella spp., Salmonella Typhi and Salmonella Typhimurium. *Trop Med Health.* 2011;39(1):9–15.

90. Hopkins KL, Lawson AJ, Connell S, Peters TM, de Pinna E. A novel real-time polymerase chain reaction for identification of *Salmonella enterica* subspecies enterica. *Diagn Microbiol Infect Dis.* 2011;70(2):278–280.

91. Gonzalez-Escalona N, Hammack TS, Russell M, et al. Detection of live Salmonella sp. cells in produce by a TaqMan-based quantitative reverse transcriptase real-time PCR targeting invA mRNA. *Appl Environ Microbiol.* 2009;75(11):3714–3720.

92. Park HJ, Kim HJ, Park SH, Shin EG, Kim JH, Kim HY. Direct and quantitative analysis of *Salmonella enterica* serovar Typhimurium using real-time PCR from artificially contaminated chicken meat. *J Microbiol Biotechnol.* 2008;18(8):1453–1458.

93. O'Regan E, McCabe E, Burgess C, et al. Development of a real-time multiplex PCR assay for the detection of multiple Salmonella serotypes in chicken samples. *BMC Microbiol.* 2008;8:156.

94. Hadjinicolaou AV, Demetriou VL, Emmanuel MA, Kakoyiannis CK, Kostrikis LG. Molecular beacon-based real-time PCR detection of primary isolates of Salmonella Typhimurium and Salmonella Enteritidis in environmental and clinical samples. *BMC Microbiol.* 2009;9:97.

95. Park SH, Ricke SC. Development of multiplex PCR assay for simultaneous detection of Salmonella genus, Salmonella subspecies I, Salm. Enteritidis, Salm. Heidelberg and Salm. Typhimurium. *J Appl Microbiol.* 2015;118(1):152–160.

96. Bugarel M, Tudor A, Loneragan GH, Nightingale KK. Molecular detection assay of five Salmonella serotypes of public interest: typhimurium, Enteritidis, Newport, Heidelberg, and Hadar. *J Microbiol Methods.* 2017;134:14–20.

97. Maurischat S, Baumann B, Martin A, Malorny B. Rapid detection and specific differentiation of *Salmonella enterica* subsp. enterica Enteritidis, Typhimurium and its monophasic variant 4,[5],12:i:- by real-time multiplex PCR. *Int J Food Microbiol.* 2015;193:8–14.

98. Ashton PM, Nair S, Peters TM, et al. Identification of Salmonella for public health surveillance using whole genome sequencing. *PeerJ.* 2016;4:e1752.

99. Galen JE, Buskirk AD, Tennant SM, Pasetti MF. Live attenuated human Salmonella vaccine candidates: tracking the pathogen in natural infection and stimulation of host immunity. *EcoSal Plus.* 2016;7(1).

100. Collaborators GBDDD. Estimates of global, regional, and national morbidity, mortality, and aetiologies of diarrheal diseases: a systematic analysis for the Global Burden of Disease Study 2015. *Lancet Infect Dis.* 2017;17(9):909–948.

101. Ries AA, Wells JG, Olivola D, et al. Epidemic Shigella dysenteriae type 1 in Burundi: panresistance and implications for prevention. *J Infect Dis.* 1994;169(5):1035–1041.

102. Keddy KH, Sooka A, Crowther-Gibson P, et al. Systemic shigellosis in South Africa. *Clin Infect Dis.* 2012;54(10):1448–1454.

103. Sansonetti PJ. Rupture, invasion and inflammatory destruction of the intestinal barrier by Shigella: the yin and yang of innate immunity. *Can J Infect Dis Med Microbiol.* 2006;17(2):117–119.

104. Lampel KA, Maurelli AT. Shigella species. In: Miliotis MD, Bier JW, eds. *Handbook of Foodborne Pathogens.* New York: Marcel Dekker; 2003:167–180.

105. Liu J, Platts-Mills JA, Juma J, Kabir F, Nkeze J, Okoi C, et al. Use of quantitative molecular diagnostic methods to identify causes of diarrhoea in children: a reanalysis of the GEMS case-control study. *Lancet.* 2016;388(10051):1291–301.

106. Liew PS, Teh CS, Lau YL, Thong KL. A real-time loop-mediated isothermal amplification assay for rapid detection of Shigella species. *Trop Biomed.* 2014;31(4):709–720.

107. Barletta F, Mercado EH, Lluque A, Ruiz J, Cleary TG, Ochoa TJ. Multiplex real-time PCR for detection of Campylobacter, Salmonella, and Shigella. *J Clin Microbiol.* 2013;51(9):2822–2829.

108. Radhika M, Saugata M, Murali HS, Batra HV. A novel multiplex PCR for the simultaneous detection of Salmonella enterica and Shigella species. *Braz J Microbiol.* 2014;45(2):667–676.

109. Lobersli I, Wester AL, Kristiansen A, Brandal LT. Molecular differentiation of Shigella spp. from enteroinvasive E. Coli. *Eur J Microbiol Immunol.* 2016;6(3):197–205.

110. Kim HJ, Ryu JO, Song JY, Kim HY. Multiplex polymerase chain reaction for identification of Shigellae and four Shigella species using novel genetic markers screened by comparative genomics. *Foodborne Pathogens Dis.* 2017;14(7):400–406.

111. Farfan MJ, Garay TA, Prado CA, Filliol I, Ulloa MT, Toro CS. A new multiplex PCR for differential identification of Shigella flexneri and Shigella sonnei and detection of Shigella virulence determinants. *Epidemiol Infect.* 2010;138(4):525–533.

112. Ojha SC, Yean Yean C, Ismail A, Singh KK. A pentaplex PCR assay for the detection and differentiation of Shigella species. *BioMed Res Int.* 2013;2013:412370.

113. Gentle A, Ashton PM, Dallman TJ, Jenkins C. Evaluation of molecular methods for serotyping Shigella flexneri. *J Clin Microbiol.* 2016;54(6):1456–1461.

114. van der Ploeg CA, Roge AD, Bordagorria XL, de Urquiza MT, Celi Castillo AB, Bruno SB. Design of Two Multiplex PCR Assays for Serotyping Shigella flexneri. *Foodborne Pathogens Dis.* 2018;15(1):33–8.

115. Kaper JB, Morris Jr JG, Levine MM. Cholera. *Clin Microbiol Rev.* 1995;8(1):48–86.

116. Mutreja A, Kim DW, Thomson NR, et al. Evidence for several waves of global transmission in the seventh cholera pandemic. *Nature.* 2011;10.

117. Weill FX, Domman D, Njamkepo E, et al. Genomic history of the seventh pandemic of cholera in Africa. *Science.* 2017;358(6364):785–789.

118. Keddy KH, Sooka A, Parsons MB, Njanpop-Lafourcade BM, Fitchet K, Smith AM. Diagnosis of *Vibrio cholerae* O1 infection in Africa. *J Infect Dis.* 2013;208(suppl 1):S23–S31.

119. Keasler SP, Hall RH. Detecting and biotyping *Vibrio cholerae* O1 with multiplex polymerase chain reaction. *Lancet (Lond Engl).* 1993;341(8861):1661.

120. Khuntia HK, Pal BB, Chhotray GP. Quadruplex PCR for simultaneous detection of serotype, biotype, toxigenic potential, and central regulating factor of *Vibrio cholerae.* *J Clin Microbiol.* 2008;46(7):2399–2401.

121. Koskela KA, Matero P, Blatny JM, et al. A multiplatform real-time polymerase chain reaction detection assay for *Vibrio cholerae.* *Diagn Microbiol Infect Dis.* 2009;65(3):339–344.

122. Hoshino K, Yamasaki S, Mukhopadhyay AK, et al. Development and evaluation of a multiplex PCR assay for rapid detection of toxigenic *Vibrio cholerae* O1 and O139. *FEMS Immunol Med Microbiol.* 1998;20(3):201–207.

123. Lyon WJ. TaqMan PCR for detection of *Vibrio cholerae* O1, O139, non-O1, and non-O139 in pure cultures, raw oysters, and synthetic seawater. *Appl Environ Microbiol.* 2001;67(10):4685–4693.

124. De K, Ramamurthy T, Ghose AC, et al. Modification of the multiplex PCR for unambiguous differentiation of the El Tor & classical biotypes of *Vibrio cholerae* O1. *Indian J Med Res.* 2001;114:77–82.

125. Barua D. Miracle cure for an old scourge. *Bull World Health Organ.* 2009;87(2):91–92.

126. Chaignat CL, Monti V. Use of oral cholera vaccine in complex emergencies: what next? Summary report of an expert meeting and recommendations of WHO. *J Health Popul Nutr.* 2007;25(2):244–261.

127. Nishibuchi M. Vibrio parahaemolyticus. In: Miliotis MD, Bier JW, eds. *International Hadnbook of Foodborne Pathogens.* New York: Marcel Dekker; 2003:237–252.

128. Ansaruzzaman M, Chowdhury A, Bhuiyan NA, et al. Characteristics of a pandemic clone of O3 : K6 and O4 : K68 Vibrio parahaemolyticus isolated in Beira, Mozambique. *J Med Microbiol.* 2008;57(Pt 12):1502–1507.

129. Hopkins RJ, Wilson RB. Treatment of recurrent *Clostridium difficile* colitis: a narrative review. *Gastroenterol Rep.* 2018;6(1):21–28.

130. Forrester JD, Cai LZ, Mbanje C, Rinderknecht TN, Wren SM. *Clostridium difficile* infection in low- and middle-human development index countries: a systematic review. *Trop Med Int Health.* 2017;22(10):1223–1232.

131. Louh IK, Greendyke WG, Hermann EA, et al. Clostridium difficile infection in acute care hospitals: systematic review and best practices for prevention. *Infect Control Hosp Epidemiol.* 2017;38(4):476–482.

132. Hryckowian AJ, Pruss KM, Sonnenburg JL. The emerging metabolic view of *Clostridium difficile* pathogenesis. *Curr Opin Microbiol.* 2017;35:42–47.

133. George RH, Symonds JM, Dimock F, et al. Identification of *Clostridium difficile* as a cause of pseudomembranous colitis. *Br Med J.* 1978;1(6114):695.

134. Willey SH, Bartlett JG. Cultures for *Clostridium difficile* in stools containing a cytotoxin neutralized by Clostridium sordellii antitoxin. *J Clin Microbiol.* 1979;10(6):880–884.

135. Burnham CA, Carroll KC. Diagnosis of *Clostridium difficile* infection: an ongoing conundrum for clinicians and for clinical laboratories. *Clin Microbiol Rev.* 2013;26(3):604–630.

136. Bai Y, Sun X, Jin Y, Wang Y, Li J. Accuracy of Xpert *Clostridium difficile* assay for the diagnosis of *Clostridium difficile* infection: a meta analysis. *PLoS One.* 2017;12(10):e0185891.

137. Surawicz CM, Brandt LJ, Binion DG, et al. Guidelines for diagnosis, treatment, and prevention of *Clostridium difficile* infections. *Am J Gastroenterol.* 2013;108(4):478–498. quiz 99.

138. O'Horo JC, Jones A, Sternke M, Harper C, Safdar N. Molecular techniques for diagnosis of *Clostridium difficile* infection: systematic review and meta-analysis. *Mayo Clin Proc.* 2012;87(7):643–651.

139. Eckert C, Jones G, Barbut F. Diagnosis of *Clostridium difficile* infection: the molecular approach. *Future Microbiology.* 2013;8(12):1587–1598.

140. Houser BA, Hattel AL, Jayarao BM. Real-time multiplex polymerase chain reaction assay for rapid detection of *Clostridium difficile* toxin-encoding strains. *Foodborne Pathogens Dis.* 2010;7(6):719–726.

141. Lemee L, Dhalluin A, Testelin S, et al. Multiplex PCR targeting tpi (triose phosphate isomerase), tcdA (Toxin A), and tcdB (Toxin B) genes for toxigenic culture of *Clostridium difficile*. *J Clin Microbiol.* 2004;42(12):5710–5714.

142. Peng Z, Jin D, Kim HB, et al. Update on antimicrobial resistance in *Clostridium difficile*: resistance mechanisms and antimicrobial susceptibility testing. *J Clin Microbiol.* 2017;55(7):1998–2008.

143. Ward SJ, Douce G, Figueiredo D, Dougan G, Wren BW. Immunogenicity of a *Salmonella typhimurium* aroA aroD vaccine expressing a nontoxic domain of *Clostridium difficile* toxin A. *Infect Immun.* 1999;67(5):2145–2152.

144. Le Guern AS, Martin L, Savin C, Carniel E. Yersiniosis in France: overview and potential sources of infection. *Int J Infect Dis.* 2016;46:1–7.

145. Robins-Browne RM, Hartland EL. Yersinia species. In: Miliotis MD, Bier JW, eds. *International Handboof of Foodborne Pathogens.* New York: Marcel Dekker; 2003:323–355.

146. Fredriksson-Ahomaa M, Stolle A, Korkeala H. Molecular epidemiology of Yersinia enterocolitica infections. *FEMS Immunol Med Microbiol.* 2006;47(3):315–329.

147. Pha K, Navarro L. Yersinia type III effectors perturb host innate immune responses. *World J Biol Chem.* 2016;7(1):1–13.

148. Honda K, Iwanaga N, Izumi Y, et al. Reactive arthritis caused by Yersinia enterocolitica enteritis. *Intern Med.* 2017;56(10):1239–1242.

149. Wang JZ, Duan R, Liang JR, et al. Real-time TaqMan PCR for Yersinia enterocolitica detection based on the ail and foxA genes. *J Clin Microbiol.* 2014;52(12):4443–4444.

150. Lambertz ST, Nilsson C, Hallanvuo S, Lindblad M. Real-time PCR method for detection of pathogenic Yersinia enterocolitica in food. *Appl Environ Microbiol.* 2008;74(19):6060–6067.

151. Arrausi-Subiza M, Ibabe JC, Atxaerandio R, Juste RA, Barral M. Evaluation of different enrichment methods for pathogenic Yersinia species detection by real time PCR. *BMC Vet Res.* 2014;10:192.

152. Rundell MS, Pingle M, Das S, et al. A multiplex PCR/LDR assay for simultaneous detection and identification of the NIAID category B bacterial food and water-borne pathogens. *Diagn Microbiol Infect Dis.* 2014;79(2):135–140.

153. Wannet WJ, Reessink M, Brunings HA, Maas HM. Detection of pathogenic Yersinia enterocolitica by a rapid and sensitive duplex PCR assay. *J Clin Microbiol.* 2001;39(12):4483–4486.

154. Kato H, Sasaki S, Sekiya N. Primary cellulitis and cutaneous abscess caused by Yersinia enterocolitica in an immunocompetent host: a case report and literature review. *Medicine.* 2016;95(26):e3988.

155. Frazao MR, Andrade LN, Darini ALC, Falcao JP. Antimicrobial resistance and plasmid replicons in Yersinia enterocolitica strains isolated in Brazil in 30 years. *Braz J Infect Dis.* 2017;21(4):477–480.

CHAPTER 13

Molecular Diagnosis of Gastrointestinal Infections

ESTHER BABADY, PHD, D (ABMM) • PETER MEAD, MD

INTRODUCTION

Gastrointestinal (GI) infections are a significant cause of mortality and morbidity worldwide. The World Health organization (WHO) estimates that in 2013, diarrheal and intestinal infectious diseases caused approximately 90 million all-age disability adjusted life years, with approximately 1.5 million deaths in 2015, ranking them in the top 10 causes of death globally.[1,2] The greatest number of GI infections occurs in regions of low to middle income countries where inadequate sanitation and hygiene are prevalent. In the United States, approximately 179 million annual cases of acute gastroenteritis are estimated to occur, resulting in 474,000 hospitalizations and 5000 deaths.[3]

Pathogens responsible for GI infections vary based on multiple factors including the patient population (e.g., immunocompetent vs. immunocompromised hosts), the socioeconomic status (e.g., high vs. low income patients), the geographic locations (e.g., Northern vs. Southern Hemisphere) or the patient location within the healthcare system spectrum at the time of diagnosis (e.g., community vs. hospitalized patients). Therefore, depending on epidemiological risks, the differential diagnosis for infectious gastroenteritis may be broad and include a variety of viruses, bacteria, or parasites (Table 13.1).[4] In the following section, diagnostic methods for GI infections including clinical presentation and methods available for the molecular diagnosis of the most important GI infections are discussed.

CLINICAL DIAGNOSIS OF GASTROINTESTINAL INFECTIONS

Clinical evaluation of any patient suspected of having a gastrointestinal infection is essential.[5,6] The successful determination of the etiology of a patient's illness depends heavily on determining the a priori likelihood of diagnoses (before microbiological testing). This determines which set of diagnostic tests are likely to yield relevant results. This set of likely diagnoses,

in turn, depends primarily on patient characteristics (including age and immune status), characterization of symptoms, and exposures (as most gastrointestinal infections are the result of acquisition of pathogenic organisms). Although some organisms (e.g., *Salmonella*) would almost always be considered a pathogen if detected,[5] many other organisms could be considered colonizers (or a false-positive result) if detected in the absence of a compatible clinical syndrome.

Many gastrointestinal infections are self-limiting and do not require antimicrobial therapy.[5,6] As such a specific diagnosis is often not necessary. Diagnosis is usually significant in two circumstances: (1) if the diagnosis has clinical implications for the patient: usually this means antimicrobial treatment is indicated, but other relevant clinical situations include where antimicrobial therapy is potentially harmful (e.g., β-lactams treatment in the setting of Shiga-like toxin producing *E. coli* O157:H7), and when the pretest differential diagnosis is sufficiently broad that making the diagnosis of a self-limited disease would stave off the need for further diagnostic testing (and eliminate the need for or curtail the use of empiric antimicrobials); (2) where the diagnosis is important for epidemiological or infection control purposes (such as in outbreak detection and investigation).

Symptomatology is the primary means for making a clinical diagnosis (and usually why the patient has come to medical attention). Symptomatology serves both to indicate that (primary) gastrointestinal disease is present and to determine the likelihood that such disease is due to an infection. Often fever is interpreted as indicating the presence of infection. Absence of fever, however, is common with certain infections (such as with Norovirus and Rotavirus). The most common set of upper GI tract symptoms is nausea and vomiting. Acute vomiting, if due to infection, typically indicates a viral (and most likely self-limited disease). Noroviruses are frequently implicated. The typical norovirus infection is also associated with watery diarrhea (typically

Gastrointestinal Diseases and Their Associated Infections. https://doi.org/10.1016/B978-0-323-54843-4.00013-1
Copyright © 2019 Elsevier Inc. All rights reserved.

TABLE 13.1
Common Causes of Gastrointestinal Infections

Bacteria	Viruses	Parasites
Clostridium difficile	Norovirus	Giardia duodenalis
Salmonella species	Sapovirus	Cryptosporidium species
Shigella species	Astrovirus	Entamoeba histolytica
Campylobacter species	Enterovirus	Cyclospora species
Toxin-producing E. coli	Parechovirus	Isospora species
Yersinia species	Rotavirus	Balantidium coli
Vibrio species	Adenovirus	Blastocystis species
Aeromonas species		Entamoeba species
Plesiomonas species		Dientamoeba fragilis
		Microsporidia species
		Nematodes
		Cestodes
		Trematodes

following the diarrhea) and may include systemic symptoms as well including fever, chills.[7] Norovirus illness typically resolves within 3 days (but immunocompromised patient may be ill and shed virus longer).[8] Asymptomatic infection occurs in about a third of (immunocompetent) patients. Rotavirus may produce a similar clinical syndrome but much more common in children than adults.

The primary (and sometimes sole) symptom of gastrointestinal infections is diarrhea. Diarrhea itself is a very common symptom of a wide array of causes beyond infection. WHO defines diarrhea as the passage of three or more loose or liquid stools per day (or more frequent passage than is normal for the individual); frequent passing of formed stools is not diarrhea. Diarrhea is further characterized by chronicity: acute diarrhea (lasting <7 days); prolonged diarrhea (lasting 7–13 days); persistent diarrhea (lasting 14–29 days); and chronic (lasting 30 or more days). Diarrhea is often further characterized as watery, fatty, or inflammatory—typically by inspection though laboratory analysis can aid in making these distinctions. Most of

gastrointestinal infections produce one of the following diarrhea syndromes: acute watery diarrhea, acute inflammatory diarrhea (otherwise known as acute invasive diarrhea or dysentery), persistent/chronic diarrhea, and enteric fever (an illness characterized by diarrhea then days to weeks of persistent fever).

Acute watery diarrhea is produced by an extensive array of pathogens including viruses (Norovirus, Rotavirus, Adenovirus, for example), bacteria (various forms of E. coli, B. cereus), and parasites (such as Cryptosporidium). In most cases of acute watery diarrhea in immunocompetent outpatients, the disease is self-limiting and no specific microbiological diagnosis is necessary (except as part of outbreak investigation or infection control efforts). However, in severe illness, certain outbreak situations, and in the immunocompromised, antimicrobial therapy may be warranted—and in these cases broad testing is recommended. A subcategory of watery diarrhea where antimicrobial therapy is more likely necessary is profuse diarrhea, often called "rice water" diarrhea—such as that produced by Vibrio cholerae, and sometimes enterotoxigenic E. coli. Guidelines recommend testing for Vibrio spp. In this setting (if patient has had a compatible exposure, see below).

Dysentery is characterized by the presence of blood and/or mucus in stool—from inflammation of the bowel due to invasive infection. The pathogens that cause this clinical syndrome may also cause acute watery diarrhea. The list of potential pathogens is extensive and includes bacteria: Shigella, Enteroinvasive E. coli, Campylobacter species, nontyphoidal Salmonella, Yersinia enterocolitica, etc. (Table 13.1). Fever usually accompanies dysentery. In the United States, the most common pathogens are Shigella, Campylobacter jejuni, and Salmonella species. Typically, antimicrobial therapy is offered for these diagnoses (and hence specific diagnosis would be desired)—particularly for the immunocompromised and/or in cases of severe illness. However, most sources would avoid treatment in the case of illness due to E. coli O157:H7 and other Shiga-like toxin producing E. coli (STEC) strains due to increased risk of treatment patients developing hemolytic-uremic syndrome. In the work-up of dysentery, guidelines recommend at least testing for Salmonella, Shigella, Campylobacter, Yersinia, C. difficile, and STEC—with a broader array of testing if the patient is immunocompromised.

Persistent or chronic diarrhea is associated with parasites (Giardia, Cryptosporidium, Cystoisospora, Cyclospora) and some bacteria (enteropathogenic E. coli, enteroaggregative E. coli)—but also may be related to the patient's immunological state. However, complicating the diagnosis in this setting is that many causes of acute infectious diarrhea may also lead to intestinal mucosa damage and/or irritable-bowel-syndrome-like functional damage such that the symptoms persist even after the infection has cleared. Thus, the significance of positive testing for acute pathogens in this setting is unclear.

Diarrhea from *Clostridium difficile* requires both an exposure (which may be nosocomial) to the organism and dysbiosis. Typically, dysbiosis may result from recent or ongoing antimicrobial therapy but other treatments, such as chemotherapy, may also precipitate *Clostridium difficile* diarrhea.[9] Postinfection irritable-bowel-syndrome may follow *C. difficile* associated illness and make judgments regarding clinical improvement and cure difficult. In addition, frequently the patient remains colonized with *C. difficile* following therapy—significantly reducing the positive-predictive value of PCR testing for *C. difficile* in these patients.

Given the wide range of infectious etiologies, timely diagnosis of gastrointestinal infections is ideal for optimal patient care.

MOLECULAR DIAGNOSTICS OF GASTROINTESTINAL INFECTIONS

The introduction of molecular methods, especially real-time PCR, in the clinical laboratory revolutionized the diagnosis of infectious diseases.[10] The need for these assays arose from the need for increased sensitivity and more rapid time to results and, in general, molecular assays have overall better performance than conventional methods (i.e., culture, antigens tests and microscopic examination). Thus, they provide diagnosis in a timeframe that allow support of clinical diagnosis as described in the previous section. Although originally limited to laboratories with significant expertise in the design and implementation of molecular tests, recent years have seen a significant increase in the number of commercially available, simple to perform molecular tests (Tables 13.2–13.4). Many of these molecular assays are cleared for in vitro *diagnostics* (IVD) and designed to amplify and detect pathogens nucleic acids directly from raw or preserved stool samples (Table 13.2). Molecular assays vary in terms of their complexity, the instruments throughput, the number and type of organisms tested on the panels and the turn-around time to results.[11] However, most assays are designed to target the most common causes of infectious diarrhea (Table 13.1) and thus, laboratory-developed tests (LDT) and assays marketed as research-use only (RUO) or using analyte specific reagents (ASR) remain relevant and necessary to fill in the molecular diagnostic gaps.

The next section will present and discuss both LDT and IVD molecular tests for diagnosis of infectious gastroenteritis.

Bacterial Infections
Campylobacter/Shigella/Salmonella

Campylobacter, *Shigella*, and *Salmonella* species represent the most common cause of infectious diarrhea worldwide. Therefore, a standard bacterial culture includes agar media designed to detect at minimum these three organisms. Although a few molecular tests, both conventional and real-time PCR, were originally developed to target each of these pathogens individually, the most recent approach has been to develop multiplex methods that target at least all three pathogens. Detection of *Campylobacter* species, particularly *C. jejuni* and *C. coli*, have targeted the *CadF* (Campylobacter adhesion to Fn), *mapA* (membrane-associated protein), and 16S rRNA genes, while *Shigella* and *Salmonella* detection targets the *ipaH* (invasion plasmid antigen H) *and invA* (invasion gene) or *ttrC-ttrA* genes, respectively.[12–14] The analytical sensitivity of molecular methods varies across studies, ranging from 16 to 1000 CFU/mL for *Campylobacter* species, 52 to 1000 CFU/mL for *Shigella* species and 990 to 5528 CFU/mL for *Salmonella* species when tested on fresh stool samples. Although in general the detection rate may be similar to culture, with a slightly higher cost, the results of these multiplexed PCR were available in less than 3–4 h compared to 2–5 days needed for culture.[13,14] With the increased availability of commercial syndromic gastrointestinal panel, all targets described in this section are routinely screened as part of a larger panel.

Toxin producing E. coli

Several toxin-producing *E. coli* (STEC) may cause infectious diarrhea. Both commercial molecular methods and LDTs have been described for rapid detection in stool samples in comparison to either enzyme immunoassays (EIA), when available, and culture methods. STECs, including *E. coli* O157:H7, are the pathogens most commonly targeted for molecular diagnosis given their frequent association with a variety of syndromes including hemolytic uremic syndrome (HUS) and food-borne gastroenteritis. LDTs for STEC commonly target both the stx_1 and stx_2 genes.[15,16] In general, when compared to EIA and culture, PCR assays, especially real-time PCR have higher sensitivity and specificity of up to 100% but differences may be observed depending on the assay design with TaqMan-based methods performing better than SYBR green in one study.[16] Of note, most assays are designed to detect the most common serotypes, without necessarily

TABLE 13.2
Select Commercially Available Molecular Methods for Detection of Gastrointestinal Pathogens

Manufacturer	Test Name	Number of Pathogens	Pathogens	Regulatory Status	Stool Specimen	Methodology
Beckton Dickson (BD)	BD MAX ™ Enteric Parasite Panel	3	*Cryptosporidium* spp. *Entamoeba histolytica* Giardia lamblia	CE-IVD US-IVD	Unpreserved Preserved	Integrated, automated nucleic acid extraction Real-time PCR
	BD MAX ™ Enteric Bacterial Panel	4	*Salmonella* spp. *Shigella* spp. *Campylobacter* spp. STEC	CE-IVD US-IVD	Unpreserved Preserved	Integrated, automated nucleic acid extraction Real-time PCR
	BD MAX ™ Extended Enteric Bacterial Panel	4	*Yersinia enterocolitica* ETEC *Plesiomonas shigelloides* *Vibrio (vulnificus, cholerae parahaemolyticus)*	CE-IVD US-IVD	Unpreserved Preserved	Integrated, automated nucleic acid extraction and Real-time PCR
BioFire Diagnostics	FilmArray Gastrointestinal Panel	22	*Campylobacter* spp. *Clostridium difficile* (toxin A/B) *Plesiomonas shigelloides* *Salmonella* species *Yersinia enterocolitica* *Vibrio (parahaemolyticus, vulnificus, and cholerae)* *Vibrio cholerae* EAEC EPEC ETEC *lt/st* STEC *stx1/stx2* *E. coli* O157 *Shigella*/EIEC Adenovirus F 40/41 Astrovirus Norovirus GI/GII Rotavirus A Sapovirus (I, II, IV and V) *Cryptosporidium* spp. *Cyclospora cayetanensis* *Entamoeba histolytica* Giardia lamblia	CE-IVD US-IVD	Preserved	Sample-to-answer Nested PCR Melt-curve analysis

TABLE 13.2
Select Commercially Available Molecular Methods for Detection of Gastrointestinal Pathogens—cont'd

Manufacturer	Test Name	Number of Pathogens	Pathogens	Regulatory Status	Stool Specimen	Methodology
Luminex	xTAG® Gastrointestinal Pathogen Panel	14	*Campylobacter* species *Clostridium difficile* (toxin A/B) *Salmonella* species *Vibrio cholerae* EPEC ETEC *lt/st* STEC *stx1/stx2* *E. coli* O157 Adenovirus F 40/41 Norovirus GI/GII Rotavirus A *Cryptosporidium* species *Entamoeba histolytica* *Giardia lamblia*	CE-IVD US-IVD	Unpreserved	Nucleic acids extraction PCR amplification Bead suspension array
	Verigene Enteric Pathogens Nucleic Acid Test	7	*Campylobacter* species *Shigella* species *Salmonella* species *Vibrio* species STEC *stx1/stx2* Norovirus GI/GII Rotavirus A	CE-IVD US-IVD	Unpreserved	PCR amplification Gold nanoparticle Probe-based endpoint detection
R-Biopharm	RIDA®GENE Parasitic Stool Panel I	4	*Cryptosporidium parvum* *Dientamoeba fragilis* *Entamoeba histolytica* *Giardia lamblia*	CE-IVD	Unpreserved	Nucleic acids extraction Real-time PCR
	RIDA®GENE Bacterial Stool Panel	4	*Campylobacter* species *Salmonella* species STEC *stx1/stx2* *Shigella*/EIEC	CE-IVD	Unpreserved	Nucleic acids extraction Real-time PCR
	RIDA®GENE Viral Stool Panel I	4	Adenovirus F 40/41 Astrovirus Norovirus GI/GII Rotavirus A	CE-IVD	Unpreserved	Nucleic acids extraction*** Real-time PCR
	RIDA®GENE Viral Stool Panel II	3	Adenovirus F 40/41 Astrovirus Rotavirus A	CE-IVD	Unpreserved	Nucleic acids extraction Real-time PCR

Continued

Manufac-turer	Test Name	Number of Patho-gens	Pathogens	Regulatory Status	Stool Specimen	Methodology
Savyon Diagnos-tics	NanoCHIP® GIP (Gas-trointestinal Panel) Combi I	8	Salmonella species Shigella species Campylobacter species C. difficile STEC Cryptosporidium species Entamoeba histolytica Giardia lamblia	CE-IVD	Unpre-served Preserved	DNA extraction PCR, microarray hybridization
	NanoCHIP® GIP (Gas-trointestinal Panel) Combi II	9	Salmonella species Shigella species Campylobacter species Blastocystis hominis Cryptosporidium species Dientamoeba fragilis Entamoeba histolytica Entamoeba dispar Giardia lamblia	CE-IVD	Unpre-served Preserved	DNA extraction PCR, microarray hybridization
	NanoCHIP® GIP Parasites Panel I	6	Blastocystis hominis Cryptosporidium species Dientamoeba fragilis Entamoeba histolytica Entamoeba dispar Giardia lamblia	CE-IVD	Unpre-served Preserved	DNA extraction PCR, microarray hybridization
AusDiag-nostics	Fecal patho-gens M	15	Campylobacter species C. difficile (toxin B) Aeromonas hydrophila Salmonella species Shigella species Yersinia species EIEC STEC Adenovirus F and G Astrovirus Norovirus GI/GII Rotavirus A Cryptosporidium species Entamoeba histolytica Giardia lamblia	CE-IVD	Unpre-served	DNA extraction Multiplex-tandem PCR

TABLE 13.2
Select Commercially Available Molecular Methods for Detection of Gastrointestinal Pathogens—cont'd

Manufacturer	Test Name	Number of Pathogens	Pathogens	Regulatory Status	Stool Specimen	Methodology
	Enteric viruses	7	Adenovirus F and G Astrovirus Norovirus GI/GII Rotavirus A Sapovirus Enterovirus types A/B/C/D	CE-IVD	Unpreserved	DNA extraction Multiplex-tandem PCR
	Parasites	7	*Blastocystis hominis* *Cryptosporidium* species *Dientamoeba fragilis* *Entamoeba histolytica* *Cyclospora cayetanensis* *Giardia* species *Giardia lamblia*	CE-IVD	Unpreserved	DNA extraction Multiplex-tandem PCR
	Faecal bacteria and parasites	7	*Campylobacter* species *Salmonella/Shigella* species STEC *stx1/stx2* *E. coli* O157 *Cryptosporidium* species *Entamoeba histolytica* *Giardia lamblia*	CE-IVD	Unpreserved	DNA extraction Multiplex-tandem PCR
Great Basin Scientific, Inc	Great Basin Stool Bacterial Pathogen Panel (SBPP)	6	*Campylobacter* species *Salmonella* species Shiga toxin 1 (stx1) Shiga toxin 2 (stx2) *E. coli* O157 *Shigella* species	CE-IVD	Preserved	DNA extraction Multiplex-tandem PCR
Diagenode S.A.	G-DiaNota™	2	Norovirus GI/GII Rotavirus A	CE-IVD	Unpreserved	Nucleic acids extraction Real-time PCR
	G-DiaBact™	2	*Salmonella enterica* *Campylobacter jejuni*	CE-IVD	Unpreserved	Nucleic acids extraction Real-time PCR
	G-DiaPara™	3	*Cryptosporidium parvum* *Entamoeba histolytica* *Giardia lamblia*	CE-IVD	Unpreserved	Nucleic acids extraction Real-time PCR

EAEC, Enteroaggregative *E. coli*; *EIEC*, Enteroinvasive *E. coli*; *EPEC*, Enteropathogenic *E. coli*; *STEC*, Shiga toxin producing *E.coli*.

TABLE 13.3
Selected Molecular Commercial Assays for Clostridium difficile

Manufacturer	Name	Target	Workflow	Methodology
BD Diagnostics	BD MAX Cdiff Assay	Toxin B	Sample to results	Real-time PCR
	BD GeneOhm Cdiff Assay	Toxin B	DNA extraction Amplification	Real-time PCR
Cepheid	Xpert *C. difficile*	Toxin B	Sample to results	Real-time PCR
	Xpert *C. difficile*/Epi	Toxin B Binary toxin tcdC nt 117	Sample to results	Real-time PCR
Diagenode Diagnostics	G-DiaDiff™	Toxin A Toxin B	DNA extraction Amplification	Real-time PCR
Focus Diagnostics, Inc.	Simplexa *C. difficile* Universal Direct Assay	Toxin B	Sample to results	Real-time PCR
GenePOC, Inc.	GenePOC CDiff	Toxin B	Sample to results	Real-time PCR
Great Basin Scientific, Inc.	Portrait Toxigenic *C. difficile* Assay	Toxin B	Sample to results	Helicase-dependent amplification
Intelligent Medical Devices, Inc.	IMDx *C. difficile* for Abbott m200	Toxin A Toxin B	DNA extraction Amplification	Real-time PCR
Luminex Molecular Diagnostics, Inc.	Aries *C. difficile* complete	Toxin A Toxin B	Sample to results	Real-time PCR
	Verigene *C. difficile* test	Toxin A Toxin B Binary toxin Tcdc nt 117	Sample to results	PCR amplification Gold nanoparticle probe-based end-point detection
Meridian Biosciences, Inc.	Illumigene *C. difficile* DNA Amplification	Toxin A Toxin B	Sample preparation Amplification	Loop mediated isothermal DNA amplification
Primera Dx	ICEPlex *C. difficile* kit	Toxin B	DNA extraction Amplification	Real-time PCR
Prodesse, Inc.	ProGastro Cd Assay	Toxin B	DNA extraction Amplification	Real-time PCR
Qiagen GmbH	Artus *C. difficile* QS-RGQ MDX kit	Toxin A Toxin B	DNA extraction Amplification	Real-time PCR
Quidel Corp.	Quidel Molecular Direct *C. difficile* Assay	Toxin A Toxin B	Sample preparation Amplification	Real-time PCR
	Solona *C. difficile* Assay	Toxin A	Sample to results	Helicase-dependent amplification
	AmpliVue *C. difficile* Assay	Toxin A Toxin B	Sample preparation Amplification	Helicase-dependent amplification
R-BioPharm	RIDA®GENE Astrovirus	16S-rDNA Toxin A Toxin B	DNA extraction Amplification	Real-time PCR

TABLE 13.3
Selected Molecular Commercial Assays for Clostridium difficile—cont'd

Manufacturer	Name	Target	Workflow	Methodology
Roche Molecular Systems, Inc	Cobas Cdiff Nucleic Acid Test For Use On The Cobas Liat System	Toxin B	Sample to results	Real-time PCR
	Cobas Cdiff Nucleic Acid Test For Use On The Cobas 4800 System	Toxin B	DNA extraction Amplification	Real-time PCR
Savyon Diagnostics	NanoCHIP *Clostridium difficile* Panel	GDH Toxin A Toxin B	DNA extraction Amplification	PCR, microarray hybridization

TABLE 13.4
Select Target Specific Commercial Assays

Manufacturer	Name	Status	Methodology
Altona	RealStar® Adenovirus PCR kit	US RUO	Real-time PCR
		CE-IVD	TaqMan probes
	RealStar® EHEC PCR kit	US RUO	Real-time PCR
		CE-IVD	TaqMan probes
	RealStar® Norovirus PCR kit	US RUO	Real-time PCR
		CE-IVD	TaqMan probes
	RealStar® Rotavirus PCR kit	US RUO	Real-time PCR
		CE-IVD	TaqMan probes
bioMerieux	Adenovirus R-Gene	US RUO	Real-time PCR
		CE-IVD	TaqMan probes
Cepheid	Xpert Norovirus	US IVD	Real-time PCR
		CE-IVD	TaqMan probes
ELITechGroup	MGB Alert Adenovirus Primer Mix MGB Alert Adenovirus Probe Mix	ASR	Real-time PCR Minor groove binder probes
	Norovirus 2.0 Detection regent mix	US RUO	Real-time PCR Minor groove binder probes
	Parechovirus Detection reagent mix	US RUO	Real-time PCR Minor groove binder probes
	Salmonella typhoid	US RUO	Real-time PCR Minor groove binder probes
	Salmonella paratyphoid	US RUO	Real-time PCR Minor groove binder probes

Continued

TABLE 13.4
Select Target Specific Commercial Assays—cont'd

Manufacturer	Name	Status	Methodology
Luminex	Adenovirus MultiCode	ASR	Real-time PCR
			Labeled primers
	Aries Norovirus	CE-IVD	Real-time PCR
		US-IVD	Labeled primers
R-BioPharm	RIDA®GENE Astrovirus	CE-IVD	Real-time PCR
			TaqMan probes
	RIDA®GENE Norovirus GI/GII	US IVD	Real-time PCR
		CE-IVD	TaqMan probes
	RIDA®GENE Rotavirus	CE-IVD	Real-time PCR
			TaqMan probes
	RIDA®GENE Sapovirus	CE-IVD	Real-time PCR
			TaqMan probes
	RIDA®GENE Enterovirus	CE-IVD	Real-time PCR
			TaqMan probes
	RIDA®GENE *Entamoeba histolytica*	CE-IVD	Real-time PCR
			TaqMan probes
	RIDA®GENE *Dientamoeba fragilis*	CE-IVD	Real-time PCR
			TaqMan probes
	RIDA®GENE EAEC	CE-IVD	Real-time PCR
			TaqMan probes
Savyon Diagnostics	Savvygen™ GI-Rotavirus	CE-IVD	Real-time PCR
			TaqMan probes
	Savvygen™ GI-Astrovirus	CE-IVD	Real-time PCR
			TaqMan probes
	Savvygen™ GI-Adenovirus	CE-IVD	Real-time PCR
			TaqMan probes
	Savvygen™ GI-Norovirus I	CE-IVD	Real-time PCR
			TaqMan probes
	Savvygen™ GI-Norovirus II	CE-IVD	Real-time PCR
			TaqMan probes
	Savvygen™ GI-Giardia	CE-IVD	Real-time PCR
			TaqMan probes
	Savvygen™ GI-Entamoeba	CE-IVD	Real-time PCR
			TaqMan probes
	Savvygen™ GI-Campylobacter	CE-IVD	Real-time PCR
			TaqMan probes
	Savvygen™ GI-Shigella/EIEC	CE-IVD	Real-time PCR
			TaqMan probes
	Savvygen™ GI-Salmonella	CE-IVD	Real-time PCR
			TaqMan probes

differentiating among serotypes, except in some instance E. coli O157:H7, in which case additional genes (e.g., rfbEO157: perosamine synthase) are targeted.[17,18]

Molecular multiplex methods have also been developed to additionally detect other diarrheagenic E. coli including enteropathogenic E. coli (EPEC), enteroaggregative E. coli (EAEC), enterotoxigenic E. coli (ETEC), enteroinvasive E. coli (EIEC), and enterohemorrhagic E. coli (EHEC).[19-22] In all assays, primers and/or probes are designed to target virulence factors unique to each strain of E. coli: aatA/aggR (EAEC), elt/est (EHEC), ipaH (EIEC), eaeA (EPEC), stIa/stIb (ETEC), followed by detection of amplified DNA by either gel electrophoresis in older studies[20,21] and more recently by melt-curve analysis or use of specific hydrolysis probes.[19,22] The reported analytical performance of molecular methods ranged from 300 CFU to 10,000 CFU/mL depending on the assay and the targets.[19,21] Molecular methods have the added advantage of facilitating the correct classification of diarrheagenic E. coli, which can be challenging using culture and serological methods. Although some commercial reagents are available for the specific molecular detection of some diarrheagenic E. coli (Table 13.4), detection of these toxins producing E. coli by commercial methods occurs primarily as part of large syndromic panel (Table 13.2) as described further in the text.

Vibrio *and* Yersinia

Fewer assays have been developed for the molecular detection of Vibrio species and Yersinia enterocolitica directly from clinical samples. Several species of Vibrio may cause gastrointestinal infections with three species including V. parahaemolyticus, V. vulnificus, and V. cholerae being responsible for most cases of gastroenteritis. Diagnosis of Vibrio gastroenteritis requires high clinical suspicion based on exposure history and thus testing for Vibrio species may not be part of routine stool culture. Molecular assays for Vibrio species have been designed to either detect the most common pathogenic Vibrio species[23,24] or focus primarily on V. cholera[25,26] with many of these assays used for both clinical and environmental testing.

Similarly, a high clinical suspicion is needed for a diagnosis of Yersinia enterocolitica. A few studies have reported assays based on the detection of various genes including the 16S rRNA, ail gene, foxA, and yst genes to identify either or both pathogenic and nonpathogenic strains of Y. enterocolitica on either bacterial isolates or directly from stool samples.[27-29] More recently, both Vibrio species (including V. cholerae) and Yersinia enterocolitica have been included as targets in most commercially available gastrointestinal pathogens molecular panels (Table 13.2).

Clostridium difficile

In the last few years, several commercial assays have become available for the molecular diagnosis of C. difficile infection (CDI) (Table 13.3). Nucleic acids amplification tests for molecular diagnosis of C. difficile infections are based on a range of techniques including PCR, real-time PCR, loop-mediated isothermal amplification and helicase-dependent amplification with many of these assays primarily target C. difficile toxin B (tcdB) gene (Table 13.3). Other gene targets used for C. difficile molecular testings includes the toxin A gene (tcdA), the cdt/tcdC gene and the nucleotide (nt) 117 deletion, which may further provide strain type information, specifically strain NAP1/027/BI.[30]

Testing by molecular methods provides the highest analytical sensitivity for the detection of C. difficile. Most studies comparing detection of C. difficile by molecular assays to detection by EIA show a significant increase in sensitivity, ranging from 77% to 100% and 90% to 100% depending on the method used as the gold standard, either toxigenic culture or cell culture cytotoxicity neutralization (CYT) assays.[31] The CYT assay, which is often considered the gold standard for CDI diagnosis, as it detects the presence of preformed toxins present in stool samples, has reported sensitivity as low as 56%[32] and is technically challenging to perform. Hence, testing algorithms are often used that take advantages of the high sensitivity of glutamate dehydrogenase (GDH), an antigen present in abundance in both toxigenic and nontoxigenic C. difficile, and/or molecular tests and the high specificity of toxin A/B antigen tests to improve the overall diagnosis of CDI. These include two-step and three-step algorithms using various combination of toxin A/B EIA, GDH EIA, CYT, and PCR.[33-36] In a study by Babady et al., a testing algorithm comprising the GDH EIA test followed by the Xpert PCR had a sensitivity of 100% compared to a sensitivity of 61% for an algorithm of GDH followed by CYT.[37] In another study, the sensitivity of an algorithm that included GDH EIA followed by PCR had a lower sensitivity at 86.1%, highlighting differences in study population and gold standard to evaluate assay performances.[38]

The clinical significance of this increased sensitivity, however, has recently been challenged given the increased detection of asymptomatic carriage or colonization.[39] Thus, the use of algorithm that includes testing for Clostridium antigens including GDH and/or toxin A/toxin B prior to testing by molecular methods is one of the approaches that is recommended in the most recent guidelines from the Infectious Diseases Society of America (IDSA).[40] Therefore, interpretation of the C. difficile molecular tests results should be done in the correct clinical presentation.

Viral Infections

Norovirus

Norovirus is a nonenveloped, RNA virus and a recognized cause of community acquired gastroenteritis. The first molecular assays for the diagnosis of Norovirus were made possible by the increased availability of Norovirus genome sequences. Many LDT for norovirus target the open reading frame 1 (ORF1) region or the ORF1-ORF2 junction regions, with the latter showing increased sensitivity and inclusivity for most norovirus genotypes.[41,42] Other targets have been used for LDTs including the nonstructural polyprotein gene.[43] Although most LDT today are based on real-time PCR to identify and or differentiate the GI and GII Norovirus genotypes, other assays have been developed for more inclusivity, identifying genotype group 4 (GIV) as well.[44,45]

Several assays and reagents are commercially available for the rapid diagnosis of gastroenteritis caused by Norovirus (Table 13.4). In the United States, two of these assays are cleared by the United States Food and Drug Administration (US FDA) for in vitro diagnostics, the Xpert Norovirus and the RIDA GENE Norovirus GI/GII assay. The Xpert Norovirus (Cepheid) is a sample-to-result, qualitative, real-time reverse transcriptase polymerase chain reaction (RT-PCR) to detect norovirus RNA on the GeneXpert instrument. The assay was FDA-cleared in 2014 and is also CE-IVD marked for the detection and differentiation of norovirus genotype I and II. The Xpert Norovirus was developed for the rapid diagnosis of norovirus gastroenteritis in both routine clinical care and during outbreak investigations. A few studies have evaluated the performance of the Xpert Norovirus compared to LDT real-time PCRs.[46–49] In a multicenter study, the performance of the Xpert Norovirus was evaluated on fresh and frozen stool samples using a combination of the CDC real-time reverse transcription PCR assays and bidirectional sequencing as the reference standard.[46] The authors reported a positive percent agreement of 98.3% and 99.4% for GI and GII respectively and a negative percent agreement of 98.1% and 98.2% for GI and GII, respectively. While the negative predictive value of the assay in that study where the prevalence of Norovirus was 9.9% was 100% and 99.9% for GI and GII, respectively, the positive predictive value was lower at 75% for GI and 86.5% for GII, suggesting that the assay is excellent to rule-out norovirus infections but a positive sample should be interpreted in the right clinical context.[46] Henningsson and colleagues evaluated the performance of the Xpert Norovirus on both stool and vomitus samples compared to an in-house RT-PCR assay in three hospitals in Sweden.[49] The sensitivity and specificity of the Xpert

Norovirus assay was 100% and 93% respectively with a median TAT of 2.4 h, a significant decrease from the median TAT of 22 h prior to the implementation of the Xpert Norovirus assay.

The RIDA GENE Norovirus GI/GII assay (R-Biopharm, Darmstadt, Germany) is a qualitative RT-PCR to detect norovirus genogroup I (GI) and II (GII) RNA. The assay is cleared for testing on the Applied Biosystems 7500 Fast Dx System and is intended for use on raw or unpreserved stool samples to diagnose norovirus gastroenteritis in both sporadic and outbreak settings. In one study, both the sensitivity and the specificity of the RIDA GENE assay were reported at 98%, however, the sensitivity of the assay was lower for the GI genotype compared to the sensitivity for the GII genotype (85% vs. 100%).[50] The RIDA GENE Norovirus GI/GII has a longer TAT to results than the Xpert Norovirus at 4 h versus 1 h. The potential drawback of molecular assays is that asymptomatic shedding of virus after clinical disease may complicate positive test results for norovirus.

Adenovirus

Molecular diagnosis of human adenovirus (HAdV) can be challenging given the high number of recognized genotypes. Based on serological and sequencing methods, up to seven species (A–G) and more than 70 types of HAdV have been characterized to date.[51] Community onset gastroenteritis are caused primarily by HAdV species F, types 40/41 (HAdV F40/41). In immunocompromised hosts, HAdV is also frequently recovered but gastrointestinal infection is not limited to genotypes 40/41.[52,53] As more adenovirus genotypes are being identified, molecular assays targeting HAdv need to be inclusive of all genotypes.[54]

There are currently no single-plex US IVD cleared tests for testing of HAdV in stool samples. LDT for HAdV detection targets primarily the hexon gene,[55–58] although other genes including the penton base gene[59] and the fiber gene[60] have been used. Achieving efficient amplifications and quantifications of all serotypes may be difficult with one set of primers and as such, some LDT methods use multiple primers and probes to ensure detection of all possible genotypes.[57]

A few kits (RUO and ASR in the United States or CE-IVD) are commercially available for the detection of HAdV.[61,62] These assays perform comparably to LDT when tested on stool samples with agreement greater than 90% in most cases but with the added advantage of standardizing performance across laboratories, which is particularly important for quantitative PCRs. Additionally, ASR reagents are available to facilitates the development of LDTs (Table 13.4). This is particularly important, as many of the new syndromic panel for GI pathogens only include the enteric HAdV genotypes F40/41, which are responsible for most but not all adenoviral gastrointestinal infections. Thus additional testing using pan-adenoviral PCR is necessary.

Rotavirus

Rotaviruses are segmented, double stranded RNA viruses that are responsible for gastroenteritis in children under 5 years of age, although infections in adults occurs as well. Until recently, diagnosis of rotavirus infections was accomplished primarily through detection of rotavirus antigens. Several molecular methods including both conventional and real-time reverse-transcription (RT) PCRs targeting either the NSP3 or VP genes have been developed over the years to increase the sensitivity and specificity of rotavirus diagnosis compared to antigens assays.[63,64] While conventional RT-PCRs were cumbersome and susceptible to amplicon contamination, real-time PCR offered the advantage of simplifying detection, significantly increasing sensitivity and specificity with the added advantage of offering strain typing if designed accordingly.[63,65,66] A couple of molecular assays are commercially available for the targeted diagnosis of rotavirus (Table 13.4) but peer-reviewed publications evaluating their performance are lacking.

Astrovirus and Sapovirus

In addition to the viruses described above, other viruses including astroviruses and sapoviruses cause viral gastroenteritis, mainly in children and immunocompromised hosts. Both viruses have single-stranded RNA genomes and molecular methods are the preferred method to detect their presence in clinical samples. Real-time RT PCR with primers and probes targeting the capsid gene (astrovirus) or the RNA polymerase/capsid genes junction (sapovirus) have been developed, with analytical sensitivity of 0.0026 IU/μL or 76 copies/100 μg for astrovirus[67,68] and 10–25 copies/reaction for sapovirus.[69,70] As is the case for rotavirus detection, a couple of molecular assays are commercially available for the targeted diagnosis of astrovirus and sapovirus (Table 13.4) but peer-reviewed publications evaluating their performance are lacking.

Parasitic Infections

Enteric parasites are detected most commonly by use of microscopic examination (ova and Parasites (OVP) Exam). In addition to OVP, rapid antigen tests that are simpler to perform, requiring only minimal manipulation and providing results in 15–30 min, are available

for a few parasites including *Cryptosporidium species, Entamoeba histolytica, Giardia lamblia.* Although parasitic infections causing gastrointestinal infections account for high morbidity, particularly in developing countries, fewer molecular methods have been developed for their rapid diagnosis, which still relies heavily on OVP exams. This may be due in part to the limited availability of specialized laboratory facilities, high costs of instrumentations and reagents and limited expertise needed to develop molecular methods in countries where these assays would have the highest impact.[71] A few commercial reagents are available to facilitate the development of molecular assays for common enteric GI parasites including *Entamoeba, Giardia* and *Cryptosporidium* species (Table 13.4). Molecular diagnosis of helminth infections however, relies primarily on laboratory-developed tests. Several targets are used for the detection of GI parasites including the small subunit ribosomal DNA, intergenic spacer (IGS) regions, β-giardin and triosephosphate isomerase.[72] Molecular methods for GI parasites offer increased sensitivity and specificity (ranges 90%–100%), especially in cases where differentiation of pathogenic and nonpathogenic organisms cannot be done solely based on microscopic examination or antigen tests (e.g., *Entamoeba histolytica* vs. *Entamoeba dispar*).

Syndromic Panels

One of the first IVD cleared gastrointestinal syndromic molecular assays was the xTAG Gastrointestinal Pathogen Panel (Luminex Corp, Austin, TX). The GPP panel includes the following 15 targets: *Salmonella* species, *Shigella* species, *Campylobacter* species, *Clostridium difficile* (toxin A/toxin B), STEC, ETEC, *Vibrio cholera, Yersinia enterolitica,* adenovirus 40/41, noroviruses (Group GI and GII), rotavirus A, *Giardia lamblia, Entamoeba histolytica,* and *Cryptosporidium* species. The xTAG GPP is a four-step process starting with pretreatment of stool samples, extraction, amplification, hybridization, and detection. A few studies have been published on various versions of the xTAG GPP assay.[73–78] In general, the detection rate in the aforementioned studies ranged between 30% and 40% with a small percentage of positive results not confirmed by alternative methods. The results of the clinical trials for the assay reported a sensitivity greater than 90% (except for *Salmonella* spp. with a sensitivity of 84.6%) and a specificity greater than 95% for all targets evaluated.[79] In one of the first study published on the xTAG GPP, the performance of the assays was evaluated against both conventional methods (culture, microscopy, and EIA) and laboratory-developed single-plex real-time PCRs.[76] The overall sensitivity and specificity of the xTAG GPP assay was greater than 94% and 98%, respectively. However, performance of the xTAG GPP varied depending on the target, ranging from 83.3% for *E. coli* O157% to 100% for many of the other targets on the panel. This first study by Claas revealed several advantages of a syndromic panels over conventional methods: (1) detection of an alternate pathogen than the one requested by the clinician in 65% of samples tested, (2) detection of coinfections in 9.5% of samples and (3) a TAT of 5 h for detecting 15 targets compared to hours to days with conventional methods.[76] Of note, the sensitivity for Adenovirus 40/41 was only 20% when compared to a pan-Adenovirus real-time PCR. The authors suggested that the low sensitivity was due to the fact the xTAG only targeted genotypes 40/41. This limitation was highlighted in a recent study showing that Adenovirus type C/2 was the most common type recovered in stool samples of an oncology patient population followed by Adenovirus type F40/41.[80] Hence, molecular tests need to be more inclusive of other Adenovirus genotypes.

The performance of the xTAG GPP has been evaluated in several other studies against conventional methods and other multiplexed gastrointestinal panels.[77,81–87] In general, the sensitivity of the xTAG GPP was higher than most conventional methods, greater than 90% for most targets with a significantly higher detection of mixed infections ranging from 10% to 35% compared to culture and EIA, especially in immunocompromised hosts and pediatric patients.

A second assay, the ProGastro SSCS assay (Gen-Probe Incorporated, San Diego, USA), which detects and differentiates between *Salmonella*, *Shigella*, *Campylobacter* (*C. jejuni* and *C. coli* only), and Shiga Toxin-producing *Escherichia coli*, was also FDA cleared in 2013. The ProGastro SSCS is a two-step assay and includes a nucleic acids extraction and an amplification by real-time PCR. In one study, the ProGastro SSCS was 100% sensitive for all targets with specificity ranging from 99.4% to 100% when compared to culture and EIA with bidirectional sequencing for discrepant analysis.[88] Similar to the xTAG GPP, the use of the ProGastro SSCS increased the overall detection of pathogens from 5.6% by culture and 8.3% by EIA. However, different from the xTAG GPP, the ProGastro SSCS only targets bacterial pathogens, requiring additional testing for the detection of viral and parasitic pathogens. As the ProGastro SSCS is a real-time PCR assay, it has advantages over the xTAG GPP including no postamplification manipulations of amplified nucleic acids and a simplified workflow. Kahlau and colleagues compared the performance of the ProGastro assay to xTAG GPP on

a few samples with high concordance, 27/29 samples, suggesting similar performance of molecular panels for common targets.[77]

Similar to the ProGastro SSCS, the BD Max Enteric Bacterial Panel (EBP, BD Diagnostics, Sparks, MD), only targets bacterial pathogens including *Salmonella* sp., *Campylobacter jejuni*, *Campylobacter coli*, *Shigella* sp., and the stx_{1a} and stx_{2a} genes in Shiga-toxin-producing *E. coli* and *Shigella dysenteriae*. The assay is based on real-time PCR and is a walkaway platform that process and amplify up to 24 samples in approximately 3 h. In a multicenter study, the BD Max EBP was compared to culture and EIA and showed an overall positive and negative percent agreement of 97.1% and 99.2% for *Salmonella* spp., 99.1% and 99.7% for *Shigella* spp., 97.2% and 98.4% for *C. jejuni* and *C. coli*, and 97.4% and 99.3% for Shiga toxins.[89] Knabl et al. reported lower positive percent agreement in their cohort for *Salmonella* spp. and Shiga toxins at 75% and 88%, respectively, while negative percent agreements were similarly high for all targets.[90] Although the BD Max EBP is IVD cleared for testing on fresh and perseuved stool samples, one study evaluated its performance on rectal swabs collected from pediatric patients compared to bacterial culture and Shiga-toxin EIA.[91] Performance characteristics were like those established on stool samples, with positive percent agreement of 100% for all targets and negative percent agreement ranging from 95.3% to 100%. An extended BD Max EBP (xEBP) panel was subsequently released, which additionally test for *Yersinia enterocolitica*, ETEC, *Vibrio* (*Vibrio parahaemolyticus*, *Vibrio cholerae*, and *Vibrio vulnificus*), and *Plesiomonas shigelloides*. The BD Max xEBP uses a separate master mix than the EBP and is essentially a second assay that can be run concurrently with the EBP on the BD Max platform. The BD Max xEBP showed a high correlation (kappa, 0.97; 95% CI, 0.95–0.98) with conventional methods (culture and/or PCR) with overall positive and negative percent agreement, respectively, of 97.6% and 99.8% for ETEC, 100% and 99.7% for *Vibrio*; 99.0% and 99.9% for *Y. enterocolitica*, and 100% and 99.8% for *P. shigelloides*.[92]

In addition to the EBP and xEBP, an Enteric Parasite Panel (EPP) that identifies *Giardia intestinalis*, *Entamoeba histolytica*, and *Cryptosporidium* spp. (*C. hominis* and *C. parvum*) is available from BD Diagnostics. The BD Max EPP allows the differentiation *Entamoeba histolytica* from *Entamoeba dispar* that cannot be accomplished by microscopy and may be challenging when using antigen assays. Several studies have evaluated the performance of the EPP using either microscopy or laboratory-developed molecular assays as the comparator methods.[93-97] In one study, the performance of the EPP compared to microscopy and LDT PCR was excellent for *E. histolytica* and *Cryptosporidium* species (100%) but sensitivity for *Giardia intestinalis* was lower at 67%.[95] A follow-up study by the same group[93] further challenged the performance of the EPP for *Giardia intestinalis* by testing a larger number of positive samples and found a higher sensitivity of 98%, a result in line with other studies that used the current version of the assay with an optimized software analysis that improved interpretation of positive samples.[94,96,97]

The Verigene Enteric Pathogens Nucleic Acid Test (EP) (Nanosphere/Luminex Inc.) targets both bacterial and viral pathogens including *Campylobacter* species (*C. coli, C. jejuni, and C. lari*), Shiga toxin producing *E coli* (STEC: Shiga toxin I gene and Shiga toxin 2), *Salmonella* species, *Shigella* species (*S. dysenteriae, S. boydii, S. sonnei, and S. flexneri*), *Vibrio* species (*V. cholerae* and *V. parahaemolyticus*) and *Yersinia enterocolitica*, Rotavirus, and Norovirus (GI/GII). The Verigene platform is an automated system, with sample-to-answer, microarray format that includes three steps: RT, PCR, and array hybridization. End-point detection of amplified nucleic acids occurs through a two-step process including first, capture of the amplified product by oligonucleotides bound to the microarray followed by binding by of a mediator oligonucleotide that subsequently binds gold nanoparticle probe. The resulting complex is enhanced through addition of silver, and the gold-silver aggregates are detected through scatter light. The EP system includes two instruments, the Processor (SP) for automated extraction, amplification, and hybridization of the amplified product to gold nanoparticles and the Reader, which analyzes data in approximately 2 h. Huang et al. compared the performance of the Verigene EP assay to that of Luminex GPP and the BioFire GP assays.[82] The sensitivities and specificities of the Verigene EP assays for each target was 83.3% and 99.3% for *Campylobacter* species; 83.3% and 100% for *Salmonella* species; 95.4% and 99.1% for *Shigella* species; 91.7% and 100% for STEC; 89.0% and 100% for Norovirus; and 71.4% and 100% for Rotavirus.

The largest multiplex gastrointestinal panel that is commercially available is the BioFire GP assay that targets 22 pathogens including 13 bacteria (*Campylobacter* species, *C. difficile, E. coli* O157, EPEC, EAEC, ETEC, STEC, *Salmonella* species and *Shigella* species/Enteroinvasive *E. coli*, *Vibrio* species, *Vibrio cholera*, *Yersinia enterocolitica*, *Plesiomonas shigelloides*), five viruses (Adenovirus 40/41, Rotavirus, Norovirus GI/GII, Astrovirus, and Sapovirus), and four parasites (*Giardia intestinalis, Entamoeba histolytica, Cyclospora cayetanensis*, and *Cryptosporidium* species).

A few studies have evaluated the performance of the Bio-Fire GPP assay,[83,98-101] including a head-to-head comparison with other multiplexed GI panels.[83,100] Overall, the BioFire GP had comparable or better performance to other panels, with results being concordant (>90%) for many of the targets common to all panels.[83,85,102] Differences may be observed across targets and across different population tested (e.g., pediatric and immunocompromised patients).

CONCLUSIONS

Molecular methods are providing rapid and more sensitive diagnostic tools for gastrointestinal infections. The increased options for commercial tests have further facilitated the implementation of these molecular methods in many clinical laboratories, not just large references laboratories. Furthermore, with the increased use of syndromic gastrointestinal panels, new knowledge on the distribution and clinical significance of many pathogens is emerging. However, some limitations of molecular assays should be noted: (1) exclusive reliance on molecular methods results in a lack of bacterial isolates needed for susceptibility testing or public health purpose including epidemiological testing, (2) given that molecular assays are targeted to specific pathogens, the current designs are not inclusive of all possible etiologies of GI infections, (3) clinical outcome studies on the impact of molecular method tests results in various patient populations are still limited, (4) compared to conventional methods, molecular methods are often more expensive. However, despite these limitations, the simplicity and increased sensitivity of molecular methods makes them useful diagnostics tools for gastrointestinal infections.

REFERENCES

1. Dalys GBD, Collaborators H, Murray CJ, et al. Global, regional, and national disability-adjusted life years (DALYs) for 306 diseases and injuries and healthy life expectancy (HALE) for 188 countries, 1990-2013: quantifying the epidemiological transition. *Lancet*. 2015;386(10009):2145–2191.
2. Organization WH. The Top 10 Causes of Death. http://www.who.int/mediacentre/factsheets/fs310/en/.
3. Scallan E, Griffin PM, Angulo FJ, Tauxe RV, Hoekstra RM. Foodborne illness acquired in the United States–unspecified agents. *Emerg Infect Dis*. 2011;17(1):16–22.
4. Shane AL, Mody RK, Crump JA, et al. 2017 infectious diseases society of America clinical practice guidelines for the diagnosis and management of infectious diarrhea. *Clin Infect Dis*. 2017;65(12):1963–1973.

5. Shane AL, Mody RK, Crump JA, et al. 2017 infectious diseases society of America clinical practice guidelines for the diagnosis and management of infectious diarrhea. *Clin Infect Dis.* 2017;65(12):e45–e80.

6. LaRocque RC, Calderwood SB. 98-Syndromes of enteric infection A2-Bennett John E. In: Dolin R, Blaser MJ, eds. *Mandell, Douglas, and Bennett's Principles and Practice of Infectious Diseases.* 8th ed. Philadelphia: Content Repository Only!; 2015.

7. Glass RI, Parashar UD, Estes MK. Norovirus gastroenteritis. *N Engl J Med.* 2009;361(18):1776–1785.

8. Bok K, Green KY. Norovirus gastroenteritis in immunocompromised patients. *N Engl J Med.* 2012;367(22):2126–2132.

9. Husain A, Aptaker L, Spriggs DR, Barakat RR. Gastrointestinal toxicity and Clostridium Difficile Diarrhea in patients treated with paclitaxel-containing chemotherapy regimens. *Gynecol Oncol.* 1998;71(1):104–107.

10. Espy MJ, Uhl JR, Sloan LM, et al. Real-time PCR in clinical microbiology: applications for routine laboratory testing. *Clin Microbiol Rev.* 2006;19(1):165–256.

11. Hanson KE, Couturier MR. Multiplexed molecular diagnostics for respiratory, gastrointestinal, and Central nervous system infections. *Clin Infect Dis.* 2016;63(10):1361–1367.

12. Van Lint P, De Witte E, De Henau H, et al. Evaluation of a real-time multiplex PCR for the simultaneous detection of Campylobacter jejuni, Salmonella spp., Shigella spp./EIEC, and Yersinia enterocolitica in fecal samples. *Eur J Clin Microbiol Infect Dis.* 2015;34(3):535–542.

13. Barletta F, Mercado EH, Lluque A, Ruiz J, Cleary TG, Ochoa TJ. Multiplex real-time PCR for detection of Campylobacter, Salmonella, and Shigella. *J Clin Microbiol.* 2013;51(9):2822–2829.

14. Cunningham SA, Sloan LM, Nyre LM, Vetter EA, Mandrekar J, Patel R. Three-hour molecular detection of Campylobacter, Salmonella, Yersinia, and Shigella species in feces with accuracy as high as that of culture. *J Clin Microbiol.* 2010;48(8):2929–2933.

15. Grys TE, Sloan LM, Rosenblatt JE, Patel R. Rapid and sensitive detection of Shiga toxin-producing *Escherichia coli* from nonenriched stool specimens by real-time PCR in comparison to enzyme immunoassay and culture. *J Clin Microbiol.* 2009;47(7):2008–2012.

16. Chui L, Couturier MR, Chiu T, et al. Comparison of Shiga toxin-producing *Escherichia coli* detection methods using clinical stool samples. *J Mol Diagn.* 2010;12(4):469–475.

17. Li B, Liu H, Wang W. Multiplex real-time PCR assay for detection of *Escherichia coli* O157:H7 and screening for non-O157 Shiga toxin-producing *E. coli*. *BMC Microbiol.* 2017;17(1):215.

18. Qin X, Klein EJ, Galanakis E, et al. Real-time PCR assay for detection and differentiation of shiga toxin-producing *Escherichia coli* from clinical samples. *J Clin Microbiol.* 2015;53(7):2148–2153.

19. Souza TB, Lozer DM, Kitagawa SM, Spano LC, Silva NP, Scaletsky IC. Real-time multiplex PCR assay and melting curve analysis for identifying diarrheagenic *Escherichia coli*. *J Clin Microbiol.* 2013;51(3):1031–1033.

20. Vidal M, Kruger E, Duran C, et al. Single multiplex PCR assay to identify simultaneously the six categories of diarrheagenic *Escherichia coli* associated with enteric infections. *J Clin Microbiol.* 2005;43(10):5362–5365.

21. Toma C, Lu Y, Higa N, et al. Multiplex PCR assay for identification of human diarrheagenic *Escherichia coli*. *J Clin Microbiol.* 2003;41(6):2669–2671.

22. Guion CE, Ochoa TJ, Walker CM, Barletta F, Cleary TG. Detection of diarrheagenic *Escherichia coli* by use of melting-curve analysis and real-time multiplex PCR. *J Clin Microbiol.* 2008;46(5):1752–1757.

23. Nhung PH, Ohkusu K, Miyasaka J, Sun XS, Ezaki T. Rapid and specific identification of 5 human pathogenic Vibrio species by multiplex polymerase chain reaction targeted to dnaJ gene. *Diagn Microbiol Infect Dis.* 2007;59(3):271–275.

24. Wei S, Zhao H, Xian Y, Hussain MA, Wu X. Multiplex PCR assays for the detection of Vibrio alginolyticus, Vibrio parahaemolyticus, Vibrio vulnificus, and *Vibrio cholerae* with an internal amplification control. *Diagn Microbiol Infect Dis.* 2014;79(2):115–118.

25. Engku Nur Syafirah EAR, Nurul Najian AB, Foo PC, Mohd Ali MR, Mohamed M, Yean CY. An ambient temperature stable and ready-to-use loop-mediated isothermal amplification assay for detection of toxigenic *Vibrio cholerae* in outbreak settings. *Acta Trop.* 2018;182:223–231.

26. Greig DR, Hickey TJ, Boxall MD, et al. A real-time multiplex PCR for the identification and typing of *Vibrio cholerae*. *Diagn Microbiol Infect Dis.* 2018;90(3):171–176.

27. Wang JZ, Duan R, Liang JR, et al. Real-time TaqMan PCR for Yersinia enterocolitica detection based on the ail and foxA genes. *J Clin Microbiol.* 2014;52(12):4443–4444.

28. Ibrahim A, Liesack W, Griffiths MW, Robins-Browne RM. Development of a highly specific assay for rapid identification of pathogenic strains of Yersinia enterocolitica based on PCR amplification of the Yersinia heat-stable enterotoxin gene (yst). *J Clin Microbiol.* 1997;35(6):1636–1638.

29. Wannet WJ, Reessink M, Brunings HA, Maas HM. Detection of pathogenic Yersinia enterocolitica by a rapid and sensitive duplex PCR assay. *J Clin Microbiol.* 2001;39(12):4483–4486.

30. Burnham CA, Carroll KC. Diagnosis of *Clostridium difficile* infection: an ongoing conundrum for clinicians and for clinical laboratories. *Clin Microbiol Rev.* 2013;26(3):604–630.

31. Carroll KC, Buchan BW, Tan S, et al. Multicenter evaluation of the Verigene *Clostridium difficile* nucleic acid assay. *J Clin Microbiol.* 2013;51(12):4120–4125.

32. Delmee M, Van Broeck J, Simon A, Janssens M, Avesani V. Laboratory diagnosis of Clostridium difficile-associated diarrhoea: a plea for culture. *J Med Microbiol.* 2005;54(Pt 2):187–191.

33. Quinn CD, Sefers SE, Babiker W, et al. C. Diff Quik Chek complete enzyme immunoassay provides a reliable first-line method for detection of *Clostridium difficile* in stool specimens. *J Clin Microbiol.* 2010;48(2):603–605.

34. Schmidt ML, Gilligan PH. *Clostridium difficile* testing algorithms: what is practical and feasible? *Anaerobe.* 2009;15(6):270–273.

35. Larson AM, Fung AM, Fang FC. Evaluation of tcdB real-time PCR in a three-step diagnostic algorithm for detection of toxigenic *Clostridium difficile*. *J Clin Microbiol.* 2010;48(1):124–130.

36. Babady NE. Hospital-associated infections. *Microbiol Spectr.* 2016;4(3).

37. Babady NE, Stiles J, Ruggiero P, et al. Evaluation of the Cepheid Xpert *Clostridium difficile* Epi assay for diagnosis of *Clostridium difficile* infection and typing of the NAP1 strain at a cancer hospital. *J Clin Microbiol.* 2010;48(12):4519–4524.

38. Novak-Weekley SM, Marlowe EM, Miller JM, et al. *Clostridium difficile* testing in the clinical laboratory by use of multiple testing algorithms. *J Clin Microbiol.* 2010;48(3):889–893.

39. Polage CR, Gyorke CE, Kennedy MA, et al. Overdiagnosis of *Clostridium difficile* infection in the molecular test Era. *JAMA Intern Med.* 2015;175(11):1792–1801.

40. McDonald LC, Gerding DN, Johnson S, et al. Clinical practice guidelines for *Clostridium difficile* infection in adults and children: 2017 update by the infectious diseases society of America (IDSA) and society for healthcare epidemiology of America (SHEA). *Clin Infect Dis.* 2018;66(7):e1–e48.

41. Vennema H, de Bruin E, Koopmans M. Rational optimization of generic primers used for Norwalk-like virus detection by reverse transcriptase polymerase chain reaction. *J Clin Virol.* 2002;25(2):233–235.

42. Kageyama T, Kojima S, Shinohara M, et al. Broadly reactive and highly sensitive assay for Norwalk-like viruses based on real-time quantitative reverse transcription-PCR. *J Clin Microbiol.* 2003;41(4):1548–1557.

43. Ramanan P, Espy MJ, Khare R, Binnicker MJ. Detection and differentiation of norovirus genogroups I and II from clinical stool specimens using real-time PCR. *Diagn Microbiol Infect Dis.* 2017;87(4):325–327.

44. Trujillo AA, McCaustland KA, Zheng DP, et al. Use of TaqMan real-time reverse transcription-PCR for rapid detection, quantification, and typing of norovirus. *J Clin Microbiol.* 2006;44(4):1405–1412.

45. Logan C, O'Leary JJ, O'Sullivan N. Real-time reverse transcription PCR detection of norovirus, sapovirus and astrovirus as causative agents of acute viral gastroenteritis. *J Virol Methods.* 2007;146(1–2):36–44.

46. Gonzalez MD, Langley LC, Buchan BW, et al. Multicenter evaluation of the Xpert norovirus assay for detection of norovirus genogroups I and II in fecal specimens. *J Clin Microbiol.* 2016;54(1):142–147.

47. Rovida F, Premoli M, Campanini G, Sarasini A, Baldanti F. Evaluation of Xpert(R) Norovirus Assay performance in comparison with real-time RT-PCR in hospitalized adult patients with acute gastroenteritis. *Diagn Microbiol Infect Dis.* 2016;85(4):426–427.

48. Cleary O, McNerney R, Yandle Z, O'Sullivan CE. Evaluation of the Xpert Norovirus assay for the rapid detection of norovirus genogroups I and II in faecal specimens within a routine laboratory setting. *Br J Biomed Sci.* 2017;74(3):144–147.

49. Henningsson AJ, Nilsson Bowers A, Nordgren J, Quttineh M, Matussek A, Haglund S. Rapid diagnosis of acute norovirus-associated gastroenteritis: evaluation of the Xpert Norovirus assay and its implementation as a 24/7 service in three hospitals in Jonkoping County, Sweden. *Eur J Clin Microbiol Infect Dis.* 2017;36(10):1867–1871.

50. Dunbar NL, Bruggink LD, Marshall JA. Evaluation of the RIDAGENE real-time PCR assay for the detection of GI and GII norovirus. *Diagn Microbiol Infect Dis.* 2014;79(3):317–321.

51. Lion T. Adenovirus infections in immunocompetent and immunocompromised patients. *Clin Microbiol Rev.* 2014;27(3):441–462.

52. Babady E. Laboratory diagnosis of infections in cancer patients: challenges and opportunities. *J Clin Microbiol.* 2016;54:2635–2646.

53. Lion T, Kosulin K, Landlinger C, et al. Monitoring of adenovirus load in stool by real-time PCR permits early detection of impending invasive infection in patients after allogeneic stem cell transplantation. *Leukemia.* 2010;24(4):706–714.

54. Kosulin K, Berkowitsch B, Lion T. Modified pan-adenovirus real-time PCR assay based on genome analysis of seventy HAdV types. *J Clin Virol.* 2016;80:60–61.

55. Gu Z, Belzer SW, Gibson CS, Bankowski MJ, Hayden RT. Multiplexed, real-time PCR for quantitative detection of human adenovirus. *J Clin Microbiol.* 2003;41(10):4636–4641.

56. Ebner K, Suda M, Watzinger F, Lion T. Molecular detection and quantitative analysis of the entire spectrum of human adenoviruses by a two-reaction real-time PCR assay. *J Clin Microbiol.* 2005;43(7):3049–3053.

57. Claas EC, Schilham MW, de Brouwer CS, et al. Internally controlled real-time PCR monitoring of adenovirus DNA load in serum or plasma of transplant recipients. *J Clin Microbiol.* 2005;43(4):1738–1744.

58. Heim A, Ebnet C, Harste G, Pring-Akerblom P. Rapid and quantitative detection of human adenovirus DNA by real-time PCR. *J Med Virol.* 2003;70(2):228–239.

59. Buckwalter SP, Teo R, Espy MJ, Sloan LM, Smith TF, Pritt BS. Real-time qualitative PCR for 57 human adenovirus types from multiple specimen sources. *J Clin Microbiol.* 2012;50(3):766–771.

60. Pehler-Harrington K, Khanna M, Waters CR, Henrickson KJ. Rapid detection and identification of human adenovirus species by adenoplex, a multiplex PCR-enzyme hybridization assay. *J Clin Microbiol.* 2004;42(9):4072–4076.

61. Jeulin H, Salmon A, Bordigoni P, Venard V. Comparison of in-house real-time quantitative PCR to the Adenovirus R-Gene kit for determination of adenovirus load in clinical samples. *J Clin Microbiol.* 2010;48(9):3132–3137.

62. Rennert H, Ramrattan G, Chen Z, et al. Evaluation of a human adenovirus viral load assay using the Altona RealStar(R) PCR test. *Diagn Microbiol Infect Dis.* 2018;90(4):257–263.

63. Gautam R, Mijatovic-Rustempasic S, Esona MD, Tam KI, Quaye O, Bowen MD. One-step multiplex real-time RT-PCR assay for detecting and genotyping wild-type group A rotavirus strains and vaccine strains (Rotarix(R) and RotaTeq(R)) in stool samples. *PeerJ*. 2016;4:e1560.

64. Katz EM, Gautam R, Bowen MD. Evaluation of an alternative recombinant thermostable thermus thermophilus (rTth)-Based real-time reverse transcription-PCR kit for detection of rotavirus A. *J Clin Microbiol*. 2017;55(5):1585–1587.

65. De La Cruz Hernandez SI, Anaya Molina Y, Gomez Santiago F, et al. Real-time RT-PCR, a necessary tool to support the diagnosis and surveillance of rotavirus in Mexico. *Diagn Microbiol Infect Dis*. 2018;90(4):272–276.

66. Tong Y, Lee BE, Pang XL. Rapid genotyping of human rotavirus using SYBR green real-time reverse transcription-polymerase chain reaction with melting curve analysis. *World J Virol*. 2015;4(4):365–371.

67. Royuela E, Negredo A, Sanchez-Fauquier A. Development of a one step real-time RT-PCR method for sensitive detection of human astrovirus. *J Virol Methods*. 2006;133(1):14–19.

68. Zhang Z, Mitchell DK, Afflerbach C, et al. Quantitation of human astrovirus by real-time reverse-transcription-polymerase chain reaction to examine correlation with clinical illness. *J Virol Methods*. 2006;134(1–2):190–196.

69. Chan MC, Sung JJ, Lam RK, Chan PK, Lai RW, Leung WK. Sapovirus detection by quantitative real-time RT-PCR in clinical stool specimens. *J Virol Methods*. 2006;134(1–2): 146–153.

70. Oka T, Katayama K, Hansman GS, et al. Detection of human sapovirus by real-time reverse transcription-polymerase chain reaction. *J Med Virol*. 2006;78(10):1347–1353.

71. Wong SS, Fung KS, Chau S, Poon RW, Wong SC, Yuen KY. Molecular diagnosis in clinical parasitology: when and why? *Exp Biol Med*. 2014;239(11):1443–1460.

72. Verweij JJ, Stensvold CR. Molecular testing for clinical diagnosis and epidemiological investigations of intestinal parasitic infections. *Clin Microbiol Rev*. 2014;27(2):371–418.

73. Zboromyrska Y, Hurtado JC, Salvador P, et al. Aetiology of traveller's diarrhoea: evaluation of a multiplex PCR tool to detect different enteropathogens. *Clin Microbiol Infect*. 2014.

74. Mengelle C, Mansuy JM, Prere MF, et al. Simultaneous detection of gastrointestinal pathogens with a multiplex Luminex-based molecular assay in stool samples from diarrhoeic patients. *Clin Microbiol Infect*. 2013;19(10):E458–E465.

75. Wessels E, Rusman LG, van Bussel MJ, Claas EC. Added value of multiplex Luminex Gastrointestinal Pathogen Panel (xTAG(R) GPP) testing in the diagnosis of infectious gastroenteritis. *Clin Microbiol Infect*. 2014;20(3):O182–O187.

76. Claas EC, Burnham CA, Mazzulli T, Templeton K, Topin F. Performance of the xTAG(R) gastrointestinal pathogen panel, a multiplex molecular assay for simultaneous detection of bacterial, viral, and parasitic causes of infectious gastroenteritis. *J Microbiol Biotechnol*. 2013;23(7):1041–1045.

77. Kahlau P, Malecki M, Schildgen V, et al. Utility of two novel multiplexing assays for the detection of gastrointestinal pathogens - a first experience. *SpringerPlus*. 2013;2(1):106.

78. Navidad JF, Griswold DJ, Gradus MS, Bhattacharyya S. Evaluation of Luminex xTAG gastrointestinal pathogen analyte-specific reagents for high-throughput, simultaneous detection of bacteria, viruses, and parasites of clinical and public health importance. *J Clin Microbiol*. 2013;51(9):3018–3024.

79. Dunbar SA, Zhang H, Tang YW. Advanced techniques for detection and identification of microbial agents of gastroenteritis. *Clin Lab Med*. 2013;33(3):527–552.

80. McMillen T, Lee YJ, Kamboj M, Babady NE. Limited diagnostic value of a multiplexed gastrointestinal pathogen panel for the detection of adenovirus infection in an oncology patient population. *J Clin Virol*. 2017;94:37–41.

81. Deng J, Luo X, Wang R, et al. A comparison of Luminex xTAG(R) Gastrointestinal Pathogen Panel (xTAG GPP) and routine tests for the detection of enteropathogens circulating in Southern China. *Diagn Microbiol Infect Dis*. 2015;83(3):325–330.

82. Huang RS, Johnson CL, Pritchard L, Hepler R, Ton TT, Dunn JJ. Performance of the Verigene(R) enteric pathogens test, Biofire FilmArray gastrointestinal panel and Luminex xTAG(R) gastrointestinal pathogen panel for detection of common enteric pathogens. *Diagn Microbiol Infect Dis*. 2016;86(4):336–339.

83. Khare R, Espy MJ, Cebelinski E, et al. Comparative evaluation of two commercial multiplex panels for detection of gastrointestinal pathogens by use of clinical stool specimens. *J Clin Microbiol*. 2014;52(10):3667–3673.

84. Onori M, Coltella L, Mancinelli L, et al. Evaluation of a multiplex PCR assay for simultaneous detection of bacterial and viral enteropathogens in stool samples of paediatric patients. *Diagn Microbiol Infect Dis*. 2014;79(2):149–154.

85. Otto CC, Chen LH, He T, Tang YW, Babady NE. Detection of gastrointestinal pathogens in oncology patients by highly multiplexed molecular panels. *Eur J Clin Microbiol Infect Dis*. 2017;36(9):1665–1672.

86. Patel A, Navidad J, Bhattacharyya S. Site-specific clinical evaluation of the Luminex xTAG gastrointestinal pathogen panel for detection of infectious gastroenteritis in fecal specimens. *J Clin Microbiol*. 2014;52(8):3068–3071.

87. Vocale C, Rimoldi SG, Pagani C, et al. Comparative evaluation of the new xTAG GPP multiplex assay in the laboratory diagnosis of acute gastroenteritis. Clinical assessment and potential application from a multicentre Italian study. *Int J Infect Dis*. 2015;34:33–37.

88. Buchan BW, Olson WJ, Pezewski M, et al. Clinical evaluation of a real-time PCR assay for identification of Salmonella, Shigella, Campylobacter (Campylobacter jejuni and C. coli), and shiga toxin-producing *Escherichia coli* isolates in stool specimens. *J Clin Microbiol*. 2013;51(12):4001–4007.

89. Harrington SM, Buchan BW, Doern C, et al. Multicenter evaluation of the BD max enteric bacterial panel PCR assay for rapid detection of Salmonella spp., Shigella spp., Campylobacter spp. (C. jejuni and C. coli), and Shiga toxin 1 and 2 genes. *J Clin Microbiol.* 2015;53(5):1639–1647.

90. Knabl L, Grutsch I, Orth-Holler D. Comparison of the BD MAX(R) Enteric Bacterial Panel assay with conventional diagnostic procedures in diarrheal stool samples. *Eur J Clin Microbiol Infect Dis.* 2016;35(1):131–136.

91. DeBurger B, Hanna S, Powell EA, Ventrola C, Mortensen JE. Utilizing BD MAX enteric bacterial panel to detect stool pathogens from rectal swabs. *BMC Clin Pathol.* 2017;17:7.

92. Simner PJ, Oethinger M, Stellrecht KA, et al. Multisite evaluation of the BD max extended enteric bacterial panel for detection of Yersinia enterocolitica, enterotoxigenic *Escherichia coli*, Vibrio, and Plesiomonas shigelloides from stool specimens. *J Clin Microbiol.* 2017;55(11):3258–3266.

93. Parčina MR-OI, Mockenhaupt FP, Vojvoda V, Gahutu JB, Hoerauf A, Ignatius R. Highly sensitive and specific detection of Giardia duodenalis, Entamoeba histolytica, and Cryptosporidium spp. in human stool samples by the BD MAX™ Enteric Parasite Panel. *Parasitol Res.* 2018;117(2):447–451.

94. Perry MD, Corden SA. Lewis white P. Evaluation of the BD MAX enteric parasite panel for the detection of Cryptosporidium parvum/hominis, Giardia duodenalis and Entamoeba histolytica. *J Med Microbiol.* 2017;66(8):1118–1123.

95. Molling P, Nilsson P, Ennefors T, et al. Evaluation of the BD max enteric parasite panel for clinical diagnostics. *J Clin Microbiol.* 2016;54(2):443–444.

96. Batra R, Judd E, Eling J, Newsholme W, Goldenberg SD. Molecular detection of common intestinal parasites: a performance evaluation of the BD Max Enteric Parasite Panel. *Eur J Clin Microbiol Infect Dis.* 2016;35(11):1753–1757.

97. Madison-Antenucci S, Relich RF, Doyle L, et al. Multicenter evaluation of BD max enteric parasite real-time PCR assay for detection of Giardia duodenalis, Cryptosporidium hominis, Cryptosporidium parvum, and Entamoeba histolytica. *J Clin Microbiol.* 2016;54(11):2681–2688.

98. Buss SN, Leber A, Chapin K, et al. Multicenter evaluation of the BioFire FilmArray gastrointestinal panel for etiologic diagnosis of infectious gastroenteritis. *J Clin Microbiol.* 2015;53(3):915–925.

99. Halligan E, Edgeworth J, Bisnauthsing K, et al. Multiplex molecular testing for management of infectious gastroenteritis in a hospital setting: a comparative diagnostic and clinical utility study. *Clin Microbiol Infect.* 2014;20(8):O460–O467.

100. Mhaissen MN, Rodriguez A, Gu Z, et al. Epidemiology of diarrheal illness in pediatric oncology patients. *J Pediatr Infect Dis Soc.* 2016.

101. Coste JF, Vuiblet V, Moustapha B, et al. Microbiological diagnosis of severe diarrhea in kidney transplant recipients by use of multiplex PCR assays. *J Clin Microbiol.* 2013;51(6):1841–1849.

102. Gu Z, Zhu H, Rodriguez A, et al. Comparative evaluation of broad-panel PCR assays for the detection of gastrointestinal pathogens in pediatric oncology patients. *J Mol Diagn J Mod Dynam.* 2015;17(6):715–721.

CHAPTER 14

Tropheryma Whipplei Agent of Self-Limiting Infections and Whipple's Disease

VERENA MOOS, PHD

TROPHERYMA WHIPPLEI

A bacterial cause of Whipple's disease has already been suspected at its first description, but only the first successful treatment with antibiotics[1] and the visualization of bacterial structures by electron microscopy[2] substantiated this assumption. In the 1990s, segments of 16S ribosomal DNA of T. whipplei were amplified by PCR from duodenal lesions of patients.[3,4] Sequencing of the PCR products allowed the phylogenetical classification of the new species. It was named Tropheryma whipplei (words "trophe" meaning food in Greek, and "eryma" meaning barrier) and later corrected to the grammatically correct form Tropheryma whipplei.

Tropheryma (T.) whipplei is a rod-shaped organism of approximately 2 μm length with a trilaminar plasma membrane surrounded by a homogeneous cell wall. Despite these structures are usually seen in Gram-negative bacteria, T. whipplei is Gram-positive and other characteristics as the central location of tubules and vesicles correspond to the typical features of Gram-positive organisms.[2,5-9]

Cultivation of T. whipplei was not possible by routine methods over many years. Only in 1997, a first short time cultivation of T. whipplei isolated from heart valves succeeded in peripheral blood mononuclear cells deactivated by dexamethasone, interleukin (IL)-4 or IL-10.[10] A stable cultivation of the organism was some years later established by shell-vial techniques in human fibroblasts cell lines.[11,12] The replication time of this first isolates of T. whipplei was as long as 18 days, and thus growth of T. whipplei can require several weeks.[11,13] Later genome analysis revealed that T. whipplei lacks several biosynthetic pathways for amino acids, and enabled the development of a special mammalian cell-free ("axenic") growth media.[14,15] The adapted strains revealed a considerably reduced doubling time. Culture from sterile fluids or tissues is easier, and a large number of strains from cardiac valves, blood, synovial fluid, cerebro-spinal fluid (CSF), duodenal biopsies, and saliva in serial cultures have been obtained.[11,13,15-20] The unique resistance of T. whipplei to glutaraldehyde also enabled the cultivation of the agent from stool specimens.[17]

T. whipplei is dependent from a host for its replication, and it has been suggested that the bacterium multiplies in the digestive lumen of the human gut, becomes phagocytized, and then degraded in macrophages. In vitro T. whipplei is able to replicate within peripheral blood mononuclear cells (which release the bacteria), and within macrophages of Whipple's disease patients. In HeLa cells, T whipplei can survive and multiply in acidic vacuoles at pH 5. The acid milieu that enables replication of the agent may impair antibiotic activity and thus may diminish the efficacy of some antibiotics.[16,21-23] By electron microscopy, T. whipplei has been detected in large amounts of macrophages of the lamina propria of the small intestine, but has also been identified among others in endothelial cells, epithelial cells, muscle cells, and cells of the immune system (e.g., in leukocytes, lymphocytes, plasma cells, mast cells).[2,5,6,8,24,25]

The complete genomic sequence of two different T. whipplei strains has been published.[13,26] The genetic structure shows some characteristics that are common to intracellular bacteria. The genetic sequences of both strains have a high guanin/cytosin (GC) content of 47%, consist of around 900 K base pairs in a unique circular chromosome, and are very similar (>99% identity). Around 800 protein-coding genes have been identified. These data and the 16S–23S intergenic sequence analysis[27] resulted in the taxonomic classification of T. whipplei between the subdivision of Gram-positive actinomycetes with B peptidoglycan and the cellulomonadacea. T. whipplei is the only known

Gastrointestinal Diseases and Their Associated Infections. https://doi.org/10.1016/B978-0-323-54843-4.00014-3
Copyright © 2019 Elsevier Inc. All rights reserved.

reduced-genome species (<1 Mb) within the actinobacteria, and is closely related to cellulomonads and nocardioforms. Distinct *T. whipplei* strains neither are associated with the location of the patients, nor the manifestation of infection.[28]

The genomic characteristics suggest a host-dependent lifestyle, requirement on external nutrients, and hint to mechanisms for evasion from the hosts immune response ("parasitic lifestyle").[13,26] The organism lacks information for biosynthetic pathways of 16 amino acids, thioredoxine, and thioredoxine reductase homologs. Genome sequence alignment revealed a large chromosomal inversion and the presence of a common repeat, highly conserved at the nucleotide level, pointing to a high genetic diversity. This results in the expression of many different subsets of cell surface proteins.

Based on the idea, that *T. whipplei* might persist in soil and thus preferentially farmers are at risk to get infected,[5] *T. whipplei* was assigned to the actinobacteria that include the actinomycetes that are essentially environmental microorganisms.[29] However, although *T. whipplei* can be identified in influxes to sewage plants,[30,31] another possible source except humans has not been identified convincingly till know.

Asymptomatic Carriage of *T. whipplei* and Transmission

T. whipplei can be detected molecular biologically in stool and saliva from healthy asymptomatic carriers.[31,32] The prevalence of healthy carriage of *T. whipplei* in the stool seems to depend mainly on the hygienic standards with very low rates in Europe (estimated to be between 1% and 11%) and a higher incidence in situations with possible enhanced exposure as in sewage plant workers (12%–26%) or shelters for homeless.[31-35] Similarly, the prevalence of *T. whipplei* in saliva is enhanced in sewage plant workers compared to the average population (2,2% vs. 0.2%).[31] In rural regions of subSaharan Africa, dependent on the accessibility of toilets, the healthy carrier rate of *T. whipplei* is much higher (31% in stool and 3.5% in saliva).[35,36] *T. whipplei* is viable in human feces and saliva and thus, a human-to-human transmission of *T. whipplei* via the fecal–oral or oral–oral route has been suggested.[17,33] This idea has further been supported by the accumulation of *T. whipplei* carriage in families with cases of Whipple's disease,[34] and the detection of identical *T. whipplei* genotypes among children during episodes of *T. whipplei* gastroenteritis,[37] among relatives of people positive for *T. whipplei*,[34] and among homeless people sleeping in the same shelter.[33]

Other sources of *T. whipplei* than human have not been identified so far. Even the extensive search for alternative sources in Senegal in dust, stool from domestic animals such as chicken, goats, donkeys, cattle, sheep, ducks, pigeons, and dogs, ixodid ticks from domestic animals, fleas collected from human dwellings, dogs, and cats, and finally human head lice, revealed any convincing contamination with *T. whipplei*.[36] From the 1002 environmental specimens only four samples, three samples from two chickens and one goat, and one household dust sample revealed a slight contamination with *T. whipplei* that was supposed to be the result of ingestion of food contaminated with human feces.[36] In intestinal samples from cattle, pigs, chickens, sheep, horses, dogs, or cats, *T. whipplei* could not be detected by PCR.[29]

As humans seem the only host of *T. whipplei* and all environmental sources might be contaminated by humans and their wastes, *T. whipplei* may be able to form spore like forms facilitating survival outside the human body that also could explain the high tenacity of the agent even against formaldehyde.[17]

Self-Limiting Infections with *T. whipplei*

In recent years, *T. whipplei* has been recognized as a cause for acute infections such as gastroenteritis, fever, cough, or pneumonia. *T. whipplei* can be found in 15% of stool samples of children with gastroenteritis.[37] Other causes may be absent, and *T. whipplei* disappears after amelioration of symptoms, thus it has been suggested as the only cause of gastroenteritis.[37] In rural Africa, patients with cough and fever may present with bacteriemia with *T. whipplei*.[38] Bronchioalveolar lavages of patients with pneumonia are contaminated with *T. whipplei* in 3% of cases, and HIV-positive patients with pneumonia even reveal a higher rate of *T. whipplei*-positive bronchioalveolar lavages.[39,40] However, these infections seem to be transient and do not result in the establishment of chronic Whipple's disease.

WHIPPLE'S DISEASE
Epidemiology of Whipple's Disease
In a review summarizing 664 patients with Whipple's disease mainly from the United States, a preferential affection of Caucasian middle-aged males was reported.[5] There occurred no familial clustering, but most of the patients were in occupational contact to soil or animals; 35% were farmers. In more recent reports of mainly German patients from 1986 to 1995, up to 22% patients were female, and the mean age at diagnosis was increasing (55,7 years for male and

61,9 years for female patients, respectively).[41] The condition affects almost exclusively the Caucasian population; it is extremely rare in Asian populations and virtually unknown in Africa.[29,42]

For many years, a genetic predisposition for Whipple's disease has been discussed, and indeed, in recent years associations of Whipple's disease with distinct human leukocyte antigen (HLA) alleles and different cytokine polymorphisms were described.[43-45]

Pathogenesis of Whipple's Disease

A healthy asymptomatic carrier status can be detected in around 2%–4% of the general European population,[32] which is in discrepancy with the low estimated prevalence of Whipple's disease of 1:1.000.000 evolving only in a minority of the affected persons.[32,37,38,46,47] Thus, host factors have been suspected to be responsible for the chronification of the infection. Several observations assist the idea of an individual predisposition for Whipple's disease: (1) a higher rate of exposure, as in sewage plant workers, does not translate in a higher incidence of Whipple's disease, (2) there has been found no correlation of genotype of the infecting strain and the manifestation of the infection,[28] (3) immune-deficiencies, such as HIV infection, may enhance the risk of carriage of T. whipplei;[40] however, up to now there is no robust evidence for an enhanced risk for immunocompromised patients to develop Whipple's disease. Thus, an underlying predisposition for Whipple's disease can strongly be suspected. Human-to-human transmission[33] seems to result in a primary infection that is asymptomatic or self-limiting[37,39] and only very rarely evolves to Whipple's disease.

In the last years, indeed, distinct genes were found to be associated with Whipple's disease. The genetic predisposition of Whipple's disease patients seems to influence the axis of antigen presentation and T-cell activation: HLA associations[43] might interfere with optimal presentation of antigens, cytokine gene polymorphisms might polarize cytokine production toward an activity of tolerogenic and T-helper cells of type 2 (Th2),[44] and polymorphisms within the IL-16 gene might be associated with dysfunctions of dendritic cells.[45,48] Thus, there is strong evidence for a specific multifactorial predisposition toward Whipple's disease that results in a lifetime susceptibility of the affected patients.[49]

The destruction of the mucosal integrity during the chronic infection with T. whipplei enables a translocation of bacterial antigens from the gastrointestinal lumen to system.[50] Diarrhea, a main symptom of Whipple's disease, seems to be the result of a leaky gut

and the translocation of pyrogens might be a cause for systemic immune activation.[50] These alterations of the duodenal mucosa persist to some degree also following successful treatment of the infection.[50]

Immunological Aberrations of Whipple's Disease Patients

After a first infection, only in predisposed patients, T. whipplei spreads systemically throughout the whole body and Whipple's disease develops in the course of many years or even decades. The extreme long replication time of T. whipplei probably is responsible for the slow course of the disease. As a hallmark of the disease is a massive accumulation of macrophages stuffed with T. whipplei in the lamina propria of the small intestinal mucosa, deficiencies of macrophages were at focus in first studies of immune deficiencies of Whipple's disease patients. A reduced phagocytotic activity and intracellular degradation of macrophages of Whipple's disease patients were described very early,[51,52] and the first in vitro cultivation of T. whipplei was achieved in macrophages deactivated by dexamethasone, IL-4 or IL-10.[10] In more recent years, several immunological aberrations of Whipple's disease patients point at an impairment of macrophages: Patients reveal reduced serum levels of IL-12,[53] monocytes produce only low levels of IL-12,[54] and macrophages present preferentially as an alternatively activated phenotype,[55,56] which is not able to induce inflammatory reactions. Apoptosis of macrophages that is induced by T. whipplei, contributes to bacterial spread[57] and reduced maturation of phagosomes favors persistence of the agent.[58-60] The cytokines IL-16 and type I interferon (IFN) are both enhanced during Whipple's disease and reduce the resistance of monocytes/macrophages against T. whipplei.[58,59,61,62] Thus, intestinal macrophages of Whipple's disease patients ingest T. whipplei, but are unable to kill the bacteria.

However, not only macrophages seem to be responsible for the persistence of T. whipplei in predisposed patients, since Whipple's disease is also characterized by the absence of an inflammatory reaction and T helper cell (Th) type 1 response against T. whipplei and the predominance of regulatory T-cells.[63-65] At first contact with T. whipplei, that is supposed to occur in early childhood, most of the infected persons develop a protective humoral and cellular immune response.[64,66,67] This specific protective immune reaction is lacking in patients with Whipple's disease, which results in an antiinflammatory cytokine milieu. Several publications describe these disturbances in the balance of inflammatory and regulatory cytokines and deficits in the specific immune reaction against *T. whipplei*: (1) there are high levels of IL-10 and transforming growth factor (TGF)-β, while amounts of IFNγ in the serum and in the gastrointestinal mucosa are low;[53,65,68] (2) The serological reaction against *T. whipplei is* reduced;[66,67] (3) the number of duodenal lymphocytes is reduced,[68] and (4) the activity of Th1 cells is dysregulated.[63,64] The reduced Th1 activity is *T. whipplei*-specific[64] and could be a consequence of inefficient antigen-presentation by macrophages and dendritic cells. Regulatory T cells are present in enhanced numbers in the duodenal mucosa and are more activated in the peripheral blood of Whipple's disease patients[65] and thus inhibit a systemic and duodenal inflammatory reaction.

CLINICAL PRESENTATION OF WHIPPLE'S DISEASE

In recent years, the clinical spectrum of *T. whipplei* infection has broadened considerably and besides the self-limiting infections mentioned earlier, also the clinical presentation of chronic Whipple's disease need to be reconsidered. Besides the rare, classical form of Whipple's disease predominantly involving the intestinal tract with diarrhea and weight loss as well as arthritis, isolated forms in extraintestinal organs with little or without involvement of the alimentary tract seem to be more frequent than previously assumed.[69,70]

The spectrum of symptoms of Whipple's disease is broad, and a lot of "atypical" cases have been reported. Thus, distinct characteristic clinical features cannot be defined, but the combination of arthropathy and diarrhea is common to many patients and has been considered as the manifestation of classical Whipple's disease. However, gastrointestinal symptoms might be absent, and thus it is important to consider Whipple's disease also in the any case of unexplained chronic inflammatory signs.[69,71]

Table 14.1 summarizes the most common manifestations of Whipple's disease. Among them are gastrointestinal symptoms such as diarrhea, malabsorption, weight loss and abdominal pain, and joint symptoms such as arthralgia or arthritis. Less common symptoms include night sweats low-degree fever, hyperpigmentation of the skin, and abdominal lymphadenopathy that may be present in around half of the cases.[5,7,8,71] Cardiac involvement presents mostly with cardiac murmurs and signs of heart failure. Pulmonary infiltration and pleural effusion have been described in 40%–50% of patients with classical Whipple's disease.[5,19,70,72]

The intestinal malabsorption leading to diarrhea and weight loss may progress to severe cachexia, found

TABLE 14.1
Major Symptoms of Classical Whipple's Disease

Symptoms	Percentage
Weight loss	85–95
Anemia	80–90
Arthropathy	70–85
Diarrhea	70–80
Abdominal pain	55–60
Lymphadenopathy	45–60
Fever	40–45
Hyperpigmentation	35–45
CNS involvement	10–40
Ocular signs	5–10

in two thirds of the patients with classical Whipple's disease. Hypoproteinemia may lead to ascites and peripheral edema.[19,73] The diarrhea of Whipple's disease is mostly watery, and only rarely patients have occult intestinal blood loss. Steatorrhea may contribute to malabsorption, but it is seen less frequently.

Central nervous system (CNS) manifestations are the most serious manifestations in Whipple's disease, often limiting recovery and prognosis even despite appropriate treatment. The proportion of the patients that show a symptomatic involvement of the CNS is variable (Table 14.1). The frequency is mostly reported at about 15% in case series, but it has been observed also in higher percentages.[5,19,74,75] Most of the CNS manifestations are difficult to recognize as symptoms of Whipple's disease. Unspecific headache, cognitive dysfunction, epilepsy, ataxia, seizures, insomnia, and meningitic symptoms or involvement of the peripheral nerves and spinal cord may occur, but are unspecific.[74-76] Only progressive supranuclear ophthalmoplegia with oculomasticatory myorhythmia or oculofacioskeletal myorhythmia are considered to be pathognomonic for Whipple's disease.[73,75] As an extension of the brain, ocular involvement such as uveitis may be observed in up to 11% of cases.[73,75,77] Sometimes the diagnosis of Whipple's disease can be established from the eye.[77] *T. whipplei* can be detected in CSF by specific PCR and a positive CSF has been reported in 40%–50% of patients,[78,79] the majority of them did nor reveal any CNS symptoms.

The first symptom of Whipple's disease arthropathy occurs in around 65% of patients. The arthropathy is typically a seronegative, nondestructive joint disease predominantly of the small peripheral joints with migratory characteristics. Joint symptoms may precede final diagnosis by several years.[5,69,80] Very often, Whipple's disease is misdiagnosed as rheumatologic disease and subsequently treated with immunosuppressive drugs.[69,71,80,81] Consequently, there is often a significant delay between onset of first symptoms of Whipple's disease and final diagnosis. In one series, the onset of arthralgia occurred in average 105 months before the establishment of diagnosis of Whipple's disease while diagnosis was established more quickly following onset of diarrhea (12 months) or weight loss (8 months).[80,81]

Localized infections with *T. whipplei* occurred in two series of 142 and 191 patients, respectively, in ca. 20% of cases.[71,81] Isolated *T. whipplei* infections most often affect the CNS[81] or present as isolated joint manifestations.[69] In addition, localized *T. whipplei* infection manifesting as adenopathy, pulmonary or pleural involvement, or uveitis might occur.[5,71,72,81]

Infective endocarditis caused by *T. whipplei* should be considered as a special condition.[70] It frequently necessitates surgical valve replacement of either the mitral or aortic valve and can be diagnosed only from the excised tissue by histology via PCR, as other organs do not reveal any affection. In a cohort of German patients, *T. whipplei* infection was the most common agent found in culture-negative endocarditis.[70] However, *T. whipplei* induced endocarditis might also occur in the context of classical Whipple's disease.

DIAGNOSIS OF WHIPPLE'S DISEASE

Once the clinical suspicion of Whipple's disease is established, diagnosis in most cases can be accomplished from duodenal biopsies. However, due to a possible lack of gastrointestinal affection, some patients need a more elaborate diagnostic algorithm that finally ensures the diagnosis of Whipple's disease.[71] An algorithm for the diagnosis of Whipple's disease is demonstrated in Fig. 14.2.

As a hallmark of classical Whipple's disease is a massive infiltration of the duodenal mucosa with macrophages stuffed with *T. whipplei*, upper endoscopy with multiple duodenal biopsies remains the first recommended diagnostic procedure if Whipple's disease is suspected. As in most cases there are no macroscopic changes of the mucosal surface, multiple biopsies should be taken from various sites of the duodenum to avoid sampling errors and subsequently examined histopathologically with Periodic acid–Schiff's (PAS) staining to detect *T. whipplei*.[71] Molecular analysis with *T. whipplei*-specific PCR is advised to identify the agent definitively.[82–84]

Despite an impressive presence of the pathogen in the lamina propria of the duodenal mucosa, the majority of cases reveal an unsuspicious appearance of the duodenum at upper endoscopy.[71] A pale yellow mucosal surface with clumsy and dilated villi and ecstatic lymph vessels may be present in some cases and has been considered as a hint for classical Whipple's disease, but is not specific (Fig. 14.1A).[71,81]

A clear diagnostic hint toward classical Whipple's disease is the detection of foamy macrophages in the lamina propria that contain large amounts of diastase-resistant PAS-positive particles in the cytoplasm (Fig. 14.1B).[9] An additional Ziehl–Neelsen staining should be performed to exclude mycobacterial infection and may be helpful particularly in immunocompromised patients. Even in the absence of gastrointestinal symptoms that are true for about 20% of patients, duodenal histology may be positive.[71,81] The absence of PAS-staining of duodenal biopsies does not completely rule out Whipple's disease, but makes it much less probable.

PAS-positive cells can be classified into subtypes: type I macrophages in untreated patients convert type II–IV macrophages in treated patients.[85] Even after appropriate treatment of *T. whipplei*, PAS-positive macrophages may persist for years within the tissues.[85] Thus, the persistence of PAS-positive material within the mucosa not automatically indicates insufficient treatment. However, the intensity of the staining and the amount of PAS-positive macrophages should reduce to ensure the success of the treatment.[85]

To assist the diagnosis of Whipple's disease, *T. whipplei*-specific immunohistochemistry may be used.[86] It seems to be more sensitive than PAS staining and detects *T. whipplei* within the tissue before the possible evidence of PAS-positive macrophages.[71,86]

T. whipplei-specific PCR is helpful for diagnosis and follow-up.[82–84] PCR enables the definite identification of *T. whipplei* in the patients and testing should be confirmed by sequencing and multiple *T. whipplei* target genes should be addressed to avoid false positive results. However, due to the existence of healthy carriers, a positive PCR from gastrointestinal tissues should be evaluated very critical and an isolated positive PCR from duodenal biopsies does not ensure a reliable diagnosis of Whipple's disease and should be confirmed by histology or from alternative tissues (Fig. 14.2).

However, if clinical suspicion for Whipple's disease is very strong but histopathological examination is unclear or difficult to evaluate, PCR may be helpful for treatment decisions. In case of negative PCR but suspicious histology, the possibility of a previous antibiotic treatment should be taken into account[7,78,79,85] and in

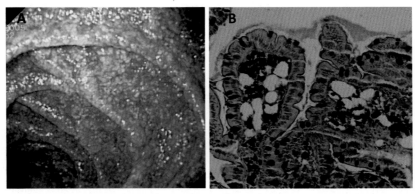

FIG. 14.1 Characteristic appearance of the duodenal mucosa and classical diagnosis of Whipple's disease from the duodenum: **(A)** Macroscopic view at endoscopy of a heavily affected case with clumsy and dilated villi with ecstatic lymph vessels that are extensively infiltrated with macrophages. **(B)** intensively PAS-positive macrophages in a biopsy of the duodenal mucosa with villous atrophy and lymphangiectasia. (Copy from Schneider T, Moos V, Loddenkemper C, Marth T, Fenollar F, Raoult D. Whipple's disease: new aspects of pathogenesis and treatment. Lancet Infect Dis:179–90, Copyright (2008), with the printable licence from Elsevier.)

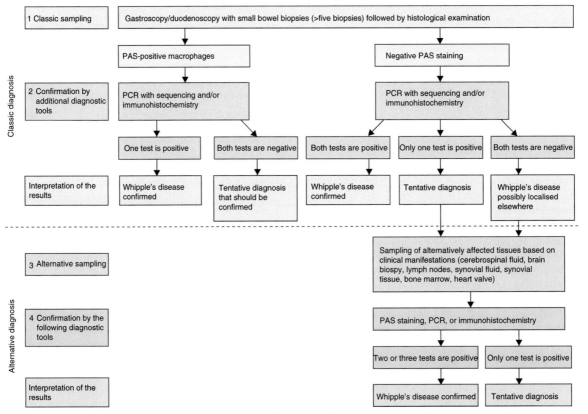

FIG. 14.2 Hierarchic scheme for the diagnosis of Whipple's disease based on clinical symptoms. (Copy from Schneider T, Moos V, Loddenkemper C, Marth T, Fenollar F, Raoult D. Whipple's disease: new aspects of pathogenesis and treatment. Lancet Infect Dis:179–90, Copyright (2008) with the printable licence from Elsevier.)

cases with positive PCR, additional specimens should be analyzed to ensure the diagnosis of Whipple's disease (Fig. 14.2).[71]

Serological diagnosis of Whipple's disease is hitherto not applicable, as healthy subjects reveal a positive serological reaction against *T whipplei* as well.[67]

Electron microscopy is suitable to detect *T. whipplei* in various stages of degradation within cells and in the extracellular space. It is often located in large numbers in macrophages of the lamina propria of the small intestine.[6,9] However, electron microscopy today is not a standard procedure for diagnosis.

In patients with a strong clinical suspicion of Whipple's disease even after negative histopathology and PCR from the small intestinal mucosa, additional tissues have to be analyzed in dependence of the clinical manifestation (Fig. 14.2).[7,8] As CNS, joints, lymph nodes, muscles, synovial sheaths, eyes, lung, or heart valves might be affected by isolated chronic infections with *T. whipplei*, specimens from clinically affected sites should be analyzed.[70,71,81] PAS-positive cells may be detected in any solid organs besides the various sites of the gastrointestinal tract. Especially lymph nodes, synovia, bone marrow, skin, or heart valves are suitable for histological analysis and may be stuffed with PAS-positive macrophages.[70,71,81] As for small intestinal specimens, a specific PCR analysis should be performed from all PAS-positive specimens for definite identification of *T. whipplei*. For any specimens from sterile body fluids such as CSF or synovial fluid, ascites or pleural effusion *T. whipplei*-specific PCR is of exceptional diagnostic value. In addition PCR is advisable for CNS biopsies, as PAS-staining may be unspecific in CNS tissue.[81]

Although PCR is of increasing importance for the diagnosis of Whipple's disease, a positive *T. whipplei*-specific PCR from oral, gastrointestinal, stool, bronchial, or lung specimens is not advisable for the ensured diagnosis due to asymptomatic carriage of *T. whipplei*.[31–33] A positive PCR from specimens with environmental contact should be confirmed by a positive histological analysis from the same or another tissue or a PCR from sterile specimens.

In addition, PAS-staining of biopsy specimens from the colon, rectum, CNS, or the eyes may be very unspecific. They do not unequivocally indicate Whipple's disease and need to be confirmed by other techniques, such as PCR, or histology from another specimen.[87,88]

Independent from the primary diagnosis of Whipple's disease and from the appearance of CNS symptoms, to complement diagnosis, in any case of classical Whipple's disease, a PCR from CSF is highly recommended. A high rate of asymptomatic CNS infection in up to 50% of patients has been described.[78,79,81] Due to severe complications that may result from CNS infection even despite appropriate antimicrobial treatment, eradication of the agent from the CNS is absolutely essential and should be monitored carefully by PCR from CSF.

TREATMENT OF WHIPPLE'S DISEASE

Whipple's disease is fatal without antibiotic treatment. Since its first use in 1952,[1] distinct antibiotic regimens were used on an empirical basis with increasing success. In the first decades of empiric antibiotic use, tetracycline was frequently applied. However, high relapse rates and severe CNS manifestations with subsequent poor prognosis were obvious in retrospective studies.[89,90] Several other treatment options such as antibiotic monotherapy with penicillin, minocycline, or chloramphenicol, antibiotic combinations in case of CNS disease,[74,91] or additional use of IFN-γ in case of refractory disease[92] have been published.

Case reports and a nonrandomized retrospective treatment trial including 30 patients indicated that trimethoprim-sulfamethoxazole (TMP-SMX) was superior to tetracycline and most importantly, more effectively cured CNS disease.[93] The preeminence of TMP-SMX was confirmed later in a retrospective analysis of 52 patients.[73]

A first prospective randomized controlled trial that analyzed the outcome of 40 previously untreated patients with Whipple's disease was published in 2010.[78] The treatment regime encompasses an induction therapy with either intravenous ceftriaxone or meropenem for 14 days and all patients received subsequently oral TMP-SMX for 12 months, patients were followed over a period of 3 years. The two treatment regimens were comparable; only one patient presented with an asymptomatic cerebrospinal infection, resistant to all treatments that finally was cleared by chloroquine and minocycline.[91] Two patients died of myocardial infarction and aspiration pneumonia in a mentally disabled patient, two conditions that have to be seen in the context of infection with *T. whipplei*.[78] This trial revealed a very high rate of prolonged clinical remission, which may reflect the predominance of the antibiotic regimen and due to good antibiotic adherence in a trial setting.[78] However, based on the results of this first prospective trial, currently a treatment with 14 days of intravenous ceftriaxone followed by 12 months of TMP-SMX is recommended (Table 14.2).

TABLE 14.2
Recommended Treatment of Whipple's Disease

Treatment	Duration	Dose	Alternative
1. *Initial therapy* ceftriaxone	2 weeks	2 g iv once daily	meropenem (1 g iv thrice daily)
2. *Long-term therapy* TMP-SMX	1 year	960 mg orally twice daily	Oral doxycycline (100 mg twice daily) plus hydroxychloroquine (200 mg thrice daily)

Alternative Treatment Options

One prospective trial of 40 patients evaluated the possibility of short-term treatment of Whipple's disease with 2 weeks of intravenous ceftriaxone followed by 3 months of TMP-SMX.[79] In this trial, one relapse and three deaths were reported. Despite a lack of significant difference to the standard long-term therapy, the currently recommended therapy remains the long-term treatment approach due to a higher safety and more validated observations.

Based on observations of antibiotic resistance to TMP-SMX in single patients and on in vitro data showing resistance of *T. whipplei* to TMP and since doxycycline in combination with hydroxychloroquine has been demonstrated to be bactericidal active against *T. whipplei*,[21,22,94,95] a retrospective series of 29 patients that were treated with doxycycline (mostly 100 mg orally twice daily) plus hydroxychloroquine (200 mg orally thrice daily) has been published recently.[96] However, the group of patients described was somehow heterogeneous: 14 patients received cotrimoxazole, some patients sulfadiazine, and seven patients received intravenous therapy. Of 29 patients, 22 were treated with long-term doxycycline.[96] In this series, 24 of 29 patients were free of relapse, three patients were lost during follow-up, one relapse occurred and one patient died.

Localized manifestations of Whipple's disease such as endocarditis or CNS affection should be treated according to the regimens suggested for systemic disease.[49,70,72,75] There is no evidence that different manifestations of Whipple's disease have distinct underlying pathomechanisms that justify differential treatment regimens, and it may be difficult to definitively assure an isolated infection, as it is not feasible to test every alternative location for infection.

In conclusion, data on the treatment of classical Whipple's disease still have limitations: Patient numbers of the randomized trials were low, and at trial start data on the genome of *T. whipplei* or its antibiotic susceptibility were not available.[22,94] Although not occurring during the randomized trials, relapses may occur during treatment with TMP-SMX, and resistance to TMP-SMX has been described.[94-96] In addition, some patients do not tolerate TMP-SMX. Thus, other treatment strategies need to be considered and should be evaluated comparatively in future.

Consequently, in Germany an oral treatment with doxycycline (100 mg orally twice daily) plus hydroxychloroquine (200 mg orally thrice daily) for 12 months is actually being tested against the standard treatment of 14 days of intravenous ceftriaxone followed by 12 months of TMP-SMX in a randomized controlled trial. The results of this trial have not been published till now.

Outcome Following Treatment

Upon antibiotic treatment, a rapid improvement usually is observed and appropriate treatment in most cases leads to clinical remission. The major symptoms diarrhea and fever often disappear within a few days or at least within weeks.[79,93] Arthropathy and other symptoms should improve during some weeks after initiation of treatment. However, in dependence from the grade of irreparable articular damage, arthropathy may persist although inflammatory reactions ameliorate and may necessitate endoprotesis. Histologically, a gradual reconstitution of the villous architecture of the small intestine occurs, and a fading of the PAS-staining can be observed.[50,78,79,85,93] PCR of infected tissues and body fluids should turn negative within some months and laboratory findings and immunologic parameters also return to normal also within some months.[78,79] However, some defects in cell-mediated immunity and the absence of *T. whipplei*-specific Th1 reactions will persist.[49,64]

Patients with CNS infection still are difficult to handle. Even upon appropriate treatment, preexisting CNS damage may proceed and even in patients in remission CNS manifestations may deteriorate till a fatal course. Thus, the treatment of CNS infections needs to be reevaluated very carefully.

Patients should be followed by duodenal biopsies after 6 months and 1 year after diagnosis. If histopathological subtyping of macrophages reveals a clear fading of PAS-positive material after 1 year and PCR is negative, antibiotic therapy can be stopped.[78,79] In all patients with a *T. whipplei* positive PCR of the CSF at time of diagnosis, CSF has to be controlled and therapy continued until PCR turns negative. For all patients, clinical follow-up is advisable lifelong. However, in asymptomatic patients, invasive controls are necessary only at rare intervals.

Complications During Treatment

In a certain percentage, side effects to antibiotics are like vomiting or rash might be observed.[19,89] In patients with intolerance to ceftriaxone, meropenem can be applied, and in patients with intolerance to TMP-SMX, doxycycline in combination with hydroxychloroquine is advisable because doxycycline has been already used more frequently.[78,79,93]

Quite rarely, a Jarisch–Herxheimer reaction with high fever within 24 h after initiation of antibiotics has been reported. A Jarisch–Herxheimer reaction seems to occur more frequently in patients receiving penicillins[5,89] and in these patients symptomatic therapy is indicated, and antibiotics may need to be changed.

Although older publications reported relapse rates in up to 30%,[5,89] two current controlled trials showed no relapse in 73 out of 80 patients over a period of 7 years.[78,79] Retrospective studies revealed a higher percentage of CNS affection in the case of clinical relapse.[5,19,75,89] However, in most cases there is no evidence that these relapses are due to bacterial reinfection or persistence of infection.[97] New reports show that relapses may occur repeatedly in individuals, and may include several T. whipplei strains.[49] Patients are livelong susceptible to repeated infection due to their immunological predisposition, and this has been used as an argument for a life-long antibiotic therapy.[49,96] However, an argument against persistent treatment is the fact that T. whipplei replicates extremely slowly and that a second infection may only get symptomatic after many years and patients that are diagnosed in their 60s will not experience this subsequent infection.

However, no systematic analysis of the treatment of relapses is currently available. In some publications, treatment of first relapse has been successful with the antibiotics used during the first treatment course.[89,93] Referring to data from newer reviews and the two prospective trials,[78,79] one would recommend a change of the primary antibiotic regimen in case of relapse. In regard to prognosis, relapsing patients reveal a poor prognosis.

As relapses of CNS infection can occur even late and may have a progressive till fatal course,[5,19,74,75,97] T. whipplei should be absolutely eradicated from the CNS at first treatment. For that, antibiotics with good penetration of the blood–brain barrier such as TMP-SMX

should be applied.[78,93] The use of penicillin, minocycline, and chloramphenicol has been reported to treat successfully CNS infection with T. whipplei as well.[5,89,91] Additional supportive therapy with Th1 cytokines (IFN-γ) has been described as beneficial[92] but should be applied only under strictly controlled conditions (e.g., in a reference center experienced in the treatment of Whipple's disease).

Untreated Whipple's disease normally has a fatal course,[1,5] but the overall or current mortality rate of treated Whipple's disease has not been evaluated.[5,19] In the two prospective trials mentioned, comprising 80 individuals, 5% of patients had a lethal outcome.[78,79] The deaths were probable Whipple's disease-related and consequences of tissue damage induced by T. whipplei.

The most frequent and often serious complication during the treatment of Whipple's disease is an immune reconstitution inflammatory syndrome (IRIS) that occurs in about 10% of patients. IRIS is characterized by the recurrence of inflammatory signs and symptoms in the absence of other definable causes.[98]

IRIS occurs following antimicrobial treatment as active T. whipplei infection induces an immunosuppression that is weakened by the antimicrobials. After the start of antimicrobial treatment, the transient immunosuppression by the pathogen dissolves, and the immune system, especially the activity of CD4+ T cells, reconstitutes.[99] However, in patients developing IRIS, the normally balanced regulatory mechanisms lag behind the inflammatory activity.[99] This leads to a flare up of unspecific inflammatory immune reactions in infiltration of activated CD4+ T cells in the tissues that are responsible for the pathogenesis of IRIS.[99] Consequently, patients under immunosuppressive therapy prior to the diagnosis of Whipple's disease are at enhanced risk to suffer from subsequent IRIS.[98,99] Therefore, patients previously treated immunosuppressively due to the misdiagnosis of a rheumatic disease need to be monitored closely following the initiation of antibiotic therapy, and immunosuppressive drugs need to be tampered very slowly. However, due to the natural immunosuppressive activity of T. whipplei, medicamentous immunosuppression is not an obligate prerequisite for the pathogenesis of IRIS.[98]

The predominant clinical manifestations of IRIS are frequently fever, arthritis, or digestive problems. However, a variety of other symptoms have been described such as erythema nodosum, pleuritis, orbitopathy, or CNS symptoms such as meningitis or brain abscess.[98] As these symptoms might be life-threatening, timely and adequate therapy for IRIS is essential. However, as the symptoms of IRIS resemble the manifestations of the active infection with *T. whipplei*, IRIS is often mistaken as refractory disease. Thus, in patients with inflammatory problems after initiation of treatment, one has to ponder carefully between IRIS and treatment failure that occurs much more rarely than IRIS.

Today, treatment of IRIS has not been evaluated prospectively. However, the rapid application of high dose oral corticosteroids has been shown to be effective against the flare up of inflammatory reactions, and thus might be lifesaving.[98] When inflammatory signs do not resolve within the first few days of treatment, the diagnosis of IRIS needs to be reconsidered.[98] In future, there is the need for prospective trials to evaluate effective treatment of IRIS.

CONCLUSION

T. whipplei is ubiquitous in the human population and occurs frequently during asymptomatic carriage or self-limiting infection. Whipple's disease evolves only rarely after contact with the agent in predisposed patients that reveal a dysregulated immune reaction against *T. whipplei*. The symptoms of Whipple's disease are very variable and in most of the cases many years pass from first symptoms to final diagnosis. However, once the suspicion of Whipple's disease is established, diagnosis can be established in most of the patients from small intestinal tissue by histology. In cases without gastrointestinal affection, symptomatic tissues need to be evaluated. Treatment with long-term antibiosis is recommended and the combination of intravenous ceftriaxone with oral TMP-SFX has been demonstrated to be effective. Alternatively, a sole oral treatment with doxycycline in combination with hydroxychloroquine may be applied. Relapses following these treatments are observed only rarely, much more frequent is IRIS that might be a life-threatening complication during the treatment of Whipple's disease. IRIS should be medicated with immunosuppressive drugs. Although Whipple's disease can be successfully treated in most of the patients, there still occur fatal courses and clinicians experienced in the management Whipple's disease should be consulted in any case.

REFERENCES

1. Paulley JW. A case of Whipple's disease (intestinal lipodystrophy). *Gastroenterology*. 1952;22:128.
2. Cohen AS, Schimmel EM, Holt PR, et al. Ultrastructural abnormalities in Whipple's disease. *Proc Soc Exp Biol Med*. 1960;105:411.
3. Relman DA, Schmidt TM, MacDermott RP, et al. Identification of the uncultured bacillus of Whipple's disease. *N Engl J Med*. 1992;327:293.
4. Wilson KH, Blitchington R, Frothingham R, et al. Phylogeny of the Whipple's-disease-associated bacterium. *Lancet*. 1991;338(474).
5. Dobbins WI. *Whipple's Disease*. Springfield, IL: Charles C. Thomas; 1987.
6. Trier JS, Phelps PC, Eidelman S, et al. Whipple's disease: light and electron microscope correlation of Jejunal mucosal histology with antibiotic treatment and clinical status. *Gastroenterology*. 1965;48:684.
7. Schneider T, Moos V, Loddenkemper C, et al. Whipple's disease: new aspects of pathogenesis and treatment. *Lancet Infect Dis*. 2008;8:179.
8. Marth T, Moos V, Muller C, et al. Tropheryma whipplei infection and Whipple's disease. *Lancet Infect Dis*. 2016;16:e13.
9. Silva MT, Macedo PM, Moura Nunes JF. Ultrastructure of bacilli and the bacillary origin of the macrophagic inclusions in Whipple's disease. *J Gen Microbiol*. 1985;131:1001.
10. Schoedon G, Goldenberger D, Forrer R, et al. Deactivation of macrophages with interleukin-4 is the key to the isolation of Tropheryma whippelii. *J Infect Dis*. 1997;176:672.
11. Raoult D, Birg ML, La Scola B, et al. Cultivation of the bacillus of Whipple's disease. *N Engl J Med*. 2000;342:620.
12. La Scola B, Fenollar F, Fournier PE, et al. Description of Tropheryma whipplei gen. nov., sp. nov., the Whipple's disease bacillus. *Int J Syst Evol Microbiol*. 2001;51:1471.
13. Fenollar F, Birg ML, Gauduchon V, et al. Culture of Tropheryma whipplei from human samples: a 3-year experience (1999 to 2002). *J Clin Microbiol*. 2003;41:3816.
14. Raoult D, Ogata H, Audic S, et al. Tropheryma whipplei Twist: a human pathogenic Actinobacteria with a reduced genome. *Genome Res*. 2003;13:1800.
15. Renesto P, Crapoulet N, Ogata H, et al. Genome-based design of a cell-free culture medium for Tropheryma whipplei. *Lancet*. 2003;362:447.
16. Raoult D, Lepidi H, Harle JR. Tropheryma whipplei circulating in blood monocytes. *N Engl J Med*. 2001;345:548.
17. Raoult D, Fenollar F, Birg ML. Culture of T. whipplei from the stool of a patient with Whipple's disease. *N Engl J Med*. 2006;355:1503.
18. Maiwald M, von Herbay A, Fredricks DN, et al. Cultivation of Tropheryma whipplei from cerebrospinal fluid. *J Infect Dis*. 2003;188:801.
19. Marth T, Raoult D. Whipple's disease. *Lancet*. 2003;361:239.
20. La Scola B, Fenollar F, Perreal C, et al. Epidemiologic implications of the first isolation and cultivation of Tropheryma whipplei from a saliva sample. *Ann Intern Med*. 2011;154:443.
21. Boulos A, Rolain JM, Mallet MN, et al. Molecular evaluation of antibiotic susceptibility of Tropheryma whipplei in axenic medium. *J Antimicrob Chemother*. 2005;55:178.
22. Boulos A, Rolain JM, Raoult D. Antibiotic susceptibility of Tropheryma whipplei in MRC5 cells. *Antimicrob Agents Chemother*. 2004;48:747.

23. Ghigo E, Capo C, Aurouze M, et al. Survival of Tropheryma whipplei, the agent of Whipple's disease, requires phagosome acidification. *Infect Immun.* 2002;70:1501.

24. Eck M, Kreipe H, Harmsen D, et al. Invasion and destruction of mucosal plasma cells by Tropheryma whippelii. *Hum Pathol.* 1997;28:1424.

25. Finzi G, Franzi F, Sessa F, et al. Ultrastructural evidence of Tropheryma whippelii in PAS-negative granulomatous lymph nodes. *Ultrastruct Pathol.* 2007;31:169.

26. Bentley SD, Maiwald M, Murphy LD, et al. Sequencing and analysis of the genome of the Whipple's disease bacterium Tropheryma whipplei. *Lancet.* 2003;361:637.

27. Maiwald M, Ditton HJ, von Herbay A, et al. Reassessment of the phylogenetic position of the bacterium associated with Whipple's disease and determination of the 16S-23S ribosomal intergenic spacer sequence. *Int J Syst Bacteriol.* 1996;46:1078.

28. Li W, Fenollar F, Rolain JM, et al. Genotyping reveals a wide heterogeneity of Tropheryma whipplei. *Microbiology.* 2008;154:521.

29. Dutly F, Altwegg M. Whipple's disease and "Tropheryma whippelii". *Clin Microbiol Rev.* 2001;14:561.

30. Maiwald M, Schuhmacher F, Ditton HJ, et al. Environmental occurrence of the Whipple's disease bacterium (Tropheryma whippelii). *Appl Environ Microbiol.* 1998;64:760.

31. Schoniger-Hekele M, Petermann D, Weber B, et al. Tropheryma whipplei in the environment: survey of sewage plant influxes and sewage plant workers. *Appl Environ Microbiol.* 2007;73:2033.

32. Fenollar F, Trani M, Davoust B, et al. Prevalence of asymptomatic Tropheryma whipplei carriage among humans and nonhuman primates. *J Infect Dis.* 2008;197:880.

33. Keita AK, Brouqui P, Badiaga S, et al. Tropheryma whipplei prevalence strongly suggests human transmission in homeless shelters. *Int J Infect Dis.* 2013;17:e67.

34. Fenollar F, Keita AK, Buffet S, et al. Intrafamilial circulation of Tropheryma whipplei, France. *Emerg Infect Dis.* 2012;18:949.

35. Keita AK, Bassene H, Tall A, et al. Tropheryma whipplei: a common bacterium in rural Senegal. *PLoS Neglected Trop Dis.* 2011;5:e1403.

36. Keita AK, Mediannikov O, Ratmanov P, et al. Looking for Tropheryma whipplei source and reservoir in rural Senegal. *Am J Trop Med Hyg.* 2013;88:339.

37. Raoult D, Fenollar F, Rolain JM, et al. Tropheryma whipplei in children with gastroenteritis. *Emerg Infect Dis.* 2010;16:776.

38. Fenollar F, Mediannikov O, Socolovschi C, et al. Tropheryma whipplei bacteremia during fever in rural West Africa. *Clin Infect Dis.* 2010;51:515.

39. Bousbia S, Papazian L, Auffray JP, et al. Tropheryma whipplei in patients with pneumonia. *Emerg Infect Dis.* 2010;16:258.

40. Lozupone C, Cota-Gomez A, Palmer BE, et al. Widespread colonization of the lung by Tropheryma whipplei in HIV infection. *Am J Respir Crit Care Med.* 2013;187:1110.

41. von Herbay A, Otto HF, Stolte M, et al. Epidemiology of Whipple's disease in Germany. Analysis of 110 patients diagnosed in 1965-95. *Scand J Gastroenterol.* 1997;32:52.

42. Yajima N, Wada R, Kimura S, et al. Whipple disease diagnosed with PCR using formalin-fixed paraffin-embedded specimens of the intestinal mucosa. *Intern Med.* 2013;52:219.

43. Martinetti M, Biagi F, Badulli C, et al. The HLA alleles DRB1*13 and DQB1*06 are associated to Whipple's disease. *Gastroenterology.* 2009;136:2289.

44. Biagi F, Badulli C, Feurle GE, et al. Cytokine genetic profile in Whipple's disease. *Eur J Clin Microbiol Infect Dis.* 2012;31:3145.

45. Biagi F, Schiepatti A, Badulli C, et al. -295 T-to-C promoter region IL-16 gene polymorphism is associated with Whipple's disease. *Eur J Clin Microbiol Infect Dis.* 2015;34:1919.

46. Wetzstein N, Fenollar F, Buffet S, et al. Tropheryma whipplei genotypes 1 and 3, central Europe. *Emerg Infect Dis.* 2013;19:341.

47. Fenollar F, Trape JF, Bassene H, et al. Tropheryma whipplei in fecal samples from children. *Senegal Emerg Infect Dis.* 2009;15:922.

48. Della Bella S, Nicola S, Timofeeva I, et al. Are interleukin-16 and thrombopoietin new tools for the in vitro generation of dendritic cells? *Blood.* 2004;104:4020.

49. Lagier JC, Fenollar F, Lepidi H, et al. Evidence of lifetime susceptibility to Tropheryma whipplei in patients with Whipple's disease. *J Antimicrob Chemother.* 2011;66:1188.

50. Epple HJ, Friebel J, Moos V, et al. Architectural and functional alterations of the small intestinal mucosa in classical Whipple's disease. *Mucosal Immunol.* 2017;10:1542.

51. Bai JC, Sen L, Diez R, et al. Impaired monocyte function in patients successfully treated for Whipple's disease. *Acta Gastroenterol Latinoam.* 1996;26:85.

52. Bjerknes R, Odegaard S, Bjerkvig R, et al. Whipple's disease. Demonstration of a persisting monocyte and macrophage dysfunction. *Scand J Gastroenterol.* 1988;23:611.

53. Kalt A, Schneider T, Ring S, et al. Decreased levels of interleukin-12p40 in the serum of patients with Whipple's disease. *Int J Colorectal Dis.* 2006;21:114.

54. Marth T, Neurath M, Cuccherini BA, et al. Defects of monocyte interleukin 12 production and humoral immunity in Whipple's disease. *Gastroenterology.* 1997;113:442.

55. Desnues B, Ihrig M, Raoult D, et al. Whipple's disease: a macrophage disease. *Clin Vaccine Immunol.* 2006;13:170.

56. Desnues B, Lepidi H, Raoult D, et al. Whipple disease: intestinal infiltrating cells exhibit a transcriptional pattern of M2/alternatively activated macrophages. *J Infect Dis.* 2005;192:1642.

57. Gorvel L, Al Moussawi K, Ghigo E, et al. Tropheryma whipplei, the Whipple's disease bacillus, induces macrophage apoptosis through the extrinsic pathway. *Cell Death Dis.* 2010;1:e34.

58. Al Moussawi K, Ghigo E, Kalinke U, et al. Type I interferon induction is detrimental during infection with the Whipple's disease bacterium, Tropheryma whipplei. *PLoS Pathog.* 2010;6:e1000722.

59. Ghigo E, Barry AO, Pretat L, et al. IL-16 promotes T. whipplei replication by inhibiting phagosome conversion and modulating macrophage activation. *PLoS One.* 2010;5:e13561.

60. Mottola G, Boucherit N, Trouplin V, et al. Tropheryma whipplei, the agent of Whipple's disease, affects the early to late phagosome transition and survives in a Rab5- and Rab7-positive compartment. *PLoS One.* 2014;9:e89367.

61. Benoit M, Fenollar F, Raoult D, et al. Increased levels of circulating IL-16 and apoptosis markers are related to the activity of Whipple's disease. *PLoS One.* 2007;2:e494.

62. Desnues B, Raoult D, Mege JL. IL-16 is critical for Tropheryma whipplei replication in Whipple's disease. *J Immunol.* 2005;175:4575.

63. Marth T, Kleen N, Stallmach A, et al. Dysregulated peripheral and mucosal Th1/Th2 response in Whipple's disease. *Gastroenterology.* 2002;123:1468.

64. Moos V, Kunkel D, Marth T, et al. Reduced peripheral and mucosal Tropheryma whipplei-specific Th1 response in patients with Whipple's disease. *J Immunol.* 2006;177:2015.

65. Schinnerling K, Moos V, Geelhaar A, et al. Regulatory T cells in patients with Whipple's disease. *J Immunol.* 2011;187:4061.

66. Bonhomme CJ, Renesto P, Nandi S, et al. Serological microarray for a paradoxical diagnostic of Whipple's disease. *Eur J Clin Microbiol Infect Dis.* 2008;27:959.

67. Fenollar F, Amphoux B, Raoult D. A paradoxical Tropheryma whipplei western blot differentiates patients with whipple disease from asymptomatic carriers. *Clin Infect Dis.* 2009;49:717.

68. Moos V, Schmidt C, Geelhaar A, et al. Impaired immune functions of monocytes and macrophages in Whipple's disease. *Gastroenterology.* 2010;138:210.

69. Glaser C, Rieg S, Wiech T, et al. Whipple's disease mimicking rheumatoid arthritis can cause misdiagnosis and treatment failure. *Orphanet J Rare Dis.* 2017;12:99.

70. Geissdorfer W, Moos V, Moter A, et al. High frequency of Tropheryma whipplei in culture-negative endocarditis. *J Clin Microbiol.* 2012;50:216.

71. Gunther U, Moos V, Offenmuller G, et al. Gastrointestinal diagnosis of classical Whipple disease: clinical, endoscopic, and histopathologic features in 191 patients. *Medicine (Baltim).* 2015;94:e714.

72. Muller C, Stain C, Burghuber O. Tropheryma whippelii in peripheral blood mononuclear cells and cells of pleural effusion. *Lancet.* 1993;341:701.

73. Durand DV, Lecomte C, Cathebras P, et al. Whipple disease. Clinical review of 52 cases. The SNFMI research group on whipple disease. Societe Nationale Francaise de Medecine interne. *Medicine (Baltim).* 1997;76:170.

74. Panegyres PK. Diagnosis and management of Whipple's disease of the brain. *Pract Neurol.* 2008;8:311.

75. Gerard A, Sarrot-Reynauld F, Liozon E, et al. Neurologic presentation of Whipple disease: report of 12 cases and review of the literature. *Medicine (Baltim).* 2002;81:443.

76. Panegyres PK, Edis R, Beaman M, et al. Primary Whipple's disease of the brain: characterization of the clinical syndrome and molecular diagnosis. *Qjm.* 2006;99:609.

77. Blessin UB, Fischer A, Schneider T, et al. More than meets the eye. *Gut.* 2018;67:69.

78. Feurle GE, Junga NS, Marth T. Efficacy of ceftriaxone or meropenem as initial therapies in Whipple's disease. *Gastroenterology.* 2010;138:478.

79. Feurle GE, Moos V, Blaker H, et al. Intravenous ceftriaxone, followed by 12 or three months of oral treatment with trimethoprim-sulfamethoxazole in Whipple's disease. *J Infect.* 2013;66:263.

80. Mahnel R, Kalt A, Ring S, et al. Immunosuppressive therapy in Whipple's disease patients is associated with the appearance of gastrointestinal manifestations. *Am J Gastroenterol.* 2005;100:1167.

81. Lagier JC, Lepidi H, Raoult D, et al. Systemic Tropheryma whipplei: clinical presentation of 142 patients with infections diagnosed or confirmed in a reference center. *Medicine (Baltim).* 2010;89:337.

82. Fenollar F, Raoult D. Molecular techniques in Whipple's disease. *Expert Rev Mol Diagn.* 2001;1:299.

83. Moter A, Schmiedel D, Petrich A, et al. Validation of an rpoB gene PCR assay for detection of Tropheryma whipplei: 10 years' experience in a National Reference Laboratory. *J Clin Microbiol.* 2013;51:3858.

84. Fenollar F, Fournier PE, Robert C, et al. Use of genome selected repeated sequences increases the sensitivity of PCR detection of Tropheryma whipplei. *J Clin Microbiol.* 2004;42:401.

85. von Herbay A, Maiwald M, Ditton HJ, et al. Histology of intestinal Whipple's disease revisited. A study of 48 patients. *Virchows Arch.* 1996;429:335.

86. Baisden BL, Lepidi H, Raoult D, et al. Diagnosis of Wihipple disease by immunohistochemical analysis: a sensitive and specific method for the detection of Tropheryma whipplei (the Whipple bacillus) in paraffin-embedded tissue. *Am J Clin Pathol.* 2002;118:742.

87. Jakobiec FA, Callahan AB, Zakka FR. Intraocular PAS-positive macrophages simulating Whipple's disease. *Graefes Arch Clin Exp Ophthalmol.* 2013;251:1033.

88. Azzopardi JG, Evans DJ. Mucoprotein-containing histiocytes (muciphages) in the rectum. *J Clin Pathol.* 1966;19:368.

89. Keinath RD, Merrell DE, Vlietstra R, et al. Antibiotic treatment and relapse in Whipple's disease. Long-term follow-up of 88 patients. *Gastroenterology.* 1985;88:1867.

90. Fleming JL, Wiesner RH, Shorter RG. Whipple's disease: clinical, biochemical, and histopathologic features and assessment of treatment in 29 patients. *Mayo Clin Proc.* 1988;63:539.

91. Feurle GE, Moos V, Schneider T, et al. The combination of chloroquine and minocycline, a therapeutic option in cerebrospinal infection of Whipple's disease refractory to treatment with ceftriaxone, meropenem and co-trimoxazole. *J Antimicrob Chemother.* 2012;67:1295.

92. Schneider T, Stallmach A, von Herbay A, et al. Treatment of refractory Whipple disease with interferon-gamma. *Ann Intern Med.* 1998;129:875.

93. Feurle GE, Marth T. An evaluation of antimicrobial treatment for Whipple's Disease. Tetracycline versus trimethoprim-sulfamethoxazole. *Dig Dis Sci.* 1994;39:1642.

94. Fenollar F, Perreal C, Raoult D. Tropheryma whipplei natural resistance to trimethoprim and sulphonamides in vitro. *Int J Antimicrob Agents.* 2014;43:388.

95. Fenollar F, Rolain JM, Alric L, et al. Resistance to trimethoprim/sulfamethoxazole and Tropheryma whipplei. *Int J Antimicrob Agents.* 2009;34:255.

96. Lagier JC, Fenollar F, Lepidi H, et al. Treatment of classic Whipple's disease: from in vitro results to clinical outcome. *J Antimicrob Chemother.* 2014;69:219.

97. Compain C, Sacre K, Puechal X, et al. Central nervous system involvement in Whipple disease: clinical study of 18 patients and long-term follow-up. *Medicine (Baltim).* 2013;92:324.

98. Feurle GE, Moos V, Schinnerling K, et al. The immune reconstitution inflammatory syndrome in whipple disease: a cohort study. *Ann Intern Med.* 2010;153:710.

99. Moos V, Feurle GE, Schinnerling K, et al. Immunopathology of immune reconstitution inflammatory syndrome in Whipple's disease. *J Immunol.* 2013;190:2354.

CHAPTER 15

Celiac Disease: Autoimmunity, Infectious Links, and the Microbiome

ARUNJOT SINGH, MD, MPH • YAEL NOBEL, MD •
SUNEETA KRISHNAREDDY, MD • PETER H. GREEN, MB, BS, MD, FRACP, FACG

INTRODUCTION/BACKGROUND

Celiac disease (CD) is an autoimmune enteropathy occurring due to aberrant immune response from dietary gluten in genetically susceptible individuals.[1] It was first described in 1888 by Dr. Samuel Gee as "the coeliac affection"; he declared that regulation of food was the root cause and any patient cure will also be from diet.[2] This theory holds true today, although advancements in the study of CD have shed light on its multifactorial pathogenesis, opening the door for future therapies. This chapter provides an overview on the epidemiology and presentation of CD, its complex pathophysiology, and the diagnostic tools and therapeutics in the pipeline. We highlight the diet–gene interactions, infectious links to immune dysregulation, and advancements in celiac microbiome research that hold great promise to finding a cure.

EPIDEMIOLOGY

Initially characterized as a rare childhood disease, the increasing diagnosis and understanding of CD has led it to be one of the most common food intolerances worldwide in both children and adults. Screening studies estimate 0.5%–1% of the population is affected in many parts of the world.[3] The National Health and Nutrition Examination Survey (NHANES) data shows a prevalence of 0.71% overall in the United States and up to 1.01% among Caucasians in the United States.[4] The rise in numbers is dramatic, as Catassi et al.[5] found the incidence to increase fivefold in 25 years from 1989–2014. The age of presentation has also changed—one retrospective analysis of patients in Ireland found the median age of presentation to be 34 years in the 1960–1985 group versus age 45 years in the 1985–2015 group.[6]

Although historically considered to have originated in Europe, epidemiologic characterization of the disease has also been seen in different ethnic and racial groups. North Africa, the Middle East, and India have all shown increased prevalence rates; in fact, the highest prevalence of CD (5.6%) is actually described in the Saharawi population in Western Sahara, Africa.[7] Despite its high prevalence worldwide, majority of individuals with CD remain undiagnosed, although the most recent analysis of the NHANES data suggested that the rate of diagnosis now exceeds 50%.[8] Given the heterogeneity in clinical presentations we will discuss, lack of provider awareness, medical access, and gaps in understanding the pathogenesis are just some variables that contribute to a significant delay and missed diagnosis.

PATHOGENESIS

The pathogenesis of CD is multifactorial, with interaction of genetics, dietary gluten exposure, and environment.[9,10] This interplay between the host genome and dietary and environmental triggers leads to immune dysregulation and subsequent intestinal inflammation, although the precise mechanism remains poorly understood.

Genetics

The genetic predisposition in CD is the first and foremost component related to disease. Apparent from early linkage and familial studies, concordance for CD in monozygotic twins is over 80% versus less than 20% in dizygotic twins—a notable difference comparable to siblings reared at different periods. A major breakthrough in the disease susceptibility and risk stratification was identified by profiling human leukocyte antigen (HLA) class II genes. Found on chromosome 7, these variant HLA genotypes are in some combination essential, but not sufficient for diagnosis or development. In fact, over 30% of the general population is estimated to carry at least one of these allele variants, yet only a small percentage (~3% of that subset)

Gastrointestinal Diseases and Their Associated Infections. https://doi.org/10.1016/B978-0-323-54843-4.00015-5
Copyright © 2019 Elsevier Inc. All rights reserved.

develop CD. This supports the notion that CD is a true polygenic disorder, with additional non-HLA genes influencing susceptibility. Nevertheless, HLA genotyping has been applied in clinical practice as an adjunct test in screening, which will be discussed in the Diagnosis section.

Advancements from next-generation sequencing and genome-wide association studies have implicated new disease-associated loci. As of today, 43 single nucleotide polymorphisms (SNPs) have been linked to CD. Unfortunately, majority of these SNPs localize to noncoding regions, suggesting a need to investigate regulatory effects and epigenetic elements that may contribute to sequences of interest. This has opened another facet in CD research, studying DNA methylation, microRNA, and long noncoding RNA effects to help elucidate biological mechanisms that cause immune-mediated intestinal damage.[11,12] One such discovery was the implication of a long noncoding RNA (lncRNA13), where the variant SNP sequence showed decreased affinity to bind and block the heterogeneous nuclear ribonucleoprotein that expresses inflammatory genes.[12]

Dietary Gluten Exposure

CD is a unique autoimmune disorder, as the central environmental or dietary precipitant is known. Characterized by small intestinal mucosal injury and nutrient malabsorption, CD is activated by dietary ingestion of proline- and glutamine-rich proteins found in wheat, rye, and barley.[13] These cereal grains are derived from the Triticeae grass family and are often widely labeled as "gluten." Nevertheless, gluten more accurately reflects disease-activating proteins found in wheat alone, namely, gliadins and glutenins. Related proteins in barley and rye that similarly activate celiac inflammation are hordeins and secalins. All four celiac activating proteins have high proline content that render these proteins resistant to proteolytic digestion by enzymes in the gastrointestinal tract, resulting in the accumulation of large peptide fragments (up to 33 amino acids) in the small intestine.[14] These large molecules enter the mucosa where they become deamidated by tissue transglutaminase and incite a T-cell–mediated immune response.[15]

The timing of gluten exposure and breastfeeding in CD has also been intensely debated with mixed results. A Swedish study found infants who were abruptly introduced to gluten later (≥7 months) had a threefold higher prevalence of CD than those with gradual introduction at 4–6 months. These findings led European Society for Paediatric Gastroenterology, Hepatology

and Nutrition (ESPGHAN) to publish a recommendation for small amounts of gluten to be gradually introduced between 4 and 7 months, although this was later revised because follow-up showed no change in total risk reduction, just a later age of onset.[16] Similarly, no significant difference was seen in studies that delay gluten ingestion to 12 months of age,[17] as with breastfeeding versus formula-fed infants, although breastmilk should continue to be promoted for its other well-established health benefits.[18]

In addition, the amount of wheat ingested may be important after the first year,[19] and through adulthood as exemplified by the regional differences seen in India. In this comparative study, CD was most prevalent in northern India (1.23%) than in southern India (0.1%) ($P<.0001$) despite similar HLA-DQ2/8 genotype rates.[20] Given that mean daily wheat intake is significantly higher in the northern Indian population, the correlation with dietary exposure appears significant, although researchers have been unable to pinpoint direct causation thus far.

Environmental Factors

In addition to gluten exposure, other environmental factors have been suggested in the cause of CD, including mode of infant delivery, socioeconomic status, season of birth, infections, and the gut microbiota. Limited to primarily observational study data, particular demographic variables are designated as associations, not causation. Nevertheless, further insight into these potential triggers may facilitate new strategies for primary prevention of CD.

One area of investigation has been the mode of infant delivery, with a significant trend toward CD in children born by cesarean delivery versus vaginally. The postnatal period is recognized as a dynamic phase in establishing host–microbe homeostasis. As such, birth in this sterile environment may alter the intestinal microbiota, which could have consequences on epithelial barrier function, establishment of the mucosal immune system, and inappropriate inflammatory response.[21]

The second major environmental aspect in CD pathogenesis is the potential link to infections. Viral and bacterial infections are the prime culprits that alter the intestinal microenvironment and set the stage for mucosal T-cell response to gluten peptides. Multiple studies have demonstrated an association between specific gastrointestinal infections and CD susceptibility. Rotavirus is one such example. It causes a common diarrheal infection that can induce inflammation, and longitudinal studies found that children with frequent rotavirus infections correlate with a nearly twofold increased risk of CD autoimmunity compared with those who had zero infections[22] by the 24-month follow-up. Similarly, risk of CD was reduced in children vaccinated against rotavirus. The mechanism of autoantibody induction and molecular mimicry is essential, as common VP7 peptide sequence in rotavirus plays a similar effect on T cells as dietary antigen.[23] Following activation, these intraepithelial cells in patients with CD transition from antigen-specific T cells to natural killer–like cells that are able to mediate epithelial cell damage through the recognition of cytokines on intestinal epithelial cells. In addition, campylobacter infections increase the risk of CD.[24] Increased risk may be the result of tissue transglutaminase activation by the infection.

The most recent discovery is the potential link to reovirus, a pathogen that we initially presumed produces protective immunity, but was later found to disrupt intestinal immune homeostasis, suppress peripheral regulatory T cells, and promote helper T-cell immunity to dietary antigens dependent on interferon regulatory factor.[25]

In contrast, infections may have protective effects. *Helicobacter pylori* is a gram-negative spiral bacteria known to cause significant gastroduodenal diseases including gastritis, peptic ulcer disease, and gastric malignancies, lymphoma and adenocarcinoma.[26] The role of *H. pylori* infection in the development of, or protection against, various autoimmune disorders is controversial. We, however, determined a decreased prevalence of CD in patients with *H. pylori* colonization: the 2008–12 cross-sectional study of over 136,000 patients found that the prevalence of CD was 4.4% in the total number of patients with *H. pylori* infection versus 8.8% in those with no *H. pylori* history.[27]

Geographic location (latitudes), seasonal patterns, and even socioeconomic status of the general population all may also have an unforeseen effect in disease susceptibility. Seasonal effects have identified a connection that typifies spring/summer birth being more common in patients with CD compared with their fall–winter counterparts in the northern hemisphere. A Swedish study examining nearly 2 million children including 6600 with CD showed a 10% greater incidence among children born in warmer seasons than in children born in the winter months (December–February).[28] This type of pattern was highest in children younger than 2 years, especially boys. Although climate may play a role, researchers have theorized that expectant mothers with increased rate of infections, those pregnant through the winter months, may have some

increased susceptibility as a result. Similarly, point latitudes show statistically significant differences in the prevalence of CD and gluten-related disorders. In a 2017 US study, adults living in the northern latitudes of the country had a greater likelihood of CD (odds ratio [OR] = 5.4) than their counterparts in the southern latitudes (OR = 3.2).[29]

Socioeconomic variations in the incidence have also been identified and may affect geographic variability. A 2008 pediatric study compared populations in adjacent Russian Karelia and Finland, an ideal epidemiologic setting because both were relatively equally exposed to grain products and partly share genetic ancestry but have completely different socioeconomic environments. These results found positive in celiac serologic tests (transglutaminase antibodies) were less frequent in the Russian group than the Finish group (0.6% vs. 1.4%, P < .0001).[30] A similar study in the United Kingdom showed a gradient of CD diagnosis across socioeconomic groups, with rates of diagnosis 80% higher in children from the least deprived areas than those from the most deprived areas (incidence rate ratio, 1.80; 95% confidence interval [CI], 1.45–2.22). Although such results open up theories to the hygiene hypothesis and microbiota changes, further studies need to be conducted to provide a mechanistic insight to disease causation.[30]

Toxic exposures including smoking and medications (e.g., antibiotics, proton pump inhibitors) have also been explored as potential links with mixed results to date. Given the increase of antisecretory medication exposure and subsequent development of CD, a population-based study in Sweden was conducted to identify such causal relationships. This study found a strong association (OR, 4.79; 95% CI, 4.17–5.51) in subjects with prior proton pump inhibitor prescription use.[31] Although this type of study may be limited for confounding protopathic bias (as early symptoms of CD may have been initially diagnosed and treated for presumed reflux), taking measures to exclude any subjects with initial proton pump inhibitor prescription within the past year continued to demonstrate a statistically significant association (OR 2.28 vs. 4.7).

Clinical presentation

CD exhibits a broad spectrum of clinical presentations, ranging from subtle to extremely prominent. However, there has been a consensus paper on the somewhat confusing terminology used in describing the presentations including classical, atypical and asymptomatic forms of CD.[32]

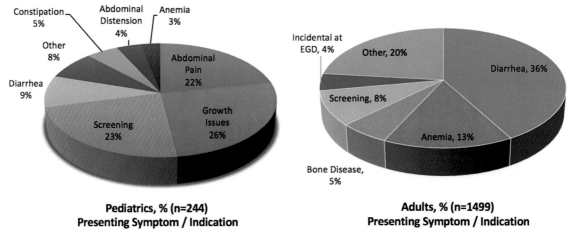

Pediatrics, % (n=244)
Presenting Symptom / Indication

Adults, % (n=1499)
Presenting Symptom / Indication

FIG. 15.1 Clinical presentation and the many faces of celiac disease. The Celiac Disease Center at Columbia University (New York, USA) studied pediatric (*n* = 244) and adult (*n* = 1499) cohorts with this autoimmune disease and the variety of gastrointestinal and extraintestinal manifestations that can lead to presentation. EGD, esophagogastroduodenoscopy. (Representative data from the Celiac Disease Center at Columbia University (New York, USA).)

The clinical presentation can also vary based on the age of the patient, with clear differences between pediatric and adult cohorts as shown in the retrospective data in Fig. 15.1. In children the major modes of presentation are recurrent abdominal pain, growth issues (short stature, failure to thrive), and screening. Diarrhea and malabsorption are actually not common, but instead constipation can be the early presentation. Those who are screen detected are typically the relatives of a patient with CD or have an autoimmune disease or Down syndrome. Even among children, there are differences according to age, with only the very young presenting with diarrhea and the older children detected by screening. Growth issues can occur at any age.[33]

In adults, diarrhea is the classic presentation, although other gastrointestinal symptoms can also occur, such as abdominal pain, bloating, and foul-smelling stools. Extraintestinal manifestations, which are considered nonclassic presentations, are increasingly common in adults with CD. These include anemia, bone disease, dermatitis herpetiformis, ataxia, liver disease, infertility, dental enamel abnormalities, and psychiatric conditions. Similarly, this can also be found during screening or incidental duodenal biopsy for an unrelated condition that required endoscopy.

Patients may be asymptomatic or have nonclassic presentation. These patients are typically detected during screening for subjects at increased risk (i.e., family members, history of diabetes, or thyroid dysfunction). Similar to patients with symptomatic disease, these patients are also at risk from long-term complications such as malignancy (e.g., small bowel adenocarcinoma, T-cell lymphoma), sequelae of malnutrition (anemia, osteoporosis), and an increased susceptibility to infections. Nevertheless, lack of overt symptoms may create a challenge for these patients to remain compliant to a gluten-free diet (GFD).

The third group is potential CD, represented by positive results in celiac serologic tests on a gluten-containing diet and normal small bowel mucosa on endoscopy. These subjects may or may not develop the disease over time. Additionally, these patients can develop minor symptoms and long-term complications such as osteoporosis, suggesting the need for close surveillance.[34]

DIAGNOSIS

Diagnosis requires an initial index of suspicion due to the patients' symptoms, presence of osteoporosis or anemia, although patients in the at-risk groups are increasingly screened. These include those with certain genetic syndromes (i.e., Down, Williams, or Turner syndrome), comorbidities (i.e., diabetes mellitus, thyroid disease), or a pertinent family history (i.e., CD or other autoimmune diseases).

TABLE 15.1
Histopathologic Classification Systems of Celiac Disease

Morphology of Duodenal Mucosa	Marsh Classification	Marsh-Oberhuber Classification	Corazza Classification
Normal	Type 0	Type 0	Normal
IEL ≥ 30/100 enterocytes, normal architecture	Type 1	Type 1	Grade A
IEL ≥ 30/100 enterocytes with crypt hyperplasia, normal architecture	Type 2	Type 2	Grade A
IEL ≥ 30/100 enterocytes, partial villous atrophy	Type 2 hyperplastic lesion	Type 3 destructive 3a: Partial villous atrophy 3b: Subtotal villous atrophy	Grade B1 atrophic, villous to crypt ratio <3:1
IEL ≥ 30/100 enterocytes, total villous atrophy	Type 3 destructive	Type 3c: Total villous atrophy	Grade B2 atrophic, villi not detectable
Normal IEL count, atrophic hypoplastic lesion	No Equivalent	Type 4	No Equivalent

Adapted from Ludvigsson et al.[32] this table categorizes celiac disease typing per classic histologic features of intraepithelial lymphocytosis (IEL), crypt hyperplasia and villous atrophy.

Serologic Testing

Serologic test is generally the initial screening tool used in patients suspected to have CD. Commercial celiac serologic tests are readily available with high sensitivity and specificity, although normal ranges can vary between different testing kits. Generally, serologic testing is most definitive when patients regularly consume gluten because on the GFD, values will normalize, irrespective of healing of the mucosa.

Based on the current evidence and practical considerations, including accuracy, reliability, and cost, the preferred screening test for individuals over the age of 2 years is the immunoglobulin A (IgA) antitissue transglutaminase antibody.[4] This enzyme-linked immunosorbent assay (ELISA)-based test has 90% sensitivity and 98% specificity in patients on a gluten-containing diet. The higher the titer, the greater the likelihood of a true-positive test result. Nevertheless, serologic test has its limitations in patients less than 2 years of age (low sensitivity)[35] as well as in those with selective IgA deficiency. To avoid reassurance of such false-negative results obtaining a baseline IgA level or additional IgG serologic testing may be warranted.

Endomysial IgA antibody test is the second major celiac serologic test and actually has the highest specificity (~99%). Determined by indirect immunofluorescence, serum endomysial IgA antibody concentration test can be expensive, can

be time-consuming, and is subject to observer variability, which may affect the sensitivity. As such, it is most often used as a supplemental test. An alternative to IgA-based serologic tests is the deamidated gliadin peptide IgG panel. This has replaced IgG antibodies against native gliadin (which lost favor, given the wide variability) and is recognized as the primary test in children less than 2 years of age.

Duodenal Biopsy and Histologic Examination

The gold standard for diagnosis remains endoscopy with histologic findings seen on duodenal biopsy. Current guidelines recommend a minimum of six biopsies from the duodenum, of which 1–2 should be taken from the duodenal bulb to potentially increase diagnostic yield. Traditionally, the diagnosis of CD required three different intestinal biopsies: first on a gluten-containing diet (initial diagnosis), follow-up after a period on GFD, and finally a repeat biopsy after gluten challenge. Subsequent studies however (particularly in children) demonstrated that initial biopsy at diagnosis is able to correctly detect CD in over 95% of patients; hence, this is no longer the standard, given its cost and procedural risks.[4]

The diagnosis of CD is based on the histologic changes of the small intestine classified according to the Marsh, Oberhuber, or Corazza classifications as reported in Table 15.1.[36] Generally, normal duodenal mucosa shows long villi with a villous-to-crypt ratio

HISTOLOGIC CLASSIFICATION OF CELIAC DISEASE

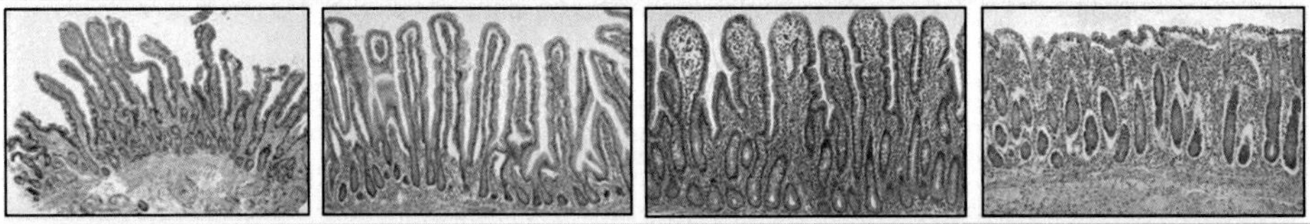

	Normal/Marsh 0	Marsh 1	Marsh 2	Marsh 3
IEL/100 enterocytes	<30	>30	>30	>30
Crypt Hyperplasia	Normal	Normal	Increased	Increased
Villous Atrophy	Normal	Normal	Normal	Mild (3a) Marked (3b) Complete (3c)

FIG. 15.2 Histologic spectrum of celiac disease as per Marsh criteria versus normal duodenal histologic examination. *IEL*, intraepithelial lymphocytosis.

of 3:1 as well as a normal number of intraepithelial lymphocytes (<30). Based on histologic changes in lymphocytic infiltration, crypt hyperplasia, and villous atrophy shown in Fig. 15.2, the spectrum of CD can be classified for diagnosis, severity, and follow-up surveillance.

ESPGHAN produced guidelines for a biopsy-sparing approach for the diagnosis of CD in symptomatic children. The criteria include a symptomatic child, tissue transglutaminase IgA >10× the upper level of normal, a repeat blood test at a later date that is positive for the endomysial antibody, and the presence of an at-risk HLA type. There is however debate about this approach.[37]

Celiac Genetics and Human Leukocyte Antigen Genotyping

As a complex polygenic disease, no single genetic test is available to diagnose CD. Nevertheless, HLA-DQ2 and HLA-DQ8 are key allele variants in disease susceptibility, making them useful adjuncts in the diagnosis of and to rule out the likelihood of CD. If a patient shows negative results for some combination of these allele variants, there is close to no likelihood for him or her to develop CD. From a diagnostic standpoint, HLA genotyping can be used to screen family members and identify patients at increased risk requiring additional surveillance.

One exception where genetic tests can actually support a CD diagnosis without needing a biopsy is presented in the 2012 ESPGHAN guidelines. In these guidelines, children with gluten-related symptoms and significantly abnormal serologic test results (tissue transglutaminase IgA >10× the upper limit of normal) can be accurately diagnosed with CD without endoscopy if the endomysial antibody is also positive and there is genetic susceptibility based on HLA genotyping (HLA-DQ2 and/or HLA-DQ8). Nevertheless, prospective data to validate the ESPGHAN recommendations are lacking and have not yet been accepted by other pediatric and adult international gastroenterology committees (Fig. 15.3).

COMPLICATIONS OF CELIAC DISEASE

Major complications classically associated with CD are malignancy, both gastrointestinal and extraintestinal; refractory CD; collagenous sprue; and ulcerative jejunoileitis. In the past decade, however, there has been increased investigation of how patients with established diagnosis of CD are impacted by systemic infections. Patients with CD have been found to have increased rates and increased severity of a variety of infections. Infections are among the leading causes of death in patients with CD, and patients with CD have higher mortality from sepsis than healthy controls.[38,39] Several hypotheses exist to explain the cause of this increased susceptibility to infections, and the pathophysiology may vary according to the individual pathogens. Other features of CD, including dysregulated adaptive and innate immunity and altered gut microbiota, likely contribute to susceptibility to

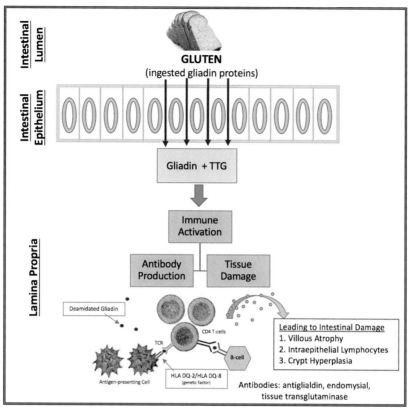

FIG. 15.3 Celiac disease pathogenesis is triggered by the dietary insult of gluten or gliadin proteins. As these pass through tight junctions into the lamina propria, gliadin is taken up by tissue transglutaminase (TTG) antibody, leading to a complex immunologic cascade and subsequent intestinal damage.[3] *HLA*, human leukocyte antigen; *TCR*, T-cell receptor.

infections in general among patients with CD, but the mechanisms remain to be elucidated (Fig. 15.4).

Pneumococcal Disease and Community-Acquired Pneumonia

Several population-based cohort studies in the United Kingdom and Sweden have demonstrated that the prevalence of infections due to *Streptococcus pneumoniae*, including bacteremia, pneumonia, meningitis, or other invasive diseases, is higher in patients with CD than that in controls, with relative rates up to twice as high as in patients with CD.[40–42] Patients with CD are also twice as likely to develop sepsis from pneumococcal infection as controls.[38] The rate of community-acquired pneumonia in general remains elevated in patients with CD regardless of whether analysis is limited to infections caused by *S. pneumoniae* alone, although pneumococcal infection accounts for the majority of bacterial pneumonia in Western countries.

A possible driving force of the disproportionately high rates and severity of pneumococcal infection among patients with CD is hyposplenism. Patients with CD have hyposplenism due to splenic atrophy and impaired splenic phagocytic function. This has been demonstrated via radiologic evidence of reduced spleen size, hallmark findings on peripheral blood smear such as target cells and Howell-Jolly bodies, and functionally by peripheral persistence of radiolabeled erythrocytes beyond the duration that would be expected with normal splenic function.[43–45] Like patients with hyposplenism or asplenia of other causes, those with hyposplenism due to CD are at risk for infections by encapsulated organisms, including *S. pneumoniae*.

Pneumococcal vaccination should be considered for all children and adults with CD and is explicitly recommended in some regions such as the United Kingdom.[46] In a UK population study by Zingone et al. of the prevalence of community-acquired pneumonia

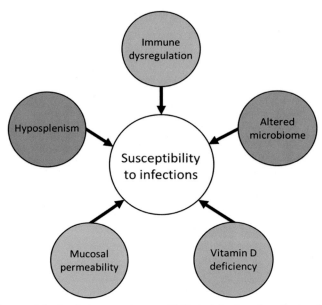

FIG. 15.4 Factors contributing to increased susceptibility to infections in patients with celiac disease.

in patients with CD, when only the subset of controls and patients with CD who had received the pneumococcal vaccine were considered, the rate of community-acquired pneumonia was actually lower among vaccinated patients with CD than in vaccinated controls.[41] However, only 27% of patients in this study received the pneumococcal vaccine in over 6 years following CD diagnosis, while other estimates demonstrated that only 53% of all patients with splenic dysfunction in the United Kingdom received pneumococcal vaccination.[47] Pneumococcal vaccination remains an important opportunity for intervention and disease prevention in patients with CD. A meta-analysis documenting increased risk of pneumococcal infection supports the use of pneumococcal vaccination for those with CD at all ages.[48]

Tuberculosis

Initial investigation of *Mycobacterium tuberculosis* in relation to CD considered intestinal tuberculosis as an alternative explanation for small bowel villous atrophy. Subsequent reports, however, identified that patients with CD have increased rates of pulmonary tuberculosis.[49,50] Population-based studies describe tuberculous disease two- to threefold more often in patients with CD than in controls.[51,52]

A leading explanation for increased susceptibility to tuberculosis is vitamin D deficiency in patients with CD. This nutritional deficiency is common among

patients with CD because of intestinal malabsorption and low levels of vitamin D in gluten-free foods.[53] Vitamin D is involved in multiple antimicrobial pathways implicated in suppressing and killing *M. tuberculosis*, including upregulation of antimicrobial peptides and increased macrophage nitric oxide synthesis; patients with either vitamin D deficiency or mutations of the vitamin D receptor have increased risk of active tuberculosis infection.[49,52,54]

Alternative hypotheses for susceptibility to tuberculosis among patients with CD relate to the polymorphisms in HLA, tumor necrosis factor, and complement factors, but the specific role of these immune variants in the development of tuberculosis in patients with CD is unknown.[49,50,52]

Influenza Infection

One national Swedish cohort study compared the rate of hospital admission for influenza A or B virus infection in patients with CD with that of matched controls and found that patients with CD were twice as likely to present with influenza compared with controls. Furthermore, patients with CD had significantly increased 28-day mortality following hospital admission for influenza. The cause of the increased rate of influenza and severity of disease in patients with CD may be multifactorial, including increased permeability of the airway mucosa[55] and malnutrition and vitamin D deficiency, leading to impaired immunity.

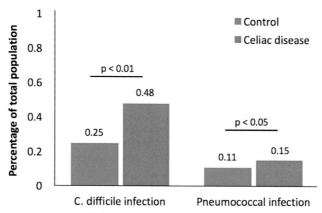

FIG. 15.5 Comparative incidence of *Clostridium difficile* infection and invasive pneumococcal infection in patients with celiac disease compared with controls. In two population-based Swedish studies, hazard ratios of two infections among patients with celiac disease compared with controls were *C. difficile* infection: 2.00 (95% confidence interval, 1.64–2.45, $P<.001$) and pneumococcal infection: 1.46 (1.05–2.03, $P=.025$).[40,57]

As with pneumococcal infection, annual vaccination against influenza should be considered in all patients with CD.

Gastrointestinal Infections

Several factors may predispose patients with CD to more frequent or severe intestinal infections specifically. First, CD is associated with altered gut microbiota; this is discussed in detail elsewhere in this chapter. Second, patients with CD have increased intestinal permeability, as demonstrated by increased intestinal excretion of a chemical probe, compared with that in controls.[56] This may reflect either sequelae of intestinal inflammation or an inherited defect in mucosal integrity, especially because permeability does not seem to correlate with the degree of CD activity.

Data regarding rates of gastrointestinal infections in patients with CD is currently limited, but several studies are ongoing regarding the prevalence of *Clostridium difficile* and other bacterial and nonbacterial diarrheal infections in this population (Fig. 15.5).[57] Given that evaluation and treatment of gastrointestinal infections is a key component of monitoring and controlling CD, further studies of these infections can provide an important therapeutic opportunity. Gastrointestinal infections are considered to predispose to the development of CD. This includes rotavirus infection in childhood[22] and campylobacter infections in adulthood.[24]

Herpes Zoster (Shingles)

A population-based study from Sweden revealed that those with CD also have an increased risk of the development of herpes zoster or shingles. In this study, there was found to be a 1.62-fold increased risk of herpes zoster (95% CI, 1.35–1.95).[58]

TREATMENTS
Dietary Gluten Avoidance

To date a GFD is the only approved therapy for patients with CD, as it reduces symptoms, lowers serologic levels, and leads to healing of damaged intestinal mucosa.[59] GFD is safe, effective, and with minimal risk if appropriately monitored with a balanced diet. Despite these pros, the major lifestyle modification required to maintain a gluten-free lifestyle can cause psychosocial stress and reduce quality of life. Low compliance can be due to a variety of reasons: poor palatability, dining outside the home, social challenges, and limited access to gluten-free options. The cost of GFD is also two to three times that of a standard diet, which can represent a significant financial hardship to the patient and family.[9]

Ingestion of gluten is common among those with CD. One study from the United Kingdom revealed that about 70% of those with CD questioned admitted to ingesting gluten either intentionally or unintentionally.[60] Patients refer to the inadvertent ingestion of gluten as cross-contamination as subjects may unknowingly ingest gluten through gluten-free foods that were processed alongside wheat products or prepared with the same utensils, frying oils, and ovens. This is in addition to the hidden gluten in foods and products (e.g., hair products, cosmetics, vitamins) that are poorly labeled or marketed as gluten free with lack of certified testing. One study of 200 commercially available "gluten-free products" in the Italian market found that 9% of those items had gluten levels higher than the standardized cutoff of 20 parts per million.[61] Often these individuals are identified as "nonresponders" but are found to have accidental gluten exposure and lapses in dietary gluten avoidance. Using a multidisciplinary care model composed of the patient, family, gastroenterologist, dietician, psychologist, and primary care provider, optimal tools are put in place for provision of GFD teaching and to achieve long-term adherence.[62]

Management of Refractory Celiac Disease

Even with the utmost compliance, there is a subset of patients resistant to treatment, labeled refractory CD. Defined by persistent villous atrophy with persistent or recurrent malabsorptive symptoms, these patients are simply unresponsive to a GFD. This is a diagnosis of exclusion and requires a minimum of 6–12 months of strict GFD adherence, with the number of such cases varying greatly between major celiac referral centers (10%–18%) and nonreferral population-based cohorts (0.7%–1.47%).[63] In refractory CD, corticosteroids are the mainstay of treatment, with budesonide having a major role.[64,65] Refractory CD, especially type II, has a poor prognosis and can be regarded as an occult T-cell lymphoma.[66] Aggressive nutritional support and parenteral nutrition is also a vital arm in the treatment of refractory disease, with newer experimental therapies using cyclosporine, infliximab, and chemotherapeutic agents showing promise.

Advances in Drug Development

New treatments and drug targets in CD are in the pipeline, many of which have advanced to phase I or II clinical trials. All therapies currently are proposed to be used to assist people maintain a GFD, which appears to be very attractive to those with the disease.[67] Targets to reduce gluten exposure are appearing with developing select proteases (endopeptidases) to degrade the toxic gluten peptides in the stomach.[68]

Theoretically, these glutenases work exclusively in the intestinal lumen avoiding the immune cascade that occurs in the lamina propria and limiting harmful side effects.[69] A small group of such dietary supplements are already marketed, although national drug agencies such as the Food and Drug Administration have yet to approve these enzymes and there is little evidence of their efficacy or value.[70] A randomized double-blinded phase II study of latiglutenase, an oral mixture of two recombinant gluten proteases, in 494 patients with CD who had been on a GFD for at least 1 year failed

to demonstrate histologic or serologic improvements including in the villous height to crypt depth ratio and the numbers of intraepithelial lymphocytes.[71] However, all groups including placebo had significant improvements in histologic and symptom scores, which has been ascribed to the Hawthorne effect. Further analysis of this study data revealed a subgroup of patients with positive serologic test results who did in fact respond to latiglutenase, indicating the potential therapeutic value of this drug.[72]

Another area in drug targets has been modifying intestinal permeability because an early action of gluten in CD is an increase in gut permeability via disruption of epithelial tight junctions between enterocytes, resulting in the entry of gliadin from the intestinal lumen into the lamina propria.[73] Larazotide acetate (AT-1001), a small intestinal tight junction regulator, is a synthetic oral peptide that has been developed as a therapeutic agent for CD to supplement a GFD.[73] It has been studied in several clinical trials, including phase I and II studies, showing overall good tolerability but mixed efficacy results. In a four-arm, double-blinded, randomized study, 184 patients with CD were randomized to three different doses of larazotide acetate or placebo after an initial run-in period of GFD and they subsequently received 2.7 g of gluten daily for 6 weeks.[74] The drug was well tolerated and patient symptoms as assessed by the Gastrointestinal Symptom Rating Scale (GSRS) showed improvement. The mean ratio of antitissue transglutaminase IgA levels over baseline was also lower in the treatment groups than those in placebo (5.78, 3.88, and 7.72 in larazotide acetate for 1-, 4-, and 8-mg groups, respectively vs. 19.0 in placebo group, $P < .05$). Interestingly, no significant differences were observed in intestinal permeability assessed by the lactulose-to-mannitol ratio.[74] Another study compared different doses of larazotide acetate and placebo in 342 adult patients with CD who had been on a GFD for 12 months or longer and showed a prolonged improvement in clinical symptoms assessed by GSRS score. The 0.5-mg dose resulted in a significant reduction in patient reported symptoms including a 26% decrease in symptomatic days, a 31% increase in improved symptom days, and a 50% reduction of the weekly average abdominal pain score.[75] Leading off this promising results, further studies are proposed with larazotide.

Researchers have also been developing a therapeutic vaccine, Nexvax2, a mixture of three peptides that include immunodominant epitopes for gluten-specific CD4-positive T cells, with the rationale of suppressing their response to antigenic stimulation. Two randomized, double-blinded, placebo-controlled phase I trials in HLA-DQ2.5-positive adult patients with CD on a GFD revealed alteration in immune responsiveness to Nexvax2 peptides assessed by an interferon-γ release assay without any worsening noticed in duodenal histologic examination. The maximum tolerated dose of the vaccine was 150 μg for twice weekly intradermal administration over 8 weeks, and following the first intradermal administration of the vaccine, the gastrointestinal symptoms resembled those associated with oral gluten challenge.[76] Given these promising results from the phase I studies, the vaccine among other potential therapeutics has begun its development in phase II trials.

MICROBIOME AND CELIAC DISEASE

The human gastrointestinal tract is a complex and dynamic environment, sheltering a vast number and variety of commensal microorganisms.[77] This balanced microecosystem is a natural defense against invasion of pathogens. Much research has focused on the role of the human microbiome in health and disease and the ability to harness the power of the microbiome for the treatment of diseases, as well as on the role of dysbiosis in autoimmunity and disease pathogenesis.

Genetic Linkage to Microbiota

CD is a complex multifactorial disorder involving both genetic and environmental factors. For many years the only securely established genetic factors contributing to CD risk were the genetic variants located within the HLA region (those encoding the HLA-DQ2/DQ8 heterodimers).[3] With the introduction of genome-wide association studies and immunochip studies identifying additional non-HLA regions of CD, there are new targets for investigation, some of which are associated with other autoimmune diseases.[78–80] Interestingly, most of the chromosome regions associated with CD predisposition contain genes with immune-related functions, and some CD susceptibility genes and/or their altered expression play a role in bacterial colonization and sensing. Studies have also shown an altered expression of nonspecific CD risk genes involved in host–microbiota interactions in the intestinal mucosa of patients with CD, such as those of toll-like receptors and their regulators.[81] Disturbances in the host–microbiota interaction and shifts in the immune balance in subjects with CD might propagate the inflammatory response by gluten that is pathognomonic to CD.

Studies of the role the microbiome play in CD are still in its infancy, and as with most studies of the microbiome, most studies have shown descriptive data, but lack cause and effect. Indeed, although CD is prevalent in both adults and children, most of the microbiome data in CD comes from studies done in children.[82–85] Studies characterizing the microbiota of adult patients with CD only began in 2012, and a single study of both children and adults reported a slight difference in the percentages of the main phyla between subjects and also a more diverse profile in duodenal biopsy specimens from adults (11). The Firmicutes are the most abundant bacteria in adults with CD, whereas Proteobacteria are present mainly in children with CD. Other phyla shared between adults and children with CD belong to the Bacteroidetes and Actinobacteria. Regarding bacterial genera, adults with CD harbor larger numbers of *Mycobacterium* spp. and *Methylobacterium* spp. While *Neisseria* spp. and *Haemophilus* spp. are more abundant in children with CD. While these studies have given us information about the general makeup of the microbiome of patients with CD, they do little to answer the questions if these changes precede disease onset, if they are a consequence of inflammation, or if the changes seen in the microbiome are associated with changes in immune cell phenotype. Future studies need to focus on causality, and possibly a specific bacterial group that could be pathogenic or protective in this group of patients, and that could be targeted for treatment.

Microbiome—Cause or Consequence of Celiac Disease

Whether the altered microbiome is a cause or consequence of CD remains unclear. Nevertheless, it is hypothesized that gram-negative bacteria in genetically susceptible individuals may contribute to the loss of gluten tolerance. If modified bacteria are a result of disease, the disrupted mucosa inundated with immature enterocytes could lead to conditions favoring gram-negative instead of gram-positive bacterial colonization. While this theory has not been proven, early studies have shown a propensity toward higher gram-negative colonization in duodenal samples of pediatric patients with CD than in healthy controls, in which case the dysbiosis seen seems to be clinically important.[86] Additionally, CD is a unique disease to study the microbiome because many other factors can be controlled for, including genetic makeup, environment, and trigger, as these are all known, and the effect of the microbiome on disease pathogenesis can be further explored. Also, since the genetic makeup can be determined prior to a subject acquiring CD, it is possible to do longitudinal studies in these patients and observing the change in microbiome to see if the alterations noted are a cause or consequence of disease.[87]

Gluten-Free Diet and Microbiome

Several studies have compared the gut microbiota of patients with CD following a GFD and on a gluten-containing diet, as well as controls. In patients with CD, even after following a GFD (for at least 2 years), the duodenal mucosa microbiota was not completely restored and showed a less abundant bacterial richness compared with healthy and untreated subjects, with a persistent imbalance of the ratio of potentially harmful/beneficial bacteria.[87] Species-specific analysis has shown that while *Escherichia coli* and *Staphylococcus* counts are restored after a GFD, *Bifidobacteria* counts remain lower in the feces of patients on a GFD than in controls. A targeted study on *Bifidobacteria* composition from patients with CD on both a gluten-containing diet and a GFD and from healthy controls showed a correlation between the levels of *Bifidobacterium* and *Bifidobacterium longum* in the fecal and tissue samples. Moreover, a generalized reduction in these bacterial populations was found in patients with CD as compared with healthy children overall.[88] Additional information from a study evaluated the effect of a GFD on healthy subjects[82] using fluorescence in situ hybridization and quantitative polymerase chain reaction. In this study, it was noted that the GFD leads to a decrease in *B. longum*, *Clostridium lituseburense*, *Lactobacillus*, and *Faecalibacterium prausnitzii* and an increase in Enterobacteriaceae and *E. coli* strains. This was thought to be due to the reduced production of proinflammatory and regulatory cytokines due to a generalized reduction in the total luminal bacterial load of the large intestine caused by the GFD. The main finding was that a GFD influenced gut microbial composition and immune activation (as measured by cytokine production) regardless of the presence of disease, and these effects were directly related to reduction in polysaccharide intake. Few studies have followed the same patients before and after GFD to test the effect of gluten on the microbiome in the presence of CD. An Italian study showed that the *Lactobacillus* community was lower before than after a GFD and was lower in patients with CD than in healthy controls. There was also a lower ratio of *Bifidobacterium* to *Bacteroides* and *Enterobacteria* as compared with healthy controls.[89]

Overall, these studies show that a GFD only partially restores fecal microbiota balances in patients with CD. The reason is still unclear, although some suggest that genetic influences in those predisposed to CD affects the colonization of the microbiome, which persists despite a GFD; furthermore, since gluten has a prebiotic action, its absence in the GFD induces a different gut microbiota even in healthy individuals.[90] These findings need to be further studied to clarify the effect of the diet on the microbiome on disease resolution, again to determine where therapeutic targets lie, and how the microbiome can be manipulated to further treat patients with CD.

CONCLUSION

CD is a widespread autoimmune disease with a unique well-known dietary antigen trigger. The only current treatment is a GFD that is often difficult to follow strictly, given its ubiquitous presence in a variety of foods. Given its broad range of intestinal and extraintestinal manifestations, including increased susceptibility to malignancies, it is paramount to develop new effective therapies for CD. Many hurdles remain in finding a cure due to its complex pathogenesis, and so far, there has been limited progress in developing innovative therapeutics. As research advancements continue in the microbiome, infectious links, and the epigenome, this knowledge will inspire novel targets for therapy both in CD and in other important autoimmune or gastrointestinal disorders.

REFERENCES

1. Parzanese IQD, Patrinicola F, Aralica M, et al. Celiac disease: from pathophysiology to treatment. *World J Gastrointest Pathophysiol*. 2017;8(2):27–38.
2. Dowd B, W-S J. Samuel gee, aretaeus, and the coeliac affection. *Br Med J*. 1974;45–47.
3. Green PH, Cellier C. Celiac disease. *N Engl J Med*. 2007;357(17):1731–1743.
4. Rubio-Tapia A, Hill ID, Kelly CP, Calderwood AH, Murray JA. American College of G. ACG clinical guidelines: diagnosis and management of celiac disease. *Am J Gastroenterol*. 2013;108(5):656–676; quiz 677.
5. Catassi C, Gatti S, Fasano A. The new epidemiology of celiac disease. *J Pediatr Gastroenterol Nutr*. 2014;59(suppl 1):S7–S9.
6. Dominguez Castro P, Harkin G, Hussey M, et al. Changes in presentation of celiac disease in Ireland from the 1960s to 2015. *Clin Gastroenterol Hepatol*. 2017;15(6):864–871. e863.
7. Lionetti E, Gatti S, Pulvirenti A, Catassi C. Celiac disease from a global perspective. *Best Pract Res Clin Gastroenterol*. 2015;29(3):365–379.
8. Choung RS, Unalp-Arida A, Ruhl CE, Brantner TL, Everhart JE, Murray JA. Less hidden celiac disease but increased gluten avoidance without a diagnosis in the United States: findings from the national health and nutrition examination surveys from 2009 to 2014. *Mayo Clin Proc*. 2016; 30634–30636.

9. Lee AR, Ng DL, Zivin J, Green PH. Economic burden of a gluten-free diet. *J Hum Nutr Diet.* 2007;20(5):423–430.

10. Lebwohl B, Ludvigsson JF, Green PH. Celiac disease and non-celiac gluten sensitivity. *BMJ.* 2015;351:h4347.

11. Withoff S, Li Y, Jonkers I, Wijmenga C. Understanding celiac disease by genomics. *Trends Genet.* 2016;32(5):295–308.

12. Castellanos-Rubio A, Fernandez-Jimenez N, Kratchmarov R, et al. A long noncoding RNA associated with susceptibility to celiac disease. *Science.* 2016;352(6281):91–95.

13. Kagnoff MF. Overview and pathogenesis of celiac disease. *Gastroenterology.* 2005;128(4 suppl 1):S10–S18.

14. Shan L, Molberg O, Parrot I, et al. Structural basis for gluten intolerance in celiac sprue. *Science.* 2002;297(5590):2275–2279.

15. Green PH, Jabri B. Coeliac disease. *Lancet.* 2003;362(9381):383–391.

16. Pinto-Sanchez MI, Verdu EF, Liu E, et al. Gluten introduction to infant feeding and risk of celiac disease: systematic review and meta-analysis. *J Pediatr.* 2016;168:132–143.e133.

17. Lionetti E, Castellaneta S, Francavilla R, et al. Introduction of gluten, HLA status, and the risk of celiac disease in children. *N Engl J Med.* 2014;371(14):1295–1303.

18. Szajewska H, Shamir R, Mearin L, et al. Gluten introduction and the risk of coeliac disease: a position paper by the European Society for pediatric gastroenterology, Hepatology, and nutrition. *J Pediatr Gastroenterol Nutr.* 2016;62(3):507–513.

19. Ludvigsson JF, Lebwohl B, Green PH. Amount may beat timing: gluten intake and risk of childhood celiac disease. *Clin Gastroenterol Hepatol.* 2016;14(3):410–412.

20. Ramakrishna BS, Makharia GK, Chetri K, et al. Prevalence of adult celiac disease in India: regional variations and associations. *Am J Gastroenterol.* 2016;111(1):115–123.

21. Decker E, Hornef M, Stockinger S. Cesarean delivery is associated with celiac disease but not inflammatory bowel disease in children. *Gut Microb.* 2011;2(2):91–98.

22. Stene LC, Honeyman MC, Hoffenberg EJ, et al. Rotavirus infection frequency and risk of celiac disease autoimmunity in early childhood: a longitudinal study. *Am J Gastroenterol.* 2006;101(10):2333–2340.

23. Dolcino M, Zanoni G, Bason C, et al. A subset of anti-rotavirus antibodies directed against the viral protein VP7 predicts the onset of celiac disease and induces typical features of the disease in the intestinal epithelial cell line T84. *Immunol Res.* 2013;56(2–3):465–476.

24. Riddle MS, Murray JA, Cash BD, Pimentel M, Porter CK. Pathogen-specific risk of celiac disease following bacterial causes of foodborne illness: a retrospective cohort study. *Dig Dis Sci.* 2013;58(11):3242–3245.

25. Bouziat R, Hinterleitner R, Brown JJ, et al. Reovirus infection triggers inflammatory responses to dietary antigens and development of celiac disease. *Science.* 2017;356(6333):44–50.

26. Garza-Gonzalez E, Perez-Perez GI, Maldonado-Garza HJ, Bosques-Padilla FJ. A review of *Helicobacter pylori* diagnosis, treatment, and methods to detect eradication. *World J Gastroenterol.* 2014;20(6):1438–1449.

27. Lebwohl B, Blaser MJ, Ludvigsson JF, et al. Decreased risk of celiac disease in patients with *Helicobacter pylori* colonization. *Am J Epidemiol.* 2013;178(12):1721–1730.

28. Namatovu F, Lindkvist M, Olsson C, Ivarsson A, Sandstrom O. Season and region of birth as risk factors for coeliac disease a key to the aetiology? *Arch Dis Child.* 2016;101(12):1114–1118.

29. Unalp-Arida A, Ruhl CE, Choung RS, Brantner TL, Murray JA. Lower prevalence of celiac disease and gluten-related disorders in persons living in southern vs northern latitudes of the United States. *Gastroenterology.* 2017;152(8):1922–1932.e1922.

30. Kondrashova A, Mustalahti K, Kaukinen K, et al. Lower economic status and inferior hygienic environment may protect against celiac disease. *Ann Med.* 2008;40(3):223–231.

31. Lebwohl B, Spechler SJ, Wang TC, Green PH, Ludvigsson JF. Use of proton pump inhibitors and subsequent risk of celiac disease. *Dig Liver Dis.* 2014;46(1):36–40.

32. Ludvigsson JF, Leffler DA, Bai JC, et al. The Oslo definitions for coeliac disease and related terms. *Gut.* 2013;62(1):43–52.

33. Rizkalla Reilly N, Dixit R, Simpson S, Green PH. Celiac disease in children: an old disease with new features. *Minerva Pediatr.* 2012;64(1):71–81.

34. Elfstrom P, Granath F, Ye W, Ludvigsson JF. Low risk of gastrointestinal cancer among patients with celiac disease, inflammation, or latent celiac disease. *Clin Gastroenterol Hepatol.* 2012;10(1):30–36.

35. Lagerqvist C, D I, Hansson T, et al. Antigliadin immunoglobulin a best in finding celiac disease in children younger than 18 Months of age. *J Pediatr Gastroenterol Nutr.* 2008;47:428–435.

36. Pena AS. What is the best histopathological classification for celiac disease? Does it matter? *Gastroenterol Hepatol Bed Bench.* 2015;8(4):239–243.

37. Reilly NR, Husby S, Sanders DS, Green PHR. Coeliac disease: to biopsy or not? *Nat Rev Gastroenterol Hepatol.* 2017;60–66.

38. Ludvigsson JF, Olen O, Bell M, Ekbom A, Montgomery SM. Coeliac disease and risk of sepsis. *Gut.* 2008;57(8):1074–1080.

39. Peters U, Askling J, Gridley G, Ekbom A, Linet M. Causes of death in patients with celiac disease in a population-based Swedish cohort. *Arch Intern Med.* 2003;163(13):1566–1572.

40. Rockert Tjernberg A, Bonnedahl J, Inghammar M, et al. Coeliac disease and invasive pneumococcal disease: a population-based cohort study. *Epidemiol Infect.* 2017;145(6):1203–1209.

41. Zingone F, Abdul Sultan A, Crooks CJ, Tata LJ, Ciacci C, West J. The risk of community-acquired pneumonia among 9803 patients with coeliac disease compared to the general population: a cohort study. *Aliment Pharmacol Ther.* 2016;44(1):57–67.

42. Thomas HJ, Wotton CJ, Yeates D, Ahmad T, Jewell DP, Goldacre MJ. Pneumococcal infection in patients with coeliac disease. *Eur J Gastroenterol Hepatol.* 2008;20(7):624–628.

43. Marsh GW, Stewart JS. Splenic function in adult coeliac disease. *Br J Haematol.* 1970;19(4):445–457.

44. Corazza GR, Bullen AW, Hall R, Robinson PJ, Losowsky MS. Simple method of assessing splenic function in coeliac disease. *Clin Sci (Lond).* 1981;60(1):109–113.

45. Robinson PJ, Bullen AW, Hall R, Brown RC, Baxter P, Losowsky MS. Splenic size and function in adult coeliac disease. *Br J Radiol.* 1980;53(630):532–537.

46. Ludvigsson JF, Bai JC, Biagi F, et al. Diagnosis and management of adult coeliac disease: guidelines from the British Society of Gastroenterology. *Gut.* 2014;63(8):1210–1228.

47. Pebody RG, Hippisley-Cox J, Harcourt S, Pringle M, Painter M, Smith G. Uptake of pneumococcal polysaccharide vaccine in at-risk populations in England and Wales 1999–2005. *Epidemiol Infect.* 2008;136(3):360–369.

48. Simons M, Scott-Sheldon LAJ, Risech-Neyman Y, Moss SF, Ludvigsson JF, Green PHR. Celiac disease and increased risk of pneumococcal infection: a systematic review and meta-analysis. *Am J Med.* 2017;83–89.

49. Sanders DS, West J, Whyte MK. Coeliac disease and risk of tuberculosis: a population-based cohort study. *Thorax.* 2007;62(1):1–2.

50. Williams AJ, Asquith P, Stableforth DE. Susceptibility to tuberculosis in patients with coeliac disease. *Tubercle.* 1988;69(4):267–274.

51. Ludvigsson JF, Wahlstrom J, Grunewald J, Ekbom A, Montgomery SM. Coeliac disease and risk of tuberculosis: a population based cohort study. *Thorax.* 2007;62(1):23–28.

52. Ludvigsson JF, Sanders DS, Maeurer M, Jonsson J, Grunewald J, Wahlstrom J. Risk of tuberculosis in a large sample of patients with coeliac disease–a nationwide cohort study. *Aliment Pharmacol Ther.* 2011;33(6):689–696.

53. Kupper C. Dietary guidelines and implementation for celiac disease. *Gastroenterology.* 2005;128(4 suppl 1):S121–S127.

54. Nnoaham KE, Clarke A. Low serum vitamin D levels and tuberculosis: a systematic review and meta-analysis. *Int J Epidemiol.* 2008;37(1):113–119.

55. Robertson DA, Taylor N, Sidhu H, Britten A, Smith CL, Holdstock G. Pulmonary permeability in coeliac disease and inflammatory bowel disease. *Digestion.* 1989;42(2):98–103.

56. Bjarnason I, Marsh MN, Price A, Levi AJ, Peters TJ. Intestinal permeability in patients with coeliac disease and dermatitis herpetiformis. *Gut.* 1985;26(11):1214–1219.

57. Lebwohl B, Nobel YR, Green PHR, Blaser MJ, Ludvigsson JF. Risk of *Clostridium difficile* infection in patients with celiac disease: a population-based study. *Am J Gastroenterol.* 2017;1878–1884.

58. Ludvigsson JF, Choung RS, Marietta EV, Murray JA, Emilsson L. Increased risk of herpes zoster in patients with coeliac disease - nationwide cohort study. *Scand J Public Health.* 2017:1403494817714713.

59. Guandalini S, Assiri A. Celiac disease: a review. *JAMA Pediatrics.* 2014;168(3):272–278.

60. Hall NJ, Rubin GP, Charnock A. Intentional and inadvertent non-adherence in adult coeliac disease. A cross-sectional survey. *Appetite.* 2013;68:56–62.

61. Verma AK, Gatti S, Galeazzi T, et al. Gluten contamination in naturally or labeled gluten-free products marketed in Italy. *Nutrients.* 2017;9(2).

62. Isaac DM, Wu J, Mager DR, Turner JM. Managing the pediatric patient with celiac disease: a multidisciplinary approach. *J Multidiscip Healthc.* 2016;9:529–536.

63. Rishi AR, Rubio-Tapia A, Murray JA. Refractory celiac disease. *Expert Rev Gastroenterol Hepatol.* 2016;10(4):537–546.

64. Mukewar SS, Sharma A, Rubio-Tapia A, Wu TT, Jabri B, Murray JA. Open-capsule budesonide for refractory celiac disease. *Am J Gastroenterol.* 2017;112(6):959–967.

65. Brar P, Lee S, Lewis S, Egbuna I, Bhagat G, Green PH. Budesonide in the treatment of refractory celiac disease. *Am J Gastroenterol.* 2007;102(10):2265–2269.

66. Rubio-Tapia A, Murray JA. Classification and management of refractory celiac disease. *Gut.* 2010;59(4):547–557.

67. Tennyson CA, Simpson S, Lebwohl B, Lewis S, Green PH. Interest in medical therapy for celiac disease. *Therap Adv Gastroenterol.* 2013;6(5):358–364.

68. Leffler D. Celiac disease diagnosis and management: a 46-year-old woman with anemia. *J Am Med Assoc.* 2011;306(14):1582–1592.

69. Kaukinen K, Lindfors K. Novel treatments for celiac disease: glutenases and beyond. *Dig Dis.* 2015;33(2):277–281.

70. Krishnareddy S, Stier K, Recanati M, Lebwohl B, Green PH. Commercially available glutenases: a potential hazard in coeliac disease. *Therap Adv Gastroenterol.* 2017;10(6):473–481.

71. Murray JA, Kelly CP, Green PHR, et al. No difference between latiglutenase and placebo in reducing villous atrophy or improving symptoms in patients with symptomatic celiac disease. *Gastroenterology.* 2017;152(4):787–798.e782.

72. Syage JA, Murray JA, Green PHR, Khosla C. Latiglutenase improves symptoms in seropositive celiac disease patients while on a gluten-free diet. *Dig Dis Sci.* 2017;2428–2432.

73. Khaleghi S, Ju JM, Lamba A, Murray JA. The potential utility of tight junction regulation in celiac disease: focus on larazotide acetate. *Therap Adv Gastroenterol.* 2016;9(1):37–49.

74. Kelly CP, Green PH, Murray JA, et al. Larazotide acetate in patients with coeliac disease undergoing a gluten challenge: a randomised placebo-controlled study. *Aliment Pharmacol Ther.* 2013;37(2):252–262.

75. Leffler DA, Kelly CP, Green PH, et al. Larazotide acetate for persistent symptoms of celiac disease despite a gluten-free diet: a randomized controlled trial. *Gastroenterology.* 2015;148(7):1311–1319.e1316.

76. Goel G, King T, Daveson AJ, et al. Epitope-specific immunotherapy targeting CD4-positive T cells in coeliac disease: two randomised, double-blind, placebo-controlled phase 1 studies. *Lancet Gastroenterol Hepatol.* 2017;2(7):479–493.

77. Kau AL, Ahern PP, Griffin NW, Goodman AL, Gordon JI. Human nutrition, the gut microbiome and the immune system. *Nature.* 2011;474(7351):327–336.

78. van Heel DA, Franke L, Hunt KA, et al. A genome-wide association study for celiac disease identifies risk variants in the region harboring IL2 and IL21. *Nat Genet.* 2007;39(7):827–829.

79. Hunt KA, Zhernakova A, Turner G, et al. Newly identified genetic risk variants for celiac disease related to the immune response. *Nat Genet.* 2008;40(4):395–402.

80. Dubois PC, Trynka G, Franke L, et al. Multiple common variants for celiac disease influencing immune gene expression. *Nat Genet.* 2010;42(4):295–302.

81. Kalliomaki M, Satokari R, Lahteenoja H, et al. Expression of microbiota, Toll-like receptors, and their regulators in the small intestinal mucosa in celiac disease. *J Pediatr Gastroenterol Nutr.* 2012;54(6):727–732.

82. De Palma G, Nadal I, Collado MC, Sanz Y. Effects of a gluten-free diet on gut microbiota and immune function in healthy adult human subjects. *Br J Nutr.* 2009;102(8):1154–1160.

83. De Palma G, Nadal I, Medina M, et al. Intestinal dysbiosis and reduced immunoglobulin-coated bacteria associated with coeliac disease in children. *BMC Microbiol.* 2010;10:63.

84. De Palma G, Capilla A, Nadal I, et al. Interplay between human leukocyte antigen genes and the microbial colonization process of the newborn intestine. *Curr Issues Mol Biol.* 2010;12(1):1–10.

85. Nadal I, Santacruz A, Marcos A, et al. Shifts in clostridia, bacteroides and immunoglobulin-coating fecal bacteria associated with weight loss in obese adolescents. *Int J Obes.* 2009;33(7):758–767.

86. Nistal E, Caminero A, Herran AR, et al. Differences of small intestinal bacteria populations in adults and children with/without celiac disease: effect of age, gluten diet, and disease. *Inflamm Bowel Dis.* 2012;18(4):649–656.

87. Collado MC, Donat E, Ribes-Koninckx C, Calabuig M, Sanz Y. Specific duodenal and faecal bacterial groups associated with paediatric coeliac disease. *J Clin Pathol.* 2009;62(3):264–269.

88. Collado MC, Donat E, Ribes-Koninckx C, Calabuig M, Sanz Y. Imbalances in faecal and duodenal Bifidobacterium species composition in active and non-active coeliac disease. *BMC Microbiol.* 2008;8:232.

89. Di Cagno R, Rizzello CG, Gagliardi F, et al. Different fecal microbiotas and volatile organic compounds in treated and untreated children with celiac disease. *Appl Environ Microbiol.* 2009;75(12):3963–3971.

90. Jackson FW. Effects of a gluten-free diet on gut microbiota and immune function in healthy adult human subjects - comment by Jackson. *Br J Nutr.* 2010;104(5):773.

CHAPTER 16

Parasitic Diarrhea

JOHN FREAN, MB BCH, MMED (PATH MICROBIOL), FFSCI RCPA, FFTM RCPS (GLASGOW), FACTM, MSC (MED PARASITOL)

INTRODUCTION

When all infectious causes of diarrhea are considered, parasites contribute a minority of causes and cases of disease. In some segments of the global community, however, parasitic infections are significant in terms of clinical impact. These vulnerable subsets of persons are generally young children, those that are immunocompromised for a variety of reasons, and those living in low-income countries with poor standards of sanitation and hygiene, and unsafe food and water supplies. Another group at risk for these parasitic causes of diarrhea is travellers from developed countries, who usually lack the same degree of acquired protective immunity as the local population, and are therefore highly susceptible to symptomatic infection.

A classification of important parasitic causes of diarrhea is shown in Fig. 16.1. The emphasis of this chapter will be on those parasitic infections in which diarrhea is the primary expression of disease. In contrast, some parasitic diseases may produce loose stools as an incidental part of the infective process, but their major pathological effects are different and/or occur elsewhere in the body (e.g., *Trichinella* spp., *Anisakis* spp.). Generally benign and asymptomatic infections such as intestinal tapeworm infections sometimes produce diarrhea. Some intestinal parasites (e.g., *Schistosoma mansoni*, *Trichuris trichiura*) only cause diarrhea or dysentery in heavily infected persons. These parasite categories will not be covered in any detail (summary in Table 16.1).

PROTOZOAN PARASITES

Cryptosporidium Species

Cryptosporidium species are apicomplexan protozoan parasites that are predominantly zoonotic pathogens, with a wide host range. Thirty-one species are currently recognized, more than 20 of which have been found in humans, but the species most frequently associated with human infections are *Cryptosporidium parvum* (broadly but not exclusively zoonotic, natural animal hosts being even-toed ungulates) and *Cryptosporidium*
hominis (anthroponotic), contributing 90% of cryptosporidiosis cases.[1] Other species that commonly affect humans are *C. meleagridis* (bird hosts) and *C. cuniculus* (rabbit hosts). Genotyping to identify and distinguish between species is usually based on 18S rRNA gene analysis, with subtyping mainly at the *gp60* gene locus. Certain subtypes of *C. parvum* are regarded as anthroponotically transmitted.[2]

Epidemiology

Infections can be acquired by direct contact with feces of infected animals or humans, but more commonly indirectly, via contaminated water or food, with the risk of producing outbreaks because of the low infective dose (10 or fewer oocysts, in adult volunteers).[3] Cryptosporidia normally undergo sexual and asexual reproduction in the enterocytes of the small intestine of infected hosts, but occasionally (predominantly in immunocompromised individuals) affect other organs, for example, respiratory, hepatobiliary, and upper gastrointestinal tracts. Thick-walled oocysts are excreted in the feces and able to persist in the environment, resisting normal levels of chlorination in drinking water and swimming pools. Exposure to surface water, typically in, but not limited to, swimming and splashing pools, is a recognized risk factor for infection, and discouraging diarrheic persons from using recreational aquatic facilities is an important measure to reduce the risk of outbreaks, although difficult to enforce.[4]

Geographically, cryptosporidiosis occurs worldwide, but its contribution to the burden of disease varies geographically. It is endemic in developing countries, where high prevalences occur predominantly in young children, a proportion of whom are asymptomatic carriers. The Global Enteric Multicentre Study (a 3-year, 7-site, case–control study of moderate to severe diarrhea in sub-Saharan Africa and South Asia (India, Pakistan, Bangladesh, Nepal, and Afghanistan)) reported that rotavirus was the only pathogen that caused more cases of severe diarrhea than *Cryptosporidium* in under-5-year-olds.[5] In under-2-year-olds, it was estimated that, respectively, 2.9 and 4.7 million cases of cryptosporidial

Gastrointestinal Diseases and Their Associated Infections. https://doi.org/10.1016/B978-0-323-54843-4.00016-7
Copyright © 2019 Elsevier Inc. All rights reserved.

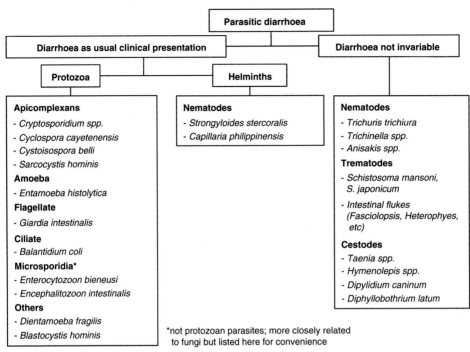

FIG. 16.1 Classification of parasitic causes of diarrhea.

TABLE 16.1
Parasitic Helminth Diseases Sometimes Associated with Diarrhea

Parasite Name	Disease	Geographic Distribution	Diagnosis	Treatment
Trichuris trichiura; some animal species can cause human infection	Trichuriasis, whipworm disease	Humid tropical and subtropical areas worldwide; some temperate regions	Microscopy of stool; molecular methods described	Albendazole, mebendazole
Trichinella spiralis, T. britovi, T. nativa, T. nelsoni, T. murrelli, T. pseudospiralis	Trichinellosis	*T. spiralis* is cosmopolitan; other species in arctic, Eurasia, N, C, S America, tropical Africa	Serological tests; muscle biopsy; indirectly, eosinophilia and raised muscle enzymes	AlbendazoleSymptomatic (analgesia, corticosteroids) for myositis stage
Anisakis spp. and *Pseudoterranova* sp.	Anisakiasis	Japan, Europe, N America	Endoscopy; biopsy of ectopic sites	Removal of worm
Schistosoma mansoni (minor species *S. intercalatum* in Africa)	Intestinal schistosomiasis	Africa, parts of Middle East, S America, Caribbean	Microscopy of stool, serology, molecular methods	Praziquantel
Schistosoma japonicum (minor sp. *S. mekongi* in SE Asia)	Intestinal schistosomiasis (acute: Katayama syn.)	China, SE Asia		
Fasciolopsis buski	Intestinal fluke disease	East & South Asia and SE Asia	Microscopy of stool	Praziquantel, triclabendazole
Heterophid flukes (*Heterophyes* spp., *Metagonimus* spp. etc)		N. Africa, Middle East, Asia, SE Asia		
Echinostoma spp.		SE Asia, East & South Asia, Egypt, C & S America		

TABLE 16.1				
Parasitic Helminth Diseases Sometimes Associated with Diarrhea—cont'd				
Parasite Name	**Disease**	**Geographic Distribution**	**Diagnosis**	**Treatment**
Taenia spp., *Hymenolepis* spp.,*Diphyllobothrium* sp.,*Dipylidium caninum*, others	Intestinal cestode infection	Cosmopolitan	Microscopy of stool; proglottid examination	Praziquantel, albendazole, niclosamide

disease occur annually in sub-Saharan Africa and South Asia, leading to about 202,000 deaths across both regions.[6] In South Africa, a lower-middle income country, 15% of diarrheic under-5 children were infected with *Cryptosporidium* spp.[2] In contrast, in developed countries, cryptosporidiosis only accounts for 1%–9% of childhood diarrheal episodes, and infections are typically distributed across all age bands. Outbreaks, involving children visiting farms and petting zoos, and veterinary students starting practical work, have been described.[7]

Individuals who are immunocompromised (due to HIV or immunosuppression for transplants or malignancy) are an important risk group for cryptosporidiosis. It is an AIDS-defining illness, and may cause life-threatening infections, typically intractable diarrhea, in these patients, but also acalculous cholangitis and respiratory infections. A systematic review and meta-analysis of global coccidian parasite prevalence among HIV-infected patients reported that the global pooled prevalence of cryptosporidiosis was 14% overall, but was 21.1% in sub-Saharan Africa.[8] On the other hand, immunocompetent persons generally experience self-limiting diarrhea lasting up to 2 weeks, often with preceding vomiting and anorexia in children, and accompanied by abdominal cramping pain, and recover without specific treatment.

Diagnosis

Cryptosporidial diarrhea stool is usually liquid or semi-solid with strands of mucus, with oocyst numbers inversely correlated with increasing solidity. Shedding may be sporadic, and more than one fecal sample may be required. The traditional method for detecting oocysts is by modified Ziehl–Neelsen (or modified Kinyoun) staining of dried and methanol-fixed stool smears, with or without prior concentrating by sedimentation (formol-ether/ethyl acetate) or flotation (e.g., Sheather's sucrose) methods, and light microscopic examination. Oocysts are characterized by bright pink to crimson staining,

5–8 μm diameter, and the suggestion of intracystic forms in the form of internal particles, or sometimes the sausage-shaped sporozoites may be seen at high magnification (Fig. 16.2). Oocysts have to be distinguished from acid-fast yeasts and nonspecific fecal matter, which requires skill and training. The sensitivity of this method has been suggested to be as low as 50,000–500,000 oocysts per gram of stool.[9] Several alternative nonfluorescence- or fluorescence-based staining methods, for example, safranin-methyleneblue, auramine-rhodamine, auramine-carbol fuchsin, or acridine orange, among others, have been used.

Immunological-based tests are widely available, in the forms of indirect immunofluorescence, or coproantigen detection by enzyme immunoassay or immunochromatographic methods, but diagnostic performance is variable (in some cases less than 50%)[10] and some may not cater well for uncommon *Cryptosporidium* species. Polymerase chain reaction (PCR)-based assays, including quantitative or real-time PCR, have been developed, with good sensitivity and specificity.[11,12] Several studies have determined the performance of multiplex qPCR assays for the simultaneous detection of *Cryptosporidium* spp. and other protozoan pathogens, usually *G. lamblia* and *E. histolytica*, in stool specimens.[13–16] In all these studies, multiplex qPCR assays outperformed microscopy in terms of sensitivity and specificity.

Treatment

Cryptosporidiosis is self-limiting in immunocompetent persons, requiring rehydration and supporting nutrition. Antimotility agents may help symptomatically. Stopping immunosuppressives, or restoring immune function with antiretrovirals in HIV-infected patients, will assist in controlling the disease. Certain protease inhibitors may have anticryptosporidial action.[17] The many antibacterial and antiparasitic drugs and other therapies tested include the aminoglycoside paromomycin, high-dose azithromycin alone or in combination with paromomycin, bovine

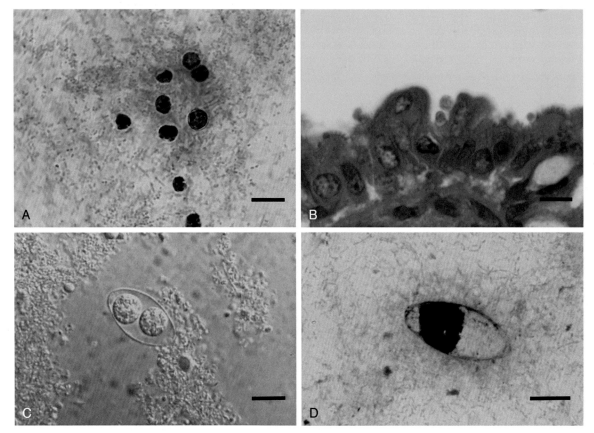

FIG. 16.2 **(A)** Oocysts of *Cryptosporidium* species. Modified ZN stain, 1000×. **(B)** *Cryptosporidium* species infecting mouse intestine; note parasites attached to the brush border of enterocytes. H&E stain, 1000×. **(C)** Oocyst of *Cystoisospora belli* containing two sporocysts. Differential interference contrast (DIC), 1000×. **(D)** Oocyst of *C. belli* containing sporoblast. Modified ZN stain, 1000×. All bars = 10 μm.

hyperimmune colostrum, or the somatostatin ana-logue octreotide, but none of these have become standard. Currently, the only FDA-approved drug for cryptosporidiosis is nitazoxanide, but it is not highly effective in immunocompromised or malnourished patients. Clearly, new, effective drugs and/or vaccines are a priority for reducing the burden of childhood cryptosporidial disease in the developing world. Limited progress in developing animal cryptosporidiosis vaccines[7] may provide some basis for future research on preventing human infection.

Cystoisospora belli

This is another apicomplexan protozoan organism, but different from *Cryptosporidium* spp., only humans are infected with this species. Other species in the genus affect nonhuman mammals.[18]

Epidemiology

Transmission is via ingestion of food or water containing the mature (sporulated) oocysts, which are resistant to environmental conditions and remain infective if kept cool and moist. The life cycle occurs in the enterocytes of the distal duodenum and proximal jejunum, with eventual passage of the oocysts in the feces. *C. belli* infections occur worldwide, but some tropical and subtropical areas are known to be more highly endemic, frequently related to the prevalence of HIV/AIDS in the population.[19]

As in the case of *Cryptosporidium*, in immunocompetent persons, the infection tends to be self-limiting in the form of watery diarrhea lasting for 6–10 days, but is occasionally severe or even fatal,[20] and sometimes chronic infections can be present for months to years or decades.[19] However, in immunocompromised persons, typically HIV/AIDS patients, long-term infections with diarrhea (up to 10 episodes per day), weight loss (ascribed to malabsorption), abdominal colic, and fever, are well described. It is one of the more common causes of HIV-associated diarrhea, predominantly in patients with CD4 counts less than 200 cells/mm.[3] A systematic review reported a pooled prevalence of *C. belli* infection for sub-Saharan Africa of 6.1% (global prevalence 2.5%). In a subset of case–control studies, the odds ratio for *C. belli* infection in HIV cases with diarrhea compared with those without diarrhea was 4.95.[8] Acute or chronic acalculous cholecystitis due to *C. belli* has been described in both immunocompromised and immunocompetent patients.[21,22]

Other immunodepressive conditions, such as HTLV-1 infection,[23] transplantation, leukemia, Hodgkin's disease, and non-Hodgkin's lymphomas, are also risk factors for prolonged infections.

Diagnosis

The characteristic spindle-shaped oocysts are readily recognizable in wet preparations of unconcentrated or concentrated (sedimentation or flotation) stool. They are also acid-fast, so the same staining methods described for *Cryptosporidium* (above) apply to *C. belli* (Fig. 16.2). Histopathological examination of small bowel or other tissue biopsy may reveal cryptic infections. Immature *Isospora* cysts have been found in extraintestinal sites such as spleen, liver, and lymph nodes, and in the biliary tract. Immunological-based or molecular assays are not commercially available, in contrast to the situation with *Cryptosporidium*, although PCR assays have been described.[24]

Treatment

Trimethoprim-sulfamethoxazole (TMP-SMX) is the standard therapy, and is effective in HIV-positive patients provided that secondary prophylaxis is continued until the CD4 count is >200 cells/µL. A subgroup of these patients respond poorly, and suffer frequent relapses, despite secondary prophylaxis, antiretroviral therapy, and immune reconstitution, with significant morbidity and mortality.[25] One reason for treatment failure and relapse may be the ability of *C. belli* to infect extraintestinal sites, forming tissue cysts that return to the intestine and reinitiate disease. It may be that the tissue phase of *C. belli* does not respond to TMP-SMX or the immune response, or that there is a general reduction in intestinal immunity, allowing relapse or reinfection. Finally, drug resistance is possible, but this has apparently not yet been studied in vitro. Second-line

drug options are ciprofloxacin, pyrimethamine, and nitazoxanide.[25]

Cyclospora cayetanensis

This is a relatively recently recognized and named (1990s) apicomplexan protozoan parasite. *C. cayetanensis* is anthroponotic, with no known susceptible animal hosts. Other species in the genus infect African monkeys.[26]

Epidemiology

The reproductive cycle is similar to that of *Cryptosporidium* and *Cystoisospora*, with environmentally resistant oocysts passed in feces being the transmission stage, although *Cyclospora* oocysts require a longer period to become infectious than for the other two coccidians, precluding direct transmission from fresh feces. The infection is endemic in developing countries, affecting mainly 2–5-year-old children during the warmer seasons, and international travellers visiting those countries.[27] Of more than 1000 sporadic infections in the United States, about one third were acquired in returned travellers, mostly from South and Central America.[28] In developed countries, most (but not all) outbreaks have been linked to imported foods such as berries, leafy greens, and herbs that are eaten raw.[29] *C. cayetanensis* is not regarded as a major opportunistic infection in HIV/AIDS, although the duration of disease may be prolonged in immunodeficient persons.

Diagnosis

Oocysts may be detected using the modified Ziehl–Neelsen method in concentrated or unconcentrated stool samples. The microscopist needs to recognize oocysts that are larger (8–10 µm) than those of *Cryptosporidium*, and that frequently have a wrinkled, refractile surface, and are variably acid-fast, some remaining unstained (Fig. 16.3). Other methods utilize blue–white autofluorescence under ultraviolet light of the right wavelength, or a modified safranin staining method. There are no commercial rapid tests; several PCR-based methods have been used to detect *C. cayetanensis* for various purposes.

Treatment

The drug of choice is TMP-SMX, given for 10 days.

Sarcocystis Species

These protozoan parasites are grouped in a subset of apicomplexans that require two hosts to maintain the life cycle, namely, a definitive host infected with the intestinal stage parasites, the oocyst and sporocyst

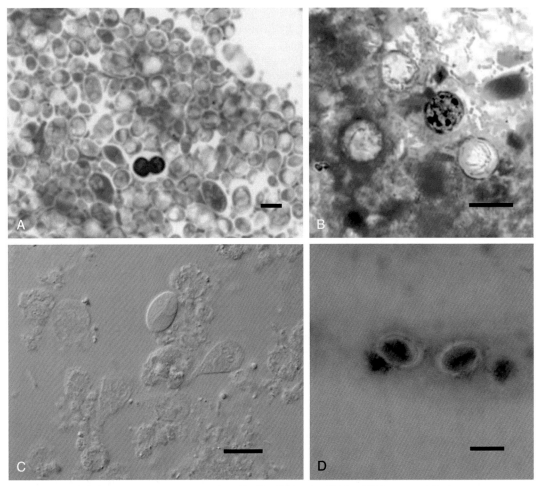

FIG. 16.3 **(A)** Oocyst of *Sarcocystis* species. Modified ZN stain, 1000×. **(B)** Oocysts of *Cyclospora cayetanensis.* Modified ZN stain, 1000×. **(C)** Cyst and trophozoites of *Giardia intestinalis.* DIC, 1000×. **(D)** Cysts of *G. intestinalis.* Iron hematoxylin stain, 1000×. All bars = 10 µm. (Image B courtesy of DPDx, Centers for Disease Control and Prevention, Atlanta, USA.)

forms of which are excreted in feces; and the intermediate host/s, that when infected by the oocysts/sporocysts, carry the tissue stage sarcocysts in muscles. The sarcocysts are infective for the definitive host. There are more than 150 *Sarcocystis* species that parasitize intermediate hosts that include herbivorous mammals, primates including humans, and other animals. Definitive hosts are carnivores or omnivores, including humans. Two species are known to utilize humans as definitive hosts: *Sarcocystis hominis* and *Sarcocystis suihominis,* the vehicles for infection being raw or undercooked beef and pork, respectively, but there may be other undefined species to which humans are susceptible.

Epidemiology

Intestinal sarcocystosis in humans has a worldwide distribution, reflecting geographic patterns of consumption of pork and beef, and regional preferences for eating meat in raw or undercooked form. Most clinical reports originate in Europe, Asia, Australia, and South America (reviewed in Ref. 30). Apparent absence from Africa and the Middle East is probably due to lack of detection and reporting. There is wide variation in incubation period, clinical severity and duration of illness, and prepatent and patent periods of excretion of oocysts/sporocysts. Many natural infections are asymptomatic or mild. The spectrum of symptoms includes fever, nausea, vomiting, acute enteritis with abdominal pain, distension, and diarrhea, and chronic enteritis. Chronic acalculous cholecystitis has been reported in a patient with AIDS.[31] Patent period of sporocyst excretion lasts from about 2 weeks to more than 120 days; exceptionally, periods of excretion of 6, 12, and 21 months have been recorded.[32] Repeated symptomatic infections have been noted in volunteer studies, suggesting that protective immunity is not acquired.

Diagnosis

Presumptive diagnosis of intestinal sarcocystosis can be made on symptoms of enteritis, and a history of consumption of raw or undercooked meat. Confirmation depends on microscopic identification of oocysts or sporocysts in fecal samples, but these may not be present during the acute phase of infection.[33] Microscopic examination of direct preparations or preferably, concentration by sedimentation (e.g., formol-ether/ethyl acetate) and flotation methods, as for other coccidian parasites, will detect the oocysts/sporocysts, which look the same in both *Sarcocystis* species. Acid-fast staining of oocysts/sporocysts is inconsistent (Fig. 16.3). Molecular techniques have been extensively applied to diagnosing and identifying the muscle form of sarcocystosis in animals (and recently in humans for the unusual *S. nesbitti* infections acquired by tourists on islands off the Malaysian coast[34,35]), but minimally so far to intestinal sarcocystosis in humans, although these assays will undoubtedly be developed and applied in future.[33]

Treatment

Intestinal infections are self-limiting; some apparently long-persisting infections may be the result of reinfection. Neither treatment nor prophylaxis for intestinal sarcocystosis has been developed.

Giardia intestinalis

This is a flagellate protozoan parasite, synonyms *G. duodenalis* and *G. lamblia*. Earlier taxonomic groupings of the genus based on morphology and apparent host preferences were confusing. Molecular genotyping has identified eight genotype assemblages and subtypes, some of which (assemblages A and B) infect animals and humans and are regarded as zoonotic.[36,37] Among these are ones that affect household companion and farm animals.

Epidemiology

G. intestinalis is a frequent cause of diarrhea and has been estimated to cause 2.8×10^8 infections per year worldwide,[38] with a preponderance of disease in developing countries. Prevalences of up to 60% have been reported in Africa (reviewed in Ref. 38). Transmission routes are direct contact (person to person, or animal to person), or ingestion of contaminated food or water. Cysts are resistant to normal drinking water-chlorination levels. As with *Cryptosporidium*, asymptomatic infections in humans and animals may occur, particularly commonly in developing countries. In Africa, *Giardia* prevalences of <6% to >30% have been found in adult cattle and calves, respectively.[38] In the developed world, waterborne and daycare-related outbreaks are frequent, and giardiasis is an important cause of travellers' diarrhea. Pet dogs and cats have been implicated as sources of human infection, acquired by close contact.

Overall, only about 40% of *Giardia* infections are symptomatic,[26] producing diarrhea, abdominal cramping, nausea, and vomiting; bloating and malabsorption are typical; intermittent and/or prolonged symptoms may occur. Infections are generally self-limiting, but some children and immunocompromised persons may develop chronic diarrhea, malabsorption, and weight loss.

Diagnosis

Giardia infections are detectable by conventional laboratory microscopy methods (Fig. 16.3), but as intestinal shedding is intermittent, several fecal samples taken at daily intervals may be required. The formol-ether/ethyl acetate method will concentrate the cysts and trophozoites. Trichrome, iron hematoxylin, or other staining methods can be used. Numerous immunological techniques like direct or indirect immunofluorescence or EIA/ELISA are commercially available (reviewed in Ref. 26). Sensitive molecular methods based on PCR are extending from research or public health laboratory applications to routine diagnostic tests often in multiplex form to detect several protozoan parasites simultaneously.[13–16]

Treatment

Metronidazole or tinidazole are standard treatment. Treatment failure is well recognized, occurring in up to 30% of cases in travellers, and drug resistance may be involved. Alternative drugs are albendazole, nitazoxanide, furazolidone, paromomycin, and quinacrine, but not all are readily available, nor always efficacious; refractory cases may require repeated or combination therapy.[39,40]

Entamoeba histolytica

Other members of this genus that infect humans (*E. dispar, E. polecki, E. coli, E. hartmannii,* and *E. moshkovskii*) are nonpathogens. Morphologically, *E. histolytica*, *E. dispar*, and *E. moshkovskii* are indistinguishable in their cyst and noninvasive trophozoite forms, hence provide a challenge in accurate microscopic diagnosis of *Entamoeba* spp. carriage and disease. Most *Entamoeba*-infected persons are colonized with *E. dispar*.

Epidemiology

Amebic diarrheal disease is estimated to have caused 55,500 deaths (upper confidence limit, 74,000 deaths) worldwide annually in 2010,[41] with the largest burden in developing countries, as for most other parasitic diarrheal disease. In the GEMS study,[5] *E. histolytica* was one of the top causes of severe diarrhea and mortality in children aged 1–2 years in Africa and Asia. It is one of the main parasitic causes of death globally, ranking third after malaria and cryptosporidiosis.[41] In developed countries, most infections are diagnosed in immigrants or travellers from less-developed endemic areas, HIV-positive or institutionalized individuals, or men who have sex with men.[42] Recently, local transmission in Western Sydney has been described, with some infections diagnosed in persons who had never travelled to endemic countries.[43] *Entamoeba* infections are acquired by ingesting the infective cysts by the fecal–oral route, usually via contaminated water or food, or directly by sexual contact. Possible transmission via colonic irrigation has been suggested.[43]

Diagnosis

Most *E. histolytica* infections are asymptomatic; the proportion progressing to invasive disease is approximately 4%–10% per year, with higher rates in males.[42] Amebic colitis is the most common clinical invasive form, presenting variously as abdominal pain and tenderness, watery diarrhea, dysentery, or ameboma (inflammatory mass in the large intestinal wall). Active colitis is usually accompanied by polymorphonuclear leukocytosis. Fulminant colitis is the most serious complication of intestinal infection, with ensuing bowel necrosis, toxic megacolon, perforation or peritonitis, and high mortality rate. Inappropriate corticosteroid treatment for presumed inflammatory bowel disease has resulted in fulminant amebic colitis.[44] Hematogenous spread to liver, lung, or brain may occur in the absence of overt intestinal disease, and the skin around the anus, genitalia, or colostomy openings may be invaded by virulent amebae from the bowel.

Microscopic identification of *E. histolytica* is confounded by inability to distinguish between pathogenic and nonpathogenic species in stool samples. The classical large, rapidly moving, hematophagous amebae in fresh, warm stools, are rarely seen in routine diagnostic laboratories. Fecal samples should ideally be concentrated (e.g., formol-ether/ethyl acetate method) before being examined microscopically for the presence of cysts. Some laboratories routinely make permanent stained preparations with trichrome or other stains (Fig. 16.4). Even if cysts that are compatible with the appearance of *E. histolytica* are observed, it is not possible to state that this pathogen is present or is the definitive cause of the patient's illness; therefore, nonmicroscopic diagnostic methods need to be considered. Culture is not a practical option for routine laboratories. Histopathological examination of large bowel biopsies may reveal characteristic morphological features of invasive amebic colitis or ameboma (Fig. 16.4), and fulminant amebic colitis has characteristic radiological features.

Some commercially available immunologically based antigen-detection tests are able to specifically identify *E. histolytica*, and may be easily and rapidly utilized with good sensitivity and specificity. Some antigen-detection tests simultaneously detect other parasitic stool pathogens such as *Giardia* and *Cryptosporidium* species. As with other intestinal parasitic infections, more sensitive and specific molecular methods like PCR and its relatives (e.g., real-time, multiplex) are becoming more frequently utilized for detecting *E. histolytica* in well-resourced diagnostic laboratories.[13–16,45] Ideally, if costs for antigen detection and molecular assays reduce sufficiently, these will become accessible to more and more laboratories that currently rely on traditional methods. Loop-mediated isothermal amplification (LAMP) is an example of a molecular technique that can be adapted for use in lower-tech settings than are suitable for traditional PCR.[46]

In nonendemic settings, serological tests are a sensitive way of detecting invasive amebic disease. A wide range of techniques (e.g., ELISA, IFA, indirect hemagglutination, latex agglutination) is commercially available. In endemic areas, up to a third of residents have antibodies, so serological testing for suspected acute disease is confounded by previous exposure in a large proportion of cases.

Treatment

Persons in whom *E. histolytica* parasites are detected should all be treated, even if asymptomatic, because of the potential for invasive infection. The standard treatment for invasive amebiasis is metronidazole. A systematic review of the treatment of amebic dysentery[47] indicated that other nitroimidazole drugs (tinidazole, ornidazole, secnidazole) have similar efficacy and fewer reported adverse effects. Luminal amebicides (paromomycin, diloxanide, diiodohydroxyquinoline (iodoquinol)), while not recommended

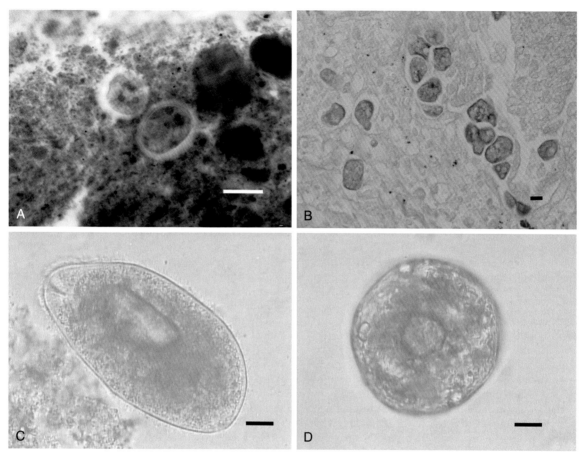

FIG. 16.4 **(A)** Cysts of *Entamoeba histolytica.* Iron hematoxylin stain, 1000×. **(B)** Amebic colitis, showing trophozoites of *E. histolytica.* PAS stain, 1000×. **(C)** Trophozoite of *Balantidium coli*, showing ciliated surface. Unstained, 400×. **(D)** Cyst of *B. coli.* Unstained, 400×. All bars = 10 μm. (Images C and D courtesy of DPDx, Centers for Disease Control and Prevention, Atlanta, USA.)

for treatment of symptomatic amebic infection, when used after a tissue amebicide like metronidazole, improve elimination of surviving parasites, and thereby reduce parasitological failure, prevent relapse, and interrupt transmission of *E. histolytica* cysts.[47]

Balantidium coli

This is the only ciliate, and the largest protozoan parasite, of humans.

Epidemiology

Pigs are the natural hosts of this parasites, and are asymptomatically infected. The parasite is found worldwide, matching the distribution of pigs.[48] The global prevalence was estimated as 0.025%–1%, depending on location. The infective stage is the environmentally resistant cyst, passed in feces, and infection is usually acquired via contaminated food or water. People keeping or living close to pigs in conditions of poor sanitation and hygiene are most at risk for infection; these are usually in tropical or subtropical developing countries, especially South America, the Philippines, Papua New Guinea, West Irian, and parts of the Middle East. Tourists and travellers to these areas may also be exposed to *B. coli*, and present with diarrhea on returning home. However, balantidiasis has also been reported in Scandinavian countries and northern Russia. In institutionalized communities (mental hospitals, prisons, orphanages, old-age homes), poor hygiene may lead to outbreaks originating in asymptomatic carriers via the fecal–oral route.

Diagnosis

Generally, the infection is asymptomatic or manifests as mild nonbloody diarrhea and abdominal pain due to colitis. A small proportion of patients may develop acute fulminating infection, presenting with dysentery, and sometimes progressing to intestinal hemorrhage, perforation, and death. Rarely, extraintestinal infections, including liver, genitourinary tract, and lungs, have been described.

B. coli trophozoites are large (up to 200 µm × 70 µm) and highly motile, and therefore easy to see in wet slide preparations of liquid stool or other infected samples (Fig. 16.4). Cysts are more likely to be found in formed stool samples, and can be confused with helminth ova due to their large size (50–70 µm).

Treatment

Metronidazole (for 5 days) or tetracycline (for 10 days). Nitazoxanide has also been suggested for treating children.[49]

Microsporidial infections

Microsporidia are obligate intracellular eukaryotic parasites (in the broad sense) that, on phylogenetic evidence, evolved from within the fungi and share some characteristics with them, for example, chitin synthesis, and certain gene arrangements.[50] It is a large and diverse group, with more than 1200 species that parasitize vertebrate and invertebrate hosts ranging from insects to fish and mammals. Two species, *Enterocytozoon bieneusi* and *Encephalitozoon intestinalis*, are predominantly enteric pathogens and cause diarrhea in immunocompetent and especially, in immunocompromised persons.

Epidemiology

In immunocompetent individuals, microsporidia may cause diarrhea that is protracted (up to a month or 6 weeks) but ultimately self-limiting. In some populations, high prevalences of pathogenic species have been reported in healthy subjects, for example, 67.5% prevalence in healthy volunteers in Cameroon.[51] The main risk group for microsporidial infections are HIV-positive and other immunocompromised persons. The global pooled prevalence of microsporidial infections in HIV-infected persons is estimated at about 12%, with sub-Saharan Africa having the highest prevalence at 15.4%.[8] When stratified by income level, countries with low incomes had a higher prevalence (25%) than middle- or high-income countries (8.4% and 14.4% prevalences, respectively).[8]

E. bieneusi was first identified in AIDS patients with diarrhea and wasting and it is still the most common species in HIV-infected individuals. There are more than 200 genotypes of *E. bieneusi* that infect humans, or animals (domestic and wild, mammals and birds), or both, indicating that there is zoonotic potential in at least some genotypes.[50] *E. intestinalis* is the second most prevalent microsporidial pathogen of humans. Although most commonly causing diarrhea, both species can cause extraintestinal disease, for example, respiratory, urinary, biliary, or disseminated infections that may variably manifest as encephalitis, keratoconjunctivitis, myositis, peritonitis, nephritis, and hepatitis.[52] Other *Encephalitozoon* species (e.g., *E. cuniculi*) may also infect the intestine. In non-HIV-infected but immunocompromised patients, organ transplants, malignancies, extremes of age, and diabetes have been identified as risk factors for infection.[52]

Contaminated food or water are the most likely vehicles for transmission of microsporidian spores to humans. Excretion of spores from infected humans and animals in urine and feces is the major source of water contamination. Microsporidia have also been found in food such as fruit, vegetables and herbs, and milk.[53] Exposure in developing countries with poor standards of sanitation and hygiene led to the recognition of microsporidia as a cause of travellers' diarrhea in people returning from tropical areas. Contact with infected insects, poultry, livestock and regional food animals such as guinea pigs and rabbits, and pets, is another potential risk factor for acquiring infection.[53]

Diagnosis

Microscopic identification of microsporidia in stool samples is challenging. The spores are small (1–4 µm) and difficult to distinguish from other fecal organisms and debris even if special stains like hot Gram-chromatrope or modified trichrome blue stains are used with ordinary microscopy; calcofluor white staining with UV epi-illumination is also difficult to interpret when applied to stool samples, because of its nonspecific nature (Fig. 16.5). In contrast, these techniques are more successful when applied to nonfecal samples such as urine, corneal scrapings, or tissue sections. Similarly, microscopy that utilizes the property of birefringence of microsporidial spores in polarized light is generally not useful for stool samples. Transmission electron microscopy can be applied to biopsy and other specimens and may assist in identification of the microsporidial species.[54] Various PCR techniques have been described that outperform microscopic examination.[55–57] Application of PCR and amplicon sequencing

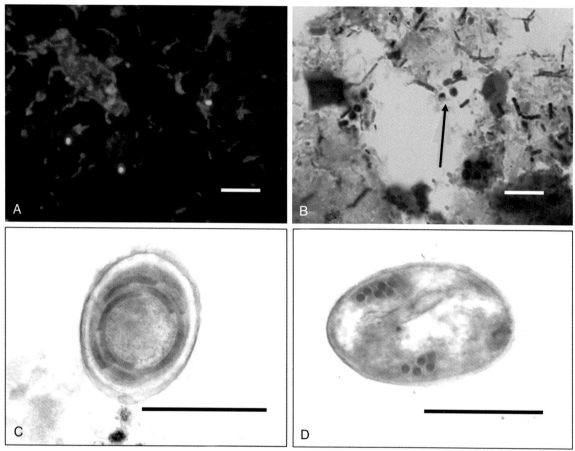

FIG. 16.5 **(A)** Spores of intestinal microsporidial species. Calcofluor white stain, untraviolet epi-illumination, 1000x. **(B)** Spores of microsporidial species; note vacuole in spore (arrow). Gram-hot chromotrope stain, 1000x. **(C)** Spore of *Enterocytozoon bieneusi*, transverse section. TEM, 30,000x. **(D)** Spore of *E. bieneusi*, longitudinal section. Note the double layer of polar filament gyres in both micrographs. TEM, 30,000x. Bars = 10 μm (A, B) and 1 μm (C, D).

has been applied to fecal spots on Whatman FTA cards to detect and identify microsporidial species in persons living in a low-resource environment.[58]

Treatment

Albendazole is effective against *Encephalitozoon* species, but *E. bieneusi* does not respond as well. Fumagillin is more active against *E. bieneusi*, but has serious side effects in the form of neutropenia and thrombocytopenia.[59] In addition to antimicrosporidial drugs, restoration of immune function with antiretroviral therapy in HIV/AIDS patients or modification of immunosuppressive drug treatment in transplant patients is important in treating microsporidiosis. The expanded access to highly active antiretrovirals in some populations has

led to a corresponding decrease in the incidence of HIV-related microsporidial infections.

Blastocystis hominis

The taxonomic position of *Blastocystis* sp. has changed several times, as it was accepted as being a protozoan, rather than a yeast, in the 1960s. Initially classified then as a sporozoan, it was moved into the Sarcodina (a since-dismantled macrotaxon accommodating the amebae). Molecular phylogenetic studies have now placed it in the Stramenopiles, a group of protists comprising slime nets, water molds, and brown algae.[60] The genus accommodates isolates from humans and a variety of animals, with *Blastocystis* species subtype 3 most frequently associated with human infections. There is some evidence of zoonotic transmission of some subtypes, for example, from pigs.[61]

Epidemiology

Blastocystis spp. found in humans and animals have a worldwide distribution. Transmission of the cystic stage is by the fecal–oral route, via contaminated food or water, or directly in situations of poor personal hygiene. In some areas, predominantly developed countries, *Blastocystis* is the most frequent enteric protozoan parasite in persons with diarrhea, but its real pathogenic potential is controversial. Presence of *Blastocystis* has been associated with diarrhea, irritable bowel syndrome, unexplained abdominal pain,[62] or other chronic gastrointestinal disease of unknown cause,[42] but many studies have found no causal link. One suggestion is that presence of *Blastocystis* is a marker of intestinal upset due to other infections. Massive *Blastocystis* proliferation in a patient with culture-proven *Vibrio cholerae* 01 (author's personal observation) would seem to support this theory, in at least some cases. As irritable bowel syndrome probably has many contributing factors, it is possible that in certain cases, *Blastocystis* has a causative role.

Diagnosis

Blastocystis organisms in stool samples are polymorphic, with granular, vacuolar, ameboid, and cystic forms, among others that have been described. Microscopic examination of wet preparations, or trichrome or other stained permanent preparations, may demonstrate the presence of the organism (Fig. 16.6). In vitro culture is possible but is not a practical method for routine diagnostic laboratories. Molecular diagnostic

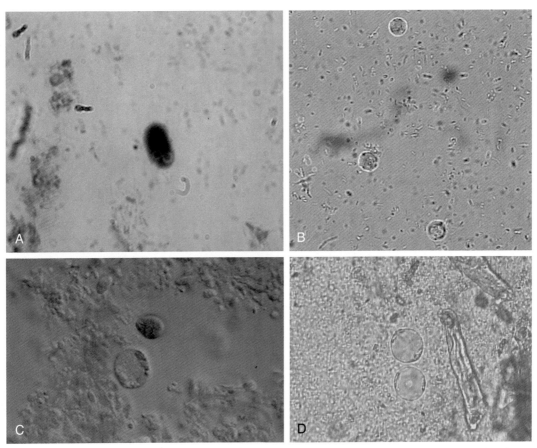

FIG. 16.6 **(A)** Trophozoite of *Dientamoeba fragilis*. Trichrome stain, 1000x. **(B)** Cysts of *Blastocystis hominis*. Unstained, 400x. **(C)** Cyst of *B. hominis*; above it is a cyst of *Chiomastix mesnili*, a nonpathogen. DIC, 400x. **(D)** Cysts of *B. hominis*. Unstained, 400x. All bars = 10 μm.

methods (PCR, sequencing) can be applied for detection and subtyping of *Blastocystis* species.

Treatment

Infection (or colonization) may be self-limiting. Treatment should be considered for persistent symptomatic *Blastocystis* infection in the absence of other pathogens, particularly if large numbers of this organism are present in the stool sample or the patient is immunocompromised.[63] Metronidazole is the drug of choice; alternatives are trimethoprim-sulfamethoxazole, nitazoxanide, and paromomycin-metronidazole combination. Drug susceptibility is variable and subtype dependent, and additional drug options that have been suggested are mefloquine, ornidazole, and furazolidone.[64]

Dientamoeba fragilis

This intestinal protozoan, now confirmed by ultrastructural and molecular studies as an ameboflagellate closely related to *Histomonas* and *Trichomonas* species, has long shared the same controversial status as a pathogen with *Blastocystis* species. There are a large number of reports indicating its association with human disease. Diagnostic difficulties with traditional microscopy may have previously contributed to failure to recognize such associations; application of molecular diagnostics is likely to bring clarity, likewise the development of an animal model of transmission. There are two major genotypes of *D. fragilis*, and genetic differences between lineages may be reflected in differences in pathogenicity and clinical features.

Epidemiology

Recent confirmation of the existence of precyst and cyst forms[65] have clarified previous speculation that *D. fragilis* is probably transmitted by the same fecal–oral routes of other intestinal protozoan parasites. There is also evidence for feasibility of an alternative transmission route, in the eggs of the intestinal helminths *Enterobius vermicularis* and possibly, *Ascaris lumbricoides*. Zoonotic transmission is considered to be unlikely, although naturally infected nonhuman primates and pigs have been found.[66,67]

D. fragilis is a highly cosmopolitan parasite. In symptomatic patients, various studies in developed and less-developed countries have shown prevalences from <1% (USA, Australia) to >80% (Germany), (reviewed in[68]), but variability of subject selection and diagnostic technique between studies precludes meaningful interpretation of such differences in prevalence. It is considered that in certain areas, *D. fragilis* infections are as common as, or more so than, giardiasis.[42] As many routine diagnostic laboratories do not use optimal methods for detecting the organism, it is likely that the true incidence is higher than reported.

The common clinical presentation of *D. fragilis* disease resembles irritable bowel syndrome, as for *Blastocystis* infections, with the spectrum of symptoms encompassing intermittent or persistent diarrhea, abdominal discomfort or pain, unexplained flatulence, anorexia, fatigue, and weight loss. Symptoms may be acute, or (commonly) chronic, with a high proportion of children or persons <20 years in some studies. About half of patients in some series had eosinophilia, which is unusual for an enteric protozoan infection.

Diagnosis

Ideally, at least three stool specimens from symptomatic patients should be submitted for laboratory investigation, to improve the chance of detecting the parasite, and although direct wet preparations may be suggestive, examination of a promptly fixed and suitably stained (trichrome or iron hematoxylin) fecal smear is required for definitive identification of the characteristic nuclear morphology of *D. fragilis* trophozoites and cystic forms, the latter being very small and scanty in number. Uninucleate forms of the trophozoites can be mistaken for *Endolimax nana* or *Entamoeba hartmanni*, which are nonpathogens. Immunological techniques such as IFA and ELISA have been successfully applied for antigen detection, and are likely to become commercially available in future. Serum antibody tests and culture of the organism, while well described, are unlikely to be widely utilized for routine diagnosis. Molecular methods in various formats are becoming the methods of choice for detecting enteric protozoan pathogens, and *D. fragilis* is likely to be added to the array of targeted organisms in multiplex PCR assays in due course, even if not commercially available at the present time.

Treatment

Drugs used to successfully treat *D. fragilis* infections are metronidazole, paromomycin, secnidazole, ornidazole, tetracycline, and iodoquinol; combination therapy may be required in some cases where metronidazole monotherapy has failed.

HELMINTH PARASITES
Strongyloides stercoralis

The parasitic nematode *Strongyloides stercoralis* is a unique pathogen. Its lifecycle allows opportunity for free-living existence, to a limited extent; it has the unusual property among helminth parasites of being able to reproduce within a single host. Under certain circumstances, this ability can produce serious or life-threatening disease. The related species *S. fülleborni fülleborni* and *S. fülleborni kellyi* infect humans in Africa and Papua New Guinea, respectively; nonhuman primates are natural hosts of the former species.

Epidemiology

The distribution of *S. stercoralis* is routinely stated as mainly tropical and subtropical areas, as its WHO designation as a neglected tropical disease suggests, but with some foci in more temperate countries. It has been pointed out that rather than climate being the main determinant of geographic location of transmission, it is primarily socioeconomically disadvantaged communities that are most at risk for the disease,[69] because they have the problems of poor living and sanitary conditions that facilitate the life cycle, as it is a soil-transmitted parasite. Evidence for this is the presence of strongyloidiasis in otherwise affluent countries, for example, parts of rural Appalachia in the United States, and in rural indigenous communities in Australia. In some relatively high-income populations, for example, on the Mediterranean coast of Spain, a high prevalence of strongyloidiasis is probably related to farming practices rather than poor living standards.[70] Certain groups are at higher risk of infection, namely war veterans, refugees, immigrants, travellers, HIV/AIDS patients (although it is not an AIDS-defining infection), HTLV-1 patients, immunosuppressed patients, and alcoholics.[71,72]

The global prevalence of *S. stercoralis* infection is usually estimated as 30–100 million persons, although the consensus is that it is probably underdiagnosed, and that a more accurate estimate is 300–370 million.[73-75] Reported country-specific prevalences are highly variable; a systematic review suggested that *S. stercoralis* infections affect 10%–40% of the population of many tropical and subtropical countries, with up to 60% prevalence in particularly resource-poor settings.[72] Dogs and nonhuman primates can harbor *Strongyloides*, and zoonotic outbreaks have been described among animal handlers.[76]

The autoinfection process maintains covert long-term strongyloidiasis, and is central to the parasite's ability to cause serious or life-threating disease if host immune mechanisms become defective. Low-grade infection is entirely asymptomatic in about a third of patients. Epigastric pain and watery diarrhea are typical symptoms; there may also be nausea and vomiting. Weight loss may result from malabsorption and protein-losing enteropathy.[77] Passage through the lungs can cause an eosinophilic pneumonitis (Löffler's syndrome). Some patients manifest a serpiginous, migratory urticarial eruption ("larva currens") related to the intradermal passage of migrating larvae, over prolonged periods of time. More common are transient nonmigratory urticarial wheals around the waist and buttocks.[77,78]

Accelerated autoinfection gives rise to the dangerous complications of strongyloidiasis, namely hyperinfection and disseminated infection. Cellular immunity is important to contain the infection, and a large number of underlying diseases or therapies that impair cellular defense mechanisms predispose to hyperinfection.[77,78] The most consistent association with hyperinfection is administration of corticosteroids. Conditions associated with hyperinfection include malignancies (lymphocytic and myeloid leukemia, lymphomas, lung, and gastric carcinoma); chronic renal disease (allografts, nephrotic syndrome, chronic glomerulonephritis); chronic infections (leprosy, tuberculosis); solid organ and hemopoietic stem cell transplants; and a miscellaneous group (autoimmune disease, protein-calorie malnutrition, hypogammaglobulinemia, achlorhydria). Although HTLV-1 infection is particularly associated with hyperinfection, the condition does not commonly complicate HIV infection, although such cases have been described.

Diagnosis

Löffler's syndrome typically produces patchy, transient lung infiltrates on X-ray. Extensive radiographic changes may be evident in complicated strongyloidiasis involving the lungs; radiographic features of obstruction, with loops of dilated bowel, may accompany severe hyperinfection.

The presence of a raised eosinophil count accompanying symptoms of diarrhea, abdominal pain, and urticarial rashes is typical of strongyloidiasis, but laboratory confirmation requires the identification of the larvae. Patients with mild or subclinical infection usually have low worm burdens and repeated stool examinations may be necessary. Culture of stool on nutrient agar (Koga agar plate culture, or its modification[79]) is more sensitive than the older Baermann technique or examination of stool by Kato-Katz or formol-ether/ethyl acetate concentration methods. The motile larvae distribute bacterial colonies on the agar surface in typical linear tracks; the plates can then be rinsed with 10% formalin, the fluid centrifuged, and sediment examined microscopically (Fig. 16.7). *S. stercoralis* larvae must be distinguished from those of hookworm

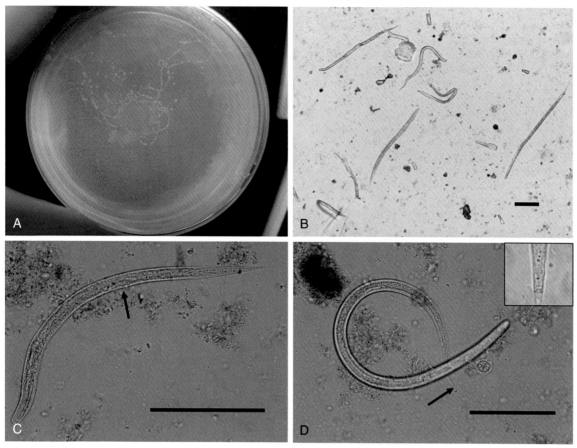

FIG. 16.7 **(A)** Agar plate culture of sputum, *Strongyloides stercoralis* hyperinfection; note trails of bacterial colonies. **(B)** Multiple larvae of *S. stercoralis* in hyperinfection. Formol-ethyl acetate stool concentrate, unstained, 100×. **(C)** Rhabditiform larva of *S. stercoralis*; note characteristic genital primordium (arrow). Stool concentrate, 400×. **(D)** Filariform larva of *S. stercoralis*; note characteristic notched appearance of end of tail (arrow and inset). Stool concentrate, 400×. All bars = 100 μm.

species hatching in a stool specimen that is not fresh. Examination of duodenal fluid obtained by aspiration or string methods is more sensitive in light infections. In the case of severe, disseminated infection, there are usually numerous larvae, and sometimes adults and eggs in stool; filariform larvae, and occasionally adults, may be detected in sputum, bronchial lavage specimens, cerebrospinal fluid, blood, and other fluids or tissues. Raised IgE and eosinophil counts are not always present, especially in patients with overwhelming infection. Eosinophil counts may be suppressed by concurrent corticosteroid administration. A clue to covert strongyloidiasis is recurrent, unexplained bacteremia due to enteric organisms. Serological diagnostic methods are generally highly sensitive and specific

(reviewed in Ref. 80). The main value of serological tests is in screening for evidence of low-level infection to identify candidates for more vigorous investigation. Capture ELISA methods have been applied to detecting *Strongyloides* coproantigen,[81] which appears to be a promising approach. Numerous PCR-based assays have been described with (usually) substantially improved sensitivity of detection of *S. stercoralis* compared with traditional methods, but their application is generally limited to reference laboratories and few commercial products are available.[80,82] Depending on whether the purpose of diagnosis is for prevalence surveys, individual diagnosis and screening, or clinical trial-related inclusion or assessment of cure, the choice of laboratory technique differs.[80]

Treatment

The ability of *S. stercoralis* infections to persist asymptomatically for long periods and potentially emerge later as serious or fatal illness, makes parasite elimination by drug treatment an important goal in all infected people. Oral ivermectin is the treatment of choice as it targets both adults and larvae. Albendazole is slightly less effective for uncomplicated infections, as it affects only adult parasites.[83] Hyperinfection is a medical emergency and ivermectin for at least 2 weeks, or until stools have been negative for 2 weeks, is recommended. Adding albendazole in this situation has been reported. Parenteral (subcutaneous) administration of ivermectin (in the form of veterinary product), because of lack of intestinal absorption due to vomiting or paralytic ileus, may be required as an emergency measure.[84,85] Reduction of immunosuppressive therapy should be considered as part of managing severe strongyloidiasis.

Capillaria (syn. *Paracapillaria*) *Philippinensis*

Infection with this nematode parasite typically presents as chronic watery diarrhea associated with weight loss and hypoalbuminemia due to malabsorption, and occasionally as chronic abdominal pain without diarrhea.[86] Similar to *Strongyloides stercoralis*, this parasite has the unusual capacity to proliferate within the host by an autoinfective process.

Epidemiology

Intestinal capillariasis was first described in 1964 during a large epidemic of disease in the Philippines, and elsewhere is found in Thailand, Iran, Japan, Egypt, Indonesia, Korea, India, and Taiwan.[87] It may be present but unrecognized in other geographic areas. The natural life cycle of the parasite involves birds as definitive hosts and fish as intermediate hosts; humans are infected by eating raw fish.

Diagnosis

Eggs, larvae, and adult worms may be detected microscopically in stools, but excretion of eggs may be intermittent, leading to low sensitivity of stool examination. Outside known endemic areas, the eggs may be mistakenly identified as those of *Trichuris trichiura*. Radiographic (barium), conventional endoscopic, and video capsule endoscopic methods have assisted definitive diagnosis of intestinal capillariasis.[86] Hypokalemia, anemia, and eosinophilia may be present.

Treatment

Albendazole is standard treatment; prolonged courses may be required. Ivermectin has also been used successfully.[86]

REFERENCES

1. Xiao L, Ryan UM. Cryptosporidiosis: an update in molecular epidemiology. *Curr Opin Infect Dis.* 2004;17:483–490.
2. Abu Samra N, Thompson PN, Jori F, et al. Genetic characterization of *Cryptosporidium* spp. in diarrhoeic children from four provinces in South Africa. *Zoonoses Public Health.* 2012;60(2):154–159. https://doi.org/10.1111/j.1863-2378.2012.01507.x.
3. Chappell CL, Okhuysen PC, Langer-Curry R, et al. *Cryptosporidium hominis*: experimental challenge of healthy adults. *Am J Trop Med Hyg.* 2006;75:851–857.
4. Ryan U, Lawler S, Reid S. Limiting swimming pool outbreaks of cryptosporidiosis – roles of regulations, staff, patrons and research. *J Water Health.* 2017;15(1):1–16.
5. Kotloff KL, Nataro JP, Blackwelder WC, et al. Burden and aetiology of diarrhoeal disease in infants and young children in developing countries (the Global Enteric Multicenter Study, GEMS): a prospective, case-control study. *Lancet.* 2013;382:209–222.
6. Sow SO, Muhsen K, Nasrin D, et al. The burden of *Cryptosporidium* diarrheal disease among children <24 months of age in moderate/high mortality regions of sub-Saharan Africa and South Asia, utilizing data from the Global Enteric Multicenter Study (GEMS). *PLoS Negl Trop Dis.* 2016;10(5):e0004729.
7. Thomson S, Hamilton CA, Hope JC, et al. Bovine cryptosporidiosis: impact, host-parasite interaction and control strategies. *Vet Res.* 2017;48:42.
8. Wang ZD, Liu Q, Liu HH, et al. Prevalence of *Cryptosporidium*, microsporidia and *Isospora* infection in HIV-infected people: a global systematic review and meta-analysis. *Parasit Vectors.* 2018;11(1):28. https://doi.org/10.1186/s13071-017-2558-x.
9. Weber R, Bryan RT, Bishop HS, Wahlquist SP, Sullivan JJ, Juranek DD. Threshold of detection of *Cryptosporidium* oocysts in human stool specimens: evidence for low sensitivity of current diagnostic methods. *J Clin Microbiol.* 1991;29(7):1323–1327.
10. Agnamey P, Sarfati C, Pinel C, et al. Evaluation of four commercial rapid immunochromatographic assays for detection of *Cryptosporidium* antigens in stool samples: a blind multicenter trial. *J Clin Microbiol.* 2011;49(4):1605–1607. https://doi.org/10.1128/JCM.02074-10.
11. Hadfield SJ, Robinson G, Elwin K, Chalmers RM. Detection and differentiation of *Cryptosporidium* spp. in human clinical samples by use of real-time PCR. *J Clin Microbiol.* 2011;49(3):918–924. https://doi.org/10.1128/JCM.01733-10.
12. Spano F, Putignani L, McLauchlin J, Casemore DP, Crisanti A. PCR-RFLP analysis of the *Cryptosporidium* oocyst wall protein (COWP) gene discriminates between *C. wrairi* and *C. parvum*, and between *C. parvum* isolates of human and animal origin. *FEMS Microbiol Lett.* 1997;150(2):209–217.
13. Verweij JJ, Blangé RA, Templeton K, et al. Simultaneous detection of *Entamoeba histolytica*, *Giardia lamblia*, and *Cryptosporidium parvum* in fecal samples by using multiplex real-time PCR. *J Clin Microbiol.* 2004;42(3):1220–1223.

14. Haque R, Roy S, Siddique A, et al. Multiplex real-time PCR assay for detection of *Entamoeba histolytica, Giardia intestinalis,* and *Cryptosporidium* spp. *Am J Trop Med Hyg.* 2007;76(4):713–717.

15. Stark D, Al-Qassab SE, Barratt JL, et al. Evaluation of multiplex tandem real-time PCR for detection of *Cryptosporidium* spp., *Dientamoeba fragilis, Entamoeba histolytica,* and *Giardia intestinalis* in clinical stool samples. *J Clin Microbiol.* 2011;49(1):257–262. https://doi.org/10.1128/JCM.01796-10.

16. Van Lint P, Rossen JW, Vermeiren S, et al. Detection of *Giardia lamblia, Cryptosporidium* spp. and *Entamoeba histolytica* in clinical stool samples by using multiplex real-time PCR after automated DNA isolation. *Acta Clin Belg.* 2013;68(3):188–192.

17. Mele R, Gomez Morales MA, Tosini F, Pozio E. Indinavir reduces *Cryptosporidium parvum* infection in both in vitro and in vivo models. *Int J Parasitol.* 2003;33(7):757–764.

18. Shrestha A, Abd-Elfattah A, Freudenschuss B, et al. *Cystoisospora suis*-a model of mammalian cystoisosporosis. *Front Vet Sci.* 2015;2:68. https://doi.org/10.3389/fvets.2015.00068.

19. Garcia LS. *Isospora (Cystoisospora) belli*. In: Khan NA, ed. *Emerging Protozoan Pathogens.* New York: Taylor & Francis; 2008:289–301.

20. Post L, Garnaud C, Maubon D, et al. Uncommon and fatal case of cystoisosporiasis in a non-HIV-immunosuppressed patient from a non-endemic country. *Parasitol Int.* 2018;67(1):1–3. https://doi.org/10.1016/j.parint.2017.10.003.

21. Agholi M, Aliabadi E, Hatam GR. Cystoisosporiasis-related human acalculous cholecystitis: the need for increased awareness. *Pol J Pathol.* 2016;67(3):270–276. https://doi.org/10.5114/pjp.2016.63779.

22. Lai KK, Goyne HE, Hernandez-Gonzalo D, et al. *Cystoisospora belli* Infection of the gallbladder in immunocompetent patients: a clinicopathologic review of 18 cases. *Am J Surg Pathol.* 2016;40(8):1070–1074. https://doi.org/10.1097/PAS.0000000000000660.

23. Shafiei R, Najjari M, Kargar Kheirabad A, Hatam G. Severe diarrhea due to *Cystoisospora belli* infection in an HTLV-1 woman. *Iran J Parasitol.* 2016;11(1):121–125.

24. ten Hove RJ, van Lieshout L, Brienen EA, Perez MA, Verweij JJ. Real-time polymerase chain reaction for detection of *Isospora belli* in stool samples. *Diagn Microbiol Infect Dis.* 2008;61(3):280–283. https://doi.org/10.1016/j.diagmicrobio.2008.03.003.

25. Boyles TH, Black J, Meintjes G, Mendelson M. Failure to eradicate *Isospora belli* diarrhoea despite immune reconstitution in adults with HIV- a case series. *PLoS One.* 2012;7(8):e42844. https://doi.org/10.1371/journal.pone.0042844.

26. Cama VA, Mathison BA. Infections by intestinal coccidia and *Giardia duodenalis. Clin Lab Med.* 2015;35(2):423–444. https://doi.org/10.1016/j.cll.2015.02.010.

27. Swaminathan A, Torresi J, Schlagenhauf P, et al. A global study of pathogens and host risk factors associated with infectious gastrointestinal disease in returned international travellers. *J Infect.* 2009;59(1):19–27. https://doi.org/10.1016/j.jinf.2009.05.008.

28. Hall RL, Jones JL, Herwaldt BL. Surveillance for laboratory-confirmed sporadic cases of cyclosporiasis – United States, 1997–2008. *MMWR Surveill Summ.* 2011;60(2):1–11.

29. Döller PC, Dietrich K, Filipp N, et al. Cyclosporiasis outbreak in Germany associated with the consumption of salad. *Emerg Infect Dis.* 2002;8(9):992–994.

30. Fayer R, Esposito DH, Dubey JP. Human infections with *Sarcocystis* species. *Clin Microbiol Rev.* 2015;28(2):295–311. https://doi.org/10.1128/CMR.00113-14.

31. Agholi M, Heidarian HR, Moghadami M, Hatam GR. First detection of acalculous cholecystitis associated with *Sarcocystis* infection in a patient with AIDS. *Acta Parasitol.* 2014;59(2):310–315. https://doi.org/10.2478/s11686-014-0243-1.

32. Laarman JJ. *Isospora hominis* (Railliet and Lucet 1891) in The Netherlands. *Acta Leiden.* 1962;31:111–116.

33. Poulsen CS, Stensvold CR. Current status of epidemiology and diagnosis of human sarcocystosis. *J Clin Microbiol.* 2014;52(10):3524–3530. https://doi.org/10.1128/JCM.00955-14.

34. Italiano CM, Wong KT, AbuBakar S, et al. *Sarcocystis nesbitti* causes acute, relapsing febrile myositis with a high attack rate: description of a large outbreak of muscular sarcocystosis in Pangkor Island, Malaysia, 2012. *PLoS Negl Trop Dis.* 2014;8(5):e2876. https://doi.org/10.1371/journal.pntd.0002876.

35. Harris VC, van Vugt M, Aronica E, et al. Human extraintestinal sarcocystosis: what we know, and what we don't know. *Curr Infect Dis Rep.* 2015;17(8):495. https://doi.org/10.1007/s11908-015-0495-4.

36. Cacciò SM, Thompson RC, McLauchlin J, Smith HV. Unravelling *Cryptosporidium* and *Giardia* epidemiology. *Trends Parasitol.* 2005;21(9):430–437.

37. Ryan U, Cacciò SM. Zoonotic potential of *Giardia. Int J Parasitol.* 2013;43(12–13):943–956. https://doi.org/10.1016/j.ijpara.2013.06.001.

38. Squire SA, Ryan U. *Cryptosporidium* and *Giardia* in Africa: current and future challenges. *Parasit Vectors.* 2017;10(1):195. https://doi.org/10.1186/s13071-017-2111-y.

39. Mørch K, Hanevik K, Robertson LJ, Strand EA, Langeland N. Treatment-ladder and genetic characterisation of parasites in refractory giardiasis after an outbreak in Norway. *J Infect.* 2008;56(4):268–273. https://doi.org/10.1016/j.jinf.2008.01.013.

40. Muñoz Gutiérrez J, Aldasoro E, Requena A, et al. Refractory giardiasis in Spanish travellers. *Travel Med Infect Dis.* 2013;11(2):126–129. https://doi.org/10.1016/j.tmaid.2012.10.004.

41. Lozano R, Naghavi M, Foreman K, et al. Global and regional mortality from 235 causes of death for 20 age groups in 1990 and 2010: a systematic analysis for the Global Burden of Disease Study 2010. *Lancet.* 2012;380(9859):2095–2128. https://doi.org/10.1016/S0140-6736(12)61728-0.

42. Fletcher SM, Stark D, Harkness J, Ellis J. Enteric protozoa in the developed world: a public health perspective. *Clin Microbiol Rev.* 2012;25(3):420–449. https://doi.org/10.1128/CMR.05038-11.

43. Domazetovska A, Lee R, Adhikari C, et al. A 12-year retrospective study of invasive amoebiasis in western Sydney: evidence of local acquisition. *Trop Med Infect Dis.* 2018;3:73. https://doi.org/10.3390/tropicalmed3030073.

44. Shirley DA, Moonah S. Fulminant amebic colitis after corticosteroid therapy: a systematic review. *PLoS Negl Trop Dis.* 2016;10(7):e0004879. https://doi.org/10.1371/journal.pntd.0004879.

45. Khairnar K, Parija SC. A novel nested multiplex polymerase chain reaction (PCR) assay for differential detection of *Entamoeba histolytica, E. moshkovskii* and *E. dispar* DNA in stool samples. *BMC Microbiol.* 2007;7:47.

46. Mwendwa F, Mbae CK, Kinyua J, Mulinge E, Mburugu GN, Njiru ZK. Stem loop-mediated isothermal amplification test: comparative analysis with classical LAMP and PCR in detection of *Entamoeba histolytica* in Kenya. *BMC Res Notes.* 2017;10(1):142. https://doi.org/10.1186/s13104-017-2466-3.

47. Marie C, Petri Jr WA. Amoebic dysentery. *BMJ Clin Evid.* 2013; pii:0918.

48. Schuster FL, Ramirez-Avila L. Current world status of *Balantidium coli. Clin Microbiol Rev.* 2008;21(4):626–638. https://doi.org/10.1128/CMR.00021-08.

49. Ochoa TJ, White Jr AC. Nitazoxanide for treatment of intestinal parasites in children. *Pediatr Infect Dis J.* 2005;24(7):641–642.

50. Mathis A, Weber R, Deplazes P. Zoonotic potential of the microsporidia. *Clin Microbiol Rev.* 2005;18(3):423–445.

51. Nkinin SW, Asonganyi T, Didier ES, Kaneshiro ES. Microsporidian infection is prevalent in healthy people in Cameroon. *J Clin Microbiol.* 2007;45(9):2841–2846.

52. Didier ES, Weiss LM. Microsporidiosis: not just in AIDS patients. *Curr Opin Infect Dis.* 2011;24(5):490–495. https://doi.org/10.1097/QCO.0b013e32834aa152.

53. Stentiford GD, Becnel JJ, Weiss LM, et al. Microsporidia - emergent pathogens in the global food chain. *Trends Parasitol.* 2016;32(4):336–348. https://doi.org/10.1016/j.pt..2015.12.004.

54. Birkhead M, Poonsamy B, Ming Sun L, du Plessis D, van Wilpe E, Frean J. Microscopy and microsporidial diagnostics – a case study. In: Méndez-Vilas A, ed. *Microscopy: Science, Technology, Applications and Education.* Vol. 7. Badajoz: Formatex Research Center; 2017:237–243.

55. da Silva AJ, Schwartz DA, Visvesvara GS, de Moura H, Slemenda SB, Pieniazek NJ. Sensitive PCR diagnosis of infections by *Enterocytozoon bieneusi* (microsporidia) using primers based on the region coding for small-subunit rRNA. *J Clin Microbiol.* 1996;34(4):986–987.

56. Da Silva AJ, Slemenda SB, Visvesvara GS, et al. Detection of *Septata intestinalis* (Microsporidia) Cali et al. 1993 using polymerase chain reaction primers targeting the small submit subunit ribosomal RNA coding region. *Mol Diagn.* 1997;2(1):47–52.

57. Visvesvara GS, da Silva AJ, Croppo GP, et al. In vitro culture and serologic and molecular identification of *Septata intestinalis* isolated from urine of a patient with AIDS. *J Clin Microbiol.* 1995;33(4):930–936.

58. Ndzi ES, Asonganyi T, Nkinin MB, et al. Fast technology analysis enables identification of species and genotypes of latent microsporidia infections in healthy native Cameroonians. *J Eukaryot Microbiol.* 2016;63(2):146–152. https://doi.org/10.1111/jeu.12262.

59. Bukreyeva I, Angoulvant A, Bendib I, et al. *Enterocytozoon bieneusi* microsporidiosis in stem cell transplant recipients treated with fumagillin. *Emerg Infect Dis.* 2017;23(6):1039–1041.

60. Tan KSW. Blastocystis spp. In: Khan NA, ed. *Emerging Protozoan Pathogens.* New York: Taylor & Francis; 2008:153–189.

61. Wang W, Owen H, Traub RJ, Cuttell L, Inpankaew T, Bielefeldt-Ohmann H. Molecular epidemiology of *Blastocystis* in pigs and their in-contact humans in Southeast Queensland, Australia, and Cambodia. *Vet Parasitol.* 2014;203(3–4):264–269. https://doi.org/10.1016/j.vetpar.2014.04.006.

62. Toro Monjaraz EM, Vichido Luna MA, Montijo Barrios E, et al. *Blastocystis hominis* and chronic abdominal pain in children: is there an association between them? *J Trop Pediatr.* 2017. https://doi.org/10.1093/tropej/fmx060.

63. Sekar U, Shanthi M. Blastocystis: consensus of treatment and controversies. *Trop Parasitol.* 2013;3(1):35–39. https://doi.org/10.4103/2229-5070.113901.

64. Mirza H, Teo JD, Upcroft J, Tan KS. A rapid, high-throughput viability assay for *Blastocystis* spp. reveals metronidazole resistance and extensive subtype-dependent variations in drug susceptibilities. *Antimicrob Agents Chemother.* 2011;55(2):637–648. https://doi.org/10.1128/AAC.00900-10.

65. Stark D, Garcia LS, Barratt JL, et al. Description of *Dientamoeba fragilis* cyst and precystic forms from human samples. *J Clin Microbiol.* 2014;52(7):2680–2683. https://doi.org/10.1128/JCM.00813-14.

66. Stark D, Phillips O, Peckett D, et al. Gorillas are a host for *Dientamoeba fragilis*: an update on the life cycle and host distribution. *Vet Parasitol.* 2008;151(1):21–26.

67. Cacciò SM, Sannella AR, Manuali E, et al. Pigs as natural hosts of *Dientamoeba fragilis* genotypes found in humans. *Emerg Infect Dis.* 2012;18(5):838–841. https://doi.org/10.3201/eid1805.111093.

68. Garcia LS. *Dientamoeba fragilis*, one of the neglected intestinal protozoa. *J Clin Microbiol.* 2016;54(9):2243–2250. https://doi.org/10.1128/JCM.00400-16.

69. Beknazarova M, Whiley H, Ross K. Strongyloidiasis: a disease of socioeconomic disadvantage. *Int J Environ Res Public Health.* 2016;13(5). pii: E517. https://doi.org/10.3390/ijerph13050517.

70. Román-Sánchez P, Pastor-Guzmán A, Moreno-Guillén S, Igual-Adell R, Suñer-Generoso S, Tornero-Estébanez C. High prevalence of *Strongyloides stercoralis* among farm workers on the Mediterranean coast of Spain: analysis of the predictive factors of infection in developed countries. *Am J Trop Med Hyg.* 2003;69(3):336–340.

71. Mascarello M, Gobbi F, Angheben A, et al. Prevalence of *Strongyloides stercoralis* infection among HIV-positive immigrants attending two Italian hospitals, from 2000 to 2009. *Ann Trop Med Parasitol.* 2011;105(8):617–623. https://doi.org/10.1179/2047773211Y.0000000006.

72. Teixeira MC, Pacheco FT, Souza JN, Silva ML, Inês EJ, Soares NM. *Strongyloides stercoralis* infection in alcoholic patients. *BioMed Res Int*. 2016;2016:4872473. https://doi.org/10.1155/2016/4872473.

73. Bethony J, Brooker S, Albonico M, et al. Soil-transmitted helminth infections: ascariasis, trichuriasis, and hookworm. *Lancet*. 2006;367(9521):1521–1532.

74. Schär F, Trostdorf U, Giardina F, et al. *Strongyloides stercoralis*: global distribution and risk factors. *PLoS Negl Trop Dis*. 2013;7(7):e2288. https://doi.org/10.1371/journal.pntd.0002288.

75. Bisoffi Z, Buonfrate D, Montresor A, et al. *Strongyloides stercoralis*: a plea for action. *PLoS Negl Trop Dis*. 2013;7(5):e2214. https://doi.org/10.1371/journal.pntd.0002214.

76. Georgi JR, Sprinkle CL. A case of human strongyloidosis apparently contracted from asymptomatic colony dogs. *Am J Trop Med Hyg*. 1974;23(5):899–901.

77. Cook GC. *Strongyloides stercoralis* hyperinfection syndrome: how often is it missed? *Q J Med*. 1987;64:625–629.

78. Grove DI. Human strongyloidiasis. In: Baker JR, Muller R, Rollinson D, eds. *Advances in Parasitology*. Vol. 38. San Diego: Harcourt Brace; 1996.

79. Pocaterra LA, Ferrara G, Peñaranda R, et al. Improved detection of *Strongyloides stercoralis* in modified agar plate cultures. *Am J Trop Med Hyg*. 2017;96(4):863–865. https://doi.org/10.4269/ajtmh.16-0414.

80. Buonfrate D, Formenti F, Perandin F, Bisoffi Z. Novel approaches to the diagnosis of *Strongyloides stercoralis* infection. *Clin Microbiol Infect*. 2015;21(6):543–552. https://doi.org/10.1016/j.cmi.2015.04.001.

81. Sykes AM, McCarthy JS. A coproantigen diagnostic test for *Strongyloides* infection. *PLoS Negl Trop Dis*. 2011;5(2):e955. https://doi.org/10.1371/journal.pntd.0000955.

82. O'Connell EM, Nutman TB. Molecular diagnostics for soil-transmitted helminths. *Am J Trop Med Hyg*. 2016;95(3):508–513. https://doi.org/10.4269/ajtmh.16-0266.

83. Nutman TB. Human infection with *Strongyloides stercoralis* and other related *Strongyloides* species. *Parasitology*. 2017;144(3):263–273. https://doi.org/10.1017/S0031182016000834.

84. Grein JD, Mathisen GE, Donovan S, Fleckenstein L. Serum ivermectin levels after enteral and subcutaneous administration for *Strongyloides* hyperinfection: a case report. *Scand J Infect Dis*. 2010;42(3):234–236. https://doi.org/10.3109/00365540903443165.

85. Zeitler K, Jariwala R, Restrepo-Jaramillo R, et al. Successful use of subcutaneous ivermectin for the treatment of *Strongyloides stercoralis* hyperinfection in the setting of small bowel obstruction and paralytic ileus in the immunocompromised population. *BMJ Case Rep*. 2018;2018. pii: bcr-2017-223138. https://doi.org/10.1136/bcr-2017-223138.

86. Limsrivilai J, Pongprasobchai S, Apisarnthanarak P, Manatsathit S. Intestinal capillariasis in the 21st century: clinical presentations and role of endoscopy and imaging. *BMC Gastroenterol*. 2014;14:207. https://doi.org/10.1186/s12876-014-0207-9.

87. Gutierrez Y. Other tissue nematode infections. In: Guerrant RL, Walker DH, Weller PF, eds. *Tropical Infectious Diseases*. 2nd ed. Philadelphia: Elsevier Churchill Livingstone; 2006:1243–1247.

CHAPTER 17

Hirschsprung-Associated Enterocolitis

JONATHAN CHER, BMED MD • CAMILLE WU, MBBS, FRACS •
SUSAN ADAMS, MBBS (HONS) FRACS (PAED)

INTRODUCTION

Hirschsprung disease (HD) is the most common congenital gut motility disorder, occurring in about 1:5000 births worldwide.[1] It is characterized by an absence of enteric nervous system ganglion cells in the myenteric and submucosal plexuses of the distal bowel.[1,2] This is due to failure of caudal migration of neural crest cells from the proximal to distal along the gastrointestinal tract, and can affect a variable distance. HD can occur as an isolated disease, or have a genetic basis.

The aganglionic segment is tonically contracted and causes obstruction to the proximal bowel. The definitive management of HD is surgical excision of the aganglionic bowel and anastomosis to reestablish intestinal continuity, via one of a range of operations termed "pull-through" procedures.

It is widely accepted that the most serious and life-threatening complication of HD is Hirschsprung-associated enterocolitis (HAEC)—an inflammatory condition of the bowel that is associated with the majority of morbidity and mortality in HD.[3–6] HAEC can occur before and/or after resection of the aganglionic bowel; it can be the presenting symptom of HD in some infants.[7–9]

This chapter aims to inform the reader of the current knowledge surrounding HAEC, including the most recent evidence-based theories on its etiology, and the current evidence surrounding its treatment and management.

INCIDENCE

Reported rates of HAEC vary widely, due to the difficulty in ascertaining a definitive diagnosis.[4] Overall rates are reported at 25%–35%,[7–12] ranging from 4.6% to 54%.[6,13–16]

The incidence has declined over the last 40 years, likely due to increased awareness leading to early diagnosis and treatment.[17]

A Japanese nationwide survey showed that overall incidence of enterocolitis had decreased over 30 years; incidence of preoperative enterocolitis fell from 29.2% to 17.3% and postoperative from 17.9% to 10.6%.[18]

Reported rates before and after definitive surgery for HD (pull-through operation) also vary widely, with pre- and postoperative rates reported in 17%–50% and 2%–35% of HD children, respectively.[3,4,11,12,19–22]

Most episodes of HAEC occur within the first 2 years of the pull-through operation,[14,17,23] but some may occur after 18 months.[11]

RISK FACTORS

All patients with HD are at risk of HAEC,[4] but there are several factors that appear to confer increased risk.

PREOPERATIVE RISK FACTORS

Older age at diagnosis—There is conflicting evidence,[24] with some reports of increased risk[8,19] and some of decreased risk[3,25] or no risk association[22] of HAEC with increased age of diagnosis. In neonates, delay in diagnosis of HD beyond 1 week of age has been reported by some to be associated with increased HAEC risk.[11,19,20,26]

Trisomy 21 is the commonest chromosomal abnormality associated with HD, and is also associated with poorer outcomes and more complications,[15,27] including increased rates of HAEC, preoperatively (OR 1.28) and postoperatively (OR 1.77).[28]

Multiple case series from around the world have reported increased incidence of HAEC in their patients with Trisomy 21 (45%–50%) compared to those without Trisomy 21 (19%–29%).[7,8,10,15,26,27] Many reviews also cite increased risk with Trisomy 21.[4,7,11,13,19]

However, this is not a uniform finding throughout the literature—some case series do not show increased risk of HAEC in Trisomy 21 patients.[12,29,30]

Family history of HD also predisposes patients to HAEC—this was found to be higher in patients with a family history of Hirschsprung (35%–57%), compared to those with no family history (16%–29%).[7,12,24]

Long-segment aganglionosis was found to be associated with higher postoperative HAEC rates in some studies,[4,11,12,16,24,31,32] but not in others.[7,26,33]

Gastrointestinal Diseases and Their Associated Infections. https://doi.org/10.1016/B978-0-323-54843-4.00017-9
Copyright © 2019 Elsevier Inc. All rights reserved.

POSTOPERATIVE RISK FACTORS

Mechanical/obstructive factors: Following the pull-through operation, stricture of the anorectum or anastomotic complications were associated with increased risk of HAEC.[3,11,22,25]

Incomplete resection of Hirschsprung-affected bowel, leaving a segment of bowel that is either aganglionic or hypoganglionic, would predispose to HAEC, constipation, or persistent obstructive symptoms.[4,34]

Other causes of obstruction that can predispose to HAEC include dysmotility, anastomotic stricture, twisted pull-through segment, or tight muscular cuff following Soave pull-through procedure.[4]

Type of pull-through operation: There are conflicting reports. The Duhamel procedure is historically associated with a lower incidence of HAEC,[7] and the Swenson procedure with an increased incidence.[16] In a recent meta-analysis, the Duhamel procedure continued to show a favorable risk profile for subsequent development of HAEC, compared to transanal endorectal pull-through procedure.[35] This was not supported by a recent Indonesian series of 100 patients, where the Soave procedure had lower HAEC rate compared to Duhamel (10% vs. 28%),[31] however a confounding factor may be that the Soave group had their operation at a significantly younger age than the Duhamel's group. In addition, a systematic review in 2010 reports transanal single-stage pull-through procedure being associated with a lower incidence of HAEC (10.2%).[6]

With the refinement of surgical technique over the years, many studies have not shown a relationship between timing and type of operation and subsequent HAEC.[6,8,10,11,14,22]

Cow's milk protein allergy was postulated by one small Japanese study[36] as a possible risk factor for developing postoperative HAEC, but the worldwide significance is not known.

There are conflicting reports on whether *preoperative episodes of HAEC* predict postoperative incidence of HAEC. Although some studies report that previous episodes of HAEC conferred increased risk,[31,32] others did not.[7,22]

High grade histological changes (ie Grade III or higher) in the bowel of Hirschsprung patients are associated with the presence or subsequent development of HAEC.[37,38] Grade III is defined as the presence of multiple crypt abscesses; Grade IV fibrinopurulent debris or mucosal ulceration; Grade V transmural necrosis or perforation.

Teitelbaum's group recommends that bowel specimens (e.g., taken at time of diagnosis or at definitive repair) are routinely assessed for histological grading of disease, as that may predict subsequent development of HAEC.[38] However this is not universal clinical practice.

Other risk factors for HAEC identified in a Chinese cohort of 181 patients included low weight at time of operation, and low levels of IgA.[32]

MORBIDITY AND MORTALITY

Postoperative HAEC is reportedly the leading cause of hospital admissions for children with HD,[6] at a substantial cost to the health system.[26,33]

Mortality rates of HD are fairly low, but HAEC accounts for a significant proportion, often quoted at 30%,[16,20] and up to 50% in some series.[5,24,39]

The mortality rate has fallen over the last 2 decades from 30% to 1%,[7,40] probably due to high index of suspicion and early treatment.[6,12,33]

The previously mentioned Japanese study of 3852 patients found that mortality rates associated with preoperative enterocolitis had significantly decreased over the years 1978–2002 (0.7% in 1998–2002, down from 6.5% in 1978–82).[18]

In Australia, the survey by the Australian Paediatric Surveillance Unit reported no HAEC-attributable mortality in 126 patients between 1997 and 2000.[20]

CLINICAL PRESENTATION

Diagnosis is predominantly clinical, and can be difficult given the nonspecific nature of the signs and symptoms, encompassing a wide clinical range from mild abdominal distension to shock.[41] In clinical practice, because of the high morbidity of a delayed diagnosis, pediatric surgeons tend to diagnose and treat suspected HAEC early.[4] There are ongoing attempts in the literature to standardize diagnostic criteria[41] and establish a grading system, and help standardize management.[4,42]

The classical signs of HAEC include abdominal distension, fever, and diarrhea,[4,26] particularly explosive diarrhea.[12]

The broad spectrum of clinical presentation includes nonspecific symptoms such as anorexia, vomiting, rectal bleed, lethargy, loose stool, and obstipation.[4] There may be a period of constipation followed by explosive diarrhea.

Mild cases can present just like viral gastroenteritis, with fever, mild distension, and diarrhea, which is very common in this age group.[4]

Severe cases can present in shock (decreased peripheral perfusion, hypotension) or with peritonitis,[4,41] and death can result albeit uncommonly.

HAEC and inflammatory bowel disease (IBD) can present with similar symptoms; Levin's series reports eight patients who were considered to have HAEC but had inflammatory bowel disease. This may be a small group

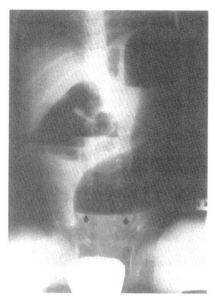

FIG. 17.1 Abdominal X-ray in HAEC: Air-fluid level in dilated bowel loop.

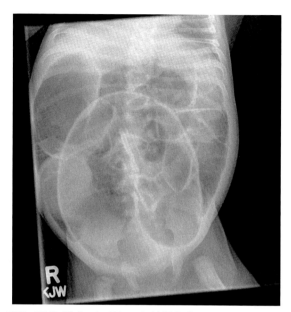

FIG. 17.2 Abdominal X-ray in HAEC: Grossly distended bowel loops, sometimes resembling free intraperitoneal air.

but further investigation for IBD should be considered in patients who appear to have recurrent or unusual HAEC.[43]

The relationship between IBD and HAEC, both inflammatory conditions, is yet to be elucidated, but there are suggestions there is some commonality, or perhaps some predisposition in HD patients to IBD.[44] Research continues in this area.

Appearances on abdominal X-ray can be non-specific, and may resemble gastroenteritis or bowel obstruction. As with clinical signs, there is a wide spectrum of severity in the findings. These include normal X-ray findings, appearances of ileus, dilated bowel loops, air–fluid levels, "cutoff" sign in the rectosigmoid (absent air distally), pneumatosis intestinalis, and even free intraabdominal air due to perforation (Fig. 17.1 and Fig. 17.2).[4,12,24,41]

The histopathology is characterized by cryptitis—neutrophils in intestinal crypts, crypt dilatation, and retained mucus—which can progress to inflammatory and ischemic and necrotic changes.[3] Teitelbaum proposed that alteration of colonic mucins in HD renders the bowel more vulnerable to enterocyte-adherent organisms, which may lead to a spectrum of histopathological changes for which he has described a grading system.[37]

Proposed Diagnostic Tools

• HAEC score—Pastor et al. sought to consensually develop a standardized definition for HAEC using the Delphi process.[41] Features on the score,

narrowed from 38 items to 16, included history, patient characteristics, physical signs, and results from laboratory, radiology, and pathology tests (see Table 17.1).[4,41] The criteria given the highest importance were *diarrhea, explosive stools, abdominal distension,* and radiological evidence of *bowel obstruction* or *mucosal edema.*[41] The resulting HAEC score is useful in research, but too cumbersome and not intended routine clinical use, also not clinically validated and not widely adopted.[4,41,42]

Frykman et al's recent multicenter study sought to evaluate Pastor's HAEC score[42] — it recognized the limitations, and sought to identify the optimal clinical criteria to diagnose HAEC. *Diarrhea with explosive stool, decreased peripheral perfusion, lethargy,* and *dilated bowel loops* were the most closely associated with HAEC episodes.[42]

In addition, the presence of any four of the following criteria maximized sensitivity and specificity of diagnosis[42]—lethargy, distended abdomen, diarrhea with explosive or foul-smelling or bloody stool, fever, explosive gas discharge on rectal examination, decreased peripheral perfusion, leucocytosis, "left shift" on FBC, previous history of enterocolitis, AXR findings of dilated bowel loops, or multiple air–fluid levels.

• "Clinical grading"[4,12]—based on degree of diarrhea, abdominal distension, and systemic signs to give an overall clinical grade—Grades I–III (mild, moderate, and severe)

TABLE 1
HAEC score[41]

History	Score
Diarrhoea with explosive stool	2
Diarrhoea with foul-smelling stool	2
Diarrhoea with bloody stool	1
History of enterocolitis	1
PHYSICAL EXAMINATION	
Explosive discharge of gas and stool on rectal examination	2
Distended abdomen	2
Decreased peripheral perfusion	1
Lethargy	1
Fever	1
RADIOLOGICAL FINDINGS	
Multiple air-fluid levels	1
Dilated loops of bowel	1
Sawtooth appearance with irregular mucosal lining	1
Cut-off sign in rectosigmoid with absence of distal air	1
Pneumatosis	1
LABORATORY RESULTS	
Leukocytosis	1
Shift to left	1
TOTAL	20
HAEC if	≥ 10

From Development of a standardized definition for Hirschsprung's-associated enterocolitis: a Delphi analysis. AC Pastor, F Osman, DH Teitelbaum, MG Caty, JC Langer. J Ped Surg 2009, 44(1):251–256. https://doi.org/10.1016/j.jpedsurg.2008.10.052.

- A guideline for diagnosis and grading, as proposed by Gosain[4] is similar to Bell's staging for necrotizing enterocolitis. There are three grades of severity based on history, physical examination and radiographic findings. This system is intended to be used as a tool to assist diagnosis and management of HAEC, rather than as a scoring system.

ETIOLOGY

The etiology of HAEC remains poorly understood. It is likely due to an interaction of multiple factors.[3,11] A variety of causes have been identified, including mucosal immunity, dysbiosis, and obstruction.[2] These factors are in interplay—the congenital anomaly of the enteric nervous system and obstruction/dysmotility are associated with dysfunctional components of gut immunity involving mucin production, immunological genes, markers and cells, and altered microbial communities.[3] Large-scale research is limited by the rarity of Hirschsprung disease itself.

OBSTRUCTION

Historically, obstruction/stasis was considered to be the cause of HAEC. However, as HAEC can present even after resection of the aganglionic bowel segment, its etiology is likely to be more complex. Recent literature indicates that obstruction may play a part, but is not the sole factor leading to enterocolitis.

The ways in which obstruction leads to HAEC have been avidly studied. Bacterial overgrowth and translocation in the setting of intestinal stasis has been reported as one such mechanism.[11,22] Similarly, postoperative anastomotic stricture has consistently been associated with increased risk for HAEC development.[3,22] In the past, successful treatment of patients with recurrent HAEC with sphincterotomy or posterior myomectomy supported functional obstruction as an etiology.[3]

Frykman's murine model study postulated that obstruction may lead to HAEC via immune system alteration (thymic involution, splenic lymphopenia, and suppression of B lymphopoeisis), perhaps via corticosterone pathway.[45]

However, HAEC can still occur in the absence of obstructive features (including after pull-through operation and in those with a defunctioning stoma). This suggests that the role of obstruction in HAEC development is more complicated. Although research tries to isolate factors for understanding the etiology of HAEC, it appears that a complex interaction of mucosal immunity, dysbiosis, and obstruction secondary to enteric aganglionosis contribute to the development of HAEC.

MUCOSAL IMMUNITY/ABNORMAL INNATE IMMUNE RESPONSE

As HD is defined by the congenital absence of the enteric nervous system (ENS), which is known to have a role in gastrointestinal immunity,[2] it is logical to investigate for pathogenesis in anomalies of the relationship between the ENS and intestinal homeostasis and immunity.[11]

Secretory IgA, the predominant immunoglobulin in the intestinal tract, has a role in preventing bacterial translocation.[3,46] Decreased levels of luminal or buccal IgA (sIgA) are seen in patients with HAEC.[11,46–48]

Other possible immunological pathways implicated include the following:[11]

- IgA, IgM, and J chain-containing plasma cells increased in HAEC[11,46]
- Abnormal distribution of IgG-containing plasma cells increased in HAEC bowel[11]
- Lamina propria CD68 positive monocyte/macrophages, and CD45RO positive leukocytes increased in HAEC patients[46]
- Increased CD57 positive NK cells in the lamina propria of ganglionated bowel of HAEC patients[46]
- Altered Tryptophan hydroxylase-2 (TPH2) expression in colonic serotonergic nerves[48a]
- Intercellular adhesion molecule-1 (ICAM-1) that allows transendothelial migration of leucocytes—stained strongly in bowel specimens from patients with HAEC, compared to those without HAEC[49]
- Splenic lymphopenia—Compared to control mice, the Hirschsprung with HAEC mouse model (Ednrb–/– mouse) had smaller spleens, abnormal splenic microarchitecture with splenic lymphopenia, and lower B cell to T cell ratio. Mice with lower total spleen and CD19+ cell counts had increased risk of HAEC.[50] Gosain found decreased mature B lymphocytes in Peyers patches in their mouse model.[47]

MUCUS DEFENSE BARRIER/INTESTINAL BARRIER DYSFUNCTION

The mucus defense barrier, along with immunoglobulins, forms an integral part of gastrointestinal mucosal immunity, by providing a physical barrier to pathogens, toxins, and foreign compounds.[51]

There are many studies in humans and animal models showing impaired intestinal barrier function in HAEC, including disturbances in mucin levels and bacterial adherence to enterocytes.[11,37,51,52]

- **Goblet Cells**
  Goblet cells secrete mucin, which traps viral and bacterial pathogens in the lumen of the gastrointestinal tract,[2] and prevents adherence of pathogens to enterocytes, thus decreasing infection risk.[9,11,37] Goblet cells are regulated by submucosal neuroendocrine cells and the enteric nervous system, which are affected in HAEC and HD, respectively.[3]
  Changes that have been discovered include altered goblet cell differentiation,[53] increase in goblet cell numbers,[53] and in the mouse model, increased goblet cell size and reduced Paneth cell function.[54]

- **Mucin**
  - *Abnormal mucin composition* in HAEC specimens– Teitelbaum found HAEC specimens contained increased neutral mucins and decreased acidic-sulfomucins.[37]
  - Mattar found that MUC-2, the predominant mucin in humans, was significantly lower in HD patients, and undetectable in HAEC patients.[52] Another study found no differences in MUC-2 levels, but MUC-4 was reduced in the distal colon of HD patients.[53]
  - *Reduced turnover* of colonic mucin was found to be associated with increased risk of HAEC.[55]
  - Abnormal mucus biosynthesis, with reduced mucin turnover, was found in ganglionic and aganglionic bowel of Hirschsprung patients.[51]
  - *Reduced mucus secretion.* Defects in neuroendocrine cells and submucosal noradrenergic neurons may result in reduced secretion of mucus.[11]

- **Neuroendocrine Cells**
  Soeda found decreased neuroendocrine cells in ganglionated bowel of HAEC patients compared to non-HAEC patients, which may represent an impaired immune response or a deficiency that can facilitate inflammation.[56]

- **Other**
  Lui et al. found that expression of CDX-1 and CDX-2 genes, which control proliferation and differentiation and hence mucosal healing of intestinal mucosal cells, were found to be reduced in patients with HAEC.[57]
  Other components under investigation include epithelial barrier and tight junctions, enteric glial cells, mast cells, and mucosal immaturity.[11]
  Ongoing research continues to investigate how the abovementioned factors interact with the innate immune system and altered luminal microbiome.

DYSBIOSIS

Infectious etiologies and an alteration of gut commensals are also associated with increased incidence of HAEC. Currently, no single specific pathogen has been identified as the causative agent in HAEC;[2,9] however, those that have received much investigative attention include *Clostridium difficile*, *Escherichia coli*, and rotavirus.[2,11,33]

Historically, *Clostridium difficile* is considered to be associated with increased risk of HAEC.[3,33,58] Some studies have correlated presence and load of *C. difficile* with the development and severity of HAEC,[58] but other studies have not supported this.[11,33] However, if pseudomembranous colitis develops, HAEC is associated with a high mortality rate.[3,39]

The infective etiology of HAEC remains to be clarified. The etiology is likely to be multifactorial and no one organism is responsible.[59] Perhaps immunological dysfunction allows commensals to become pathogenic.[59]

GUT FLORA

Disruption in normal gut flora may also be implicated in the pathogenesis of HAEC.

Studies show changes in the composition of gut flora during episodes of HAEC, compared with when there is no HAEC.[9,40,60,61] New genomic techniques (including rNA metagenomic signatures and amplified rDNA restriction analysis) are being employed to study bacterial communities.[40]

HD patients have a more stable community of intestinal microbiome compared to HAEC and HAEC-in-remission patients, suggesting that enterocolitis is associated with disruption of intestinal flora.[60]

Gut bacteria produce short chain fatty acids (SCFA) that are required for intestinal homeostasis and colonic mucosal preservation.[62] Demehri et al. found that children with a history of HAEC had fecal SCFA levels one quarter that of that in children who have never had HAEC;[62] acetate was the most markedly reduced.[62] They suggest that the HAEC-associated alteration in gut flora reduces production of SCFAs that are required for mucosal integrity.

Although differences in gut flora are described, findings are not consistent. Li et al. found that *Proteobacteria* was prevalent in HAEC intestinal flora, while *Bacteroidetes* was prevalent in HD patients without HAEC.[60]

Frykman et al. however, found increase in both *Bacteroidetes* and *Proteobacteria* in their HAEC group.[63] These differences may be accounted for by the different countries in which the studies were performed (China vs. United States), and the relatively small sample sizes.

Other differences in microbiome patterns that have been described include the following:
- HAEC patients have decreased fungal diversity, with increased *Candida* spp., and reduced *Malassezia* and *Saccharomyces* spp.[63]
- HAEC patients have markedly decreased bifidobacteria and lactobacilli.[64]
- A shift toward dysbiosis occurs prior to an episode of HAEC in the mouse model.[54] Before HAEC, *Lactobacillus* decreases, and *Bacteroidetes* and *Clostridium* spp. increase.

These findings lend theoretical support to the use of probiotics in reducing HAEC. (See later under "Prevention.")

GENETIC PREDISPOSITION

A genetic predisposition for HAEC has been sought, as HD has a strong but complex genetic component.[1,11,65]

Mutations of ret proto-oncogene (RET) and endothelin receptor B (EdnrB), which have a role in the enteric nervous system, are the two most commonly identified gene defects in HD.[9,66] RET mutations and their associations are studied with regard to HD and possible role in HAEC. Murine models with EdnrB mutations are used to study the pathogenesis of HAEC.[9]

Although a genetic cause for HAEC has not been found, there are some genetic variations associated with HAEC.[3]
- Trisomy 21 is associated with increased risk of HAEC, which may be partly due to intrinsic immunodeficiency[11,33] (decreased cytotoxic T cells and abnormal humoral function).
- Variations in the (integrin subunit beta 2) ITGB2 (CD18) immunomodulatory gene have been identified in samples from patients with HD and HAEC.[3,11,65]
  - The ITGB2 gene codes for the β-subunit of leukocyte adhesion molecule lymphocyte function-associated antigen 1, which is associated with T-cell development and function.[67]
  - ITGB2 is involved in cell-surface mediated signaling and is required for leucocyte extravasation into tissues, associated with chronic colitis conditions and participates in T-cell development.[9]
  - Impaired CD18 leucocyte and T-cell regulation can probably be linked to a genetic (ITGB2) predisposition to HAEC in 66% of cases—possible genetic link to HAEC patient selection.[65]
- RET mutation[11]—has significant implications for HD in general, but with regard to HAEC, it may be associated with autonomic dysfunction that can affect intestinal motility.
- Attempts to identify a susceptibility gene akin to that found in Crohns enterocolitis (NOD2) have not been successful.[68]

The Hirschsprung Disease Research Collaborative continues genetic analysis, enrolling families globally.[9] The concept of genetic predisposition to impaired immunity is becoming a viable hypothesis.[65]

MANAGEMENT

Treatment of HAEC remains empiric, as the cause is still not clearly elucidated. Given the difficulty in making a definitive diagnosis, and the potential high morbidity, pediatric surgeons tend to treat early for presumed HAEC.[24,41] The acute symptoms are addressed with fluids, antibiotics and rectal decompression, followed by any factors that may contribute to the cause of HAEC. Consideration is also given to the prevention of recurrent episodes.

Parents are educated on HAEC; they are taught to recognize the symptoms, to perform rectal washouts and to present to their treating team in a timely fashion.

TREATMENT

Treatment of acute HAEC depends on the severity of presentation.[4]

- **Fluid resuscitation**
- **Decompression**
  - Rectal washout[4] to evacuate retained stool or gas, using 10–20 mL/kg saline, via a large bore soft tube, and repeated 2–4 times per day.[3,24]
    - In fulminant disease, due to risk of perforation, instead of washouts, gently pass rectal tube to decompress.[3]
  - Bowel rest—ranging from clear liquids in mild cases to nil by mouth and nasogastric decompression in more severe cases. Parenteral nutrition may be required in the most severe and prolonged cases.[3]
- **Antibiotics**
  - Severity of episode will dictate what to use[3,4]
    - Mild cases—oral metronidazole[24]
    - Severe cases—IV broad spectrum antibiotics including ampicillin, gentamicin and metronidazole,[24] or piperacillin/tazobactam[4]
- **Operative intervention**
  - When above mentioned treatments are unsuccessful, proximal diversion via a stoma may be required.[3]
  - Or in the rare case of pneumoperitoneum, urgent laparotomy.[4]

PREVENTION

In the large part, we have been unable to completely prevent HAEC. Measures we have used in attempt to prevent HAEC include the following:

- **Preoperatively**:
  In the time leading up to the pull-through procedure, *rectal washouts* are commonly used to prevent fecal stasis and abdominal distension.[3,24]
- **Postoperatively**:
  - Routine postoperative *rectal washouts* have been shown in some studies to decrease the incidence and severity of HAEC.[3,24,69]

- Routine daily *anal dilatations* not shown to be useful in reducing HAEC in the absence of anastomotic stricture.[3,24,70] Nevertheless they continue to be used by many to prevent stricture formation.
- Prophylactic *antibiotics* are not useful.
- *Probiotics*: Many studies have been conducted to assess the efficacy of probiotics in the prevention of HAEC, including randomized controlled trials,[71,72] with mixed results. A 2017 meta-analysis of significant studies conducted in the last 15 years did not show statistical significant reduction in HAEC risk with the use of probiotics for Lactobacillus, Bifidobacterium, Streptococcus, and Enterococcus.[21] Further high-quality studies are required.
- Topical *isosorbide dinitrate* to relax the smooth muscle of the anal sphincter was successful in a very small case series,[73] but further studies are required to confirm the validity[24]
  The studies have had limitations and further studies are required.

RECURRENT HAEC

The reported incidence of recurrent HAEC varies from 5.2% to 41%.[11,19] The frequency of episodes tend to resolve with time,[19] and can occur in varying degrees of severity.

Some patients may have chronic or low-grade HAEC symptoms, including ongoing loose stool, soiling, intermittent abdominal distension, and failure to thrive.[3]

Risk factors for recurrent HAEC:

- Children with Trisomy 21 seem to be at increased risk of recurrent or chronic HAEC.[74,75] A meta-analysis reported recurrent episodes of HAEC occurred in 22%–57% of Trisomy 21 patients.[28]
- Total colonic aganglionosis[75]—rates reportedly 20%–40%, and even as high as 55% in one series.

The **management** of recurrent HAEC is first to manage the acute episode, then to exclude and treat any structural cause of outlet obstruction,[13] including anastomotic stricture, kinked or twisted anastomosis, retained aganglionic bowel, Duhamel spur or pouch, or tight Soave muscular cuff.[4,24] These are investigated for via anorectal examination, contrast enema, and/or rectal biopsies.[24]

If a structural cause has been excluded, management of recurrent episodes can be challenging.

Options to manage recurrence include the following:

- *Dietary* management—Rintala's group use low residue lactose-free diet,[74] but admits that this is not widely accepted treatment guideline.
- *Enteral antibiotics*—commonly used despite no evidence of efficacy.[24]

- *Sodium cromoglycate*, a mast cell stabilizer, was reported to have good results in treating chronic or recurrent HAEC in 2001.[74] It was a small study, with no further follow-up studies.[3,24]
- *Preventing outlet obstruction*:
  - Anal dilatations and/or rectal washouts—not easily sustainable as the children get older.
  - Therapies targeted at the internal anal sphincter (IAS)—Botulinum toxin injections, internal anal sphincterotomy. The evolving view is that the irreversible sphincterotomy should not be required, as repeated Botulinum toxin injections can be used as a temporizing measure until the child "grows out" of IAS achalasia. This can take some years.
- *Surgical options* aim to decrease obstruction[3]
  - Botulinum toxin injections to the internal anal sphincter—IAS achalasia may also be a cause of recurrent HAEC[13]—in HD the IAS is devoid of ganglion cells and so may be tonically contracted. Many patients respond well, and some studies show reduced hospital admissions,[24] but the degree of response is not always predictable.[24] Repeated doses may be required,[13] but is less invasive than myectomy.[24]
  - Sphincterotomy—mixed results.[24] Not shown to show significant long-term improvement,[3,24] also consider risk of fecal incontinence.
  - Posterior myotomy/myectomy (POMM)—mixed long-term results, as some reports of long-term incontinence.[3,24]
  - Redo pull-through operation, particularly if there is retained aganglionosis or hypoganglionosis or anastomotic problem.
  - Excision of Soave muscular cuff causing obstruction.[13]
  - End ileostomy or colostomy[24] may be considered for temporary diversion or as a last resort.

LONG-TERM OUTCOME

Most cases of postoperative HAEC will improve over time[6,76] with standard management (rectal washouts and antibiotics). A small proportion eventually requires operative management (e.g., stoma).[14] The course is often difficult for patients and their families.

HAEC patients have a worse functional outcome, lower bowel function score than healthy controls,[76] with less social continence, particularly if there are recurrent episodes of HAEC.[76] However there appears to be no difference after 12 years.[76]

Although there are long-term bowel problems in HD,[23] chronic or long-term HAEC is uncommon,[75] as episodes tend to reduce over time.[76] The majority of patients with HAEC continue to have problematic bowel function for many years,[10,23] and may take several years to achieve continence.[10]

Malignancy risk: 2.5%–5% of HD patients have multiple endocrine neoplasia (MEN-2) RET-mutations[75] that are associated with increased risk of medullary thyroid carcinoma.[1,77] Risk of other cancers does not appear to be increased.[75] Many centers perform routine RET mutation screening.

CHALLENGES FOR THE FUTURE

There is ongoing research into a complex area, with the aim to identify at-risk patients and develop prevention strategies.

Clinically, providing ongoing care of these patients into adulthood is a challenge—HD may be surgically corrected but the ongoing risk of bowel dysfunction and enterocolitis may be complex and unfamiliar to adult practitioners, including general surgeons and gastroenterologists.[78] Development of transitional care services would be of great benefit.

REFERENCES

1. Chhabra S, Kenny SE. Hirschsprung's disease. *Surgery (Oxford)*. 2016;34(12):628–632.
2. Gosain A, Brinkman A. Hirschsprung's associated enterocolitis. *Curr Opin Pediatrics*. 2015;27(3):364–369.
3. Demehri FR, Halaweish IF, Coran AG, Teitelbaum DH. Hirschsprung-associated enterocolitis: pathogenesis, treatment and prevention. *Pediatric Surg Int*. 2013;29(9): 873–881.
4. Gosain A, Frykman PK, Cowles RA, et al. Guidelines for the diagnosis and management of Hirschsprung-associated enterocolitis. *Pediatric Surg Int*. 2017;33(5): 517–521.
5. Pini Prato A, Rossi V, Avanzini S, Mattioli G, Disma N, Jasonni V. Hirschsprung's disease: what about mortality? *Pediatric Surg Int*. 2011;27(5):473–478.
6. Ruttenstock E, Puri P. Systematic review and meta-analysis of enterocolitis after one-stage transanal pull-through procedure for Hirschsprung's disease. *Pediatric Surg Int*. 2010;26(11):1101–1105.
7. Carneiro PMR, Brereton RJ, Drake DP, Kiely EM, Spitz L, Turnock R. Enterocolitis in Hirschsprung's disease. *Pediatric Surg Int*. 1992;7(5):356–360.
8. Surana R, Quinn FMJ, Puri P. Evaluation of risk factors in the development of enterocolitis complicating Hirschsprung's disease. *Pediatric Surg Int*. 1994;9(4): 234–236.

9. Gosain A. Established and emerging concepts in Hirschsprung's-associated enterocolitis. *Pediatric Surg Int.* 2016;32(4):313–320.

10. Menezes M, Puri P. Long-term outcome of patients with enterocolitis complicating Hirschsprung's disease. *Pediatric Surg Int.* 2006;22(4):316–318.

11. Austin KM. The pathogenesis of Hirschsprung's disease-associated enterocolitis. *Semin Pediatr Surg.* 2012;21(4):319–327.

12. Elhalaby EA, Coran AG, Blane CE, Hirschl RB, Teitelbaum DH. Enterocolitis associated with Hirschsprung's disease: a clinical-radiological characterization based on 168 patients. *J Pediatric Surg.* 1995;30(1):76–83.

13. Frischer JS, Rymeski B. Complications in colorectal surgery. *Semin Pediatric Surg.* 2016;25(6):380–387.

14. Thakkar HS, Bassett C, Hsu A, et al. Functional outcomes in Hirschsprung disease: a single institution's 12-year experience. *J Pediatric Surg.* 2017;52(2):277–280.

15. Quinn FMJ, Surana R, Puri P. The influence of trisomy 21 on outcome in children with Hirschsprung's disease. *J Pediatric Surg.* 1994;29(6):781–783.

16. Kleinhaus S, Boley SJ, Sheran M, Sieber WK. Hirschsprung's disease a survey of the members of the surgical section of the American Academy of pediatrics. *J Pediatric Surg.* 1979;14(5):588–597.

17. Engum SA, Grosfeld JL. Long-term results of treatment of Hirschsprung's disease. *Semin Pediatric Surg.* 2004;13(4):273–285.

18. Suita S, Taguchi T, Ieiri S, Nakatsuji T. Hirschsprung's disease in Japan: analysis of 3852 patients based on a nationwide survey in 30 years. *J Pediatric Surg.* 2005;40(1):197–202.

19. Vieten D, Spicer R. Enterocolitis complicating Hirschsprung's disease. *Semin Pediatric Surg.* 2004;13(4):263–272.

20. Singh SJ, Croaker GDH, Manglick P, et al. Hirschsprung's disease: the Australian paediatric surveillance unit's experience. *Pediatric Surg Int.* 2003;19(4):247–250.

21. Nakamura H, Lim T, Puri P. Probiotics for the prevention of Hirschsprung-associated enterocolitis: a systematic review and meta-analysis. *Pediatric Surg Int.* 2018;34(2):189–193. https://doi.org/10.1007/s00383-017-4188-y.

22. Hackam DJ, Filler RM, Pearl RH. Enterocolitis after the surgical treatment of Hirschsprung's disease: risk factors and financial impact. *J Pediatr Surg.* 1998;33(6):830–833.

23. Wester T, Granström AL. Hirschsprung disease—bowel function beyond childhood. *Semin Pediatric Surg.* 2017;26(5):322–327.

24. Frykman PK, Short SS. Hirschsprung-associated enterocolitis: prevention and therapy. *Semin Pediatric Surg.* 2012;21(4):328–335.

25. Haricharan RN, Seo J-M, Kelly DR, et al. Older age at diagnosis of Hirschsprung disease decreases risk of postoperative enterocolitis, but resection of additional ganglionated bowel does not. *J Pediatric Surg.* 2008;43(6):1115–1123.

26. Teitelbaum DH, Qualman SJ, Caniano DA. Hirschsprung's disease. Identification of risk factors for enterocolitis. *Ann Surg.* 1988;207(3):240–244.

27. Travassos D, van Herwaarden-Lindeboom M, van der Zee DC. Hirschsprung's disease in children with down syndrome: a comparative study. *Eur J Pediatric Surg.* 2011;21(04):220–223.

28. Friedmacher F, Puri P. Hirschsprung's disease associated with Down syndrome: a meta-analysis of incidence, functional outcomes and mortality. *Pediatric Surg Int.* 2013;29(9):937–946.

29. Kwendakwema N, Al-Dulaimi R, Presson AP, et al. Enterocolitis and bowel function in children with Hirschsprung disease and trisomy 21. *J Pediatric Surg.* 2016;51(12):2001–2004.

30. Hackam DJ, Reblock K, Barksdale EM, Redlinger R, Lynch J, Gaines BA. The influence of Down's syndrome on the management and outcome of children with Hirschsprung's disease. *J Pediatric Surg.* 2003;38(6):946–949.

31. Parahita IG, Makhmudi A, Gunadi. Comparison of Hirschsprung-associated enterocolitis following Soave and Duhamel procedures. *J Pediatric Surg.* 2017. https://doi.org/10.1016/j.jpedsurg.2017.07.010.

32. Huang W-K, Li X-L, Zhang J, Zhang S-C. Prevalence, risk factors, and prognosis of postoperative complications after surgery for Hirschsprung disease. *J Gastrointest Surg.* 2017. https://doi.org/10.1007/s11605-017-3596-6.

33. Murphy F, Puri P. New insights into the pathogenesis of Hirschsprung's associated enterocolitis. *Pediatric Surg Int.* 2005;21(10):773–779.

34. Wu X, Feng J, Wei M, et al. Patterns of postoperative enterocolitis in children with Hirschsprung's disease combined with hypoganglionosis. *J Pediatric Surg.* 2009;44(7):1401–1404.

35. Mao Y-z, Tang S-t, Li S. Duhamel operation vs. transanal endorectal pull-through procedure for Hirschsprung disease: a systematic review and meta-analysis. *J Pediatric Surg.* 2017. https://doi.org/10.1016/j.jpedsurg.2017.10.047.

36. Umeda S, Kawahara H, Yoneda A, et al. Impact of cow's milk allergy on enterocolitis associated with Hirschsprung's disease. *Pediatric Surg Int.* 2013;29(11):1159–1163.

37. Teitelbaum DH, Caniano DA, Qualman SJ. The pathophysiology of Hirschsprung's-associated enterocolitis: importance of histologic correlates. *J Pediatric Surg.* 1989;24(12):1271–1277.

38. Elhalaby EA, Teitelbaum DH, Coran AG, Heidelberger KP. Enterocolitis associated with Hirschsprung's disease: a clinical histopathological correlative study. *J Pediatric Surg.* 1995;30(7):1023–1027.

39. Bagwell CE, Langham MR, Mahaffey SM, Talbert JL, Shandling B. Pseudomembranous colitis following resection for Hirschsprung's disease. *J Pediatric Surg.* 1992;27(10):1261–1264.

40. De Filippo C, Pini-Prato A, Mattioli G, et al. Genomics approach to the analysis of bacterial communities dynamics in Hirschsprung's disease-associated enterocolitis: a pilot study. *Pediatric Surg Int.* 2010;26(5):465–471.

41. Pastor AC, Osman F, Teitelbaum DH, Caty MG, Langer JC. Development of a standardized definition for Hirschsprung's-associated enterocolitis: a Delphi analysis. *J Pediatric Surg.* 2009;44(1):251–256.

42. Frykman PK, Kim S, Wester T, et al. Critical evaluation of the Hirschsprung-associated enterocolitis (HAEC) score: a multicenter study of 116 children with Hirschsprung disease. *J Pediatric Surg.* 2018;53(4):708–717.

43. Levin DN, Marcon MA, Rintala RJ, Jacobson D, Langer JC. Inflammatory bowel disease manifesting after surgical treatment for Hirschsprung Disease. *J Pediatric Gastroenterol Nutr.* 2012;55(3):272–277.

44. Pontarelli EM, Ford HR, Gayer CP. Recent developments in Hirschsprung's-associated enterocolitis. *Curr Gastroenterol Rep.* 2013;15(8):340.

45. Frykman PK, Cheng Z, Wang X, Dhall D. Enterocolitis causes profound lymphoid depletion in endothelin receptor B- and endothelin 3-null mouse models of Hirschsprung-associated enterocolitis. *Eur J Immunol.* 2015;45(3):807–817.

46. Imamura A, Puri P, O'Briain DS, Reen DJ. Mucosal immune defence mechanisms in enterocolitis complicating Hirschsprung's disease. *Gut.* 1992;33(6):801–806.

47. Gosain A, Barlow-Anacker AJ, Erickson CS, et al. Impaired cellular immunity in the murine neural crest conditional deletion of endothelin receptor-B model of Hirschsprung's disease. *PLoS One.* 2015;10(6):e0128822.

48. Wilson-Storey D, Scobie WG. Impaired gastrointestinal mucosal defense in Hirschsprung's disease: a clue to the pathogenesis of enterocolitis? *J Pediatric Surg.* 1989;24(5):462–464.

48a. Coyle D, Murphy JM, Doyle B, O'Donnell AM, Gillick J, Puri P. Altered tryptophan hydroxylase 2 expression in enteric serotonergic nerves in Hirschsprung's-associated enterocolitis. *World J Gastroenterol.* 2016;22(19):4662–4672.

49. Kobayashi H, Hirakawa H, O'Briain DS, Puri P. Intercellular adhesion molecule-1 (ICAM-1) in the pathogenesis of enterocolitis complicating Hirschsprung's disease. *Pediatric Surg Int.* 1994;9(4):237–241.

50. Cheng Z, Wang X, Dhall D, et al. Splenic lymphopenia in the endothelin receptor B-null mouse: implications for Hirschsprung associated enterocolitis. *Pediatric Surg Int.* 2011;27(2):145–150.

51. Aslam A, Spicer RD, Corfield AP. Children with Hirschsprung's disease have an abnormal colonic mucus defensive barrier independent of the bowel innervation status. *J Pediatric Surg.* 1997;32(8):1206–1210.

52. Mattar AF, Coran AG, Teitelbaum DH. MUC-2 mucin production in Hirschsprung's disease: possible association with enterocolitis development. *J Pediatric Surg.* 2003;38(3):417–421.

53. Thiagarajah JR, Yildiz H, Carlson T, et al. Altered goblet cell differentiation and surface mucus properties in Hirschsprung disease. *PLoS One.* 2014;9(6):e99944.

54. Pierre JF, Barlow-Anacker AJ, Erickson CS, et al. Intestinal dysbiosis and bacterial enteroinvasion in a murine model of Hirschsprung's disease. *J Pediatric Surg.* 2014;49(8):1242–1251.

55. Aslam A, Spicer RD, Corfield AP. Turnover of radioactive mucin precursors in the colon of patients with Hirschsprung's disease correlates with the development of enterocolitis. *J Pediatric Surg.* 1998;33(1):103–105.

56. Soeda J, O'Briain DS, Puri P. Regional reduction in intestinal neuroendocrine cell populations in enterocolitis complicating Hirschsprung's disease. *J Pediatric Surg.* 1993;28(8):1063–1068.

57. Lui VCH, Li L, Sham MH, Tam PKH. CDX-1 and CDX-2 are expressed in human colonic mucosa and are down-regulated in patients with Hirschsprung's disease associated enterocolitis. *Biochim Biophys Acta - Mol Basis Dis.* 2001;1537(2):89–100.

58. Thomas DFM, Fernie DS, Bayston R, Spitz L, Nixon HH. Enterocolitis in Hirschsprung's disease: a controlled study of the etiologic role of *Clostridium difficile*. *J Pediatric Surg.* 1986;21(1):22–25.

59. Wilson-Storey D. Microbial studies of enterocolitis in Hirschsprung's disease. *Pediatric Surg Int.* 1994;9(4):248–250.

60. Li Y, Poroyko V, Yan Z, et al. Characterization of intestinal microbiomes of Hirschsprung's disease patients with or without enterocolitis using illumina-MiSeq high-throughput sequencing. *PLoS One.* 2016;11(9):e0162079.

61. Yan Z, Poroyko V, Gu S, et al. Characterization of the intestinal microbiome of Hirschsprung's disease with and without enterocolitis. *Biochem Biophys Res Commun.* 2014;445(2):269–274.

62. Demehri FR, Frykman PK, Cheng Z, et al. Altered fecal short chain fatty acid composition in children with a history of Hirschsprung-associated enterocolitis. *J Pediatric Surg.* 2016;51(1):81–86.

63. Frykman PK, Nordenskjöld A, Kawaguchi A, et al. Characterization of bacterial and fungal microbiome in children with Hirschsprung disease with and without a history of enterocolitis: a multicenter study. *PLoS One.* 2015;10(4):e0124172.

64. Shen DH, Shi CR, Chen JJ, Yu SY, Wu Y, Yan WB. Detection of intestinal bifidobacteria and lactobacilli in patients with Hirschsprung's disease associated enterocolitis. *World J Pediatrics.* 2009;5(3):201–205.

65. Moore SW. Genetic impact on the treatment & management of Hirschsprung disease. *J Pediatric Surg.* 2017;52(2):218–222.

66. Amiel J, Sproat-Emison E, Garcia-Barcelo M, et al. Hirschsprung disease, associated syndromes and genetics: a review. *J Med Genet.* 2008;45(1):1–14.

67. Moore SW, Sidler D, Zaahl MG. The ITGB2 immunomodulatory gene (CD18), enterocolitis, and Hirschsprung's disease. *J Pediatric Surg.* 2008;43(8):1439–1444.

68. Lacher M, Fitze G, Helmbrecht J, et al. Hirschsprung-associated enterocolitis develops independently of NOD2 variants. *J Pediatric Surg.* 2010;45(9):1826–1831.

69. Marty TL, Seo T, Sullivan JJ, Matlak ME, Black RE, Johnson DG. Rectal irrigations for the prevention of postoperative enterocolitis in Hirschsprung's disease. *J Pediatric Surg.* 1995;30(5):652–654.

70. Temple SJ, Shawyer A, Langer JC. Is daily dilatation by parents necessary after surgery for Hirschsprung

disease and anorectal malformations? *J Pediatric Surg.* 2012;47(1):209–212.

71. El-Sawaf M, Siddiqui S, Mahmoud M, Drongowski R, Teitelbaum D. Probiotic prophylaxis after pullthrough for Hirschsprung disease to reduce incidence of enterocolitis: a prospective, randomized, double-blind, placebo-controlled, multicenter trial. *J Pediatric Surg.* 2013;48(1):111–117.

72. Wang X, Li Z, Xu Z, Wang Z, Feng J. Probiotics prevent Hirschsprung's disease-associated enterocolitis: a prospective multicenter randomized controlled trial. *Int J Colorectal Dis.* 2015;30(1):105–110.

73. Messina M, Amato G, Meucci D, Molinaro F, Nardi N. Topical application of isosorbide dinitrate in patients with persistent constipation after pull-through surgery for Hirschsprung's disease. *Eur J Pediatric Surg.* 2007;17(1):62–65.

74. Rintala RJ, Lindahl H. Sodium cromoglycate in the management of chronic or recurrent enterocolitis in patients with Hirschsprung's disease. *J Pediatric Surg.* 2001;36(7):1032–1035.

75. Rintala RJ, Pakarinen MP. Long-term outcomes of Hirschsprung's disease. *Semin Pediatric Surg.* 2012;21(4): 336–343.

76. Neuvonen MI, Kyrklund K, Rintala RJ, Pakarinen MP. Bowel function and quality of life after transanal endorectal pull-through for Hirschsprung disease. *Ann Surg.* 2017;265(3):622–629.

77. Kenny SE, Tam PKH, Garcia-Barcelo M. Hirschsprung's disease. *Semin Pediatric Surg.* 2010;19(3):194–200.

78. Muise E, Cowles R. Transition of care in pediatric surgical patients with complex gastrointestinal disease. *Semin Pediatric Surg.* 2015;24(2):65–68.

CHAPTER 18

Fecal Microbiota Transplantation: Treatment of the Gut Microbiome

THOMAS BORODY, MD, PHD, DSC, FRACP, FACP, FACG, AGAF

INTRODUCTION

Fecal microbiota transplantation (FMT) is the accepted terminology used to describe the infusion of distal fecal material from a healthy donor into the GI tract of a recipient to reestablish healthy intestinal flora.[1] With a level of complexity similar to an organ, the gut is home to a complex mix of more than 1000 microbial species, which collectively harbor a 100 times more genes than the human genome.[1,2] As such the gastrointestinal microbiome (GIM) may be subject to developmental/dietary compositional differences, antibiotic damage, and superinfections, e.g., *Clostridium difficile* infection (CDI). Diet, antibiotics, probiotics, or FMT may be employed in an attempt to restore dysbioses or eradicate infectious pathogens, such as *C. difficile*. This chapter will therefore focus on FMT as a therapeutic method for CDI and commonly treated GIM conditions.

FMT use dates back to 4th-century China[3] and has been used in veterinary science since the 17th century,[4] although the administration methods and indications differ from the current use. In modern medicine, FMT was initially employed as a treatment of last resort for pseudomembranous colitis (PMC) in the 1950s.[5,6] After treating the first patient, Eiseman et al. noted the "immediate and dramatic response by this critically ill patient to a fecal retention enema"." In the same paper, it was predicted that "enteric-coated capsules might be both more aesthetic and more effective" than standard FMT in future. It was quickly recognized that this novel treatment was highly effective, with subsequent publications reporting successful use of FMT in 19 more patients.[7–10] However, between 1958 and 1989, only 35 case results were published in 31 years, whereas thousands of FMT treatments were carried out over the next 28 years after the CDI epidemic started in the early 2000s, initially in Canada,[11] followed by the United States, Europe, and to a lesser extent, Australia.[12] This was due in large part to the emergence of hypervirulent strains, including BI/NAP1/027, associated with higher rates of infection and relapse, increased mortality,

resistance to fluoroquinolones, and increased toxin production.[10–14] In this setting, FMT use dramatically increased, and it soon earned a reputation as an effective rescue therapy, consistently achieving cure rates of >90%.[15,16] Furthermore, FMT rapidly returned patients to health, often within a matter of days, and corrected the underlying deficiencies of Firmicutes and Bacteroidetes to help prevent further relapses.[17,18] Since then, thousands of patients have been treated with FMT, predominantly for CDI,[19,20] and nearly 4000 articles have been indexed by PubMed, with more than 90% published in the past 5 years,[21] firmly establishing FMT as a routine therapy for relapsing CDI. Several exhaustive reviews have been published on this topic.[13–16]

FECAL MICROBIOTA TRANSPLANTATION–BEYOND *CLOSTRIDIUM DIFFICILE* INFECTION

Rationale for Use in Other Gastrointestinal Conditions

"You need just one Martian to prove there is life on Mars."

With the success of treating PMC[5–7,9] and later CDI,[8] FMT has increasingly been used to treat other microbiome-mediated gastrointestinal (GI) conditions, including ulcerative colitis (UC),[10,17,18] Crohn's disease (CD),[10,19] irritable bowel syndrome (IBS),[10,20] and idiopathic constipation.[10,21] Additionally, extraintestinal conditions, once considered outside the realm of GI disorders, such as Parkinson's disease,[22] multiple sclerosis,[23] chronic fatigue syndrome,[24] autism,[25] and the metabolic syndrome,[26] have been reported to respond to FMT in small case reports. Such observations, coupled with the discovery that such conditions possess dysbiotic GIM, led to the notion that the GIM may be involved in the pathogenesis of a number of non-GI disorders. This chapter will focus on the application of FMT in GI conditions.

Gastrointestinal Diseases and Their Associated Infections. https://doi.org/10.1016/B978-0-323-54843-4.00018-0
Copyright © 2019 Elsevier Inc. All rights reserved.

The rationale for the therapeutic expansion of FMT to UC originated with our reading of the Eiseman paper.[5] The reason was that if CDI can cause pseudomembranous "colitis", which can be reversed by FMT[5] then it should theoretically work in the treatment of inflammatory bowel disease (IBD).[27] Because of clinical need, the authors successfully treated a patient with UC in their clinic using repeated FMT.[27] The UC went into prolonged remission and has not relapsed since the 1988 FMTs. Later, more FMT cases were reported to achieve both endoscopic and histologic remission of the UC.[28] In 1989, Bennet and Brinkman[17] reported on Bennet's self-treatment with FMT for UC, and he remains symptom-free more than 20 years later.

CDI is arguably one of the best studied examples of a GIM disease resulting in altered ecology. Studies have consistently demonstrated marked loss of bacterial diversity, decreased abundance of Bacteroidetes and Firmicutes phyla, and relative increases in Enterobacteriaceae and Proteobacteria in patients with CDI,[13,29] which correspond with increased cycles of relapses.[30,31] Patients with IBD similarly exhibit a decreased abundance of Bacteroidetes and Firmicutes, including clostridial clusters XIVa and IV (e.g., *Clostridium coccoides, Clostridium leptum* clusters [particularly *Faecalibacterium prausnitzii*] *and Roseburia intestinalis*), *Bifidobacterium*, and *Lactobacillus*, and an increase in pathogenic organisms such as enteroadherent *Escherichia coli, Campylobacter* species, *Fusobacterium* spp., and *Mycobacterium avium* subsp *paratuberculosis* (in CD) relative to healthy controls.[18,32–36] Following FMT, durable reestablishment of bacterial diversity can be observed, with an increase in Firmicutes and Bacteroidetes and a decrease in Enterobacteriaceae and Proteobacteria.[37,38] Other mechanisms by which commensal organisms contribute to the anti-inflammatory response may include induction of regulatory CD4 T-cell activation and production of anti-inflammatory metabolites.[39,40] Analysis of the microbiota composition in patients with IBS reveals a decrease in the relative abundance of *Bacteroides, Bifidobacterium, Lactobacillus*, and *Faecalibacterium*, as well as particularly butyrate- and methane-producing bacteria, and a corresponding increase in the numbers of Firmicutes (including *Clostridium* species) and Proteobacteria compared with those in healthy individuals.[41,42] Alterations in intestinal microbiota are also reported in chronic constipation and are characterized by a relative decrease in *Lactobacillus, Bifidobacterium*, and *Bacteroides* and a corresponding increase in potentially pathogenic microorganisms (e.g., *Pseudomonas aeruginosa* and *Campylobacter jejuni*).[43,44]

The exact mechanisms by which FMT may work sporadically in other GIM-related diseases is less clear but, again, preliminary FMT case experience[10,45] in these conditions pointed to potential beneficial effects that may be reproduced more frequently with greater understanding of GIM ecology and improved methods of FMT use. It needs to be clearly and unequivocally understood that cases reported by Bennet and Brinkman et al.,[17] Borody et al.,[10] Andrews et al.,[46] Borody et al.,[27,28] and Borody et al.[47] each represent a visible "Martian" that proves that sporadic cure of IBD and IBS is possible and such observations should not be disregarded or disproven. Only when we discover the mechanisms that led to these cures, randomized controlled trials (RCTs) should be used to compare the "discovered treatment/s" and the "standard of care" therapies in UC, CD, IBS, or constipation.

Given the aforementioned dysbioses, the dominant hypothesis is that FMT may work in these conditions by correcting the underlying dysbiosis and returning the GIM to its normal ecology, and the patient to health.

Ulcerative colitis

The first clinical evidence suggesting that FMT may be successful for the treatment of UC was unwittingly provided by Eiseman's group[5] when they used FMT to treat PMC. This led in May of 1988 to our first FMT treatment—a patient with UC rather than CDI—and resulted in durable clinical and histologic cure of the UC now lasting more than 20 years in the absence of all other therapy.[48] In January of 1989, Bennet reported his self-treatment using large-volume retention enema FMTs in his chronic UC.[17] He documented complete reversal of his UC symptoms for the first time in over a decade in the absence of other subsequent therapy and he continues to be asymptomatic more than 20 years later. In May of 1989, in a letter to the *Medical Journal of Australia*, we described the "cure" of 20 patients and symptom reduction in a further 9 patients out of 55 patients with UC, CD, and IBS after receiving FMT.[10] Since then, a number of case reports, cohort studies, and RCTs have been published on the use of FMT in IBD (predominantly UC). Although individual results have been variable, meta-analyses of these publications typically report remission rates between 30% and 40%.[10,17,18,28,49–61]

To date, the strongest evidence for FMT *reducing inflammation* in UC has been provided by four RCTs.[18,59–61] In the first trial by Moayyedi et al.,[60] 75 patients with active UC were randomized to weekly FMT or water enemas (50 mL) for 6 weeks, with a significantly greater proportion of patients in the FMT arm achieving remission than the controls (24% [9/38] vs.

5% [2/37]; P = .03). However, in a second trial conducted in 48 patients using suboptimal FMT in patients with mild to moderate UC, no significant difference was observed between the proportion of patients achieving the composite primary endpoint of clinical remission and ≥1-point decrease in the Mayo endoscopic score at 12 weeks following two nasoduodenal FMT infusions or placebo (41.2% [7/17] vs. 25% [5/20]; P = .29).[59] By contrast, the faecal microbiota transplantation in ulcerative colitis (FOCUS) trial adopted a more intensive FMT regimen tailored toward UC, consisting of an induction FMT using colonoscopy, followed by five FMT enemas per week for 8 weeks or placebo FMT in 85 patients with active UC.[18] Using this approach, a significantly higher proportion of patients in the FMT arm achieved the composite primary endpoint of steroid-free clinical remission and endoscopic remission or response at 8 weeks compared with placebo (27% [11/41] vs. 8% [3/40]; P = .021). Furthermore, 27% (10/37) of controls who subsequently received FMT in the 8-week open-label extension arm also went on to achieve the primary endpoint. Similarly Costello et al.[61] treated 73 patients with active UC using low-intensity FMT, consisting of induction FMT by colonoscopy plus two enema infusions within 7 days, or placebo, and reported that at 8 weeks a significantly higher proportion of patients in the FMT arm achieved steroid-free remission (32% vs. 9%; P = .02), clinical response (55% vs. 20%; P < .01), clinical remission (50% vs. 17%; P < .01), and steroid-free endoscopic remission (55% vs. 17%; P < .01).

The differing results in these trials of FMT in UC must be viewed in light of important differences in their study design.[18,59–61] For example, Rossen et al.[59] employed a suboptimal dosing regimen more suited for patients with CDI, rather than using multiple recurrent infusions better suited to UC treatment.[18,62] Furthermore, numerous studies have shown that the route of FMT administration has a significant influence on the rate of clinical efficacy, at least in CDI, with nasoduodenal infusion generally recognized as having inferior efficacy to colonoscopic infusion.[13,15,63] This discrepancy favoring distal administration may be particularly pronounced in patients with UC.[15,64] Despite the trial being halted prematurely following an interim futility analysis, the trial by Moayyedi et al. ultimately showed a greater response to FMT, likely because of the use of recurrent infusions and the power of the "single donor" effect (where most patients achieving remission had received FMT from the same donor), in spite of using low enema volumes (50 mL) known to result in poorer outcomes.[65] Costello et al., despite

employing a lower frequency dosing schedule associated with inferior response, may have partially offset this effect by using an anaerobic method of donor stool handling and preparation, which likely preserved species, such as *F. prausnitzii*, known to possess potent anti-inflammatory properties and be depleted in patients with IBD.[39,66]

Although a clear statistical benefit in reducing UC inflammation with repeated FMT was observed in UC, the fundamental difference between using FMT in CDI and in UC appears to have gone unnoticed. In CDI the measure of FMT success is generally a cure that includes marked improvement in diarrhea and eradication of *C difficile*, rather than measuring a reduction in inflammation using the Mayo Score. In UC, we do not treat an infection driving the "colitis" as we do in CDI. Rather we measure symptomatic improvement, as we are unable to eradicate an underlying infection and must therefore continue infusing the stool suspensions in order to reduce inflammation, as measured by the Mayo Score. Indeed, an infectious cause of UC has long been suggested, including some *Fusobacterium* strains.[67] However, whatever the infective agent/s may be, when the FMT infusions are ceased, clinically the patient's UC symptoms generally relapse. Therefore while such short infusion duration trials may show "statistically significant" reductions in inflammation, they are of little clinical utility for the patient. Hence, there is a clear and urgent need to conduct trials that *achieve cure or prolonged remission in the absence of medication*, as listed previously,[10,17,47,68] rather than merely seeking a reduction in inflammation. The occasional sustained remissions or cures of UC listed by some authors following FMT are crucial as, unlike trials, they point to the fact that:

a. UC needs to be treated with FMT in a different manner to that of CDI,
b. an infective cause of UC needs to be sought,
c. pretreatment with antibiotics may be required to achieve optimal implantation,
d. planning a UC FMT trial with Mayo Score endpoints is now redundant and repetitive and unless new methodology is being trialed, such studies should be discouraged and perhaps not be funded.

Crohn's disease
Although most documented cases of FMT outside CDI have focused on UC,[64,69] the role for FMT in CD is less clear, with most published evidence derived from small case series and cohort studies.[19,56,68,70] In a small open-label pilot study of FMT in CD, Vermeire and colleagues[70] reported that none of their 6 patients with

refractory CD had a significant improvement within 8 weeks after two nasojejunal infusions of FMT. In contrast, another small open-label study conducted in 10 patients with moderately active CD reported clinical response in 62% of patients following a single colonoscopic FMT.[71] Other case reports have demonstrated similarly dramatic results in some patients with CD after FMT,[19,56,68,72] whereas others have reported minimal benefit.[73] Based on our experience gained over 30 years of FMT use, our clinical impression is that CD is less responsive to FMT than UC and requires specialized antibiotic and anti-inflammatory pretreatment, followed by multiple infusions, for the vast majority of patients.[74] Nevertheless, a distinct subset is capable of losing all evidence of CD with profound, prolonged remission of CD off all therapy.[75] Again, the aim should be profound clinical and histologic remission in the absence of all other therapy, rather than an improvement in inflammation only.

Other gastrointestinal conditions

Numerous case reports and retrospective case series have shown the benefit of FMT in patients with functional bowel disorders, including IBS and idiopathic constipation,[46,76–80] with the first RCTs also completed.[21,81,82] However, each of these conditions is comparatively more complex than CDI and should therefore be treated using an optimized FMT protocol, similar to that used in IBD. In a systematic review of nine publications including 48 patients with IBS, 58% of patients experienced an improvement in IBS symptoms following FMT.[20] Similarly, the results of two recent RCTs evaluating the efficacy of FMT in IBS (N = 106) reported a significant improvement in IBS scores following a single colonoscopic infusion of FMT.[81,82]

The efficacy of FMT in constipation has been demonstrated in several case reports[10,46,79] and in prospective trials.[21,83,84] In a randomized trial conducted in 60 patients with idiopathic constipation, the addition of six FMT infusions to conventional therapy resulted in a significantly higher rate of clinical improvement (53% vs. 20%; $P = .009$) and clinical cure (37% vs. 13%; $P = .04$) as well as a significantly higher mean number of complete spontaneous bowel movements per week (3.2 ± 1.4 vs. 2.1 ± 1.2; $P = .001$), stool consistency score (3.9 vs. 2.4; $P < .001$), and colonic transit time (58.5 vs. 73.6 h; $P < .001$) compared with conventional therapy alone.[21] Taken together, the results suggest that FMT may have a prominent place in the treatment armamentarium for IBS.

Another potential application of FMT that has shown promise is the eradication of pathogenic and multiresistant enteric microorganisms, including vancomycin-resistant enterococcus colonization,[85] and sepsis.[86]

EVOLVING LANDSCAPE OF MICROBIOTA-BASED THERAPEUTICS

Thousands of patients have now been treated with FMT worldwide,[13,23] with numerous resulting publications. In this review, CDI has been summarized, FMT treatment for GIM dysbioses has been introduced, and extraintestinal GIM-related conditions have been mentioned. The most important aspect raised is the differentiation between FMT use in CDI and in IBD. We stress the point that research outcomes need to be durably effective GIM therapies. To that end, we need to move away from current RCT designs (e.g., FMT vs. placebo in UC) and emulate cases reports and trials that showed *profound, prolonged remissions.*

Trying to keep pace with the growing numbers of clinical applications for FMT beyond CDI, new innovative FMT products have been developed and continue to be intermittently announced by biotechnology companies working in the microbiome field. From crude, homogenized full-spectrum feces, highly filtered fresh[87] and filtered frozen[87] FMT materials have been reported and some have become available, e.g., via OpenBiome (www.openbiome.org). From here, sterile filtrates,[88] frozen encapsulated products of partially filtered feces,[89] lyophilized encapsulated products,[90,91] and finally, encapsulated narrow-spectrum cultured products (Fig. 8.1) are being developed. The aim of these products is to preserve bacterial viability, long-term physical stability, and portability in order to facilitate daily dosing to maintain remission in chronic conditions such as UC.

Despite its proven efficacy, crude suspensions of homogenized human feces, traditionally employed during FMT, possess a number of drawbacks that both patients and physicians would prefer to avoid. If carried out by the treating physician, these include the unappealing nature of handling and preparing stool suspension, protracted donor screening procedures, lack of standardization, limited shelf-life, and theoretic safety concerns. Establishment of commercial stool banks[13] and development of next-generation microbiota-based therapeutics (Fig. 8.1) have already improved physician and patient access to FMT and will continue to even more so once lyophilized encapsulated products become approved by the US Food and Drug Administration for CDI.

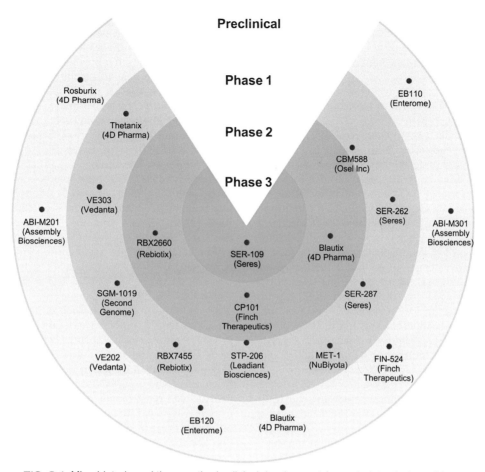

FIG. 8.1 Microbiota-based therapeutics in clinical development for gastrointestinal conditions.

Highly Filtered and Frozen Stool Preparations

The use of highly filtered stool products, prepared by extensive filtration and centrifugation of homogenized fecal slurry, was first reported by Hamilton et al.[87] and others[92] for the treatment of recurrent CDI. Using this method of preparation, a clear, virtually odorless solution was produced with reduced viscosity and volume, which was then combined with a cryoprotectant such as glycerol or trehalose to enable storage at −80 °C for up to 5 months.[92] In a study by Hamilton et al.[87] a 92% resolution rate was demonstrated using this frozen product in recurrent CDI compared with a 90% resolution rate with fresh material. Detailed microbiologic analysis using 16S ribosomal RNA (rRNA) gene sequencing showed stable "engraftment" of donor microbiota using frozen FMT product, similar to that seen using fresh donor material.[38,93] Similarly, in a randomized, open-label feasibility study by Youngster

et al.[92] a single colonoscopic or nasogastric infusion of frozen FMT inoculum, prepared using Hamilton method as a guide,[87] resulted in resolution of diarrhea in 90% of cases. These findings demonstrated that frozen and fresh FMT products are equally efficacious in treating CDI, with need for −80° C for long-term storage, a disadvantage for portability.

Commercial Stool Banks

In an effort to provide ready–to-use, safe, and high-quality frozen donor fecal products at a national or regional level, several centralized, registered stool banks have been established around the world, including the United States,[94–96] United Kingdom,[94,96] Netherlands,[94] France,[94,97] Germany,[94,97] Spain,[94] Austria,[94] Hong Kong, and Australia.[96] The majority of these supply frozen stool samples that are capable of being stored at between −20°C and −80°C for up to 6 months. An analysis of 2050 consecutive patients treated with FMT material from the OpenBiome public stool bank, the largest cohort to date, showed an overall CDI cure rate of 84%, or 87% when reanalyzed by lower GI delivery,[13] which is lower than the published rates with fresh FMT products.[37]

Encapsulated Frozen and Lyophilized (Freeze-Dried) Preparations

Although the bulk of FMT to date has been performed via enema or nasogastric/nasojejunal routes, oral administration is preferable for a number of reasons including patient convenience, reduced procedural costs and associated risks, and portability. However, given the increasing use of FMT in non-CDI conditions, the prime advantage of encapsulated FMT material is that it permits continual dosing, e.g., daily dosing, for maintenance of remission in conditions such as UC, which rarely achieve prolonged remission with a 1–2 day course of FMT. However, the first cases of UC treated in such a way are instructive because it appears that some efficacy of FMT was lost during lyophilization such that induction of remission in UC required 426 capsules,[98] suggesting that it is currently easier to achieve remission with enema FMT. Nevertheless, capsules may be used for maintenance of remission.

Studies have shown equivalent efficacy between oral FMT capsules and colonoscopic FMT, but only for the treatment of CDI. For example, in a study of 19 patients with recurrent CDI, Hirsch et al. reported a cumulative clinical cure rate of 89% following single administration of 6–22 capsules of frozen FMT products.[99] Subsequently Youngster et al., building on their previous work describing the successful use of frozen FMT inoculum in CDI,[92] prospectively followed up a cohort of 180 patients treated with frozen encapsulated FMT material for their recurrent or refractory CDI.[89] After the first administration of FMT capsules, 82% (147/180) of patients reported resolution of diarrhea, which increased to 91% (164/180) after retreatment of failures.

As the practicality of frozen liquid capsules is limited by issues relating to shelf-life, the number of capsules required (≥30 in some studies),[89,100] and uniformity, freeze-dried (lyophilized) encapsulated formulations have been devised to be stable at a range of different temperatures without apparent loss of viability. Furthermore, lyophilization concentrates the product, thereby reducing the number of capsules required for treatment. In a 2014 proof-of-concept study led by Drs. Alexander Khoruts and Michael Sadowsky at the University of Minnesota, an orally administered lyophilized FMT preparation successfully prevented

CDI recurrence over 2 months in 88% (43/49) of patients.[90] Furthermore, patients' microbial communities achieved near normalization of the fecal microbial community by 1 month following treatment. In a small case series, Borody et al. treated three patients with CDI using 6 or 8 capsules of highly filtered, dry, concentrated, low-volume, high-viability FMT material over 1 or 3 days and reported eradication of CDI in 85% (2/3) of cases.[91] Similarly Hecker et al. treated 20 patients with recurrent CDI using freeze-dried oral FMT capsules and reported resolution of diarrhea without CDI recurrence in 85% (17/20) of patients,[101] which is consistent with the results reported by others.[102,103] Given that transcolonoscopic FMT has been shown to cure 100% (29/29) of CDI cases upon its first diagnosis,[104] it is likely that the equivalent capsule CDI treatment will be used as first-line treatment in future as well as in relapsing CDI.

Sterile Fecal Filtrates

Although the majority of research to date has focused on the bacterial component of fecal suspensions used in FMT, a number of therapeutically active substances distinct from the microbiota are transferred during the FMT process (Fig. 8.2). This is perhaps best illustrated by Ott et al. who reported use of a sterile filtrate in five patients with symptomatic relapsing CDI.[88] The product was considered sterile, as bacteria had been filtered out and no organisms grew on culture. However, it did contain small bacterial debris, viruses including

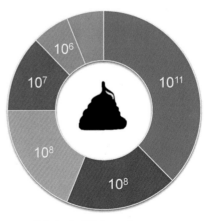

FIG. 8.2 Composition of fecal microbiota transplantation. (From Bojanova DP, et al. *PLoS Biol.* 2016;14(7):e1002503; with permission.)

bacteriophages, and various components such as antimicrobial products, proteins, metabolic products, and microbial DNA only, and presumably numerous other active and inactive substances. After a single nasogastric instillation, restoration of normal stool habits and elimination of symptoms were reported in all five patients. Analysis of the filtrate using 16S rRNA gene sequencing revealed the presence of diverse bacterial DNA signatures and viruslike particles that showed a complex signature of bacteriophages, suggesting that bacterial components were present, and metabolites, or bacteriophages mediated most of the positive effects seen. Although the filtrate was used in CDI in this instance, its potential application in various formats (e.g., enema, capsules) may extend to IBD and IBS, but our preliminary in vitro studies showed the filtrate had no antibacterial effect.

NEXT-GENERATION MICROBIOTA-BASED THERAPEUTICS

The therapeutic pipeline is currently rich with a number of next-generation microbiota-based products in clinical development; over half of the products are in early development (preclinical and phase 1), while several are in advanced stages (phase 2 and above) of development (Fig. 8.1). Numerous biotechnology companies are additionally active in the field or engaged in the development of undisclosed microbiome therapeutics in GI disease, including Assembly Biosciences, Biose, HOST Therabiomics, Janssen/Johnson & Johnson, Merck, Novartis, Pfizer, Roche, Second Genome, and Siolta Therapeutics. These therapeutics can be broadly classified as "full-spectrum" or "narrow-spectrum" microbiota-based products or microbiota-derived molecules.

"Full-Spectrum" Products in Development

As the name implies, full-spectrum microbiota products attempt to retain the entire functioning gut ecosystem including bacteria, archaea, bacteriophages, colonocytes, fungi, protists, and their metabolites (Fig. 8.2) for transplantation. RBX2660 is a full-spectrum microbiota-based suspension currently in phase 3 development by Rebiotix Inc. for the prevention of recurrent CDI. Each suspension contains $\geq 10^7$ live organisms/mL derived from 50 g of human stool (from four donors) mixed with 150 mL of 0.9% saline/polyethylene glycol 3350 in a single-dose ready-to-use enema format that can be stored at $\leq -80\,°C$.[105] In the phase 2B Punch CD 2 study in recurrent CDI, patients receiving a single dose of RBX2660 had a significantly higher rate of response, defined as an

absence of CDI-associated diarrhea at 8 weeks, compared with placebo (67% vs. 46%; $P = .048$), which was maintained over 12 months.[106] Furthermore, RBX2660 durably shifted patient's intestinal microbiomes toward that of a healthy microbiome, with a relative increase in microbiome densities, including Bacteroidia and Clostridia, and a decrease in Gammaproteobacteria abundance.[107]

Orally administered full-spectrum microbiota capsules are also in clinical development. Crestovo, in a joint venture with Finch Therapeutics Group, is currently evaluating CP101, an orally administered full-spectrum microbiota capsule, in a phase 2, randomized, placebo-controlled trial (PRISM 3) in ~240 patients with recurrent CDI, with top-line data expected in 2018. The not-for-profit stool bank, OpenBiome, has also initiated large-scale production of an FMT capsule, G3, using a novel, patent-pending approach that is designed to preserve bacterial viability while ensuring long-term physical stability. In a dose-finding pilot study in 17 patients with recurrent CDI, high-dose (30 capsules daily for 2 days) and low-dose (30 capsules at once) G3 treatment resulted in resolution of diarrhea in 71% and 70% of patients, respectively, at 8 weeks.[100] Nonresponders in both arms were treated with 30 capsules for 2 consecutive days, which resulted in a secondary clinical cure rate of 94%. Rebiotix Inc. is also evaluating RBX7455, a lyophilized, nonfrozen oral capsule formulation for the treatment of recurrent CDI in a phase 1 trial. Beyond CP101, Crestovo has developed full-spectrum lyophilized capsules for daily use in UC to maintain remission.[108]

"Narrow-Spectrum" Products in Development

In an attempt to make a safe, reproducible preparation that simulates the beneficial effects of FMT, "narrow-spectrum" or "defined consortia" FMT products have also been designed that contain a mixture of defined stool-derived microbes. The first attempt at using a narrow-spectrum extract was reported in 1989 by Tvede and Rask-Madsen who used a consortium of 10 facultative aerobic and anaerobic bacteria strains cultured from healthy donor stool for the treatment of recurrent CDI.[109] Following the enema infusion, all patients experienced prompt eradication of their CDI and associated symptoms within 24 h, which persisted for the duration of the 12 months' follow-up period, and restoration of missing GIM components. Pearce et al.[77] reported the successful use of 16 cultured bacteria (mainly *Bacteroides*) in 51 patients with IBS at our clinic. After a single endoscopic instillation into the jejunum or caecum, a highly significant improvement in symptom score was noted ($P < .001$), particularly for nausea, constipation, diarrhea, and flatulence, which persisted for the duration of the 3-month observation period in 65% of cases.

Despite the preliminary success reported by Tvede et al. in 1989[109] and Pearce et al. from our clinic in 1997,[77] the notion of cultured narrow-spectrum preparations was largely abandoned until 2012, when Jorup-Ronstrom et al.[110] described the use of a mixture of uncharacterized fecal microbes isolated and repeatedly recultured from a single Scandinavian donor 10 years earlier for the treatment of relapsing CDI. Of the 32 patients, 22 (69%) were durably cured of their recurrent CDI, with nonresponders retreated, which resulted in a cumulative cure rate of 81%. Shortly after, Petrof et al.[111] detailed a mixture of 33 nonpathogenic strains of bacteria derived from the stool of a single donor for the treatment of CDI. Termed "RePOOPulate," the strains were chosen based on their antibiotic susceptibility profiles, reliable culturability, and robustness under conditions mimicking the distal intestine, with a single colonoscopic administration resulting in durable cure of recurrent CDI in 100% (2/2) of patients.

Following a resurgence in interest in microbiota-based therapeutics, a number of narrow-spectrum products have entered clinical trials (Fig. 8.1). Vedanta's lead microbiome candidate, VE303, is an oral formulation of defined bacterial consortia that have been selected based on their activity against *C. difficile* and potentially other bacterial infections. The company is also developing VE202, an oral formulation consortium consisting of 17 cluster IV and XIVa clostridial strains for the treatment of IBD. In preclinical models, administration of VE202 was shown to induce regulatory T cells via a number of mechanisms and attenuate symptoms of experimental allergic diarrhea and colitis.[112] Fin-524 (Finch Therapeutics), a microbial cocktail of strains identified as being responsible for the efficacy of FMT, is also in preclinical development for the treatment of UC. Similarly, 4D Pharma are also producing a series of single-strain live bacterial therapeutics that are known to possess specific properties of interest, including Blautix (undisclosed strain) for the treatment of IBS, Thetanix (*Bacteroides thetaiotaomicron*) for the treatment of pediatric CD, and Rosburix (*Roseburia hominis*) for the treatment of pediatric UC.[113] For example, Blautix has been shown to consume gases inside the GI tract that are known to cause bloating, abdominal pain, and changes in bowel frequency, while Thetanix and Rosburix each possess distinct anti-inflammatory properties that make them suitable candidates for IBD.

Advantages and Disadvantages of Full-Spectrum Versus Narrow-Spectrum Products

Full-spectrum products are associated with several advantages over narrow-spectrum microbiota-based products. Unlike narrow-spectrum products, broad-spectrum products do not require characterization of the specific microbial deficiencies that require restoration, making them a potential universal therapeutic that is effective in correcting imbalances in a wide range of conditions. The safety record of human-origin microbiota, having resided within the healthy donor for decades, has no parallel in safety testing of a narrow-spectrum product for adverse effects for say 12 months, which may in part explain why virtually no documented bacterial infection has been transmitted via FMT worldwide. Nevertheless, there are some advantages to synthetic narrow-spectrum products or microbial communities. For example, the set composition of defined synthetic mixtures can theoretically be controlled, tested extensively for the absence of undesired pathogens and viruses, and reproducibly manufactured, which makes them attractive for large-scale production. However, contamination of cultured probiotics, even in Good Manufacturing Practice–certified facilities, has been reported, as demonstrated by the fatal case of mucormycosis in a commercial infant probiotic product.[114] Furthermore, the success rate reported by Jorup-Ronstrom et al. (69%) using a mixture of bacterial strains falls far short of that achieved with standard FMT, highlighting the unique challenges associated with developing narrow-spectrum therapeutics from conventional full-spectrum FMT. Perhaps the greatest challenge is that we are only beginning to realize the full potential of the human microbiome, with the vast majority of this so-called "dark matter" largely unaccounted for and therefore nonreproducible. The study by Ott et al.[88] demonstrated that a number of therapeutically active substances distinct from the microbiota are transferred during the FMT process, which could be almost entirely lost with narrow-spectrum therapeutics. It is therefore conceivable that a significant reduction in the complexity or loss of beneficial strains will translate into a corresponding reduction in efficacy of similar magnitude. This is perhaps best illustrated by Seres Therapeutics' SER-109, a mix of bacterial spores, which failed to meet its primary endpoint of reducing the risk of recurrent CDI infection in a phase 2 trial.[113] Even if this restrained therapeutic approach may work in relatively uncomplicated infections such as CDI, where the compositional deficiencies have been clearly delineated, the same cannot be presumed for other more complex conditions such as IBD, where even repeated infusions of standard FMT are required to maintain response.[18,62] The phenomenon of "passaging," which refers to the decreased viability and potency of recultured commercial probiotics and their virtual inability to implant, is well recognized in the field of commercial probiotics, whereas the "wild types" present in full-spectrum FMT durably implant in the recipient.[93] Given the sheer complexity of this recognized "virtual organ," currently it appears unlikely that a small, select number of organisms have the capacity to independently accomplish more than a few of the myriad of functions known to be performed by the full-spectrum microbiome,[115,116] suggesting that a full-spectrum product may still be required in some conditions to achieve optimal therapeutic benefit.

AVENUES FOR FUTURE DEVELOPMENT

The human gut is home to a diverse community of symbiotic, commensal, and pathogenic bacterial, viral, and eukaryotic organisms and their associated genes, gene products, and genomes.[117] Research to date has focused primarily on the bacterial component within our gut. However, the human gut virome and mycobiome, which comprise the total population of viruses (and virus-like particles) and fungi associated with the underlying gut microbiota, respectively, are less well understood. As our understanding of the gut microbiome deepens, it is anticipated that these new avenues of research may be further explored in future and exploited in the development of novel treatment strategies.

Driven in part by the emerging threat of antibiotic resistance, particularly in treating GIM infections, our attention has turned to the mechanisms that bacteria have employed to maintain or restore a host's normal gut homeostasis. Probiotic bacteria can successfully outcompete undesired species via production of metabolic products, e.g., bacteriocins, and also via stimulating the production of bacteriophages, which are viruses that infect bacteria. In contrast to antibiotics, these mechanisms selectively target bacterial pathogens, sparing the resident bacterial populations from unintended damage. For example, *Bacillus thuringiensis* is known to secrete thuricin CD, a bacteriocin with a narrow spectrum of antimicrobial activity against *C. difficile*.[118] Bacteriophages have also received renewed interest as possible therapeutic agents. For example, specific bacteriophage cocktails have been shown to completely lyse *C. difficile* in vitro,[101] significantly reduce *C. difficile* biofilms,[119] and prevent the appearance of resistant colonies.[101] Other important functions of the GIM include the synthesis of short-chain fatty acids, such as butyrate, which have been shown to suppress colonic inflammation, primarily via inhibition of nuclear factor κβ activation in human colonic epithelial cells.[120] Furthermore, in patients with IBD, enema treatment with butyrate or a cocktail of short-chain fatty acids ameliorated colonic inflammation in early case reports.[108,121] Engineered probiotics with enhanced functional properties (including for targeted control of enteric pathogens) have also been developed, with potential therapeutic applications in future.[122] For example, ViThera Pharma have developed two food-grade strains of lactic acid bacteria engineered to deliver elafin, an elastase-specific inhibitor that is deficient in IBD,[123] to sites of mucosal inflammation for the treatment of IBD.[124] While it is expected that these and other microbiota-based products will continue to be developed, as our knowledge unfolds, it is anticipated that entirely new avenues of research will also be explored, including mining of microbiota metabolites for novel and effective therapeutic agents. The full potential of FMT-based therapeutics is only beginning to be realized. Encapsulated FMT products represent the next generation of GIM therapeutics, which afford the opportunity of continual dosing. However, a wealth of increasingly exciting GIM therapies are expected to become available in future.

ACKNOWLEDGMENTS

The author had full editorial control of the chapter and provided final approval of all content.

Contributors
The author participated in the drafting, critical revision, and approval of the final version of the chapter.

Declaration of Interests
Prof. Thomas J. Borody has a pecuniary interest in the Centre for Digestive Diseases, where fecal microbiota transplantation is a treatment option for patients. He has filed patents in this field. He is on the Scientific Advisory Board of, and has a shareholding in, the Finch Therapeutic Group.

REFERENCES

1. Shreiner AB, Kao JY, Young VB. The gut microbiome in health and in disease. *Curr Opin Gastroenterol.* 2015;31:69–75.
2. Thursby E, Juge N. Introduction to the human gut microbiota. *Biochem J.* 2017;474:1823–1836.
3. Zhang F, Luo W, Shi Y, et al. Should we standardize the 1,700-year-old fecal microbiota transplantation?. *Am J Gastroenterol.* 2012;107(11):1755. https://doi.org/10.1038/ajg.2012.251. author reply pp.1755–6.

4. DePeters EJ, George LW. Rumen transfaunation. *Immunol Lett*. 2014;162:69–76.

5. Eiseman B, Silen W, Bascom GS, et al. Fecal enema as an adjunct in the treatment of pseudomembranous enterocolitis. *Surgery*. 1958;44:854–859.

6. Collins DC. Pseudomembranous enterocolitis. Further observations on the value of donor fecal enemata as an adjunct in the treatment of pseudomembranous enterocolitis. *Am J Proctol*. 1960;2:389–391.

7. Fenton S, Stephenson D, Weder C, et al. Pseudomembranous colitis associated with antibiotic therapy - an emerging entity. *CMA J*. 1974;111:1110–1114.

8. Schwan A, Sjolin S, Trottestam U, et al. Relapsing *Clostridium difficile* enterocolitis cured by rectal infusion of homologous faeces. *Lancet*. 1983;2(8354):845.

9. Bowden Jr TA, Mansberger Jr AR, Lykins LE. Pseudomembranous enterocolitis: mechanism for restoring floral homeostasis. *Am Surg*. 1981;47:178–183.

10. Borody TJ, George L, Andrews P, et al. Bowel-flora alteration: a potential cure for inflammatory bowel disease and irritable bowel syndrome? *Med J Aust*. 1989;150(10):604.

11. Labbe AC, Poirier L, Maccannell D, et al. *Clostridium difficile* infections in a Canadian tertiary care hospital before and during a regional epidemic associated with the bi/nap1/027 strain. *Antimicrob Agents Chemother*. 2008;52:3180–3187.

12. He M, Miyajima F, Roberts P, et al. Emergence and global spread of epidemic healthcare-associated *Clostridium difficile*. *Nat Genet*. 2013;45:109–113.

13. Osman M, O'Brien K, Stoltzner Z, et al. Safety and efficacy of fecal microbiota transplantation for recurrent *Clostridium difficile* infection from an international public stool bank: results from a 2050-patient multicenter cohort. *Open Forum Infect Dis*. 2016;3:2120.

14. Kelly CR, Kahn S, Kashyap P, et al. Update on fecal microbiota transplantation 2015: indications, methodologies, mechanisms, and outlook. *Gastroenterol*. 2015;149:223–237.

15. Quraishi MN, Widlak M, Bhala N, et al. Systematic review with meta-analysis: the efficacy of faecal microbiota transplantation for the treatment of recurrent and refractory *Clostridium difficile* infection. *Aliment Pharmacol Ther*. 2017;46:479–493.

16. Moayyedi P, Yuan Y, Baharith H, et al. Faecal microbiota transplantation for *Clostridium difficile*-associated diarrhoea: a systematic review of randomised controlled trials. *Med J Aust*. 2017;207:166–172.

17. Bennet JD, Brinkman M. Treatment of ulcerative colitis by implantation of normal colonic flora. *Lancet*. 1989;1(8630):164.

18. Paramsothy S, Kamm MA, Kaakoush NO, et al. Multidonor intensive faecal microbiota transplantation for active ulcerative colitis: a randomised placebo-controlled trial. *Lancet*. 2017;389:1218–1228.

19. Zhang FM, Wang HG, Wang M, et al. Fecal microbiota transplantation for severe enterocolonic fistulizing Crohn's disease. *World J Gastroenterol*. 2013;19:7213–7216.

20. Halkjaer SI, Boolsen AW, Gunther S, et al. Can fecal microbiota transplantation cure irritable bowel syndrome? *World J Gastroenterol*. 2017;23:4112–4120.

21. Tian H, Ge X, Nie Y, et al. Fecal microbiota transplantation in patients with slow-transit constipation: a randomized, clinical trial. *PLoS One*. 2017;12:e0171308.

22. Ananthaswamy A. Faecal transplant eases symptoms of Parkinson's disease. *N Sci*. 2011;209:8–9.

23. Borody TJ, Khoruts A. Fecal microbiota transplantation and emerging applications. *Nat Rev Gastroenterol Hepatol*. 2011;9:88–96.

24. Borody T, Nowak A, Finlayson S. The gi microbiome and its role in chronic fatigue syndrome: a summary of bacteriotherapy. *Australas Coll Nutr Env Med*. 2012;31:3–8.

25. Aroniadis OC, Brandt LJ. Fecal microbiota transplantation: past, present and future. *Curr Opin Gastroenterol*. 2013;29:79–84.

26. de Groot PF, Frissen MN, de Clercq NC, et al. Fecal microbiota transplantation in metabolic syndrome: history, present and future. *Gut Microb*. 2017;8:253–267.

27. Borody TJ, Campbell J. Fecal microbiota transplantation: techniques, applications, and issues. *Gastroenterol Clin N Am*. 2012;41:781–803.

28. Borody TJ, Warren EF, Leis S, et al. Treatment of ulcerative colitis using fecal bacteriotherapy. *J Clin Gastroenterol*. 2003;37:42–47.

29. Chang JY, Antonopoulos DA, Kalra A, et al. Decreased diversity of the fecal microbiome in recurrent *Clostridium difficile*-associated diarrhea. *J Infect Dis*. 2008;197:435–438.

30. Pérez-Cobas AE, Moya A, Gosalbes MJ, et al. Colonization resistance of the gut microbiota against *Clostridium difficile*. *Antibiotics*. 2015;4:337–357.

31. Vincent C, Manges AR. Antimicrobial use, human gut microbiota and *Clostridium difficile* colonization and infection. *Antibiotics*. 2015;4:230–253.

32. Matsuoka K, Kanai T. The gut microbiota and inflammatory bowel disease. *Semin Immunopathol*. 2015;37:47–55.

33. Ott SJ, Musfeldt M, Wenderoth DF, et al. Reduction in diversity of the colonic mucosa associated bacterial microflora in patients with active inflammatory bowel disease. *Gut*. 2004;53:685–693.

34. Kostic AD, Xavier RJ, Gevers D. The microbiome in inflammatory bowel disease: current status and the future ahead. *Gastroenterol*. 2014;146:1489–1499.

35. Prosberg M, Bendtsen F, Vind I, et al. The association between the gut microbiota and the inflammatory bowel disease activity: a systematic review and meta-analysis. *Scand J Gastroenterol*. 2016;51:1407–1415.

36. Bull TJ, McMinn EJ, Sidi-Boumedine K, et al. Detection and verification of Mycobacterium avium subsp. paratuberculosis in fresh ileocolonic mucosal biopsy specimens from individuals with and without Crohn's disease. *J Clin Microbiol*. 2003;41:2915–2923.

37. van Nood E, Vrieze A, Nieuwdorp M, et al. Duodenal infusion of donor feces for recurrent *Clostridium difficile*. *N Engl J Med*. 2013;368:407–415.

38. Hamilton MJ, Weingarden AR, Unno T, et al. High-throughput DNA sequence analysis reveals stable engraftment of gut microbiota following transplantation of previously frozen fecal bacteria. *Gut Microb.* 2013;4:125–135.

39. Quevrain E, Maubert MA, Michon C, et al. Identification of an anti-inflammatory protein from *Faecalibacterium prausnitzii*, a commensal bacterium deficient in Crohn's disease. *Gut.* 2016;65:415–425.

40. Kosiewicz MM, Dryden GW, Chhabra A, et al. Relationship between gut microbiota and development of T cell associated disease. *FEBS (Fed Eur Biochem Soc) Lett.* 2014;588:4195–4206.

41. Pozuelo M, Panda S, Santiago A, et al. Reduction of butyrate- and methane-producing microorganisms in patients with irritable bowel syndrome. *Sci Rep.* 2015;5:12693.

42. Hong SN, Rhee P-L. Unraveling the ties between irritable bowel syndrome and intestinal microbiota. *World J Gastroenterol.* 2014;20:2470–2481.

43. Gerritsen J, Smidt H, Rijkers GT, et al. Intestinal microbiota in human health and disease: the impact of probiotics. *Genes Nutr.* 2011;6:209–240.

44. Kirgizov IV, Sukhorukov AM, Dudarev VA, et al. Hemostasis in children with dysbacteriosis in chronic constipation. *Clin Appl Thromb Hemost.* 2001;7:335–338.

45. Andrews PJ, Borody TJ. "Putting back the bugs": bacterial treatment relieves chronic constipation and symptoms of irritable bowel syndrome. *Med J Aust.* 1993;159(9):633–634.

46. Andrews PJ, Barnes P, Borody TJ. Chronic constipation reversed by restoration of bowel flora. A case and a hypothesis. *Eur J Gastroenterol Hepatol.* 1992;4:245–247.

47. Borody T, Wettstein A, Campbell J, et al. Fecal microbiota transplantation in ulcerative colitis: review of 24 years experience. *Am J Gastroenterol.* 2012;107:S665.

48. Borody TJ, Campbell J. Fecal microbiota transplantation: current status and future directions. *Expet Rev Gastroenterol Hepatol.* 2011;5:653–655.

49. Ren R, Sun G, Yang Y, et al. A pilot study of treating ulcerative colitis with fecal microbiota transplantation. *Zhonghua Nei Ke Za Zhi.* 2015;54:411–415.

50. Kunde S, Pham A, Bonczyk S, et al. Safety, tolerability, and clinical response after fecal transplantation in children and young adults with ulcerative colitis. *J Pediatr Gastroenterol Nutr.* 2013;56:597–601.

51. Kump PK, Grochenig HP, Lackner S, et al. Alteration of intestinal dysbiosis by fecal microbiota transplantation does not induce remission in patients with chronic active ulcerative colitis. *Inflamm Bowel Dis.* 2013;19:2155–2165.

52. Kellermayer R, Nagy-Szakal D, Harris RA, et al. Serial fecal microbiota transplantation alters mucosal gene expression in pediatric ulcerative colitis. *Am J Gastroenterol.* 2015;110(4):604–606. https://doi.org/10.1038/ajg.2015.19.

53. Damman CJ, Brittnacher MJ, Westerhoff M, et al. Low level engraftment and improvement following a single colonoscopic administration of fecal microbiota to patients with ulcerative colitis. *PLoS One.* 2015;10:e0133925.

54. Damman C, Brittnacher M, Hayden H, et al. Single colonoscopically administered fecal microbiota transplant for ulcerative colitis-a pilot study to determine therapeutic benefit and graft stability. *Gastroenterol.* 2014;146:S460.

55. Cui B, Li P, Xu L, et al. Step-up fecal microbiota transplantation strategy: a pilot study for steroid-dependent ulcerative colitis. *J Transl Med.* 2015;13:015–0646.

56. Cui B, Feng Q, Wang H, et al. Fecal microbiota transplantation through mid-gut for refractory Crohn's disease: safety, feasibility, and efficacy trial results. *J Gastroenterol Hepatol.* 2015;30:51–58.

57. Angelberger S, Reinisch W, Makristathis A, et al. Temporal bacterial community dynamics vary among ulcerative colitis patients after fecal microbiota transplantation. *Am J Gastroenterol.* 2013;108:1620–1630.

58. Costello SP, Soo W, Bryant RV, et al. Systematic review with meta-analysis: faecal microbiota transplantation for the induction of remission for active ulcerative colitis. *Aliment Pharmacol Ther.* 2017;46:213–224.

59. Rossen NG, Fuentes S, van der Spek MJ, et al. Findings from a randomized controlled trial of fecal transplantation for patients with ulcerative colitis. *Gastroenterol.* 2015;149:110–118.

60. Moayyedi P, Surette MG, Kim PT, et al. Fecal microbiota transplantation induces remission in patients with active ulcerative colitis in a randomized controlled trial. *Gastroenterol.* 2015;149:102–109.

61. Costello SP, Waters O, Bryant RV, et al. Short duration, low intensity, pooled fecal microbiota transplantation induces remission in patients with mild-moderately active ulcerative colitis: a randomised controlled trial. *Gastroenterol.* 2017;152:S198–S199.

62. Borody T, Campbell J, Leis S, et al. Reversal of inflammatory bowel disease (IBD) with recurrent faecal microbiota transplants. *Am J Gastroenterol.* 2011;106:S366.

63. Furuya-Kanamori L, Doi SA, Paterson DL, et al. Upper versus lower gastrointestinal delivery for transplantation of fecal microbiota in recurrent or refractory *Clostridium difficile* infection: a collaborative analysis of individual patient data from 14 studies. *J Clin Gastroenterol.* 2017;51:145–150.

64. Paramsothy S, Paramsothy R, Rubin DT, et al. Faecal microbiota transplantation for inflammatory bowel disease: a systematic review and meta-analysis. *J Crohns Colitis.* 2017;11:1180–1199.

65. Gough E, Shaikh H, Manges AR. Systematic review of intestinal microbiota transplantation (fecal bacteriotherapy) for recurrent *Clostridium difficile* infection. *Clin Infect Dis.* 2011;53:994–1002.

66. Cao Y, Shen J, Ran ZH. Association between *Faecalibacterium prausnitzii* reduction and inflammatory bowel disease: a meta-analysis and systematic review of the literature. *Gastroenterol Res Pract.* 2014;2014:872725.

67. Ohkusa T, Sato N, Ogihara T, et al. *Fusobacterium varium* localized in the colonic mucosa of patients with ulcerative colitis stimulates species-specific antibody. *J Gastroenterol Hepatol*. 2002;17:849–853.

68. He Z, Li P, Zhu J, et al. Multiple fresh fecal microbiota transplants induces and maintains clinical remission in Crohn's disease complicated with inflammatory mass. *Sci Rep*. 2017;7:4753.

69. Colman RJ, Rubin DT. Fecal microbiota transplantation as therapy for inflammatory bowel disease: a systematic review and meta-analysis. *J Crohns Colitis*. 2014;8:1569–1581.

70. Vermeire S, Joossens M, Verbeke K, et al. Donor species richness determines faecal microbiota transplantation success in inflammatory bowel disease. *J Crohns Colitis*. 2016;10:387–394.

71. Vaughn BP, Vatanen T, Allegretti JR, et al. Increased intestinal microbial diversity following fecal microbiota transplant for active Crohn's disease. *Inflamm Bowel Dis*. 2016;22:2182–2190.

72. Bak SH, Choi HH, Lee J, et al. Fecal microbiota transplantation for refractory Crohn's disease. *Int Res*. 2017;15:244–248.

73. Goyal A, Yeh A, Siebold L, et al. Clinical efficacy and microbiome findings following fecal microbiota transplant in children with refractory inflammatory bowel disease. *Gastroenterol*. 2017;152:S959.

74. Borody TJ, Finlayson S, Paramsothy S. Is Crohn's disease ready for fecal microbiota transplantation? *J Clin Gastroenterol*. 2014;48(7):582–583.

75. Agrawal G, Jayewardene AF, Leis S, et al. Prolonged endoscopic remission with mucosal healing in Crohn's patients: treatment cessation for 3–23 years. *Am J Gastroenterol*. 2017;112:S754.

76. Pinn D, Aroniadis OC, Brandt LJ. Follow-up study of fecal microbiota transplantation (FMT) for the treatment of refractory irritable bowel syndrome (IBS). *Am J Gastroenterol*. 2013;108:S563.

77. Pearce L, Bampton P, Borody T, et al. Modification of the colonic microflora using probiotics: the way forward? *Gut*. 1997;41(suppl 3):A63.

78. Cruz Aguilar R, Buch T, Bajbouj M, et al. Fecal microbiota transplantation as a novel therapy for irritable bowel syndrome with predominant diarrhea. *Neuro Gastroenterol Motil*. 2015;27:110.

79. Andrews PJ, Borody T, Shortis NP, et al. Chronic constipation (CC) may be reversed by "bacteriotherapy". *Gastroenterol*. 1994;106:A459.

80. Huang Y, Wang X, Li X, et al. Successful fecal bacteria transplantation and nurse management for a patient with intractable functional constipation: a case study. *Holist Nurs Pract*. 2016;30:116–121.

81. Holster S, Brummer RJ, Repsilber D, et al. Fecal microbiota transplantation in irritable bowel syndrome and a randomized placebo-controlled trial. *Gastroenterol*. 2017;152:S101–S102.

82. Johnsen PH, Hilpusch F, Cavanagh JP, et al. Faecal microbiota transplantation versus placebo for moderate-to-severe irritable bowel syndrome: a double-blind, randomised, placebo-controlled, parallel-group, single-centre trial. *Lancet Gastroenterol Hepatol*. 2017;31. 30338–30332.

83. Tian H, Ding C, Gong J, et al. Treatment of slow transit constipation with fecal microbiota transplantation: a pilot study. *J Clin Gastroenterol*. 2016;50:865–870.

84. Ge X, Zhao W, Ding C, et al. Potential role of fecal microbiota from patients with slow transit constipation in the regulation of gastrointestinal motility. *Sci Rep*. 2017;7:441.

85. Eysenbach L, Allegretti JR, Aroniadis OC, et al. *Clearance of Vancomycin-resistant enterococcus Colonization with Fecal Microbiota Transplantation Among Patients with Recurrent Clostridium difficile Infection ID Week*; 2016. New Orleans, LA, USA.

86. Li Q, Wang C, Tang C, et al. Therapeutic modulation and reestablishment of the intestinal microbiota with fecal microbiota transplantation resolves sepsis and diarrhea in a patient. *Am J Gastroenterol*. 2014;109:1832.

87. Hamilton MJ, Weingarden AR, Sadowsky MJ, et al. Standardized frozen preparation for transplantation of fecal microbiota for recurrent *Clostridium difficile* infection. *Am J Gastroenterol*. 2012;107:761–767.

88. Ott SJ, Waetzig GH, Rehman A, et al. Efficacy of sterile fecal filtrate transfer for treating patients with *Clostridium difficile* infection. *Gastroenterol*. 2017;152:799–811. e797.

89. Youngster I, Mahabamunuge J, Systrom HK, et al. Oral, frozen fecal microbiota transplant (FMT) capsules for recurrent *Clostridium difficile* infection. *BMC Med*. 2016;14:016–0680.

90. Staley C, Hamilton MJ, Vaughn BP, et al. Successful resolution of recurrent *Clostridium difficile* infection using freeze-dried, encapsulated fecal microbiota; pragmatic cohort study. *Am J Gastroenterol*. 2017;112:940–947.

91. Borody T., Mitchell S.W., Wong C., et al. Encapsulated lyophilized fecal microbiota therapy for the treatment of *Clostridium difficile* infection. Program No. P589. ACG 2016 Annual Scientific Meeting Abstracts. Las Vegas, NV: American College of Gastroenterology. Available at: https://www.eventscribe.com/2016/ACG/TwitterPoster.asp?PosterID=64980.

92. Youngster I, Sauk J, Pindar C, et al. Fecal microbiota transplant for relapsing *Clostridium difficile* infection using a frozen inoculum from unrelated donors: a randomized, open-label, controlled pilot study. *Clin Infect Dis*. 2014;58:1515–1522.

93. Grehan MJ, Borody TJ, Leis SM, et al. Durable alteration of the colonic microbiota by the administration of donor fecal flora. *J Clin Gastroenterol*. 2010;44:551–561.

94. Terveer EM, van Beurden YH, Goorhuis A, et al. How to: establish and run a stool bank. *Clin Microbiol Infect*. 2017;19:30275–30276.

95. Smith M, Kassam Z, Edelstein C, et al. Openbiome remains open to serve the medical community. *Nat Biotechnol.* 2014;32:867.

96. Bolan S, Seshadri B, Talley NJ, et al. Bio-banking gut microbiome samples. *EMBO Rep.* 2016;17:929–930.

97. Amirtha T. Banking on stool despite an uncertain future. *Science.* 2016;352:1261–1262.

98. De Zoysa P., Kingston-Smith H., Maistry P., et al. Treatment-naive ulcerative colitis patient treated with lyophilized full spectrum microbiota: A case study. World Congress of Gastroenterology at ACG2017 Meeting Abstracts. Orlando, FL. Program No. P1316. Available at: https://www.eventscribe.com/2017/wcogacg2017/ajaxcalls/PosterInfo.asp?efp=S1lVTUxLQVozODMy&PosterID=117081&rnd=0.7210039.

99. Hirsch BE, Saraiya N, Poeth K, et al. Effectiveness of fecal-derived microbiota transfer using orally administered capsules for recurrent *Clostridium difficile* infection. *BMC Infect Dis.* 2015;15:015–0930.

100. Fischer M, Allegretti JR, Smith M. A multi-center, closter randomized dose-finding study of fecal microbiota transplantation capsules for recurrent *Clostridium difficile* infection. *United Eur Gastroenterol J.* 2015;3:561–571.

101. Nale JY, Spencer J, Hargreaves KR, et al. Bacteriophage combinations significantly reduce *Clostridium difficile* growth in vitro and proliferation in vivo. *Antimicrob Agents Chemother.* 2016;60:968–981.

102. Tian H, Ding C, Gong J, et al. Freeze-dried, capsulized fecal microbiota transplantation for relapsing *Clostridium difficile* infection. *J Clin Gastroenterol.* 2015;49(6):537–538.

103. Stollman N, Smith M, Giovanelli A, et al. Frozen encapsulated stool in recurrent *Clostridium difficile*: exploring the role of pills in the treatment hierarchy of fecal microbiota transplant nonresponders. *Am J Gastroenterol.* 2015;110(4):600–601.

104. Jaworski A, Borody T, Leis S, et al. Treatment of first-time *Clostridium difficile* infection with fecal microbiota transplantation. *Am J Gastroenterol.* 2015:S1354.

105. Orenstein R, Dubberke E, Hardi R, et al. Safety and durability of RBX2660 (microbiota suspension) for recurrent *Clostridium difficile* infection: results of the Punch CD study. *Clin Infect Dis.* 2016;62:596–602.

106. Blount K, Jones C, Shannon B, et al. *Changing the microbiome: Patients with a successful outcome following microbiota-based RBX2660 treatment trend toward human microbiome project healthy subjects' profile. Presented at: ASM Microbe 2017*; June 1–5, 2017. New Orleans, LA. Available at: http://www.rebiotix.com/scientific-evidence/microbiota-restoration-therapy-posters/changing-the-microbiome-patients-successful-outcome-following-microbiota-based-rbx2660-treatment-healthy-subjects-profile/.

107. Khanna S, Blount K, Jones C, et al. Successful response to microbiota-based drug rbx2660 in patients with recurrent *Clostridium difficile* infection is associated with more pronounced alterations in microbiome profile. *Open For Infect Dis.* 2017;4:S387.

108. Scheppach W, Sommer H, Kirchner T, et al. Effect of butyrate enemas on the colonic mucosa in distal ulcerative colitis. *Gastroenterol.* 1992;103:51–56.

109. Tvede M, Rask-Madsen J. Bacteriotherapy for chronic relapsing *Clostridium difficile* diarrhoea in six patients. *Lancet.* 1989;1:1156–1160.

110. Jorup-Ronstrom C, Hakanson A, Sandell S, et al. Fecal transplant against relapsing *Clostridium difficile*-associated diarrhea in 32 patients. *Scand J Gastroenterol.* 2012;47:548–552.

111. Petrof EO, Gloor GB, Vanner SJ, et al. Stool substitute transplant therapy for the eradication of *Clostridium difficile* infection: 'RePOOPulating' the gut. *Microbiome.* 2013;1:2049–2618.

112. Narushima S, Sugiura Y, Oshima K, et al. Characterization of the 17 strains of regulatory T cell-inducing human-derived clostridia. *Gut Microb.* 2014;5:333–339.

113. Carlucci C, Petrof EO, Allen-Vercoe E. Fecal microbiota-based therapeutics for recurrent *Clostridium difficile* infection, ulcerative colitis and obesity. *EBioMedicine.* 2016;13:37–45.

114. Centers for Disease Control and Prevention. Fatal gastrointestinal mucormycosis in an infant following use of contaminated ABC dophilus powder from Solgar Inc. Available from: https://www.Cdc.Gov/fungal/outbreaks/rhizopus-investigation.Html.

115. Jandhyala SM, Talukdar R, Subramanyam C, et al. Role of the normal gut microbiota. *World J Gastroenterol.* 2015;21:8787–8803.

116. Belkaid Y, Hand T. Role of the microbiota in immunity and inflammation. *Cell.* 2014;157:121–141.

117. Proctor Lita M. The human microbiome project in 2011 and beyond. *Cell Host Microbe.* 2011;10:287–291.

118. Rea MC, Sit CS, Clayton E, et al. Thuricin CD, a post-translationally modified bacteriocin with a narrow spectrum of activity against *Clostridium difficile*. *Proc Natl Acad Sci U S A.* 2010;107:9352–9357.

119. Nale JY, Chutia M, Carr P, et al. 'Get in early'; biofilm and wax moth (*Galleria mellonella*) models reveal new insights into the therapeutic potential of *Clostridium difficile* bacteriophages. *Front Microbiol.* 2016;7.

120. Canani RB, Costanzo MD, Leone L, et al. Potential beneficial effects of butyrate in intestinal and extraintestinal diseases. *World J Gastroenterol.* 2011;17:1519–1528.

121. Harig JM, Soergel KH, Komorowski RA, et al. Treatment of diversion colitis with short-chain-fatty acid irrigation. *N Engl J Med.* 1989;320:23–28.

122. Mathipa MG, Thantsha MS. Probiotic engineering: towards development of robust probiotic strains with enhanced functional properties and for targeted control of enteric pathogens. *Gut Pathog.* 2017;9:017–0178.

123. Zhang W, Teng G, Wu T, et al. Expression and clinical significance of elafin in inflammatory bowel disease. *Inflamm Bowel Dis.* 2017;23:2134–2141.

124. Motta JP. Elafin-secreting lactic acid bacteria for treating inflammatory bowel disease (IBD). *SciBX.* 2012;5. https://doi.org/10.1038/scibx.2012.1174.

Index

Note: Page numbers followed by "f" indicate figures, "t" indicate tables.

Printed in the United States
By Bookmasters